Behavioral Medicine

A Guide for Clinical Practice

Third Edition

Edited by

Mitchell D. Feldman, MD, MPhil
Professor of Medicine
Director of Faculty Mentoring
University of California, San Francisco
San Francisco, California

John F. Christensen, PhD
Director of Behavioral Medicine Training
Department of Medicine
Legacy Health System
Portland, Oregon

D1301135

Medical

New York   Chicago   San Francisco   Lisbon   London   Madrid   Mexico City   Milan
New Delhi   San Juan   Seoul   Singapore   Sydney   Toronto

Behavioral Medicine: A Guide for Clinical Practice, Third Edition

4 5 6 7 8 9 0   DOC/DOC   14 13 12 11

ISBN 978-0-07-143860-5
MHID 0-07-143860-2
ISSN 1093-3468

This book was set in Adobe Garamond by International Typesetting and Composition.
The editors were James F. Shanahan and Robert Pancotti.
The production supervisor was Thomas Kowalczyk.
Project management was provided by Preeti Longia Sinha, International Typesetting and Composition.
The cover designer was Mary Mckeon.
Cover Photos: Health care worker with an aged patient. (Credit: © Index Stock/Alamy.)
A group of doctors in consultation. (Credit: © Jupiterimages/Brand X /Alamy.)

RR Donnelley was printer and binder.

This book is printed on acid-free paper.

Contents

III. HEALTH-RELATED BEHAVIOR

IV. MENTAL & BEHAVIORAL DISORDERS

V. SPECIAL TOPICS

VI. TEACHING BEHAVIORAL MEDICINE IN MEDICAL SETTINGS

Authors

Garrick A. Applebee, MD
Assistant Professor of Neurology and Pediatrics,
University of Vermont College of Medicine;
Attending Physician, Vermont Regional Sleep
Center, Fletcher Allen Health Care, Burlington,
Vermont
garrick.applebee@vtmednet.org
Sleep Disorders

Robert B. Baron, MD, MS
Professor of Medicine Associate Dean for Graduate
and Continuing Medical Education; Vice Chief,
Division of General Internal Medicine, University of
California, San Francisco, San Francisco, California
baron@medicine.ucsf.edu
Obesity

Howard Beckman, MD, FACP, FFCH
Clinical Professor of Medicine and Family Medicine,
University of Rochester School of Medicine and
Dentistry; Medical Director, Rochester Individual
Practice Association, Rochester, New York
hbeckman@ripa.org
Difficult Patients, Difficult Situations

Donald W. Brady, MD
Associate Dean for Graduate
Medical Education,
Vanderbilt University School of Medicine
Nashville, Tennessee
donald.w.brady@vanderbilt.edu
Lesbian, Gay, Bisexual, & Transgender (LGBT) Patients

David G. Bullard, PhD
Clinical Professor of Medicine and Clinical Professor
of Medical Psychology (Psychiatry), University of
California, San Francisco; Private Practice,
San Francisco, California
dgbullard@yahoo.com
Sexual Problems

Lisa Capaldini, MD, MPH
Assistant Clinical Professor, Department of
Medicine, University of California, San Francisco,
San Francisco, California
castromedical@aol.com
HIV/AIDS

Harvey Caplan, MD
Former Co-Director of Clinical Training, Human
Sexuality Program, University of California, San
Francisco; Private Practice, San Francisco, California
hcaplan@ix.netcom.com
Sexual Problems

John F. Christensen, PhD
Director of Behavioral Medicine Training
Department of Medicine, Legacy Health System,
Clinical Assistant Professor,
Department of Medicine, Oregon Health and
Science University
Portland, Oregon
jchriste@lhs.org
*Suggestion & Hypnosis; Depression; Stress & Disease;
Mistakes in Medical Practice; Trainee Well-being*

William D. Clark, MD
Lecturer in Medicine, Harvard Medical School;
American Academy on Communication in
Healthcare, Boston, Massachusetts
wdclark@gwi.net
Alcohol & Substance Use

Henry Cohen, MS, PharmD, FCCM, BCPP, CGP
Associate Professor of Pharmacy Practice, Arnold &
Marie Schwartz College of Pharmacy and Health
Sciences, Long Island University; Chief
Pharmacotherapy Officer, Director of Pharmacy
Residency Programs, Departments of Pharmacy and
Medicine, Kingsbrook Jewish Medical Center,
Brooklyn, New York
Hcohenliu@aol.com
Depression

Mary Raju Cole, RN, MS, APRN, BC
Contributing Editor, *The Nursing Spectrum*; Faculty,
Institute for Healthcare Communication,
New Haven, Connecticut
mrajucole@aol.com
Depression

Steven A. Cole, MD
Professor of Psychiatry, Department of Psychiatry and Behavioral Science, School of Medicine, State University of New York at Stony Brook, Stony Brook, New York
stcole@notes.cc.sunysb.edu
Depression

Thomas D. Denberg, MD, PhD, FACP
Associate Professor of Medicine, University of Colorado at Denver and Health Sciences Center, Denver, Colorado
tom.denberg@uchsc.edu
Cross-cultural Communication

Christine M. Derzko, MD
Associate Professor, Obstetrics & Gynecology and Internal Medicine (Endocrinology), Faculty of Medicine, University of Toronto, Toronto, Ontario, Canada
derzkoc@smhitoronto.on.ca
Sexual Problems

M. Robin DiMatteo, PhD
Department of Psychology, University of California, Riverside, Riverside, California
robin.dimatteo@ucr.edu
Patient Adherence

Elizabeth Eckstrom, MD, MPH
Associate Professor of Medicine and Director of Geriatrics Programs, Oregon Health and Science University, Portland, Oregon
eckstrom@ohsu.edu
Older Patients

Barry Egener, MD
Medical Director, The Foundation for Medical Excellence; Faculty, Legacy Portland Internal Medicine Training Program, Portland, Oregon
begener@lhs.org
Empathy

Stuart J. Eisendrath, MD
Professor of Clinical Psychiatry, University of California, San Francisco; Director of Clinical Services, Langley Porter Psychiatric Hospital and Clinics, San Francisco, California
stuarte@lppi.ucsf.edu
Somatization

Michael H. Eisman, MD
Medical Director, Seneca View Skilled Nursing Facility, Burdett, New York
eisman@capital.net
Palliative Care, Hospice, & Care of the Dying

Ronald M. Epstein, MD
Professor of Family Medicine, Psychiatry, and Oncology, Associate Dean for Educational Evaluation and Research; Director, Rochester Center to Improve Communication in Health Care, University of Rochester School of Medicine and Dentistry, Rochester, New York
ronald_epstein@urmc.rochester.edu
Mindful Practice

Mitchell D. Feldman, MD, MPhil
Professor of Medicine, Director of Faculty Mentoring, University of California, San Francisco, San Francisco, California
mfeldman@medicine.ucsf.edu
Families; Cross-cultural Communication; Depression; HIV/AIDS; Intimate Partner Violence; Trainee Well-being

Susan Folkman, PhD
Osher Center for Integrative Medicine, University of California, San Francisco, San Francisco, California
folkman@ocim.ucsf.edu
Complementary & Alternative Medicine

Richard M. Frankel, PhD
Professor of Medicine and Geriatrics, Senior Research Scientist, Regenstrief Institute, Indiana University School of Medicine, Research Sociologist, Center for Implementing Evidence Based Practice, Roudebush Veterans Affairs Medical Center, Indianapolis, Indiana
rfrankel@iupui.edu
Professionalism; Connections & Boundaries in Clinical Practice

Lawrence S. Friedman, MD
Medical Director, Ambulatory and Primary Care, Professor of Pediatrics, University of California, San Diego, San Diego, California
lsfriedman@ucsd.edu
Adolescents

Jennifer Gafford, PhD
Clinical Psychologist, Private Practice, Clayton Sleep Institute; Consulting Psychologist, Family Care Health Centers; Consulting Psychologist, St. Louis, Missouri
jengafford@aol.com
Training of International Medical Graduates

Geoffrey H. Gordon, MD, FACP
Pain management Clinic, Kaiser Permanente, West Interstate Medical Office, Portland, Oregon
ghgordon@aol.com
Giving Bad News

Steven R. Hahn, MD
Professor of Clinical Medicine and Instructor in Psychiatry, Albert Einstein College of Medicine, Jacobi Medical Center, Bronx, New York
steveroost@aol.com
Families

Kelly B. Haskard, PhD
Assistant Professor
Department of Psychology, Texas State University, San Marcos, San Marcos, Texas
kelly.haskard@email.ucr.edu
Patient Adherence

Eric S. Holmboe, MD
Senior Vice President for Quality Research and Academic Affairs, American Board of Internal Medicine; Adjunct Professor, Yale University School of Medicine, New Haven, Connecticut
eholmboe@abim.org
Education for Competencies in the Social & Behavioral Sciences

Ellen Hughes, MD, PhD
Clinical Professor of Medicine, Director for Education, Osher Center for Integrative Medicine, University of California, San Francisco, San Francisco, California
ehughes@medicine.ucsf.edu
Complementary & Alternative Medicine

Thomas S. Inui, ScM, MD
President and Chief Executive Officer, Regenstrief Institute, Inc.; Associate Dean for Health Care Research and Regenstrief Professor of Medicine, Indiana University School of Medicine, Indianapolis, Indiana
tinui@iupui.edu
Education for Competencies in the Social & Behavioral Sciences

Susan L. Janson, DNSc, RN, NP, FAAN
Department of Community Health Systems and Department of Medicine, University of California, San Francisco, San Francisco, California
susan.janson@nursing.ucsf.edu
Chronic Illness & Patient Self-Management

Martina J. Jelley, MD, MSPH
Associate Professor, Department of Internal Medicine, University of Oklahoma College of Medicine, Tulsa, Oklahoma
martina-jelley@ouhsc.edu
Women

C. Bree Johnston, MD, MPH
Associate Professor of Medicine, Division of Geriatrics, University of California, San Francisco; San Francisco Veterans Affairs Medical Center, San Francisco, California
bree.johnston@ucsf.edu
Dementia & Delirium

Mack Lipkin, Jr., MD
Professor of Medicine, Department of Medicine, Co-Director, Section of Primary Care, New York University School of Medicine, New York, New York
mack.lipkin@med.nyu.edu
The Medical Interview

Debra K. Litzelman, MA, MD
Associate Dean for Medical Education and Curricular Affairs, Indiana University School of Medicine; Richard Powell Professor of Medicine, Indiana University Medical Center, Indianapolis, Indiana
dklitzel@iupui.edu
Education for Competencies in the Social & Behavioral Sciences

Jay S. Luxenberg, MD
Medical Director, Jewish Home, San Francisco; Clinical Professor, University of California, San Francisco, San Francisco, California
jay@luxenberg.net
Older Patients

Stephen J. McPhee, MD
Professor of Medicine, Division of General Internal Medicine, University of California, San Francisco; Attending Physician, Moffitt/Long Hospitals, San Francisco, California
smcphee@medicine.ucsf.edu
Mistakes in Medical Practice

Vishnu Mohan, MD
Associate Program Director, Internal Medicine
Residency Program, Legacy Emanuel and Good
Samaritan Hospitals, Portland; Clinical Assistant
Professor of Medicine, Oregon Health and Science
University, Portland, Oregon
vmohan@lhs.org
Training of International Medical Graduates

Diane S. Morse, MD
Clinical Associate Professor of Medicine, University
of Rochester School of Medicine and Dentistry;
General Medicine Unit, Rochester General Hospital,
Rochester, New York
diane.morse@viahealth.org
Women

Daniel O'Connell, PhD
Clinical Instructor, University of Washington School
of Medicine; Consulting Psychologist, Private
Practice, Seattle, Washington
danoconn@mindspring.com
Behavior Change

Roberta K. Oka, RN, ANP, DNSc
Associate Professor, Department of Community
Health Systems, School of Nursing, University of
California, San Francisco, San Francisco, California
roberta.oka@nursing.ucsf.edu
Chronic Illness & Patient Self-Management

Timothy E. Quill, MD
Professor of Medicine, Psychiatry and Medical
Humanities, Director, Center for Ethics, University
of Rochester School of Medicine and Dentistry,
Rochester, New York
timothy_quill@urmc.rochester.edu
Palliative Care, Hospice, & Care of the Dying

Gita Ramamurthy, MD
Attending Psychiatrist, Cambridge Hospital;
Instructor, Harvard Medical School, Cambridge,
Massachusetts
murthg@comcast.net
Practitioner Well-being

Nancy A. Rigotti, MD
Professor of Medicine, Harvard Medical School;
Associate Physician and Director, Tobacco Research
& Treatment Center, Massachusetts General
Hospital, Boston, Massachusetts
nrigotti@partners.org
Smoking

Bruce L. Rollman, MD, MPH
Associate Professor of Medicine and Psychiatry,
Center for Research on Health Care, Division of
General Internal Medicine, University of Pittsburgh
School of Medicine, Pittsburgh, Pennsylvania
rollmanbl@upmc.edu
Anxiety

Steven J. Romano, MD
Clinical Associate Professor of Psychiatry, New York
University School of Medicine; Vice President,
Neuroscience, Pain and Inflammation, GI/Hepatology,
Global Medical, Pfizer, Inc., New York,
New York
steve.romano@pfizer.com
Eating Disorders

George W. Saba, PhD
Professor of Clinical Family and Community
Medicine, Vitamin Settlement Endowed Chair in
Community Medicine, University of California, San
Francisco, San Francisco, California
gsaba@fcm.ucsf.edu
Vulnerable Patients

Jason M. Satterfield, PhD
Associate Professor of Clinical Medicine, University
of California, San Francisco, San Francisco, California
jsatter@medicine.ucsf.edu
Anxiety

Dean Schillinger, MD
Associate Professor of Clinical Medicine, University
of California, San Francisco; Director, Center for
Vulnerable Populations, San Francisco General
Hospital, San Francisco, California
dschillinger@medsfgh.ucsf.edu
Vulnerable Patients

Jason S. Schneider, MD
Assistant Professor, Division of General Medicine,
Department of Medicine, Emory University School
of Medicine; Associate Medical Director, Primary
Care Center, Grady Memorial Hospital, Atlanta,
Georgia
jsschne@emory.edu
Lesbian, Gay, Bisexual, & Transgendered (LGTB) Patients

H. Russell Searight, PhD, MPH
Associate Professor of Psychology, Department of
Psychology, Lake Superior State University, Sault
Sainte Marie, Michigan
russellsearight@msn.com
*Attention Deficit Hyperactivity Disorder; Training of
International Medical Graduates*

J. Jewel Shim, MD
Assistant Clinical Professor of Psychiatry, Langley
Porter Psychiatric Institute, University of California,
San Francisco, San Francisco, California
jewels@lppi.ucsf.edu
Somatization

Clifford M. Singer, MD
Associate Professor, Department of Psychiatry,
College of Medicine, University of Vermont,
Burlington, Vermont
clifford.singer@vtmednet.org
Older Patients; Sleep Disorders

Gregory T. Smith, PhD
Clinical Psychologist and Director, Progressive
Rehabilitation Associates, Portland, Oregon
greg@progrehab.com
Pain

Anthony L. Suchman, MD, MA
Relationship Centered Health Care,
Rochester, New York
asuchman@rchcweb.com
Practitioner Well-being

Howard L. Taras, MD
Professor, Medical Consultation to Schools,
University of California, San Diego, La Jolla,
California
htaras@ucsd.edu
Children

Teresa J. Villela, MD
Director, Family and Community Medicine
Residency Program, San Francisco General Hospital;
Associate Clinical Professor, Department of Family
and Community Medicine, University of California,
San Francisco, San Francisco, California
tvillela@fcm.ucsf.edu
Vulnerable Patients

Judith Walsh, MD, MPH
Associate Professor of Medicine, University of
California, San Francisco, San Francisco, California
judith.walsh@ucsf.edu
Women

Jocelyn C. White, MD, FACP
Department of Medicine, Oregon Health and
Science University; Medical Director, Palliative &
Hospice Care, Legacy Good Samaritan Hospital &
Medical Center, Portland, Oregon
jwhite@lhs.org
Lesbian, Gay, Bisexual, & Transgendered Patients

Sarah Williams, MD
Instructor in Psychiatry, New York University
School of Medicine; Director, Physicians Resource
Network, North Shore-Long Island Jewish Health
System, New York, New York
swillia2@nshs.edu
Connections & Boundaries in Clinical Practice

Summer L. Williams, MA
Department of Psychology, University of California,
Riverside, Riverside, California
summer.williams@email.ucr.edu
Patient Adherence

Albert W. Wu, MD, MPH
Professor, Department of Health Policy &
Management, Johns Hopkins Bloomberg School of
Public Health, Johns Hopkins Medical Institutions,
Baltimore, Maryland
awu@jhsph.edu
Mistakes in Medical Practice

Kristine Yaffe, MD
Professor, Departments of Psychiatry, Neurology,
and Epidemiology and Biostatistics, University of
California, San Francisco, San Francisco, California
kristine.yaffe@ucsf.edu
Dementia & Delirium

John Q. Young, MD, MPP
Assistant Director, Adult Psychiatry Clinic; Associate
Director, Residency Training Program, Langley
Porter Psychiatric Hospitals and Clinics;
Department of Psychiatry, University of California,
San Francisco, San Francisco, California
jqyoung@lppi.ucsf.edu
Personality Disorders

Foreword

Since the first edition of this important book was published in 1997, it has become increasingly evident that it is impossible to practice effective medicine without attention to the nuanced interaction between mind and body. Long discredited as a doctrine but less so as a practice, mind/body dualism still characterizes the way in which many patients who seek medical care are treated. But change is taking place. During the past five years (since the second edition of this book was published), the lessons learned from research and practice have led to a heightened interest in and recognition of the importance of integrating the medical and behavioral components of patient care. The evidence that medical and behavioral problems are reciprocally related is persuasive. There is a symbiotic relationship between the two, and it is clear that attention to behavioral issues facilitates quality medical care. Further, it is well documented that most medical patients with behavioral problems talk first with their physicians about these problems rather than with a mental health specialist.

There is a growing expectation that physicians and other practitioners in both outpatient and hospital settings pay attention to behavioral problems through such practices as screening and treatment for depression, motivating patients to change health risk behaviors, prescribing appropriate psychotropic medications, and counseling patients to promote self-management of chronic illness. Of course, this requires greater expertise and additional time added to the already full agenda, busy practices, and other responsibilities of general practitioners and specialists. Taking on this additional work with no added resources can easily be seen by physicians, even those who believe in its value, as difficult if not impossible.

However, incorporating the principles and processes of behavioral medicine into practice can offer considerable help. It can enrich medical practice by providing a new perspective to patient care and the tools to implement it. Paying greater attention to the body/mind connection, the effects of emotions on physical health, and the psychological impact of illness can enhance physician and patient satisfaction, produce better treatment outcomes, and reduce the excessive and inappropriate use of medical care. Patients whose emotional needs are not addressed are far more likely to return for multiple visits, often with no discernible medical problems, thereby adding to the physician's already difficult workload.

A behavioral medicine orientation can also help physicians to look at themselves and to better understand the ways in which their own behavior may be affecting that of their patients and the quality of their care. The ways in which physicians relate to their patients—what they say and how they say it as well as their nonverbal messages—affect patient adherence to treatment and consequently the course and outcome of the treatment itself. Behavioral medicine expertise is a complement to biomedical competence; both are necessary.

With this third edition of their fine and important book, Drs. Feldman and Christensen continue to do a good and important service for those who practice medicine, those who teach it, and those who learn it. It remains for all of them to open their minds and their work to the ideas and practical suggestions provided in this book.

Steven A. Schroeder, MD
Professor in Residence
University of California, San Francisco
San Francisco, California

Preface

Since the first edition of *Behavioral Medicine* was published in 1997, there have been considerable advances in medical diagnosis and treatment, as well as changes in the ways in which health care is organized and delivered. The science of genetics is revolutionizing the understanding of disease and the design of therapies targeted to specific diseases. New medications are available for treatment of a variety of health problems, including heart disease, hypertension, and depression. Hospital medicine has arisen as an area of expertise within general internal medicine, and palliative care has emerged as the care of the dying has developed into an array of therapies requiring special knowledge and skills. There are new models of chronic care and patient self-care that increase effectiveness in the treatment of those with chronic illness.

This new edition of *Behavioral Medicine* addresses these and other developments in the integration of social and behavioral science with health care. We have broadened the scope of our chapters to include the hospital as well as ambulatory settings, and case examples are drawn from both domains of practice. We have added reference to themes such as the relation of religion and spirituality to health, the practice of mindfulness both in addressing health outcomes for patients and in promoting the well-being of clinicians, and the evidence base for behavioral interventions. Chapters from the previous editions have been updated to reflect advances in pharmacotherapy and evidence on the relationship between psychosocial factors and disease. For example, we have included new evidence on depression as a risk factor for heart disease and diabetes. New chapters on mindfulness, attention deficit hyperactivity disorder, vulnerable patients, and chronic illness have enhanced our coverage of topics useful to clinicians.

The training of physicians and other health professionals has also evolved during the past decade. Education for professionalism—embodying the core values motivating patient care and the quality of interactions with patients, colleagues, and staff—has taken root in many training institutions. Medical educators are beginning to attend consciously to the "hidden curriculum," the set of implicit verbal and nonverbal messages that may enhance or erode the highest ideals of the health care professions. Another growing phenomenon is the increased number of international medical graduates entering training in U.S. residencies. Many of these graduates have trained previously in settings that have not emphasized the social and behavioral aspects of health care, and their needs for additional training and support in the relational aspects of patient care are evident. Finally, helping trainees in the health professions to find balance in their lives and to develop the life skills for a sustainable career has challenged medical schools and residencies to create curricula and educational experiences to promote well-being. To address these developments, we have added a new section on teaching behavioral medicine.

Although the term "behavioral medicine" is used widely in both medical and social science literature, there is little agreement as to its exact definition. We broadly define it as an interdisciplinary field that aims to integrate the biological and psychosocial perspectives on human behavior and to apply them to the practice of medicine. Our perspective includes a behavioral approach to somatic disease, the mental disorders as they commonly appear in medical practice, issues in the clinician-patient relationship, and other important topics that affect the delivery of medical care, such as motivating behavior change, maximizing adherence to medical treatment, complementary and alternative medicine, and care of the dying.

We hope that general internists, hospitalists, family practitioners, pediatricians, nurse practitioners, physician assistants, and other clinicians will find that this book helps them to better understand and care for persons with a wide variety of mental and behavioral problems. For residents and students in health care settings, *Behavioral*

Medicine: A Guide for Clinical Practice can function as a valuable resource for understanding the psychosocial dimensions of medicine in much the same way that *Current Medical Diagnosis & Treatment* helps them to understand the biomedical domain.

It is our intent that medical educators will find this book to be a clinically relevant text that forms a basis for developing a comprehensive curriculum in behavioral medicine. Training in the core competencies required by the Accreditation Council for Graduate Medical Education (ACGME) will be enhanced by inclusion of topics covered thoroughly in this book, including clinician-patient communication, professionalism, and cultural competence. For faculty and students who wish to explore a topic in greater depth, the suggestions for further reading and web-based resources provided at the end of each chapter will be helpful.

The principles of behavior change discussed in this book may be applicable beyond the behavior of individuals; they apply to whole societies as they move through the "stages of change" to alter lifestyles that adversely impact the environment and human health. The health and well-being of our personal lives and of the organizations where we work are intertwined with the health of our planet. Being mindful of the factors that promote environmental health can give us insights into the sustainability of our lives and careers in medicine. Land use planners use the equation $C - L = M$ (*Capacity – Load = Margin*) when determining sustainable human population growth. *Capacity* refers to the carrying capacity of the land, which includes available water, natural resources, transportation corridors, and the ability of the land to absorb the wastes of human activity. *Load* refers to the impact or "ecological footprint" of that human activity upon the land. When the carrying capacity of the natural environment is greater than the additional load of human activity, then there will be a *positive margin* and population growth is *sustainable*. Conversely, when the load exceeds the capacity of the land, then there is a *negative margin* and growth is *unsustainable*.

This same equation, $C - L = M$, can be applied to our own lives and the organizations where we work. When work, family, and other commitments chronically overload our own capacity, then we are in a negative margin state, another way of defining *burnout*. Conversely, when our capacity exceeds the load, we are in a positive margin state, and our lives are sustainable and healthy. Restoring the proper relationship of humans with the earth in a way that promotes sustainability in the whole system is what Thomas Berry has called "the great work" of our generation. Physicians and other health professionals have a vital role to play in this work, for our own health and well-being will only be as good as the health of the planet.

Acknowledgments

This book would not have been possible without the support and mentorship of a number of people. We are indebted to Stephen J. McPhee, MD, for recognizing the need for such a book over a decade ago and for continually providing encouragement and advice. We thank James Shanahan, our senior editor at McGraw-Hill, for providing the practical and personal support for this third edition. We are very grateful to our contributing authors who, despite busy schedules as clinicians and teachers, have been generous and conscientious in going the distance with us. We are indebted to Linda Pham for her superb administrative support.

Countless friends and colleagues at our own institutions, as well as the residents we have been privileged to teach and mentor, have contributed to our own learning and the selection of material for this book. We are especially indebted to our colleagues in the Society of General Internal Medicine and the American Academy on Communication in Healthcare, many of whom have contributed chapters for this book, for being the learning community that has helped us grow professionally.

We are grateful to Judy Colligan and Jim Marshall, who loaned us their house on the Oregon coast for the final phases of editing. The warmth and ambience of their place allowed us to spend some productive days while the spring rain and wind played through the surrounding forest.

Jane Kramer and Julie Burns Christensen and our children, Nina and Jonathan Kramer-Feldman and Jake and Hank Christensen and Hank's wife Kerry, have continued to be a renewing and cherished presence in our lives. This book would not have been possible without their love and support.

Mitchell D. Feldman, MD, MPhil
John F. Christensen, PhD
San Francisco, California and Portland, Oregon
November 2007

SECTION I
The Doctor & Patient

The Medical Interview

Mack Lipkin, Jr., MD

INTRODUCTION

The medical interview is the major medium of patient care and is therefore of central importance to practitioners. The interview principally determines the accuracy and completeness of data elicited from the patient. It is the most important factor in determining patient adherence to the plans agreed on—whether to take a medication, undergo a test, or change a diet. The interview is the keystone of patient satisfaction. More than 80% of diagnoses derive from the interview. Interview-related factors have been shown to impact major outcomes of care such as physiologic responses, symptom resolution, pain control, functional status, and emotional health. Quality factors influenced or determined by the medical interview include malpractice suits and their resolution, completeness and accuracy of elicited information, time efficiency, elimination of "doorknob" questions at the closing of the interview, and patient satisfaction.

The interview is therefore a major determinant of professional success, yet fewer than 10% of medical practitioners have spent any time since medical school working on their interviewing ability. When asked, most physicians indicate that they have no plan or approach to monitoring, maintaining, or improving this critical skill. Can you imagine a professional athlete, musician, or pilot not practicing or planning to do so? One would question their commitment and their competence.

The interview, which is also centrally important to practitioners' sense of well-being in their work, is the factor that most influences practitioner satisfaction with each individual encounter. Physicians with high career dissatisfaction attribute this to a great extent to unsatisfactory relationships with patients. Physicians with high job satisfaction have a significant interest in the psychosocial aspects of care, relate effectively with patients, and are capable of managing difficult patient situations.

The Ubiquitous Interview

The central importance of the interview derives from its epidemiology. For most physicians (except noninterventional radiologists, pathologists, and some surgeons), it is more prevalent than any other activity in their work or their lives. The average lengths of time per patient visit for internists, average family practitioners, and pediatricians are 15, 12, and 8 minutes, respectively, and these groups account for 75% of visits. The average overall time for physicians is 6 minutes per visit, a rate curiously constant in the United States, the United Kingdom, The Netherlands, and elsewhere. Some other physicians, who are bringing the average down to 6 minutes, are obviously moving too quickly.

Making conservative assumptions about how many hours a practitioner will work over a 40-year professional lifetime, a generalist will have around 250,000 patient encounters. Each interview can be the source of satisfaction or distress, of learning or apathy, of efficiency or wasted effort (Table 1-1), of personal growth and inspiration or of dispiriting discouragement. Few physicians, however, plan, or even think about, how to improve the balance of the desirable goals of satisfaction, learning, and efficiency for themselves.

Each discipline or special interest, such as psychiatry, occupational health, women's health, or domestic violence, has a special set of questions that must be asked of every patient for the interview to be complete and to elicit that patient's particular problems. (If an interviewer

Table 1-1. Gains from improved interviewing techniques.

- Increased efficiency in use of time
- Increased accuracy and completeness of data
- Improved diagnosis
- Fewer tests and procedures
- Increased compliance
- Increased physician satisfaction
- Increased patient satisfaction
- Decreased dissatisfaction
- Increased mutual learning from each encounter

were to ask all the questions recommended by each of the disparate interests, the interview would go on for hours.) In most cases, these question sets have neither been validated nor shown to be sensitive or specific. Notable exceptions include the CAGE Questionnaire (Table 1-2), which is highly specific, sensitive, and efficient as a screening test for alcoholism (see Chapter 21); the two-question depression screen (see Chapter 22), and the one-question domestic violence screen (see Chapter 35).

Rather than using a series of over-specific questions, the most efficient approach is to be patient centered, first by eliciting the patient's complete set of concerns and questions, followed by open-to-closed cones of questions to encourage elaboration on the information and complete the needed data about each concern. Open-ended questions elicit information more efficiently than do lists of closed-ended questions. A patient-centered approach also ensures that the patient's concerns are understood and agreed on—a predictor of increased compliance.

This approach is most efficient for several reasons. First, patients usually have a sense of what is relevant and will include some key information and data not anticipated by the interviewer. If the physician is thinking of the next question rather than listening to what is being said, the ability to attend and hear at multiple levels is compromised. If the interviewer is talking, the patient is not and so is not providing data. The physician can always refer back to specific items later to round out the data once the patient's story is told. If the same basic format is used for each interview, the variations in responses can be attributed to the patient and provide significant information.

Table 1-2. The CAGE Questionnaire.

C: Have you ever tried to **C**ut down on your drinking?
A: Do you feel **A**nnoyed when asked about your drinking?
G: Do you feel **G**uilty about your drinking?
E: Do you ever take an **E**ye opener in the morning?

The evidence favoring a patient-centered approach goes beyond its practical advantages in the interview. Outcomes of care are also favorably affected. More complete and higher quality information—with the attendant reduction in procedures and tests—reduces cost, needless side effects, and complications. Increased patient adherence to diagnostic and therapeutic plans leads to greater clinical efficiency and effectiveness. Patients take a more active role in their own care.

Active Listening & Efficiency

A number of factors enhance the interview's efficiency. Efficiency is currently of special concern as the "corporatization" of health care leads both doctors and patients to experience care as more rushed. Actual visit lengths have remained constant. As knowledge and regulation grow exponentially, however, the tasks to accomplish in a given visit multiply—more diseases and risks to evaluate, more treatments to choose among and explain, and more bureaucratic hoops to negotiate. These trends will undoubtedly prove short-sighted: when the visit is significantly cut in length or jammed with too much to do, psychosocial discussion is the first thing omitted, which can lead to unnecessary testing, patient dissatisfaction, and hazardous and needless procedures and treatments. These challenges to efficiency and effectiveness are exacerbated when behavioral medicine is removed from the benefits provided by the clinician and is provided instead by an external company. Then both sides compete not to care for the patient and predictably the relationship and quality of care deteriorate.

Because cost effectiveness and time efficiency are paramount, certain techniques can be helpful. Open-ended questions, as noted earlier, allow patients to elaborate on their responses and thus provide additional information. Active listening refers to listening to all that is being said at multiple levels—how it is being said, what is included and what is left out, and how what is said reflects the person's culture, personality, mental status, affect, conscious and unconscious motivation, cognitive style, and so on. "Active" listening also refers to acknowledging or repeating back to patients the essence of the information they have shared, whether clinical or emotional, thus allowing them to feel understood. A skilled active listener acquires such information and other data quickly and continuously. Like a jazz musician, the active listener can create a harmonious flow in synch with the other person's themes, rhythms, and style that enhances the ability of each to contribute to the complex, shifting composition of the interview. The experienced listener gives these observations their appropriate weight as clear data, hypotheses, or biases. This enables the efficient creation of a complex and textured portrait of the patient that can be used in generating hypotheses, crafting replies, giving information, relating behaviors, and further questioning to test hypotheses.

THE STRUCTURE OF THE INTERVIEW

The recent literature on the interview runs to roughly 8500 articles, chapters, and books. Although only a modest portion of these derive from empirical bases, sufficient work has been done to describe the interviews' conceptual framework as having **structure** and **functions**. Behavioral observations and analyses of interviews have related specific behaviors and skills to both structural elements and functions; performance of these behaviors and skills improves clinical outcomes. The following description of essential structural elements and their associated behaviors or techniques, although comprehensive, is not so exhaustive as to be impractical. Key behaviors are summarized in Table 1-3. One comprehensive application of this approach developed by the Macy Initiative in Health Communication is shown in Figure 1-1.

Preparing the Physical Environment

Just as some architects and designers believe that form follows function, so the way in which practitioners organize their physical environment reveals characteristics of their practice: how they view the importance of the patient's comfort and ease, how they want to be regarded, and how they as practitioners control their own environment. This last is a key point, as providers often exhort patients to control theirs. Does the patient have a choice of seating? Are both patient and provider seated at a comparable eye level? Is the room easily accessible, quiet, and private?

Preparing Oneself

Humans can process about seven bits of information simultaneously. How many of these bits are consumed because of distractions or trivia in a clinical encounter? The hypnotic concept of focus or the recently accepted psychological concepts of centering or flow apply to the clinical encounter (see Chapter 5). If thoughts about the last or next patient, yesterday's mistake, last night's argument, passion, or movie intrude, concentration lapses and information and opportunity are lost. In contrast, if the practitioner is focused, without external or internal distractions, and expects the interview to be a challenging, fascinating, and unique experience, chances are it will be.

How to achieve such a state of mind is a personal process and is related to each situation. Nevertheless, a few things are common to successful centering: eliminating outside intrusion by having someone else answer the beeper and take phone calls; tuning out other sounds; eliminating internal distractions and intrusive thoughts by resolving not to work on other matters and letting disturbing thoughts simply pass out of consciousness for the moment; and controlling distracting reactions to what is occurring in the interview by noting them, thinking about their origins, and putting them aside if they are not helpful.

These skills do not just happen. I teach my residents self-hypnosis and when they get routinely and efficiently able to get to a place of heightened, relaxed focus, I encourage them to use this together with the suggestions in Table 1-4 to enhance their chances of making something wonderful happen in each encounter.

Observing the Patient

A great deal can be learned by thoughtfully observing the patient's behavior and body language both before and during the encounter. Although such initial behavioral observations are purely heuristic—used to generate testable hypotheses about the patient—nonverbal behavior can sometimes reveal as much about the patient's state of mind as do the patient's verbal responses. Clinicians who are unaware of being influenced by initial reactions and observations in the patient interview may note that when they themselves get on a bus or an airplane, they instantly recognize the person next to whom they would prefer—or prefer not—to sit. Such responses result from integrating a considerable number of nonverbal cues. Similar input about patients can relate to their overall state of health, vital signs, cardiac and pulmonary compensation, liver function, and more. Observations about grooming, state of rest, alertness, and style of presentation can reveal much about the patient's self-confidence, the presence of psychosis, depression, or anxiety, the patient's personality style, and important changes from prior visits. The physician may also detect signs of possible alcohol or drug use. Escorting patients from the waiting area, letting them walk slightly ahead into the office, allows the practitioner to observe how patients have used their waiting time, to notice their gait, to see who accompanies them, and to find clues to their relationship with these escorts.

Developing the ability to make and use such clinical observations starts with the intention to do so. A decision to systematically retain and integrate initial observations will provide the physician with important data that have been easily available, but typically overlooked. Asking pertinent questions about behavioral cues, keeping in mind the kinds of observations that are possible and refining these skills through practice will increase the physician's speed and comprehensiveness of observing. By practicing in crowds, at rounds or in lectures, on the airplane or at parties, it is possible to train oneself to become a more astute observer. It is the clinician's equivalent of practicing scales on the piano or batting practice.

Greeting the Patient

The greeting serves to identify each party to the interaction, to set the social tone, to telegraph intentions concerning equality or dominance, and to prevent mistaken identity. It also allows the practitioner to establish an

Table 1-3. Structural elements of the medical interview.

Element	Technique or Behavior
Prepare the environment	Create a private area. Eliminate noise and distractions. Provide comfortable seating at equal eye level. Provide easy physical access.

Prepare oneself	Eliminate distractions and interruptions.
	Focus on:
	    Self-hypnosis
	    Meditation
	    Constructive imaging
	Let intrusive thoughts pass.

Observe the patient	Create a personal list of categories of observation. Practice in a variety of settings. Notice physical signs. Notice patient's presentation and affect. Notice what is said and not said.
Greet the patient	Create a flexible personal opening. Introduce oneself. Check the patient's name and how it is pronounced. Create a positive social setting.
Begin the interview	Explain one's role and purpose. Check patient's expectations. Negotiate about differences in perspective. Be sure expectations are congruent with patient's.

Detect and overcome barriers to communication	Be aware of and look for potential barriers:
	    Language
	    Physical impediments such as deafness, delirium
	    Cultural differences
	    Psychological obstacles such as shame, fear, and paranoia

Survey problems	Develop personal methods to elicit an accounting of problems. Ask "what else" until problems are described.
Negotiate priorities	Ask patient for his or her priorities. State own priorities. Establish mutual interests. Reach agreement on the order of addressing issues.

Develop a narrative thread	Develop personal ways of asking patients to tell their story:
	    When did patient last feel healthy?
	    Describe entire course of illness.
	    Describe recent episode or typical episode.

Establish the life context of the patient	Use first opportunity to inquire about personal and social details. Flesh out developmental history. Learn about patient's support system. Learn about home, work, neighborhood, and safety issues.
Establish a safety net	Memorize complete review of systems. Review issues as appropriate to specific problem.
Present findings and options	Be succinct. Ascertain patient's level of understanding and cognitive style. Ask patient to review and state understanding. Summarize and check. Tape interview and give copy of tape to patient. Ask patient's perspectives.
Negotiate plans	Involve patient actively. Agree on what is feasible. Respect patient's choices whenever possible.
Close the interview	Ask patient to review plans and arrangements. Clarify what patient should do in the interim. Schedule next encounter. Say good-bye.

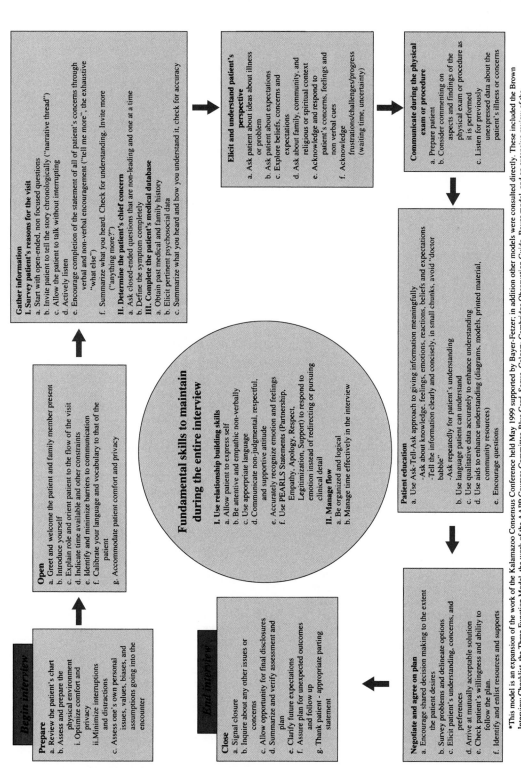

Figure 1-1. The medical interview. (Developed by the Macy Initiative in Health Communication.)

Table 1-4. Self-hypnotic suggestions to enhance interview outcomes.

In this encounter I will:
Focus on the patient and his or her concerns
Not hear outside distractors
Let intrusive thoughts pass through unheeded
Connect meaningfully with this person
Learn something new and surprising about him or her
Have a positive encounter
Leave feeling energized
Help the patient grow, change, and heal
Help the patient leave the interview feeling hopeful and committed

immediate connection with patients, showing them that they are entrusting themselves to a confident, compassionate professional. It enables the clinician to learn how patients assert their own identity and how to pronounce their names. Using a standard greeting—saying virtually the same thing each time—provides a basis for evaluating a variety of patient responses.

Beginning the Interview

The introductory phase of a medical encounter provides an opportunity for both parties to express their understanding of the purposes and conditions of the encounter, to check each other's expectations, and to negotiate any differences. For example, the patient expects to be seen by the head of the clinic, but the physician is only a year out of residency. The patient wants relief of his back pain and the practitioner is worried about his high blood pressure. The practitioner expects the consultation to lead to cardiac catheterization, whereas the patient thinks the cardiologist's opinions will be sent to his primary care physician for a decision. Or perhaps the physician can spare only 15 minutes, but the patient feels a full hour is needed.

Because one of the best predictors of the outcome of a dyadic relationship is the expectations of each person, clarifying and reconciling these is extremely valuable before beginning the main part of the interview.

Detecting & Overcoming Barriers to Communication

Many factors can interfere with communication between people, and these place even more barriers between doctor and patient. Sometimes there are tangible barriers in patient care: delirium, dementia, deafness, aphasia, intoxication on the part of patient or physician, and ambient noise. Psychological barriers can include depression, anxiety, psychosis, paranoia, and distrust. Social barriers often involve language, cultural differences, and fears about immigration status, stigma, or legal problems. It is essential to detect such barriers early in an encounter; failure to do so not only wastes time but also can seriously and sometimes dangerously mislead the physician. In addition, detecting a barrier is the first step toward its correction, whether by waiting until delirium or intoxication has cleared; finding a professional interpreter or signer; moving to a quiet, private place; or waiting to deal with difficult issues until trust is established.

Surveying Problems

Because patients come to medical encounters with multiple problems and may not lead with the most pressing issue, and because physicians typically interrupt very quickly (23 seconds on average), it is vitally important that clinicians not jump in at the first important-sounding problem, but instead survey all problems first. For example, the clinician might ask, "What problems are you having?" or "What issues would you like to work on first?" After getting the initial answer or series of answers, the clinician can then ask what else is bothering the patient until the list of problems ends.

Negotiating Priorities

Once the clinician and the patient clearly understand the full list of problems, the clinician should then ask, "Which of these would you like to work on first?" If the physician believes that something else is more important, there should be negotiation about this difference: "Our time is limited today, and I think your shortness of breath is potentially more dangerous than your back pain. Suppose we deal with that first and, if we have time, go on to your back pain. If not, we'll take that up on your next visit."

The appropriate and understandable resentment resulting when the physician does not ascertain and acknowledge the patient's priorities can lead to treatment adherence problems or failure to return to the office.

Developing a Narrative Thread

Once clinician and patient have decided which problem has priority, exploration of that problem begins. Note the term "exploration." All too often the approaches are either to jump into a review of systems ("you have rectal bleeding; . . . are your gums bleeding; . . . ?") or to elicit the seven cardinal features of the sign or symptom ("where is it, does it radiate, what makes it better or worse . . . ?" and so on). The most efficient method is to explore the problem by asking the patient to tell the story of the problem, as in "Tell me about your rectal bleeding." Although many persons will begin at an appropriate point and move toward the present, some patients may need or wish to be guided as to where to start. The physician may choose to ask when the patient last felt healthy, when the current episode began, or when the patient thinks the problem started. The patient may not have a feel for the necessary level of detail and may be either too inclusive or too superficial. It may therefore be necessary for the physician to interrupt and indicate a desire to hear more or less about the problem. Clarifying questions will show the patient what is needed, and most persons will thereafter provide the appropriate level of detail.

Establishing the Life Context of the Patient

Once the narrative thread is in place, the physician can take the opportunity, when it arises, to inquire about specific points. Such inquiries help the physician learn about and understand in more detail the context of the patient's life—spouse, family, neighborhood, job, culture. When enough information has been supplied, simply saying, "You were saying . . . " or "What happened next?" returns the patient to the narrative. This approach works because everyone understands how to tell a story and remembers the key points because they are intrinsically organized by what actually happened.

Creating a Safety Net

Once the problems the patient wishes to discuss have been explored, areas or questions may remain that have not been covered. For these, the physician may choose to ask a series of specific questions or to use a review of systems not already covered. These questions may take the form of the seven dimensions of symptoms described as the location, duration, severity, quality, associations, radiation, and exacerbants and ameliorants, or a subset of these dimensions. Such final closed-ended questions tie up the loose ends and provide the safety of completeness.

Talking During the Physical Examination & Procedures

During the physical examination, there is a tension between the quiet focusing of the senses and mutually necessary talk. Practitioners need to use their senses of smell, sight, touch, and hearing to examine the patient. They need to heighten sensory awareness and to think about what they are encountering. Patients need an explanation of what is being done and what to expect (this may hurt), instruction about what to do (please sit here, bring up your knees, hold your breath), and checking on how the patient is doing and responding (does this hurt?). The examination often stimulates patients' memories of relevant experiences and problems they had forgotten to mention.

Some physicians like to explain in detail what is happening (I am looking in the back of your eye because it is the one place in the body where blood vessels can be seen). Others do the review of systems during the physical. In general, it is probably wise to minimize distractions during the physical or a procedure by confining talk to what is necessary for the task and is needed by the patient. Then, at the end, the process of explaining what has been found can benefit from the ability of the clinician to observe and respond to the patient's reactions and questions.

Presenting Findings & Options

After the history-taking and physical examination have been completed, it is time for the physician and patient to discuss what the problems appear to be, related findings, the physician's hypotheses or conclusions, and possible approaches to further diagnostic evaluation and treatment. This should be done in language free of jargon and at a level of abstraction that the patient can understand.

It is very valuable to foreshadow any bad or potentially upsetting news (see Chapter 3). This preparation helps the patient hear and retain the information better. When bad news is a certainty, it is useful to tape record the explanation and any discussion and give the tape to the patient. These days, having a digital-recorder set up in the room allows you to copy the file and provide it by e-mail or on a CD in a common format such as MP3 which everyone can find a way to play. This way the patient can review it later, when out of shock. It has been documented that listening to the recording allows the patient to better understand the situation and improves outcomes of care. It is essential not to underestimate the potential impact of both positive and negative findings on the patient. After presenting each item the physician should explore the patient's understanding and reactions. The presentation itself should be problem oriented and systematic—and as simple and succinct as possible. Although the dictum is to be brief, content and empathy should not be sacrificed to brevity.

Negotiating a Plan

Once patients have been factually informed of the diagnosis and prognosis, it is crucial to involve them actively in making choices and in developing diagnostic and therapeutic plans. Such "activation" of patients has been shown to increase their adherence to plans and improve their medical outcomes and quality of life.

When physician and patient disagree in emphasis or choice, negotiation is necessary. The principles of negotiation can be summarized as finding the areas of mutual interest, emphasizing them, and avoiding the adoption of inflexible positions that can lead only to conflict and defeat. If physicians take the time to understand patients' positions and respect their concerns, the issues can usually be worked out, for example, by agreeing to do a procedure after a grandchild's graduation or agreeing to do noninvasive tests first in the hope they will suffice.

Closing the Interview

The closing should include reviewing the principal findings, plans, and agreements; making arrangements for the next visit and giving the patient instructions for the intervening time; making sure outstanding issues have been covered; and saying good-bye.

THE FUNCTIONS OF THE INTERVIEW

The three functions of the interview describe the major purposes of the interview and associated skills and behaviors that improve the interview process and outcomes. The three functions—(1) gathering information and monitoring progress; (2) developing, maintaining, and concluding the therapeutic relationship; and (3) educating the patient and implementing treatment plans—are interdependent. For example, patients cannot be expected to reveal personal or humiliating information unless they have developed considerable trust in their physicians. The physician cannot educate a patient effectively without knowing what level of language and which concepts to use, how to frame things for clarity, and which formulations will interpose needless barriers to acceptance—all data derived during information gathering. Therefore, the three functions cannot be pursued sequentially but must be integrated.

Gathering Information & Monitoring Progress

Many physicians consider these medical activities to be the dominant function of the interview. The tasks associated with this first function are to acquire a knowledge base of diseases and disorders and of psychosocial issues and illness behavior; to elicit the data relevant to each problem; to perceive the relevant data; and to generate and test hypotheses relevant to the elicited data. Skills useful in these tasks include starting with open questions such as "Tell me about it" and gradually narrowing the queries down to more specific questions; use of minimal encouragers (e.g., "Uh huh," "Hmmm") to facilitate flow; gentle use of direction to steer without dominating; and summarizing and checking ("I think you have said point a, point b, point c; is that right?").

Developing & Maintaining the Therapeutic Relationship

The second function of the interview includes defining the nature of the relationship (short or long term,

consultation, primary care, disease-episode oriented); demonstrating professional expertise; communicating interest, respect, empathy, and support; recognizing and resolving relational barriers to communication; and eliciting the patient's perspective. A relationship that engenders trust and safety is pivotal, as it is necessary to gather intimate information in order to enable a patient actively to make lifestyle changes or difficult medical decisions.

The belief that relationships cannot be improved, worked on, or manipulated has been disproved by the empirical psychotherapy literature. It is clear that use of appropriate relationship-building skills significantly improves interview outcomes in terms of satisfaction, compliance, data disclosure, quality of life, biological outcomes, and personal growth. These issues are particularly germane in cases involving mental disorders, in which skill in managing the patient in a manner compatible with the disorder is essential.

In general, naming feelings, communicating unconditional positive regard, expressing empathy and understanding, and being emotionally congruent (what you say is actually what you mean and feel) produce the best outcomes. Other skills include reflection, legitimization, partnership, the nonverbal skills of touch and eye contact, and the avoidance of shame or humiliation (see Chapter 2).

Educating the Patient

Patient education and implementation of treatment plans require being aware of the patient's current level of knowledge, understanding, and motivation and the patient's cognitive style and level; having a receptive patient who is neither in shock nor in disagreement; and using plain language that avoids jargon or undue complexity. The tasks associated with this third function include communicating the diagnostic significance of the problems; negotiating and recommending appropriate diagnostic and treatment options and appropriate prevention and lifestyle changes; and enhancing the patient's ability to cope by understanding and communicating the psychological and social impacts of the illness. Involving the patient in making choices, clarifying uncertainties, and expressing fears and concerns markedly improve outcomes. Having the patient actively review what has been discussed and decided is critical to check for understanding, to reinforce memory, and to be sure the patient can and will do what has been agreed (see Chapter 17).

Sometimes, the patient problem is a bad habit or addiction such as overeating, smoking, gambling, or forgetting to take pills. Two approaches have been demonstrated to be helpful in such situations—(1) using the stages of change model and (2) motivational interviewing (see Chapter 16).

Assessing the patient's stage of change uses the scheme described by Prochaska and DiClemente. This involves ascertaining if patients have thought of changing or not (precontemplative or contemplative). If they have thought of changing, then it is appropriate to move them to an action plan by setting key milestones such as a quit date for smokers. When a plan is made, the model includes discussing barriers and how to respond when relapse occurs. Thus, the notion of change as involving several cycles which eventually lead to success unloads the weight of the probable first failures, reframes them as learning experiences, and may actually improve the likelihood of eventual success.

Motivational interviewing, developed by Miller and colleagues, is an approach that increases treatment retention, adherence, and patient self-perceived motivation when it is introduced at the beginning of treatment. Developed initially for use with addicts, it reframes resistance as motivation by using such devices as the "readiness ruler," which asks the patient to rate on a scale of 1 to 10 (10 highly, 1 very little) how motivated he or she is to change the subject behavior. Even if the patient says her motivation to lose weight is a 2, you can get a motivational fingernail under that by asking, "Why wasn't that a 1?" and building on whatever slim reeds of motivation there are. The approach emphasizes collaboration with the patient, exploration of ambivalence, management of resistance, and shifts the clinician-patient approach from confrontation to partnership.

SPECIAL CIRCUMSTANCES & INTERVIEW MODIFICATIONS

Although the preceding principles are applicable to most situations, many circumstances require a modified approach to maximize the usefulness and durability of the interview and relationship. Early detection of special situations is crucial, so that the appropriate changes in technique can be made as soon as possible. In most special situations, meticulous attention to the particular relationship needs of the patient is paramount, as, for example, with the paranoid or psychotic patient.

Aids to Diagnosing Mental Disorders

Physicians currently have a variety of aids to use in diagnosing and monitoring mental disorders. The simplest aids have relatively high sensitivity (they detect most of the real cases) but lower specificity (they register as positive cases that do not meet the diagnostic criteria). Among the screening devices for depression are the Beck, Zung, and Hamilton scales. Recently, a two-question screen and a nine-question quantitative scoring method, the Patient Health Questionnaire, have also been shown to be useful in primary care settings (see Chapter 22). Some physicians administer these as part of a packet of materials to be filled out prior to the initial visit. As with other questionnaires, however, these create the additional problem of having to deal with a large number of false positives, which can be extremely time consuming. One recently developed instrument (with pharmaceutical company support) can screen for the most common mental disorders at the same time. The Primary Care Screen for Mental Disorders (PRIME-MD) is reasonably sensitive and specific and is available for telephone use and for computerized administration. However, empathic physicians have two problems with its use: the program asks about feelings but cannot respond to their expression and scoring it takes several minutes. The role of such devices is still evolving.

SUGGESTED READINGS

Back A, Baile W. Communication skills: myths, realities, and new developments. *J Support Oncol* 2003;1:169–171.

Duffy DF, Gordon GH, Whelan G, et al. Assessing competence in communication and interpersonal skills: the Kalamazoo II report. *Acad Med* 2004;79:495–507.

Haidet P. Jazz and the art of medicine: improvisation in the medical encounter. *Annuals Fam. Med.* 2007; 5:164–169.

Lipkin M, Putnam SM, Lazare A, eds. *The Medical Interview: Clinical Care, Education, and Research.* New York, NY: Springer-Verlag, 1995.

Rao JK, Anderson LA, Inui TS, Frankel RM. Communication interventions make a difference in conversations between physicians and patients. *Med Care* 2007;45:340–349.

Yedidia MJ, Gillespie C, Kachur E, et al. Effect of communications training on medical student performance. *JAMA* 2003;290: 1157–1165.

OTHER RESOURCE

Novack DH, Clark W, Saizow R, et al., eds. *Doc.com: An Interactive Learning Resource for Healthcare Communication.* American Academy on Communication in Healthcare Web site. www.aachonline.org/doccom/. Accessed September, 2007.

ORGANIZATIONS AND WEB SITES

American Academy on Communication in Healthcare Web site. www.aachonline.org. Accessed September, 2007.

Institute for Healthcare Communication (IHC) Web site. http://healthcarecomm.org. Accessed September, 2007.

Motivational Interviewing Web site. www.motivationalinterview.org. Accessed September, 2007.

Northwest Center for Physician-Patient Communication. The Foundation for Medical Excellence Web site. www.tfme.org. Accessed September, 2007.

Empathy

Barry Egener, MD

INTRODUCTION

The concept of empathy dates from the early years of this century, when discussions of the topic were restricted to psychotherapists' analyses of their interactions with patients. More recently, the concept has received renewed attention from a wide spectrum of health practitioners and educators. They believe that empathy can positively affect communication with patients and thus lead to improved therapeutic outcomes. Many of the lay public regard empathy as an avenue to the restoration of compassion and humanism to the doctor–patient relationship, which has been threatened by and has become increasingly impersonal due to technology and financial pressures.

The power of empathy lies in its ability to help us cross, if only for a moment, the divide between clinicians and patients created by their very different circumstances. To briefly bridge that divide and to become simply two humans sharing an experience can help in accomplishing professional diagnostic and therapeutic tasks. We have all experienced the gratitude of patients, isolated by depression or family loss, for our expressed understanding of their sadness.

Succeeding at the greater challenge of putting aside our disagreement with a patient requesting chronic narcotics or perhaps our negative judgment of a patient unable to quit smoking can have proportionally greater rewards. Being willing to imagine what it must be like for these more challenging patients can provide us with insight into what motivates them or what might help them. That's diagnostic information. Communicating that insight may encourage patients to change their behavior. That's therapeutic. Our disclosure also allows us to check the accuracy of what we think we know about the patient's state. We relinquish nothing of ourselves or our role in that moment, we simply expand our perspective.

Empathy can be defined as an intellectual identification with, or vicarious experiencing of, the feelings, thoughts, or attitudes of another. Some have described empathy as a momentary identification with another person in which our human capacity to feel what another feels erodes the boundaries of self. If we in fact temporarily lose awareness of self, the process might better be termed "sympathy for" or "feeling with" someone else. Remaining aware that we are experiencing empathy prevents total dissolution of ego boundaries and permits a more salutary stance. **Empathy skills** are behaviors that demonstrate empathy. They may be the clinician's most powerful therapeutic tool.

Research suggests that empathy skills can be taught. This chapter will describe how to develop and improve these skills. Research has recently shed light on the frequency of empathic opportunities in clinical practice, on how physicians respond to or neglect these opportunities, and the implications of such choices. Empathic opportunities occur in more than half of surgical and primary care visits, although on average there are more opportunities per visit in primary care (2.6) than in surgical care (1.9). Patients initiate most of the opportunities. Contrary to common belief, surgeons respond empathically at least as frequently as primary care physicians, but both miss opportunities to respond more frequently. Empathic behaviors enhance the effectiveness of care as well as patient satisfaction, and their absence may predispose patients to initiate malpractice suits.

There are numerous barriers to discussing emotions with patients, from the impersonal office setting to the disinclination of both physician and patient to address particularly sensitive topics. Nonetheless, appropriate skilled communication can break through these barriers.

OVERCOMING BARRIERS TO EMPATHY

Understanding the feelings, attitudes, and experiences of the patient is the first step toward a more potent therapeutic alliance. Many patients, however, may not be skilled in revealing their feelings to their providers. They need to be made aware that their doctor is interested in their feelings and values them, and that feelings are a legitimate topic for discussion in a medical interview.

Table 2-1. Barriers to discussing emotions.

Doctor
1. Takes too much time
2. Too draining
3. Will lose control of interview
4. Can't fix patient's distress
5. Not my job
6. Perceived conflicts of interest

Patient
1. Cultural taboo about discussing emotions
2. Preference for interpreting distress in a biomedical model
3. Somatization disorder
4. Desire to meet doctor's expectations
5. Worry about being emotionally overwhelmed
6. Lack of language for emotions

Emotions can be difficult for both doctors and patients (Table 2-1), and doctors particularly may prefer the certainty of science. From the patient's point of view, if difficult emotional issues are manifested as a somatic complaint, denial might be the first reaction to a psychological interpretation of the symptoms. The physician must appreciate and mirror the terms in which a patient will speak about illness. In many cultures, emotions are simply not discussed. In the United States, where the biomedical model of disease still predominates over the biopsychosocial model, patients may feel that it is more acceptable to have physical rather than emotional complaints. Because this expectation is often reinforced by their physicians, it behooves physicians to establish a climate conducive to the expression of emotional material and a language useful to that end. Physicians often mention the following barriers to discussing emotions with patients.

1. **It takes too much time**. In a busy practice, concerns about time are legitimate. Given an organized framework, however, it takes only a few minutes to deal effectively with emotion, and the strategies discussed later in this chapter can prove time efficient for the physician. Recent studies suggest that interviews in which physicians respond to emotions may actually be shorter than those in which they do not. An explanation of this finding is that it may be more time consuming to deal with the indirect effects of unaddressed emotions during the rest of the interview. Moreover, it may be useful to distinguish between "acute efficiency" and "chronic efficiency." "Efficiency" should take into consideration not only the duration of a particular visit, but also the total amount of time required to address the patient's concerns. Even if it were to take a few extra minutes to address emotions, that time is more than compensated by fewer phone calls and fewer unscheduled visits.

2. **It's too draining**. It is unrealistic to expect all providers to be emotionally available at all times to all their patients. A physician who has been awake all night or is emotionally needy may be justified in putting off a discussion of emotions that should otherwise occur. If the physician chooses to defer, it would be wise to return to the topic at another time. Primary care providers sometimes exert a tremendous amount of energy avoiding emotions in the belief that dealing directly with them will be draining. However, it can be far more efficient to make an emotional connection than to expend so much energy in resisting it.

   At times, patients may inadvertently raise issues that are emotionally difficult for their providers. Sometimes the clinician can discuss the difficulty with friends, family, or colleagues; at other times it may be most fruitfully addressed in the physician's own therapy. (A longer discussion of this area is beyond the scope of this chapter, but difficult encounters with patients offer physicians an opportunity for personal growth; see Chapter 4.)

3. **The interview will get out of control**. Although many doctors worry that addressing emotions will cause feelings to escalate, the opposite is often true. Addressing emotions helps diffuse them. Learning a language to handle emotions creates a comfortable distance from the emotions themselves, so that neither the doctor nor the patient becomes overwhelmed.

4. **I can't fix it for the patient**. Primary care providers are used to "fixing" things. Feelings, however, simply exist, and can't be "fixed." Patients do not expect their feelings to be eliminated; they just want them to be understood.

5. **It's not my job**. Some doctors believe that their job is to address disease and the psychotherapist's job is to address mental illness. There are several problems with this attitude. Although it is certainly true that collaboration with mental health practitioners may at times be useful, about 65% of mental illnesses are cared for exclusively by primary care physicians. About 26% of primary care patients have mental health diagnoses, and even a higher percentage have important psychiatric comorbidities. Physicians who insist on interpreting the physical symptoms of psychiatric disease such as panic disorder or depression in purely biomedical terms miss the point—and their patients will not get better. Telling a patient who develops chest pain on the anniversary of his father's death (see "The Therapeutic Language of Empathy," below) that there is nothing wrong with him will help the patient only briefly. Moreover, many physical illnesses have psychosocial sequelae that must also be addressed.

When a patient keeps returning with the same complaint, unimproved by a physician's interventions, the patient is trying to communicate a message. Physicians are often frustrated by these patients; this frustration can be alleviated and the doctor's satisfaction improved by the progress that comes with addressing the underlying problem.

6. **Perceived conflicts of interest**. Although the more apparent financial conflicts of interest presented by managed care may have diminished in recent years, it is likely that new potential conflicts of interest will continue to arise even as the field upon which these play out changes. Physicians have always needed to balance the needs of the patients in front of them with those of society at large. Research has now demonstrated that patients prefer having their concerns acknowledged and validated rather than the physician blaming an external party for shared constraints. Physicians who feel challenged by patients' questioning their motives are likely to act defensively. The empathy skills offer an alternative that makes the physician a partner again.

THE ROLE OF EMPATHY IN DIAGNOSIS

Feelings that arise in the provider during an encounter may be useful in forming a diagnostic hypothesis about the patient. For example, a doctor who feels burdened, heavy, or "down" during an interview might consider the possibility that the patient is depressed.

All clinicians have had the experience of trying to help a patient with a behavior change, such as weight loss, only to have each suggestion rejected: "I've already tried that, Doc; it doesn't work." The physician's own feelings of frustration and powerlessness in trying to motivate the patient are often mirrored by the patient's sense of frustration and powerlessness in attempting to accomplish the change in behavior. The physician can confirm the hypothesis that the patient is frustrated, as with any other diagnosis, by testing: "I'm feeling frustrated with this problem, and I'm wondering if you're feeling the same way."

Some patients consistently elicit dislike and rejection from their providers. It may seem that the patient is intentionally trying to manipulate the provider into becoming angry. This may in fact be true. When providers become aware of these feelings, they should consider the possibility that their own impulses to punish the patient may be playing into the patient's self-image as deserving of punishment. This pattern may be consistent with a borderline personality disorder (see Chapter 26).

The physician's experience does not invariably reflect the patient's experience. Rather, physicians should notice their feelings and ask, "Does the way I feel tell me something about the patient or something about myself?" For example, a physician who has recently seen a number of patients seeking drugs begins to feel angry and defensive on noticing that the nurse has recorded "low back pain" as the next patient's chief complaint; these negative feelings indicate more about the physician's recent experiences than they do about the next patient. Feelings are primary data about the person in whom they arise and indirect data about others. The next section clarifies how to test the hypothesis that a patient is feeling a particular emotion and outlines how to respond.

THE THERAPEUTIC LANGUAGE OF EMPATHY

Although empathy is not generally considered a therapeutic tool, discussion of emotional issues can be therapeutic. An empathic relationship is crucial in psychotherapy and enhances the power of all therapeutic relationships. The following sections show how to talk about emotions using specific skills. A premise of this discussion is that biomedical aspects of disease cannot be effectively addressed without considering their emotional consequences. Emotions, whether related to physiological dysfunction or psychosocial issues, color the discussion in the examining room and may be so distracting that the patient cannot fully concentrate on other issues until the emotions are addressed.

A clinical scenario helps to illustrate the usefulness of the emotion-handling skills described here.

 CASE ILLUSTRATION 1

While you are on call for admissions from the emergency room for patients without a primary care physician, a 45-year-old man is admitted because of concern that his 2-week history of chest pain may represent unstable angina. Although the emergency room physician acknowledges that it's a "soft admission," the patient has a history of elevated lipids, a family history of cardiac disease, and his blood pressure in the emergency room is 180/95. The patient describes a sharp substernal chest pain that occurs at rest, when working in the yard, and while trying to fall asleep at night. He does not smoke or have diabetes. On examination, he appears anxious, his blood pressure on the cardiac floor is 160/90, and he is 5% over ideal body weight. The rest of his examination, laboratory tests, electrocardiogram, and chest x-ray are normal, except for his low-density lipoprotein cholesterol, which is 160 mg/dL.

You greet the patient with outstretched hand:

Doctor: *Good morning, Mr. Swenson, my name is Dr. Bergen. I'll be taking care of you while you're in the hospital.*

Patient: *Well, Doctor, am I having a heart attack?*

Doctor: *You haven't had a heart attack. I can tell from your blood tests and electrocardiograms.*

Patient: *Well is the pain coming from my heart?*

Doctor: *I don't think so.*

Patient: *But you're not sure?*

Doctor: *Nothing in medicine is certain, but your age, the character of your pains, and the fact that antacids help somewhat reassure me that the problem is most likely acid indigestion or muscular pain.*

Patient: *Don't you think we should do more tests to be sure?*

Doctor: *Although you are at low risk for having coronary artery disease, I think it would be prudent to do an exercise stress test as an outpatient just to be sure.*

Patient: *What if I have a heart attack in the meantime? I'm still worried.*

Doctor: *You don't need to be. Besides, you were admitted under "observation status" to make sure you didn't have an unstable cardiac condition, and we have done that. By standard protocols, you fall into the low risk category, and your insurance will not allow you to remain an inpatient for further risk stratification. Don't worry, you'll be all right.*

Patient: *Well, okay, if you say so.*

Despite a probably accurate diagnosis of noncardiac chest pain, providing good information, and attempts to reassure the patient, something goes awry in this interaction. The patient still doesn't seem satisfied. Let's look at the effect empathic skills might have.

The techniques discussed in the following sections are adapted from a three-function model of the medical interview developed by Bird and Cole. The goals of the interview are described as gathering medical data, building a relationship with the patient, and educating and motivating the patient (see Chapter 1). The following emotion-handling skills are related to the second function, building relationships with patients (Table 2-2).

REFLECTION

Reflection refers to naming the emotion the doctor sees and reflecting it back to the patient. Reflection communicates the physician's understanding of the patient's experience. It also has the effect of making the feelings behind the patient's behavior or words explicit, so that they can be dealt with directly.

Table 2–2. The empathic skills.

Skill	Example
Reflection	"You seem upset."
Validation	"I can understand your anger with the callous way you were treated."
Support	"You are doing very well handling your grief."
Partnership	"Perhaps we can work together to make you feel better."
Respect	"You have tremendous compassion for your siblings."

For example, when a patient greets a doctor who is 20 minutes late with, "My time is as valuable as yours," the doctor might say, "I'm sorry I'm late. You seem pretty angry with me." The patient might then ventilate about the doctor's lateness or his treatment at the hands of doctors. He might even deny his anger, since many patients might view an expression of anger at their physicians as unacceptable. In any case, the doctor has a chance to deal with the emotion directly and then proceed with the interview, rather than trying to work with a patient who is angry and has not had a chance to express his anger.

After reflecting an emotion, the doctor should stop talking and see how the patient responds. Although the patient will usually elaborate, if the physician keeps talking, the exploration may be prematurely ended.

Sometimes it is clear that a patient is feeling a strong emotion, but it is not clear what that emotion is. It is perfectly acceptable (and perhaps preferable) to treat the emotion as having a differential diagnosis and test a hypothesis as one would for any other medical entity: "I'm wondering if you're upset," or, more tentatively, "It seems that you're feeling something strongly, but I'm not sure what it is. Can you help me out?"

VALIDATION

Validation informs the patient that you understand the reason for the emotion. This has the effect of normalizing the emotion and making the patient feel less isolated. For example, to a somatizing patient who has been to several doctors who have been unable to find a cause for her abdominal pain, you might say, "I can understand how frustrating it's been to be no better after seeking so much help." Some physicians are reluctant to validate emotions in difficult patients for fear of adding fuel to the fire. If reflection is the empathy skill that opens Pandora's Box, validation is the skill that closes it—it is difficult to remain upset with a person who understands how you feel. You don't have to agree with patients to express understanding of their feelings. For example, to a patient with chronic low back pain who has responded angrily when informed that you will not prescribe narcotics, you might say, "Even though I see it differently, I can understand why you would be angry with me." Although disagreeing with the patient such a statement allows you to offer support and enhances your chances of continuing a therapeutic relationship. Validation of feelings emphasizes that the patient and doctor are equals in the human condition, although they have different roles in the therapeutic relationship.

SUPPORT

An expression of support tells patients that the physician cares about them and is willing to be present to their emotion. The expression can be verbal or nonverbal. Examples of nonverbal expression are handing the tearful patient a tissue or touching the patient. In judging whether touching a patient will be perceived as supportive, invasive, or inappropriate, the physician should consider such factors as culture, age, gender, sexual orientation, previous experience of abuse, and the presence or absence of psychiatric symptoms, such as paranoia. In general, putting a hand on the patient's hand or arm will not be misinterpreted. Many physicians prefer to take the lead from the patient by matching the patient's nonverbal behavior.

Some verbal expressions of support are "It's pretty normal to get angry with children when they act out" and "A spouse's death is one of the most difficult life transitions." Again, these responses are not an attempt to suppress, eliminate, or fix the emotion, but rather an offer to help patients, to reassure them that they are not alone with an uncomfortable emotion. These three skills—reflection, validation, and support—are the most important of the emotion-handling skills and will be involved in most of the work physicians do in this area.

PARTNERSHIP

Partnership implies a team approach, in which the patient and doctor work together toward the same goal. Doctors support and are partners with patients in many ways, but in the context of this chapter the word *partnership* makes it explicit that you would like to help the patient with the troubling emotion. An advantage of partnership is that it may help motivate patients to take an active role in their improvement and may lay the foundation for a contract for behavior change. This is consistent with the notion, especially important when illness results from patient behaviors, that physicians facilitate the patient's healing rather than curing disease in the passive patient. The physician's use of the pronouns *we* and *us* expresses partnership, as in "Perhaps we can make a plan to help you feel better" or "Let's figure out a way to help you deal with this difficult diagnosis."

RESPECT

This skill honors the emotional resources within a patient. The doctor might say "You've been through a lot"

or "I'm impressed with how well you're holding up under the circumstances."

Physicians may not always know what it would be like to be the patient, but they can acknowledge the patient's experience nonetheless: "I'm not a parent, so I can only imagine what it would be like to lose a child. I can see you're feeling the loss quite deeply." On a happier occasion, she might say "What a joy it must be for you to see your grandchild's birth!"

Although it often makes sense to use reflection or validation first when addressing emotion, these skills can be used in any order, and it may be best to go through the sequence several times at different points in an interview.

CASE ILLUSTRATION 1 (CONTD.)

Let us return now to the scenario of the 45-year-old man with chest pain to see how that interaction might be improved with a physician who uses empathic skills. The empathic skills used are listed in parentheses.

Doctor: *Good morning, Mr. Swenson, my name is Dr. Bergen. I'll be taking care of you while you're in the hospital.*

Patient: *Well, Doctor, am I having a heart attack?*

Doctor: *You're understandably worried. (validation) I can tell from your lab tests and electrocardiogram that you haven't had a heart attack.*

Patient: *Then why do I have this pain?*

Doctor: *Our tests don't seem to have reassured you very much. (reflection)*

Patient: *Wouldn't you still be worried if you thought you were working up to a heart attack?*

Doctor: *I certainly would be. So you're worried you're going to have a heart attack. (reflection)*

Patient: *That's what happened to my father. He was raking leaves and just keeled over. I'm the one who found him.*

Doctor: *That must have been horrible. (support)*

Patient: *You can't imagine how awful it was. Every time I think of it I get upset. Sometimes it even brings on this chest pain. I've been thinking about him more and more lately, especially when I go to sleep at night. It makes me afraid to fall asleep. I'm afraid I'm not going to wake up.*

Doctor: *Is there a reason why you've been thinking about him more lately?*

Patient: *Yeah. I thought I got over his death. But this is the time of year he died. Just raking leaves, which I do every weekend, makes me think of him. Then I get this chest pain and worry about myself. Heart disease runs in families, I don't have to tell you.*

Doctor: I'm sorry about your father (support). It sounds as though there's a pretty strong connection between thinking about your father and the chest pain.

Patient: Yeah. I thought maybe being upset stressed my heart. Do you think maybe this is all in my head?

Doctor: I'm sure you really feel the pain, and I suspect your heart still aches for your father—even if only figuratively. It's pretty hard to lose a father. Now, you know there's a pretty strong connection between the body and the mind, and if you've been worrying about your own health, this could be your way of making sure you take care of yourself. (respect)

Patient: I never thought of it that way. What you say makes a lot of sense, and I think you're probably right. But I still have this nagging worry in the back of my mind.

Doctor: That's understandable. (validation) How about this? Let's work together to reduce whatever risk factors you do have for heart disease to make sure you don't have a problem down the line. (partnership) Although you are at low risk for having coronary artery disease, I think it would be prudent to do an exercise stress test as an outpatient just to be sure. I'm going to give you my card so that you can call my office to set it up when you get home. Any time in the next few weeks would be fine. And in the meantime, if the pain gets worse or changes in any way, give me a call. Right now you're having some pretty strong feelings about your father, and if that is the source of your chest pain, it may not go away right away. We'll talk more about it when I see you in the office.

Patient: That seems reasonable to me. I appreciate your listening to me.

Doctor: Okay, then, I'll see you in a few weeks. And remember, if the pains get worse or you get new symptoms along with them, call me immediately; don't wait til the next day.

Patient: Thanks, Doc. See you in a few weeks.

Patient satisfaction, as indicated by the patient's responses toward the end of the interview, seems much greater than in the first scenario. Although this scenario is longer than the first, using empathic skills added only approximately 1 minute to the interview, and if that additional minute prevents unnecessary visits by allaying the patient's concerns, the time is well spent. Early in the interview the doctor does very little talking, and what he does say primarily addresses the patient's charged emotional state. He initially resists the patient's

invitation to confirm conclusively that this is all in his head and instead allows the patient to continue to explore his feeling state. There is uncertainty at the end of the medical interview, but it seems to be an uncertainty that both the doctor and patient can accept comfortably, with a sense of partnership.

IMPLICATIONS FOR PROFESSIONAL DEVELOPMENT

Suppose the content of what the patient reveals is upsetting, distasteful, or even abhorrent to the physician. In the previous example of the patient with chest pain, suppose that the doctor's mother has just died and his father is scheduled for triple-bypass surgery. The mere contemplation of losing his father is so threatening that the physician withdraws into himself. Psychological defense mechanisms may cause the physician to become distracted from the patient's visit and think about his own concerns.

Suppose, on the other hand, that the patient describes a situation that is emotionally charged, but is so alien to the physician's experience that he cannot empathize. If, for example, a homosexual patient reveals that his partner has become HIV positive, the heterosexual physician may pity (feel sorry *for*) the patient but may be unable to relate to the patient's grief and fears. On the other hand, the physician may be so repelled by the concept of homosexuality that his body language betrays his negative feelings. The patient, feeling judged and embarrassed, is likely to withhold relevant information. Or suppose the physician must present certain treatments to a patient that he considers disgusting or repulsive. His own obvious feeling may prevent the patient from making a truly informed decision.

Finding just the right therapeutic stance is essential; it may be partly intuitive and partly learned, and it may vary from patient to patient—or even with the same patient over time—depending on the patient's needs. Opportunities may be lost when the physician is unable to empathize with the patient, or when the loss of ego boundaries makes a therapeutic stance impossible. The most effective physicians are those whose repertoire permits a rapid interplay of objectivity and emotion.

Calibrating responses to patients requires noticing and understanding when clinicians' own emotional issues prevent them from being maximally effective with patients. The first clue may be that a specific patient or type of patient particularly irks a physician. These "irksome patients" are our teachers. They teach us about ourselves. Personal barriers to effectiveness with patients usually originate in the physician's own family of origin. Numerous tools are available to help physicians overcome these barriers: speaking with a trusted colleague, Balint or other support groups, courses that focus specifically on personal awareness, and personal psychotherapy.

Empathy in Medical Training

Viewing empathy in this way may have special applications to medical training. There is evidence that empathy correlates with the fluctuation of mood state during residency. It is remarkable how the fresh enthusiasm and caring of medical students can quickly devolve into the wry cynicism of residents. What accounts for this withdrawal? The usual explanation is that insulating oneself in this way is an act of self-preservation in the face of overwhelming demands. It can be torturous to feel another's pain, and if the self is already stressed because of long hours and the other exigencies of training, it may be more difficult to sustain an open posture.

The ways in which doctors withdraw depend on both their personalities and their environment. If the culture around the resident tolerates derogatory labels for patients, it can be easy to see patients as *other*, as not sharing some element of humanity with *us*. Even if such labels are not tolerated and caring for patients is a highly preserved value, dark humor may surface as a means of insulation. To take care of others, one must first take care of oneself. Finding the right balance is a major developmental task of the health care professions. Perhaps by attending to the well-being of trainees, we will make them better doctors (see Chapter 42). Since empathy directly correlates with well-being in internal medicine residents, it is important that training programs demonstrate that caring for others is valuable. Experienced physicians can attend to trainees' growth, help them develop effective and healthy working styles, model those styles, and draw attention to the importance of being aware of one's own development. There is a huge contrast between the concept of residency training as nurturing or mentoring and the concept of residency as "trial by fire." And fire, we know, steels metal, making it harder.

Empathy in the Practice of Medicine

What happens after training? For some practitioners, the pressure becomes less, healthy coping styles develop, and the caring physician re-emerges. Far too many, however, are casualties of the training process—or their families are. Physicians' compulsive personality styles are susceptible to a pattern of delayed gratification. Constantly nurturing others, physicians may have no time left for themselves. Family relationships may atrophy. The most effective physicians may be those who attend to their own needs as well as those of their patients, who understand their own unique struggles, so that these struggles—by making physicians aware of their own humanity—can enhance, rather than detract from, their relationships

with patients. Studies suggest that women and those specializing in psychiatry, emergency medicine, and primary care specialties are more empathic than those specializing in the surgical subspecialties.

Because the culture of an institution strongly influences the practice of medicine within its purview, physicians who practice together have a unique opportunity to enhance each other's empathic skills. Patient-care conferences can incorporate psychosocial issues into the discussions of difficult cases. Videotaped interviews with difficult patients are a powerful tool that allows physicians to examine their own contributions to the difficulty of such interactions.

Regular videotaped conferences, in which physicians take turns presenting cases, allow them to feel at ease in front of the camera, demonstrate collaboration and mutual support, and reinforce the importance and value of empathy to the group. Balint groups or other types of support groups, which may include nonphysician office staff, can help health practitioners cope with collegial interactions or family relationships that have become stressed by practice. Such groups also show that a psychosocial perspective can benefit both physicians and their patients.

Understanding the interaction between illness and emotion helps us become more effective physicians. Familiarity and practice with the skills in this chapter can make us more comfortable discussing this interaction with our patients. Becoming aware of our own personal response to patients promotes personal growth as well. The emotional demands of the medical profession can be enriching or impoverishing. Using skills of empathy, we may become more satisfied and effective clinicians; our patients may become more satisfied and healthier.

SUGGESTED READINGS

Bellini LM, Shea JA. Mood change and empathy decline persist during three years of internal medicine. *Acad Med* 2005;80:164–167.

Branch WT, Malik TK. Using "windows of opportunity" in brief interviews to understand patients' concerns. *JAMA* 1993;269:1667–1668.

Brothers L. A biological perspective on empathy. *Am J Psychiatry* 1989;146:10–19.

Cohen-Cole S, Bird J. Building rapport and responding to the patient's emotions (relationship skills). In: Cohen-Cole S, ed. *The Medical Interview: The Three Function Approach*. St. Louis, MO: Mosby Year Book, 1991.

Halpern J. What is clinical empathy? *J Gen Intern Med* 2003;18:670–674.

Hojat M, Gonnella JS, Nasca TJ, et al. Physician empathy: definition, components, measurement, and relationship to gender and specialty. *Am J Psychiatry* 2002;159:1563–1569.

Jordan JV. Empathy and self boundaries. In: *A Developmental Perspective*. Wellesley, MA: Wellesley College Press, No. 16, 1984.

Levinson W, Gorawara-Bhat R, Lamb J, et al. A study of patient clues and physician responses in primary care and surgical settings. *JAMA* 2000;284:1021–1027.

Levinson W, Kao A, Kuby AM, et al. The effect of physician disclosure of financial incentives on trust. *Arch Intern Med* 2005;165:625–630.

Novack DH, Suchman AL, Clark W, et al. Calibrating the physician: personal awareness and effective patient care. *JAMA* 1997;278:502–509.

Roter D, Hall JA, Kern DE, et al. Improving physicians' interviewing skills and reducing patients' emotional distress: a randomized clinical trial. *Arch Intern Med* 1995;155:1877–1884.

Shanafelt TD, West C, Zhao X, et al. Relationship between increased personal well-being and enhanced empathy among internal medicine residents. *J Gen Intern Med* 2005;20: 559–564.

Spiro H. What is empathy and can it be taught? *Ann Intern Med* 1992;116:843–846.

Suchman AL, Markakis K, Beckman HB, et al. A model of empathic communication in the medical interview. *JAMA* 1997;277: 678–682.

Wilmer HA. The doctor-patient relationship and the issues of pity, sympathy, and empathy. *Br J Med Psychol* 1968;41:243–248.

Zinn W. The empathic physician. *Arch Intern Med* 1993;153:306–312.

OTHER RESOURCE

Egener B. Responding to strong emotions. *Web-based Learning Module in Doc.com: An Interactive Learning Resource for Healthcare Communication.* American Academy on Communication in Healthcare (www.aachonline.org). Accessed October, 2007.

WEB SITES

American Academy on Communication in Healthcare Web site. www.aachonline.org. Accessed October, 2007.

The Foundation for Medical Excellence. www.tfme.org. Accessed October, 2007.

Giving Bad News

3

Geoffrey H. Gordon, MD, FACP

INTRODUCTION

A debilitating or terminal illness, a catastrophic injury, an unexpected death—these are situations both patients and physicians face, and they are all situations in which the physician must break the news to patients, partners, and family members. How physicians deliver bad news can affect patient outcomes. For example, how parents are told that their child has a developmental disability affects their emotional state, attitudes, and coping. How patients are given a new diagnosis of cancer affects their satisfaction and subsequent symptoms of anxiety and depression. Despite strong emotional experiences when bad news is received, patients and families are able to distinguish between effective and ineffective communication skills, and up to a third report problems with how they received bad news.

Giving bad news is hard. Most physicians struggle to find the proper balance between honest disclosure and providing encouragement, hope, and support. Physicians giving bad news may experience feelings of sadness, anger, guilt, or failure. Most find it stressful and wish they had more training or guidelines. Patients' and relatives' views on how bad news should be delivered include the need for privacy; for a clear, concise, and unambiguous message; for a caring and concerned manner; for attention to the patient's emotional state; and for the opportunity to ask questions. These views are congruent with expert opinion and the published guidelines adapted for this chapter. The guidelines have face validity but the evidence supporting their adoption into practice, and their impact on patient care, remains preliminary.

TECHNIQUES FOR GIVING BAD NEWS

A systematic approach to giving bad news (Table 3–1) can make the process more predictable and less emotionally draining for the physician. The process of giving bad news can be divided into six categories: preparing for the discussion, maximizing the setting, delivering the news, offering emotional support, providing information, and closing the interview.

Case Study: "This Could be Cancer"

PREPARING FOR THE DISCUSSION

When cancer or other serious illness is a strong diagnostic possibility, consider discussing it with the patient early in the workup:

> **Doctor:** That shadow on your x-ray worries me. It could be an old scar, a patch of pneumonia, or even a cancer. I think we should do some more tests to find out exactly what it is. That way, we'll be able to plan the best treatment.

Discuss with the patient how he or she would like to receive the news:

> **Doctor:** Whatever the biopsy shows, I'll want to explain it carefully—is there someone you'd like to have with you when I go over this?

Before giving bad news, review what you plan to say about the disease and its treatment, and how the patient might respond. Knowing the patient's prior reactions to bad news can be useful but is not necessarily predictive of the patient's response. Ideally, primary and specialist physicians should decide in advance who will give bad news and arrange follow-up.

MAXIMIZING THE SETTING

Patients should have the opportunity to dress before receiving bad news. Whenever possible, establish privacy, sit comfortably at eye level with the patient, and minimize physical barriers such as desks and tables. Avoid watching the clock, the chart, or the computer screen. Give the patient your full attention and concern.

If family members are present, introduce yourself and your role, and ask for a few moments alone with the patient. Use this time to ask permission to talk with family members. You can also ask which family members best understands their views, and if anyone important to them is absent. When meeting with families, acknowledge each person individually and learn their relationship to the patient. In large families it may be useful to identify one

Table 3–1. Techniques for giving bad news.

Category	Technique
Preparation	Forecast possibility of bad news
	Clarify who should attend the bad news visit
	Clarify who should give the bad news
Setting	Give bad news in person
	Give bad news in private
	Sit down and make eye contact
Delivery	Identify what the patient already knows
	Give the news clearly and unambiguously
	Identify important feelings and concerns
Emotional support	Remain with the patient and listen
	Use empathic statements
	Invite further dialogue
Information	Use simple, clear words and concepts
	Summarize and check patient's understanding
	Use handouts and other resources
Closure	Make a plan for the immediate future
	Ask about immediate needs
	Schedule a follow-up appointment

individual who will coordinate communication between the health care team and the family.

DELIVERING THE NEWS

The next step is testing the patient's readiness to hear the news. Review the work-up to date:

> **Doctor:** You know we saw that shadow on your chest x-ray. When we did the computed tomography (CT) scan of your chest, we saw a mass in your lung, and then we looked down your windpipe and took a small sample of your lung. We have the results of that biopsy now.

Some patients immediately ask for their test results. Others indicate, verbally or nonverbally, that they want to go more slowly. If this is the case, consider an introductory phrase or "warning shot" to prepare the patient for the bad news:

> **Doctor:** I'm afraid I have bad news for you....This is more serious than we thought....There were some cancer cells in the biopsy.

The main challenge with this approach is to finish with a clear, unambiguous statement that the patient has cancer. Alternatively, you can present the positive message first:

> **Doctor:** The main message I want to give you is that the situation is serious, but there's plenty we can do. We'll have to work closely together over the next several months. I wish I had better news, but your tests show that you have a type of lung cancer.

Once the news sinks in, the patient will typically react with a mixture of emotions, concerns, and requests for information and guidance. Pause and ask about feelings and concerns and assess if the patient is ready for more information.

OFFERING EMOTIONAL SUPPORT

Receiving bad news is usually more an emotional than a cognitive event. Common immediate emotional reactions are fear, anger, grief, and shock or emotional numbness. An important challenge for many physicians is to remain with patients having strong emotional reactions and to tolerate their distress. There are no magic words or correct responses. Sit near the patient and use empathic statements (see Chapter 2):

> **Doctor:** I can see you're upset, and that's understandable. I wish I had different news to tell you. I want you to know that I'll continue to be your doctor and work with you on this.

Some patients find a touch on the hand or shoulder to be supportive and reassuring. It is also helpful to ask unaccompanied patients if there is anyone who should be called after they receive the news.

Some patients direct anger at the physician:

> **Patient:** You'd better check again—you doctors are always making mistakes!

or

> **Patient:** I've always come in for check-ups; why didn't you find this sooner?

Rather than becoming defensive, acknowledge that many people in this situation feel cheated and angry. It is important to emphasize that the disease, not the doctor, is the problem and that doctor and patient must work together to deal with it.

Patients who are very reserved or too stunned to communicate their feelings may be challenging to evaluate because their degree of distress is not always obvious. They may express their grief alone or with a friend or spiritual counselor, before sharing their feelings with a doctor. The physician can acknowledge the difficult nature of the news and legitimize future expression of feelings:

> **Doctor:** I know this is hard to believe. You may have some feelings later that you'd like to talk with me about—I'm always ready to listen.

PROVIDING INFORMATION

Remember that most patients consult an informal health advisor (a family member, friend, book, or web site) at some point during the illness and may have some ideas about what is wrong, what it means, and what can be done. Asking about these ideas shows respect for the patient's coping efforts and helps the physician put new information into a familiar context.

> **Doctor:** What have you already learned about this? Do you know anyone who's had something like this? What concerns you most about it?

Physicians tend to resist full disclosure of patient concerns with questions, explanations, or premature reassurance. This may help reduce physician anxiety but is rarely helpful for patients who are hearing bad news for the first time.

Even with careful explanations, many patients are unable to assimilate much information at the time bad news is given. Effective strategies include using simple, clear words; providing information in small, digestible chunks; and checking the patient's understanding of what has been said ("What message will you take to others at home?"). About a third of the time, physicians and patients have a different understanding of the extent of the disease and the intent of treatment; progress notes in the form of stage-specific treatment plans may help.

Patients often want to know if they really have cancer, if it has spread, if it is treatable or curable, and what treatments are available. Some patients also want to know whether they are going to die and, if so, how much time they have left. Difficult questions should be addressed directly and honestly:

> **Doctor:** First, you're not in any immediate danger, and we have time to plan your treatment together. There are statistics on how long people with this condition are likely to live, and I can share them with you if you'd like, but they are just statistics. No one can say for sure how long you will live. Can you tell me what's on your mind with that question?

CLOSING THE INTERVIEW

The most effective way to reach closure is to create a plan for the immediate future. This includes asking patients if anyone else needs to know the news and if they want help sharing it. Generalists should reassure patients that they will coordinate care with specialists. A follow-up appointment should be scheduled soon after giving bad news, and patients should be asked to write down questions that arise between visits.

Some patients have transient anxiety, sadness, or trouble sleeping. A short course of medication for sleeplessness or anxiety may be helpful, but patients should also be told that it is normal to feel upset or to have trouble sleeping after receiving bad news.

A special type of bad news delivery arises when the disease progresses despite all available and appropriate treatment. Over 20% of oncologists report difficulty with these conversations. They are more likely to experience patient death as a personal failure, to regard palliative care

as "giving up" or "taking away hope," and to give patients overly optimistic prognoses. In this special case of bad news, aim for a clear understanding of comfort care as the active treatment of suffering (physical, psychological, social, and spiritual) with the goal of improving or maintaining quality of life. As care takes on more palliative goals and methods, your roles and relationships with patients become more flexible, the resources you can draw on expand, and your work often becomes more personally meaningful and rewarding (see Chapter 37). Practical tips for approaching difficult communication tasks in oncology are available online (see "Suggested Reading," below).

DEATH NOTIFICATION

Some additional considerations apply when notifying family members of the death of a loved one. Unexpected or traumatic deaths are most difficult because families are unprepared and rarely have a prior relationship with the notifying physician. Begin by introducing yourself and explaining your role in the deceased person's care. While it is always preferable to deliver the news in person, telephone discussion will sometimes be necessary. In choosing between revealing that the patient has died, versus requesting that the family come to the hospital as soon as possible, weigh the benefits and risks of telephone disclosure. Factors to consider include whether the death was expected or not, how well you know the patient or family, the relationship of the person contacted to the patient, whether or not they are alone when receiving the information, their level of understanding, and the distance from the hospital, availability of transportation, and time of day. Generally, families should be told that the patient has worsened and they should have someone bring them to the hospital as soon as possible. If they ask whether the patient has died, or if they are unable to come to the hospital in a timely way, it is best to disclose the death by telephone and encourage them to call someone to be with them.

Once given the news, families often want to view the body. This is an important part of the grieving process and should not be discouraged. Families are often concerned about whether their loved one suffered or was alone at the time of death and whether they could have done anything to prevent it. Usually, they can be truthfully told that the patient was unconscious prior to death, there was no evidence of suffering, and that maximal efforts were made to help. Families may also need to be reassured that none of their actions hastened the patient's death.

Depending on the cause of death and co-morbid conditions, the deceased may be a candidate for organ donation. Although some families object, most find comfort in making an anatomic gift. Many states inquire about and record anatomic donor permission on drivers' licenses, and families may discover that the deceased did, in fact, give such consent. Permission for autopsy can also be requested at this time. Once the notifying physician has brought up these topics, many hospitals have specially trained staff to work further with families. Some hospitals and physicians routinely send sympathy cards or make follow-up calls to recently bereaved survivors.

PROBLEM AREAS

Acceptance

DON'T TELL ME IF IT'S CANCER

Some patients specifically ask not to be told their diagnosis. Patients who exercise their autonomy by delegating it to someone else should not have unwanted information forced on them. However, if they are willing to talk further, they can be asked what the bad news would mean to them, and what they are afraid might happen if they were to receive it. These questions can help patients disclose concerns that inhibit their participating in care. Patients can also be told the potential benefits of knowing the diagnosis.

> **Doctor:** One of the ways you can help is to create the best environment for our medicines and treatments to work. Your attitude and interest are important parts of your treatment; they can help you feel better, and in some cases, the treatment may even work better. Please feel free to ask questions about what is happening—any question at all. If you'd like to talk with someone who's been through this already, please let me know.

DON'T TELL HIM OR HER IT'S CANCER

Family members sometimes ask that patients not be told the diagnosis if it is cancer. This may be the norm for patients and families from Asia, and other immigrant communities. Families should be respected for their values, thanked for their concern and reassured that information will not be forced on the patient. They should also be told that patients' questions about their conditions will be answered truthfully, that patients usually know or suspect more than they let on, and that keeping secrets in health care settings may be difficult. Explain the rationale for the patient to know the diagnosis, and ask what they are concerned might happen if the patient does know. Some families may benefit from referral to a social worker for help to support the patient and each other.

I DON'T BELIEVE IT'S CANCER

Some patients are unable to accept the diagnosis, offering such statements as "I just *know* I don't have cancer, I run every day, I feel fine." This is most frustrating when it delays the early implementation of potentially curative treatment. Physicians often use logical arguments and dire predictions to persuade patients to agree to evaluation and treatment. Paradoxically, this approach makes many patients more resistant. Instead, explain that patients are often of two minds:

> **Doctor:** Many patients find this kind of diagnosis hard to believe. I can see that part of you wants to look on the bright side and stay hopeful, but I wonder if you don't also have times when you realize that problems might arise. I think we can hope for the best, and at the same time be prepared for the worst, just in case. How does that sound?

Offer to answer any future questions the patient might have and expect day-to-day variation in the patient's ability to acknowledge the accuracy of the diagnosis. Document conversations in the medical record to notify others of the patient's reaction. Sometimes anticipating future needs helps patients accept the reality of the diagnosis:

> **Doctor:** Let's take a few minutes to think about what to do if your condition worsens. For example, is there someone who can make decisions for you if at some point you become too ill to speak for yourself?

Different Cultural Values

Attitudes and beliefs about bad news, death, and the expression of grief are determined in part by cultural norms (see Chapter 12). For example, in some cultural groups, bad news about health-related matters is routinely withheld from patients; in other groups, bad news is traditionally given to an entire family group, including the patient. When death is near, some cultural traditions and practices can be problematic in Western health care settings. For example, requests to open windows and burn candles as patients are dying may be difficult to accommodate in an intensive care unit.

> **Doctor:** Are there any family or other traditions I should know about for your medical care?

Cultural differences between physicians and patients or families should be recognized as such and not attributed to uncooperativeness or psychopathology. Ethical and role conflicts may arise when physician's cultural backgrounds differ from those of their patients and colleagues. Consultation with a colleague more experienced in cultural diversity can be very useful.

HOPE & REASSURANCE

Patients and families are fearful of losing hope. Unfortunately, many physicians have never learned how to offer hope and reassurance along with bad news. To physicians, hope and reassurance bring to mind cure, or, at the very least, prolonged survival. To patients and families, hope may initially mean cure but later can mean performing usual roles despite the disease, and still later finishing favorite projects, attending a special event, staying out of the hospital, reconciling strained relationships, or being free of pain.

There are several ways physicians can provide hope and reassurance at the time of bad news:

- Avoid "medical hexing." If all of your patients with a particular type of cancer did poorly, you're more likely to assume that the next patient with the same condition will also do poorly. While this may be true generally, your negative expectations or "hex" can unwittingly become a self-fulfilling prophecy. Be prepared to recognize the unexpectedly positive outcome, and to acknowledge and celebrate it.
- Pay attention to patients' values and goals. Ask patients what they are hoping for now, how close they can get to reaching it, and what they will need. Then work with your team to help them to make it happen.

 CASE ILLUSTRATION

A woman with spinal epidural spread of lymphoma began palliative radiation therapy to avoid leg weakness so she could travel to see her granddaughter graduate from high school. Instead, she became too weak to travel. When her physician asked her what she hoped to achieve by making the trip, she said she hoped to deliver a special message to her granddaughter. Together they decided to help her make a videotape of her message and arranged for its delivery in time for the graduation.

- *Listen for and acknowledge underlying emotions. Try responding to questions about prognosis and impending death in ways that also address the underlying feelings of loss, grief, and distress (Back et al., 2005). For example, in response to a patient asking how long he has to live, the physician might wonder out loud if it's frightening not knowing what will happen next, or when. In response to a patient asking if he is going to die, the physician might state that she wishes that were not the case, but that it is likely in the near future, and could ask the patient how he would want to spend his remaining time if it were limited. Physician clarification and support are powerful therapeutic tools against grief, anger, and worry.*
- *Work to improve patients' function and participation in their health care. Help them understand that their thoughts, attitudes, and activities affect how they feel, and emphasize the importance of learning to relax, identifying new sources of pleasure and self-esteem, and accepting help from others.*

- *Help patients learn how to face and deal with their illness realistically. Patients who focus exclusively on positive approaches may delay and inhibit their own grieving or feel guilty if they can't "laugh or love their cancer away." These patients, and their families, may need permission to accept and grieve their losses. Other patients cope best by consistently fighting the disease and maintaining a positive focus, in the face of all odds, to the very end. Many patients describe alternating days of "giving in" to the disease versus "putting it in its place" and living as normally as possible under the circumstances. Patients can be important sources of information and support for each other individually, in groups, or on the web.*

THE HEALTH CARE TEAM

Although it is usually the physician's role to deliver the bad news, other team members play important roles.

Nurses are trained to evaluate patients' emotional and physical responses to treatment, their levels of comfort and activity, and their progress toward expected goals. They can be a witnessing presence when bad news is given, help interpret it if necessary, assist patients in verbalizing feelings and questions, and provide emotional support. Nurses are also skilled at ensuring that treatment decisions are congruent with the overall direction and goals of care.

Social workers are skilled at identifying resources, enhancing coping skills, and working with patients' families. Chaplains can help patients identify and meet spiritual needs, and reconnect them with a faith tradition or community if appropriate.

Patients and families may benefit from screening and referral for counseling or other mental health services. Some indications for referral include prolonged or atypical grief, concern about a patient's suicide potential if given bad news; and problems communicating with the health care team. Mental health referrals are most successful when the referring physician explains the goals of the referral to the patient and tells the patient what to expect:

Doctor: I'll do everything I can to work on the disease and symptoms, but Dr. Jones is an expert on helping people manage the impact of this disease on their lives. She will talk to you and then advise me on the best care plan.

It is important to ensure follow-up care:

Doctor: I'd like you to make an appointment to see me after you've seen Dr. Jones so we can make some plans together.

Self-awareness as a Skill

For physicians, awareness of one's own feelings is an essential and invaluable skill. For example, physicians' feelings can be useful clues to what patients are feeling. Patients often sense how physicians are feeling when giving bad news, and they value demonstrations of personal caring: "I knew the doctor really cared about Jimmy when I saw tears in his eyes as he talked with us."

One might think that avoiding painful feelings increases physicians' objectivity. However, recognizing and acknowledging our emotional "blind spots" and "hot buttons" can reduce feelings of guilt and sadness, promote compassion and connection, and restore objectivity. Most physicians benefit from talking about their feelings with a trusted colleague before or after giving bad news.

TEACHING HOW TO GIVE BAD NEWS

Most physicians first give bad news as students and residents, when they have the least experience or training, and are haunted by their experiences. With the advent of competency-based learning and certification, a growing literature describes courses, clinical evaluation exercises (CEX), and objective structured clinical examinations (OCSE) on giving bad news for students, residents, and practitioners. Program evaluations demonstrate improvements in self-rated knowledge, skills, and attitudes but few studies demonstrate changes in practice or improvements in patient outcomes. Fallowfield described a 3-day intensive course on giving bad news for oncologists that includes specific time for didactics, skills practice, and personal reflection; improvement in skills in the clinical setting persisted after a year with no further intervention.

SUGGESTED READINGS

Ambuel B, Weissman DE. Fast Fact and Concept #006 and #011: Delivering Bad News. Parts I and II. Available at: http://www.eperc.mcw.edu/fastFact/ff_006.htm and 011.htm. Accessed October, 2007.

Amiel GE, et al. Ability of primary care physicians to break bad news: a performance based assessment of an educational intervention. *Patient Educ Couns* 2006;60:10–15. PMID: 16122897.

Back AL, Arnold MR, Baile WF, et al. Approaching difficult communication tasks in oncology. *CA Cancer J Clin* 2005;55(3):164–177. Available at: http://CAonline.AmCancerSoc.org. Accessed October, 2007.

Emanuel LL, von Gunten CF, Ferris FD, eds. Module 2: communicating bad news. *The Education in Palliative and End-of-life Care (EPEC) Curriculum.* © The EPEC project, The Robert Wood Johnson Foundation, 1999. Available at: http://www.epec.net/EPEC/mespages/ph.cfm.

Fallowfield L, Jenkins V. Communicating sad, bad, and difficult news in medicine. *Lancet* 2004;363:312–319. PMID: 14751707.

Han PK, Keranen LB, Lesci DA, et al. The palliative care clinical evaluation exercise (CEX): an experience-based intervention for teaching end-of-life communication skills. *Acad Med* 2005;80(7):669–676. PMID: 15980083.

Osias RR, Pomerantz DH, Brensilver JM. Telephone Notification of Death. Parts I and II. Available at http://www.eperc.mcw.edu/fastFAct/ff_76.htm and ff_77.htm. Accessed October, 2007.

Schofield PE, Butow PN, Thompson JF, et al. Psychological responses of patients receiving a diagnosis of cancer. *Ann Oncol* 2003;14:48–56. PMID: 12488292.

Ury WA, Berkman CS, Weber CM, et al. Assessing medical students' training in end-of-life communication: a survey of interns at one urban teaching hospital. *Acad Med* 2003;78:530–537. PMID: 12742792.

WEB SITES

CurrMIT (the AAMC Curriculum Management & Information Tool) is a password-protected, online database, available only to faculty and administrators of LCME-accredited AAMC-member medical schools in the United States and Canada, through their respective offices of medical education and by special arrangement, for osteopathic medical schools that are members of the American Association of Colleges of Osteopathic Medicine (AACOM). Faculty with access to CurrMIT who wish to look for other sources or other faculty delivering this content may wish to review one of the "Existing Reports" in CurrMIT, titled, "ALL_Session_Topic: Breaking bad news." For information on CurrMIT, see http://www.aamc.org/meded/curric/. From this site, AAMC-member faculty who wish to receive access can follow a link to their main CurrMIT contact in the office of medical education. Accessed October, 2007.

The End-of-life Physician Education Resource Center (EPERC) is a peer-reviewed clearinghouse for educational materials for physicians on all aspects of end of life care, including giving bad news. Available at: http://www.eperc.mcw.edu. Accessed October, 2007.

Communicating Bad News. URMC ACGME Competency Project Web site.http://www.urmc.edu/smd/education/gme/acgme_competency_modules. One of six teaching modules from the University of Rochester; includes learning objectives, pretest questions, written text, slides with embedded videos, role plays, readings, and evaluation forms. Accessed October, 2007.

Difficult Patients/Difficult Situations | 4

Howard Beckman, MD, FACP, FAACH

INTRODUCTION

Whenever and wherever health professionals congregate, it doesn't take long for the topic of difficult patients to emerge. Patients and families we experience as difficult increase the personal frustration of delivering care, decrease our satisfaction with work, and make it difficult to deliver the person-centered care that is at the heart of high-quality, satisfying, effective health care. Why, we ask, would someone come to the office, emergency department, or hospital and harass, abuse, demean, or lie to us?

Fortunately, most difficult interactions are both diagnosable and repairable. Aside from the unusual person who is determined to be difficult, many problematic situations are created by unsatisfactory communication between practitioners and patients or by personal issues the practitioner or patient unknowingly bring into these important interactions. Such issues can mirror similar problems within the practitioner's own world and provoke negative reactions to the patient's physical condition, sexual orientation, or personality.

Increasingly, medical educators are finding that practitioners consider patients difficult based on their similarity to others, often family members, with whom they have had interpersonal problems. For example, a physician whose uncle used anger to control her may now have problems with an older male patient who responds angrily when she refuses to prescribe an antibiotic for an upper respiratory infection. Another common situation is the practitioner who is unusually intolerant of patients who won't stop smoking. This practitioner may well have had a close relative whom he or she could not convince to stop smoking who later died from lung cancer. Developing the self-awareness to separate one's own past experience from a patient's current behavior can significantly moderate ones aversive response and reduce interactions that create difficult patients. The key to dealing with such situations is to carefully examine how visits are progressing while monitoring ones's own responses to the patient and the interaction. Greater self-awareness about one's own feelings, experiences,

and beliefs can help practitioners offer more nonjudgmental care to their patients. The case illustrations that follow focus on some of the common challenging situations practitioners encounter, and offers specific approaches to dealing with them. Table 4-1 summarizes some general guidelines for working with difficult patients. Table 4-2 recommends practical strategies for approaching specific situations.

THE ANGRY PATIENT

 CASE ILLUSTRATION 1

Dr. Swanson enters the room to see her fourth of the 12 patients scheduled for her Thursday morning session. Her patient, Ms. B., a 35-year-old social worker, is sitting with arms crossed, refusing to make eye contact. Dr. Swanson greets the patient by asking, "Ms. B., how are you?" She responds, "I've been waiting 35 minutes! This is no way to run an office." The doctor, who is emotionally drained after spending the last 50 minutes talking with a patient about breast cancer, wonders why she's chosen medicine as a career.

Diagnosis

Even without the explicit expression of anger, an angry patient is not difficult to recognize. Harsh nonverbal communication such as rigid posturing, piercing stare, a refusal to shake hands, gritting the teeth, and confrontational or occasionally abusive language provide unmistakable evidence. More subtle patient behaviors include refusing to answer questions; failing to make eye contact; or constructing nonverbal barriers to communication such as crossed arms, turning away from the provider, or increasing the physical distance between them.

Table 4-1. General guidelines for working with difficult patients.

- Seek broader possibilities for the patient's emotion or problems.
- Respond directly to the patient's emotions.
- Solicit the patient's perspective on why there is a problem.
- Avoid being defensive.
- Seek to discover a common goal for the visit.

All too often, practitioners assume that the patient is angry with *them*, and, as a result, feel blamed for something they must have done or forgot to do. Although that certainly is one possibility, other important reasons must be considered as the cause for a patient's or family member's anger. These include, but are not limited to those listed in Table 4-3.

Psychological Mechanisms

Many patients come to rely on the special relationship they develop with their medical practitioners. When successful, these relationships are anchored in trust and safety. It is therefore quite common for patients to share emotions they would never consider revealing or discussing with others. Patients want to have their concerns evaluated with compassion and interest. Any perception that their concerns are not taken seriously or are viewed as mundane, may be considered a violation of their trust and result in their feeling violated, vulnerable, and angry.

Patients have lofty expectations of practitioners. They expect timely service, relevant and up-to-date information about evaluations and treatments offered, and advice on how to cope with their illness. From their point of view, interactions that fall short can result in feelings of shame and rejection. The resulting humiliation can easily turn to anger.

From the practitioner's point of view, the patient's expression of anger may trigger feelings as diverse as guilt at having failed the patient, to feeling insulted by the patient's disrespectful behavior. As a result, practitioners often become defensive. This expresses itself as reciprocal anger, withdrawal from the relationship, or a denial of the practitioner's own behavior that may have prompted the anger in the first place. The difficulties are magnified if the expression of anger is or has been problematic in the practitioner's own family. After recognizing the contributions of one's own experiences, openly exploring a patient's anger can help

Table 4-2. Tips for approaching difficult situations or patient behaviors.

Situation	Recommended Techniques
Angry patients	Elicit the patient's reason for being angry: *You seem angry; tell me more about it.* Empathize with the patient's experience: *I can understand why you would be angry.* Solicit the patient's perspective: *What can we do to improve the situation?* If appropriate, apologize: *I'm sorry you had to wait so long.*
Silent patients	Point out the problem: *You're being very quiet.* Elicit the patient's reason for silence: *Why are you being so quiet?* Explain the need for collaboration: *For me to help you, I really need you to talk to me more about your problem.* Respond to cues of hearing impairment or language barriers: *Are you having trouble hearing or understanding me?*
Demanding patients	Take a step back from the demand: *You seem adamant about the MRI. Why do you think it's so important?* Solicit the goal of the demand: *Is there a particular problem you think the MRI will help us diagnose?* Acknowledge emotions unexpressed at the time of the demand: *It must be very frustrating that your back still hurts.* Solicit the patient's perspective: *What do you think is causing your problem? In what way had you hoped I could help you?*

Table 4-3. Possible causes of patient anger.

- Difficulty in getting to the office
- Problems with the office staff
- Anger toward the illness from which the person suffers
- Anger at the cost of health care
- Problems with consultants to whom the practitioner referred the patient
- Unanticipated problems from a procedure or medication recommended by the practitioner
- Previous unsupportive or condescending treatment by a physician
- Anger directed at family members' responses—whether inadequate or overemotional—to the patient's illness
- Other significant news or problems unrelated to medical service, such as work- or family-related conflicts

create a more honest relationship, define the problem more explicitly, and facilitate an accurate and timely response.

Management

In most anger situations, evaluation and understanding should begin the therapeutic process. Responding calmly, without judgment or projection, with "You seem angry" tests whether the practitioner has correctly identified the emotion. Failing to confront anger informs the patient that the practitioner is impervious to or unsettled by anger, discourages any meaningful sharing of feelings, and ensures eliciting superficial information. On the other hand, constructively confronting anger is both efficient and medically appropriate.

Although many patients in this situation respond with, "You bet I'm angry," some deny their anger. Nonetheless, their body language or tone of voice betrays the denial. In this case, the practitioner can address the denial: "Maybe 'angry' is too strong a word. It seems to me that you're upset by something; if you'd like to tell me about it, I might be able to help." This invitation to explain offers patients the opportunity to explicitly express their feelings. As a result, the practitioner develops a more complete understanding of the patient's point of view. Armed with this, the practitioner and patient can reach a deeper agreement on the nature and magnitude of the problem. At this point in the encounter there is usually a reduction in the patient's anger, relief on the part of the practitioner, and the restoration of a positive collaboration that facilitates a solution to the identified problem. Understanding the particular cause of the anger will help manage the problem in the future.

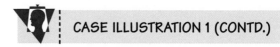

CASE ILLUSTRATION 1 (CONTD.)

In response to the question, "Why are you angry?" Ms. B. replies, "You said that when I went to the Emergency Room last week with back pain, you would call and tell them I was coming. When I got there, no one knew why I was there or anything about my medical history. It was very embarrassing."

In response, the doctor apologized, saying that the office had gotten busy and that he had simply forgotten to make the call. To prevent problems like that in the future, the staff decided at a recent meeting to put up a "follow-up" board so that process errors could be reduced. The doctor again apologizes. Ms. B. feels better understood, accepts the apology, and ends by saying, "I hope this doesn't happen again; I have enough stress at work as it is." Remembering the same patient's earlier complaint about waiting 35 minutes in the office to be seen, the practitioner says, "I should have asked the receptionist to tell you that I was running late—I'm sorry about that. We're really trying hard to make sure that we communicate more effectively with our patients and our consultants." The whole exchange took 50 seconds—time that is certainly worthwhile.

Patient Education

It is important for patients to understand that it is not only permissible but also important for them and their families to express their feelings. Encouraging the expression of anger helps to identify unresolved conflicts that can interfere with providing appropriate care. Encouraging patients and their families to express concerns or disappointments actually offers the practitioner an opportunity to become more effective by identifying and then removing significant barriers to effective, honest collaboration. Encouraging the hospital, emergency department, or office staff to use this approach can do the same.

Summary

Too often we assume that angry patients are angry with us. Sometimes this is so, but often there are much more complex reasons for the anger. The patient's reasons must be sought directly before mistakenly projecting our own beliefs onto the patient. By working hard to avoid being defensive, practitioners can acknowledge and then constructively resolve the cause of the anger. Confronted with such a responsive approach, most angry people are satisfied and resume an effective collaborative relationship with their practitioner.

THE SILENT PATIENT

CASE ILLUSTRATION 2

Dr. Cren begins his afternoon office hours with Mr. K., a 47-year-old man who has recently relocated to the area. On entering the room, Mr. K. fails to make eye contact and fiddles with a piece of paper folded over many times. In response to "Good afternoon; I'm Dr. Cren," Mr. K. quietly says, "Good afternoon." When asked what problems he is having, Mr. K. answers, "I've been really tired." After waiting a few seconds, the patient is asked to tell him more. Mr. K. responds, "I don't know what to say."

Diagnosis

Silent patients offer little but there are a number of important nonverbal cues that deserve attention. The patient may seem withdrawn, as indicated by sitting a greater distance from the physician than usual, failing to make eye contact, avoiding the physician's gaze, seeming distracted, or not acknowledging the physician's attempts at interaction. Alternatively, the patient may seem anxious, evidenced by nervous or repetitive habits such as nail-biting, pacing, or folding and refolding papers. Finally, the patient may exhibit signs of sadness like deep sighs, red eyes, or tears. Some of the more common etiologies of silence in patient visits are provided in Table 4-4.

Psychological Mechanisms

In many families, authority figures may demand "silence unless spoken to." This may be transferred to the practitioner–patient relationship. This deference may also extend to interactions in which differences in gender or social class exist. A history of humiliation or percieved mistreatment in previous medical relationships may also contribute to withdrawn silent behavior.

Table 4-4. Possible causes of silence in patients.

Cause	Discussion
Adverse reaction to prescription medication (e.g., sedation)	Check for overdose or drug interactions.
Alcohol or other drug intoxication	Screen with CAGE Questionnaire and elicit history of substance abuse.
Alzheimer or other dementia	Age-dependent; although some dementias strike as early as the mid-40s, most occur in the 65+ age group. Silence is usually a sign of advanced disease associated with withdrawal from the environment.
Anger	The patient is feeling wronged or slighted and is trying to elicit an emotional reaction.... (see Table 4-3).
Cultural or language barrier	Ask whether the patient can understand; use an interpreter or bilingual staff member, if available.
Depression, dysthymia, or adjustment disorder with depressed mood	Name the feelings; request elaboration.
Distraction secondary to depression	Associated with drawn features, sad affect, lack of eye contact.
Fear of being told that serious disease is causing the presenting problem	State clearly that, regardless of the outcome, the practitioner will be there to help.
Fear of physician authority	Family background, other experience with domineering authority figures may have demanded submissiveness; a gentle demeanor, reassurance, and an explicit request for collaboration can help win the patient's confidence.
Hearing impairment	Use the whisper test.
Passive or shy personality	Change to a more direct, closed-ended pattern of questions; encourage descriptions and elaboration.
Preoccupation with auditory or visual hallucinations	Request additional information from family or attendant.
Quiet person	Usually responds to encouragement, offers to elaborate.
Stroke, TIA (transient ischemic attack), mass lesion	Conduct thorough neurologic examination for focal findings.

When patients feel that they have a serious or potentially life-threatening illness, silence may represent denial and serve as a protective function. For example, a woman can avoid confronting her fears about having breast cancer if she does not mention feeling a breast lump while in the shower. Silence may also be a sign of a passive personality. These individuals want the interviewer to take control and direct the flow. Perhaps most important, silence may be a profound indicator of a depressed mood or an adverse effect from a psychoactive medication. Those struggling with depression or dysthymia may find it difficult to express their concerns or even find the energy to initiate conversation.

Management

When confronted with a silent patient, exploring the behavior is usually best begun by reflecting, "You seem very quiet." This offers the patient the opportunity to acknowledge the behavior and share the reason for it. Providing time for a response may encourage a tentative, frightened, or passive patient to begin speaking. When a patient seems passive, it is appropriate to explain the need for the patient to collaborate in the visit: "In order for me to help you, I really need you to tell me about what you are experiencing in more detail." If the patient seems distracted, it is fair to ask, "Are you hearing voices or seeing things you think might not be real?" If the patient appears angry, commenting on that would be appropriate. Particularly with older patients, if the patient responds with "What?", the most likely diagnosis may be hearing impairment and the practitioner needs only to speak louder. One of the most common complaints by older patients is that their practitioners do not speak as clearly or as loudly as needed.

CASE ILLUSTRATION 2 (CONTD.)

In response to "You seem quiet," Mr. K. responds, "Today is 3 months since my favorite aunt died." When Dr. Cren says, "I'm sorry to hear that; would you like to reschedule the visit?" The patient thanks him for the offer, adding that he's concerned about the fatigue and would like to talk about it. With that, the patient becomes more animated and discusses his fatigue. It is subsequently diagnosed as being related to depression.

Patient Education

By explaining that silence creates additional barriers to effective care, practitioners can invite patients to be more involved in evaluation and treatment decisions. Emphasizing the importance of this involvement underscores the value of their taking an active role in decision making. It also discourages the patient from making the practitioner solely, and inappropriately, responsible for evaluation or treatment plans.

Summary

There are many reasons for a patient's silence during the visit. Openly acknowledging it and then asking for an explanation offers patients the chance to express a feeling, an extenuating circumstance, fear of an outcome, or fear of the practitioner. Further questioning can also result in the diagnosis of an anatomic cause, like an acoustic neuroma, or a psychiatric condition. Testing a hypothesis too early runs the risk of insulting patients and worsening the relationship.

Silent patients are always distressing, particularly for practitioners who value the social and interpersonal aspects of their work. Learning to respectfully encourage more verbal collaboration is usually beneficial and rewarding. As with anger, the reason for struggling with silent patients may be that they remind us of others from our previous or personal experiences. These reminders can evoke strong negative responses. For example, a practitiner easily and strongly frustrated by silent patients may be reminded of a parent who died and didn't reveal that he was having exertional chest pain. Recognizing the sources of these intense personal responses can be most helpful in assisting practitioners to focus on the patients and avoid unproductive replays of unsettling past experiences.

THE DEMANDING PATIENT

CASE ILLUSTRATION 3

Dr. Hartwick is seeing her fifth patient of the afternoon. Mr. G. is a 48-year-old bricklayer, who is being seen for back pain that began after a day of particularly heavy work on the job. In the initial visit, after excluding historical points suggestive of an underlying cancer or spinal cord injury, Doctor H. prescribed limited activity, exercise as tolerated, analgesics, and a heating pad. Two weeks later, Mr. G. returns, and when asked how things have gone in the last 2 weeks, responds, "I'm no better. I've checked into a web-based back pain chat room and everyone agreed I should have an MRI." The doctor leans back in her chair, anticipating a frustrating encounter.

Diagnosis

Although a patient's demand is usually tied to dissatisfaction with the current plan, there are many other possible causes of dissatisfaction. As a rule, if there is disagreement about the recommended evaluation or treatment, it results from a concern about the accuracy of the diagnosis or a failure to solicit important aspects of the history. On the other hand, a recommended test or treatment may trigger a memory of a family member or friends' similar and unpleasant experience. The consequence is that the patient projects an undesirable outcome on the recommended plan.

Sometimes the reason for an unexpected demand involves secondary gain, such as workers' compensation, a disability claim, or lawsuit. Another possibility is that the patient has found something on the Internet, talked to a friend, or read something in the press.

In managed-care settings, the patient also may be concerned that the practitioner is withholding a more expensive test or treatment in order to limit cost at the expense of quality medical care. The demand then becomes a struggle to wrestle needed services from the gatekeeper/practitioner. Finally, it may be that the patient is frustrated with the lack of relief because additional treatment is actually indicated. By listening carefully to a patient's concerns, the practitioner may rethink the diagnosis and/or seek alternatives to the current treatment plan.

Patients who are isolated from family and friends during times of illness may begin to doubt that the practitioner is sufficiently interested in their problem to ensure the best possible outcome. If the distrust grows, the patient may feel increasingly responsible and seek alternative sources of care. The patient may become fearful and demanding. On the other hand, if secondary gains are associated with the illness, the patient may demand testing to demonstrate greater levels of disability or to prove that the problem is sufficiently severe. This is especially true in pain syndromes for which testing is generally unrevealing. The employer, lawyer, or insurance company may begin to feel that the problem is "all in the patient's head" leading the patient to seek further evidence of a "real" condition capable of causing incapacitating symptoms.

Practitioners often experience feelings of rejection, distrust, blame, or humiliation in response to demanding patients leading them to become defensive. By doing so prematurely, the clinician loses the opportunity to explore the patient's subtle reasons for the demands. For example, casual asides; postural shifts in response to a topic; and expressions of fear, agitation, and grief are often ignored. Possible reasons for demanding additional interventions are listed in Table 4-5.

Management

Rather than respond to the presumed cause, the first step in evaluating or re-evaluating the demand is to identify the patient's affect. Let us consider case illustration 3. Because Mr. G. seems frustrated, the practitioner reflects the feeling: "You seem frustrated." The patient responds, "I am frustrated. My father had a similar condition, and 2 years later they found he had a herniated disk which was successfully treated surgically. I don't want to wait that long to find out what I have."

In response to the practitioner's comment about frustration, the patient usually confirms or denies it. If the patient responds affirmatively (e.g., "I am angry, frustrated, sad, nervous"), the practitioner would ask, "Why are you. . . ." This permits the patient to explain and share the experience behind the emotion. Often, this prompts an interaction between practitioner and patient that provides important information. In Mr. G.'s case, a better understanding of what prompted the request for an MRI helps to determine to what extent education, a redescription of the results of evaluation or treatment, another examination, or questions about possible secondary gain might be most appropriate. As all aspects of a demand are explored, an appropriate response can usually be constructed.

When this approach is less successful, more probing questions may be useful. One is to ask patients what

Table 4-5. Possible reasons for demanding additional interventions.

Feeling	Discussion
Anger	The patient is feeling wronged or is re-experiencing a previous bad outcome (see Table 4-3).
Fear	The patient may be afraid that the illness is terminal, serious, horrible, disfiguring, and so on, if not attacked quickly.
Frustration	The patient may feel that no—or insufficient—progress has been made.
Personal responsibility for health outcome	Previous experience may have convinced the patient that physicians are not trustworthy, competent, or interested.
Doubt	The patient may wonder if economic reasons are driving decision making or if the practitioner is skilled enough or up-to-date with current evaluation and treatment technologies.

they think is causing their problem; often patients do not offer their opinions without being asked. Given the opportunity, patients frequently say that after an evaluation they were told the test results were all negative, but they believe that the cause of the problem was not addressed. This point cannot be stressed enough: *In order to provide meaningful reassurance, the patient's feelings about what caused the symptom must be elicited and confronted.*

Another useful question is: "How had you hoped I could help you?" This gives the patient the opportunity to express dissatisfaction with the extent of evaluation, treatment, or commitment by the practitioner; it often lightens the practitioner's burden, since the patient's request may be significantly less difficult than what the practitioner anticipated. A typical example might be the arthritic patient who complains bitterly about the pain in his hip. When the physician asks, "How had you hoped I could help you?" the patient responds, "I'd like a prescription for a cane." The physician had anticipated a request for additional imaging and narcotics.

CASE ILLUSTRATION 3 (CONTD.)

In response to Dr. Hartwick's question, Mr. G. says, "I want to know how I can find out exactly what I have and make sure I don't have any problems with my disk." The practitioner then describes recently updated back pain guidelines that support the use of MRI testing only for determining operability in patients with prolonged pain or defined neurologic syndromes, such as radiculopathy or cauda equina syndrome.

By offering alternatives to the MRI demand that would accomplish the same goal while taking into account the patient's reason for the demand, the practitioner has begun the process of collaborative negotiating. Respecting the patient's point of view generally provides the basis for constructing a mutually satisfactory plan.

The practitioner further explains to Mr. G.: "I've examined you again and I find no evidence of nerve involvement. From what you've said about your father's symptoms, his back problem was quite different from what you're experiencing. Let's put off doing any tests for now. What I would like to do is continue our present course of treatment, since in 90% of cases the symptoms you describe resolve within several weeks. If at the end of that time you're still having these symptoms, I'll refer you to a specialist for another opinion on what we might do. I appreciate your telling me about your dad

because it's obviously causing you some distress and making you wonder whether I was doing the right thing. Looking at things from your perspective helps me do a better job." The time cost of this explanation is less than 1 minute; the re-examination adds only 2 minutes.

When practitioners believe that the demand is related to secondary gain (e.g., a desire to remain away from work for an extended period), they can gently confront the patient and offer a plan that provides ample time for recovery.

Patient Education

Patients respond to instruction when they believe it will be helpful in solving their problems. Until there is agreement on the need for education by practitioner and patient however, the patient might perceive education as the practitioner's way to control the visit. The patient's usual response in such an encounter is either to tune out the information or to construct mental barriers to implementing the recommendation. On the other hand, once the patient's concerns have been successfully addressed and a partnership formed, the patient often asks for and benefits from information supporting the practitioner's point of view. In case illustration 3, recent web-based guidelines that support the practitioner's plan served to educate and reassure the patient that the plan was consistent with best medical practice.

Summary

Exploring the reasons for a patient's demands in a non-judgmental fashion allows most demands to be understood and addressed. Knowing the cause of the demand, a plan that is mutually agreeable can then be negotiated. If such a negotiation is not possible, the patient should be informed of realistic limits to what the practitioner can offer. The patient can then decide whether he or she is willing to accept the practitioner's boundaries or should seek alternative services.

THE "YES, BUT ..." PATIENT

CASE ILLUSTRATION 4

Mrs. M. is a 58-year-old woman being followed for obesity and poorly controlled high blood pressure. Her doctor is frustrated because his continued attempts to get Mrs. M. to lose weight have been unsuccessful. As a result, he is pessimistic about their ability to work together to treat her hypertension, which he feels is a clear risk to her health. When the doctor notes that Mrs. M.'s blood pressure is still elevated, he asks whether she is still taking her medication.

She responds, "Oh, I'm sorry doctor, I ran out of my medicine 3 days ago and didn't want to bother you for a refill." Later in the visit the doctor asks, "Did you join that exercise program you said you would last time?" Mrs. M. replies, "I've been so busy. I'll do it next week." The doctor pulls back in his chair, thinking to himself, "This will never go anywhere."

Diagnosis

When problems are being discussed, this type of patient's nonverbal behavior is usually engaged and active: leaning forward, bright affect, and dynamic gestures. As recommendations for evaluation and treatment are made, however, the patient typically becomes withdrawn, eye contact diminishes, and language becomes significantly less animated. Verbally, during the discussion of evaluation and treatment, the patient becomes quiet, volunteers little, and characteristically offers no solutions to problems. In fact, as the practitioner makes recommendations, the patient often responds with the classic, "I'd like to do that but . . . . "

Frequently, this behavior indicates a passive-aggressive personality. The practitioner initially feels encouraged to offer the patient suggestions, who then invariably rejects the offer or agrees to the plan but does not carry it out.

There are other possibilities, however, that are often not explored. Probably most important is that the practitioner's plan has not taken the patient's perspective into account and is therefore unrealistic or economically or logistically impossible. Another consideration is that the patient comes from a highly controlling family and is attempting to follow the recommendations but for psychosocial reasons is unable to.

Lastly, the patient's previous experiences with practitioners may have been so hierarchical and paternalistic that the thought of disagreeing or negotiating a position does not come to mind, even when the suggested approach is not acceptable.

Psychological Mechanisms

Passive-aggressive behavior is used by persons who do not feel capable of asserting themselves directly. They become skilled in positioning themselves so that others feel they want to, or must, save them. The practitioner's attempt to solve the problem is invariably followed by the patient's frustrating failure to collaborate. The patient successfully transfers responsibly for his or her problem to the practitioner and then rejects each solution offered. Continued failure results in repeated visits, offering the patient continuing attention while increasing the practitioner's frustration.

Other patients who are unable to fully collaborate may have been emotionally, verbally, or physically abused or may have had family or other personal experiences that taught unquestioning submission to authority.

Most people who enter the healing professions have a desire, even a need, to be helpful. Passive-aggressive patients' solicitations for practitioners to save them can be extremely seductive, luring practitioners into believing that these patients will singularly benefit from their expertise. The extent to which practitioners use a patient's recovery to validate their competence or professional value may determine how frustrated and angry they will become when treatment is unsuccessful. Rather than focusing initially on outcomes, the practitioner is better served answering the questions "Am I encouraging patients to take a more active role in their care?" and "Am I giving patients the chance to say why they're not using the treatments I thought we agreed on?"

Management

In working with people who would like their practitioner to take responsibility for solving their health problems, it is important to clearly communicate that only the patient can do so. To help differentiate patients who are dependent and unable to carry out plans from those who cannot because of a definable personality disorder, the practitioner can confront the patient and say, "I'm frustrated with how things are going. Let's start again and see if what I see as a problem is really a problem for you."

Treatment is dependent on an agreement about the diagnosis of the problem. If there is disagreement, the practitioner should ask such questions as "What do you think the problem is?" or "What do you think should be done?" If agreement is not reached, practitioner and patient must work to resolve the conflict.

If the patient agrees with the problem statement, the next step is to ask what he or she thinks would be helpful in solving the problem. One can ask, "Do you really think you can do this?" If the question is asked in a supportive fashion, most patients who initially agreed to fulfull an unrealistic plan (perhaps to please the practitioner), respond more honestly, acknowledging that they are unable to do so. Again, if asked respectfully, patients will share their reasons. Once this is done, the practitioner can encourage collaboration by saying, "Let's explore what we *can* do to solve this problem together. As we discuss options, it will really help if you tell me what's possible for you and what's not." The approach to patients with personality disorders, for whom this approach will often not work well, is covered in Chapter 26.

If the patient displays passive-aggressive behavior, the practitioner can seek agreement on the nature of the problem and then make very specific contracts for what the patient will do. They can be as direct as, "So, until our next visit, you will remain abstinent from alcohol," or

"Between now and our next visit, you'll keep a diary and record when, and under what conditions, your headaches occur." The practitioner's support and enthusiasm can be directly tied to the degree to which both parties carry out the contract. In this way, the practitioner can promote patient autonomy and offer support, without taking full responsibility for the patient's behavior.

Over time, patients learn to respond to the support offered and begin to take a more active role in their care. Of course, there is always the risk that a passive-aggressive individual attempting to control the relationship will choose to seek another practitioner who can be more easily manipulated.

Patient Education

Patients who are unfamiliar with a collaborative model can be given specific information about the practitioner's understanding and particular style of collaborating. Explicit requests for patients' opinions about collaboration can be extremely useful. Over time, given the opportunity to state opinions and formulate plans, most people find such an approach satisfying, engaging, and motivating. Indeed, there is convincing evidence that patients taught to be more assertive improve their health outcomes, such as lowering blood pressure and controlling diabetes.

Educating patients who exhibit passive-aggressive behavior about such behavior can begin a process of introspection and self-awareness. Encouraging patients to explore the origins of these behaviors and consider a therapeutic relationship that facilitates the process can be rewarding for both patient and practitioner. Descriptions of behavior that hit home can provoke emotional responses in patients, but penetrating long-held psychological defenses can spur growth. The practitioner might say, for example, "You say your mother was overbearing and controlling and withheld praise. Isn't that what your children are telling you?" In most instances, the benefits outweigh the risks.

 CASE ILLUSTRATION 4 (CONTD.)

The practitioner leans forward and says, "Mrs. M., your actions tell me I'm pushing you to do something you don't want to do. I'm concerned about your weight, what are your thoughts on this?" Mrs. M.'s eyes moisten and she responds, "I want to lose weight, but I can't do it. I've tried for years, and it's so frustrating." The practitioner nods and says, "Let's hold off on the weight control for now. How about taking one thing at a time and focusing on your blood pressure?"

Mrs. M. agrees to take her medication and to return for a blood pressure check in 2 weeks. The practitioner gives her a card so that she can record her own blood pressure when she checks it at the drug store or the mall.

Summary

Setting limits and providing explicit feedback can teach patients to collaborate more effectively. Being aware of yes-but patterns can help promote a strategy of shared responsibility, and prevent the ultimately unhelpful rescuing behaviors that interfere with successful treatment.

INDICATIONS FOR REFERRAL

Indications for referral of patients whose interactions are difficult include inability to make a diagnosis, negative personal feelings that create a barrier to a therapeutic relationship, an objective assessment that the patient is not benefiting from evaluation or treatment, or the practitioner's feeling of being threatened or in danger.

With particular reference to a practitioner's negative feelings, when an inability to work together significantly impairs the provision of effective care, outside assistance and advice is required. Interestingly, since negative feelings often relate to a practitioner's previous family and life experiences, a patient who is difficult for one physician is often not difficult for another.

Once the decision to refer is made, framing the referral in a positive way is particularly valuable. One strategy is to acknowledge the need for assistance in managing difficult situations or problems. The dialogue might take the following form:

Doctor: Mrs. S., for the last 2 months I've been trying to figure out how to help make your headaches better. I think it would help me if you were evaluated by a psychologist; I might be able to get a better handle on what else I could do to assist you in improving the problem.

Mrs. S.: Are you saying that I'm imagining this? Do you think it's all in my head?

Doctor: No, not at all. But nothing we've tried has stopped your headaches. It often helps me to have another person listen to the story and maybe find a new direction to take. Dr. F. has helped me with a number of people in the past, and I'm hopeful she can help us also.

Mrs. S.: What do I have to do? I really do want these headaches to end.

Doctor: Great. In addition to the referral, I'll schedule you for two visits with me over the next 12 weeks to see how things are going and see what else I can do.

Proposing a positive outcome from the referral can be remarkably useful. In addition, scheduling a visit for the person to return after the referral reassures the patient that the referring physician is truly seeking assistance rather than simply "dumping" the problem on someone else.

Learning to understand the patient's perspective, negotiating for realistic evaluation and treatment plans, and being aware of and responsive to verbal and nonverbal evidence that a recommendation was misunderstood or rejected creates a collaboration that can be satisfying for both participants. Underused skills such as soliciting the patient's attribution for a problem, offering praise and support, listening carefully to the patient's description of a problem, and explicitly confronting problematic or confusing behavior inform the patient that a serious attempt is underway to understand and successfully manage the patient's concerns.

By exploring one's own expectations and feelings, practitioners become more self-aware and recognize who else is in the room. To the extent practitioners become more self-aware and address their feelings, they become more effective.

Finally, in the last few years, there has been increasing recognition of the role the work environment plays in a physician's effectiveness. As we ask practitioners to be more aware of their feelings and influences, manage the complexities of chronic and life-threatening illnesses and recognize both verbal and nonverbal clues to overlying psychosocial components of disease, the medical establishment has a responsibility to create caring, responsive practice settings that nurture practitioners as we ask them to nurture patients.

SUGGESTED READINGS

Beach MC, Inui T. Relationship-centered care: a constructive reframing. *J Gen Intern Med* 2006;21:S3–S8.

Beckman HB, Markakis KM, Suchman AL, et al. The doctor-patient relationship and malpractice: lessons from plaintiff depositions. *Arch Intern Med* 1994;154:1365–1370.

Lazare A. Shame and humiliation in the medical encounter. *Arch Intern Med* 1987;147:1653–1658.

Levinson W, Gorawara-Bhat R, Lamb J. A study of patient clues and physician responses in primary care and surgical settings. *JAMA* 2000;284:1021–1027.

Quill TE. Partnerships in patient care: a contractual approach. *Ann Intern Med* 1983;98:228–234.

Safran DG, Miller W, Beckman H. Organizational dimensions of relationship-centered care: theory, evidence and practice. *J Gen Intern Med* 2006;21:S9–S15.

Suchman AL, Markakis K, Beckman HB, et al. A model of empathic communication in the medical interview. *JAMA* 1997;277:678–682.

Suggestion & Hypnosis

5

John F. Christensen, PhD

INTRODUCTION

The history of hypnosis as a healing art has varied from acceptance as a treatment modality to dismissal as a parlor trick. Discredited in 1784 by a French royal commission appointed to investigate the healing techniques of Mesmer (although commission chairman Benjamin Franklin did note that belief might influence bodily effects), hypnosis has since regained respectability. Hypnosis appears to be a special manifestation of the mind–body system's ability to process information by transforming it from a semantic to a somatic modality. Its therapeutic effectiveness is supported by both research and clinical experience. Today, hypnosis is widely used to treat a variety of conditions—pain, airway restriction, gastrointestinal disorders, skin lesions, burns, and anxiety—as well as to prepare patients for surgical procedures and to facilitate habit change (such as smoking cessation or dieting).

Trance and suggestion occur naturally throughout human experience and are a function of how the mind works. Becoming absorbed in a novel and being unaware of surrounding sounds, or daydreaming while driving and not remembering the last few miles, are common experiences that illustrate the ubiquitous nature of trance. Responding to subliminal messages in advertising by thinking about purchasing a product—or actually doing so—represents ordinary reactions to suggestions made in a carefully crafted trance. These common experiences of trance and suggestion also occur with patients in health care. The power of certain somatic sensations (e.g., abdominal pain) to evoke a trance (a restriction of the field of the patient's awareness to the abdominal region), coupled with autosuggestion as to the meaning of the symptom (e.g., "I wonder if that could be cancer"), increases attention to the sensation and may prompt a visit to the doctor.

The medical encounter can be considered to be similar to a trance phenomenon; patients are naturally absorbed in their somatic symptoms, and the clinical environment concentrates their focus of awareness. Because patients in this naturally occurring trance may be in a suggestible state, it is important for clinicians to avoid making negative suggestions and to be alert to opportunities for making positive, health-promoting suggestions. Because clinicians, too, can be induced into a trance in which they focus narrowly on biomedical pathology, they must be alert to finding ways of shifting their awareness to the larger context of the clinician–patient relationship.

This chapter will describe the therapeutic use of suggestion within the context of the patient's naturally occurring trance states and in the course of clinician–patient discourse. This application can be used routinely by clinicians in all patient encounters. We will also describe the role of therapeutic hypnosis, usually provided by a specialist trained in this procedure, in treating a variety of medical conditions.

DEFINITIONS

Derived from a Greek word meaning "sleep," hypnosis is in fact a therapeutic procedure that requires active cooperation on the part of the patient. The following definitions, used in this chapter, describe the states and processes involved:

- **Trance:** A state of focused attention, in which a person becomes uncritically absorbed in some phenomenon and defocused on other aspects of reality. Trance states can be positive or negative.
- **Suggestion:** A communication that occurs in trance, with special power to elicit a particular attentional, emotional, cognitive, or behavioral sequence of events.
- **Hypnosis:** A communicative interaction that elicits a trance in which other-than-conscious processes affect therapeutic changes in the subject's mind–body system. Hypnosis can be other- or self-induced.
- **Induction:** The process by which a trance is initiated. This can occur naturally or as the first phase of hypnosis.
- **Utilization:** The therapeutic use of trance to achieve desired outcomes and the phase of hypnosis following induction in which this occurs.

TRANCE & SUGGESTION IN THE MEDICAL ENCOUNTER

Both patient and clinician may undergo a mutual trance induction that, depending on the self-awareness of the participants, can leave either more susceptible to suggestion by the other. This state is neither pathologic nor unwarranted, but part of the natural pattern of human awareness in this environment. Generally, because of the power imbalance inherent in help-seeking situations, the patient is more vulnerable to suggestion. Being cognizant of trance and suggestion can give clinicians greater flexibility and influence in leading their patients to more positive outcomes.

Many patients waiting in an examining room are in a trance that has developed through a series of events that started with the onset of the symptom. The patient's awareness of this stimulus then leads to an internal search for meaning. Prior beliefs, personal experience, or the prompting of family or friends may lead the patient to attribute a particular meaning to the symptom. This attribution constitutes the initial suggestion, which in turn increases awareness of the sensation and further restricts the patient's attentional field. Increased absorption in the symptom and decreased awareness of other sensations are the essence of the trance.

The decision to see the doctor further deepens the trance, and this process continues as the patient, waiting first in the doctor's office and then in the examining room, rehearses how to describe the symptom and discuss it with the doctor. As noted earlier, this process of trance induction around a symptom is not pathologic, but is part of the natural unfolding of awareness surrounding a medical visit.

By the time the physician enters the examining room, the patient is in a trance and consequently susceptible to suggestion. Whatever the clinician says or does not say in the course of the interview can, because of the power generated by the patient's suggestibility, further develop the patient's trance, shift its focus, augment or diminish the patient's somatic awareness, and influence ongoing patient emotions, cognitions, and behaviors surrounding the symptom.

The clinician is also susceptible to trance. Patients can sometimes unwittingly induce a trance in the clinician through a combination of verbal and nonverbal techniques such as the initial verbalization of the problem, hand gestures, grimacing, and changes in voice tone and tempo. These all contribute to focusing the attention of the clinician on the problem or on what hurts. This narrowing of the physician's focus (even while a differential diagnosis is being developed) may preclude other internal images, such as the future good health of the patient or a positive doctor–patient relationship that could otherwise give rise to helpful discussions. A too-rapid response by the physician results in premature closure on the nature of the patient's problem and solidifies the clinician's initial trance. However, attending to and eliciting the whole story from the patient (see Chapters 1 and 2) keeps that focus fluid. Sometimes patients induce a recurrent negative trance in the provider, leading to antagonism or aversion for the patient or to feelings of powerlessness in the face of the patient's problem (see Chapter 4).

 CASE ILLUSTRATION

A 55-year-old single woman was being followed by her primary care physician for chronic chest pain after a thoracotomy. The pain affected the patient's life by causing her to withdraw from social activities. The complaints, which continued for several months, appeared inconsistent with the progress of healing around the surgical wound, however. Various pain-management strategies that the physician proposed, including physical therapy, acetaminophen, and a tricyclic antidepressant, had little effect on the complaints. Both patient and doctor became frustrated, with the patient feeling that nothing new was being done for her pain and the physician feeling powerless to alleviate the patient's suffering.

Eventually, seeing this patient's name on the appointment schedule would produce a sinking feeling and tightness in the physician's stomach, and his breathing would become more shallow. As he walked into the examining room and observed the patient's slumped posture and grim facial expression, he could predict how the discussion would go:

Doctor: How have you been doing since our last visit?

Patient: (*pointing to her chest, and responding with slow speech and long latencies*) This pain really has hold of me, and I can't escape it.

Doctor: (*anticipating a negative answer*) Did you try any of the exercises the physical therapist recommended?

Patient: (*grimacing, shifting position, looking down and then back at doctor*) I've tried that before, and it only makes the pain worse. (*eyes filling with tears*) Can't you do something for me?

This case illustrates several components of trance in both patient and doctor. The patient's recurring chest pain induces a trance in which her attention becomes narrowly focused on her suffering and disability. Anticipation of a visit to her doctor further restricts her focus, and her rehearsal of how she can convince the doctor of how bad it really is further heightens the trance. She has learned to associate the image of her doctor's face and the sound of his voice with frustrating discussions about the intractable nature of her pain. Her continued presence at these appointments corresponds with a belief that the power to alleviate her suffering lies outside of herself—this doctor, if only he knew everything there was to know about her pain, would be able to help. This expectation keeps her in a suggestible state.

The doctor, too, has shifted into a negative trance by the time he enters the examining room. The induction begins as he anticipates seeing the patient and continues as his accompanying somatic responses shift him from his habitual openness to the field of possibilities to absorption in his own powerlessness to effect change. His trance is deepened by the patient's nonverbal and verbal communications about her continuing pain. The doctor becomes more vulnerable to suggestion, and the patient's plea to do something for her creates the expectation in him that he must. This expectation, in the face of the patient's persistent pain, deepens his sense of powerlessness.

Therapeutic Uses of Trance & Suggestion in the Medical Encounter

The clinician can use the patient's trance to make specific suggestions that enhance therapeutic outcomes. The language used in medical encounters can lead to unintended patient beliefs and behaviors that influence both illness and healing. For example, the prediction of continued problems for a patient with a weak knee—"You'll probably always be bothered by some pain in that joint"—in the first postsurgical visit has an enhanced power to influence negatively the patient's future awareness of and belief in the knee's integrity. The warning becomes a self-fulfilling prophecy as the patient unwittingly guards the knee and develops a compensatory gait. A positive suggestion—"Whatever residual discomfort you feel, in time you will notice more freedom of motion and activity"—can create expectations that are more likely to enhance healing and the resumption of activity.

A more subtle consideration is the use of positive images and avoidance of negative modifiers. Consider the following statement to a patient after surgery:

Doctor: Your ankle ought to hurt less in a few weeks.

The unconscious mind tends to delete negative modifiers, in this case "less." The embedded suggestion becomes: "Ankle . . . hurt . . . in a few weeks." A positive suggestion would be:

Doctor: You will notice much more comfort within a few weeks.

Because the primary words of the sentence are positive, the suggestion might be incorporated as:

Doctor: You will notice . . . comfort . . . within a few weeks.

In the context of discussing sleep hygiene with an insomniac patient, the well-intended suggestion, "When you go to bed, try not to worry about staying awake," might contain several unintended messages leading to disturbed sleep. The word "try" connotes effort; it becomes associated with "bed"; the negative modifier "not" is deleted by the unconscious mind, leaving the additional message to "worry about staying awake." The suggestion could be positively restated:

Doctor: After you get into bed, I want you to enjoy a few minutes of deep relaxation before falling soundly asleep.

Clinicians can also use temporal clauses to embed suggestions that lead to positive patient expectations. For example, linking pain with expectations for healing can be accomplished by the following statement:

Doctor: When you first experience postoperative pain, it is important to realize that the healing has already begun.

Predicting positive change that precedes the patient's awareness of it can build positive expectations—even if the discomfort continues. For example, the physician might predict the course of recovery as a patient responds to antidepressant medication:

Doctor: Your spouse and others close to you will notice the changes in you long before you begin to feel better.

The implied suggestion is that you will begin to feel better, and when you do, positive changes will already have occurred.

The clinician can also reframe uncomfortable side effects of some medications as an indicator of their potency, thus enhancing the placebo effect. In prescribing an antidepressant, a physician could disclose the anticipated side effects:

Doctor: If you notice this kind of discomfort as you begin to adjust to the medication, keep in mind that this is a potent drug that has the capability of achieving the results we want.

The message contains two positive associations with the side effects: adjustment to the medication and movement toward the desired outcome.

The clinician who appreciates the trance-like nature of the medical encounter can use the patient's openness to suggestion not only to present positive suggestions and avoid those that are negative, but also to promote healing. This is true for both the clinician's own trance and that of the patient.

Shifting from a Negative to a Positive Trance

Clinicians have several options to shift a dysfunctional trance that runs counter to the goals of healing in a more open direction.

CHANGING BODY POSITION

This works directly with the somatic configuration that maintains a trance state. A depressed patient may have a frozen, slumped posture, downcast eyes, and shallow breathing. This frozen posture amplifies negative images and self-statements and inhibits any focus on possibilities for change. The physician can comment on this posture and suggest modifications, such as raising the eyes while walking outside to observe cloud formations, birds, or airplanes, and shifting breathing to the abdomen. The clinician might also suggest that the patient occasionally put on some music and dance—even alone—at home. Clinicians, too, can use a shift of physical position to break an unwanted trance in themselves. A physician who feels ineffectual in the face of an inordinately blaming or demanding patient and reacts physically with chest tightness and throat constriction can stand up, say "Excuse me while I adjust the light," walk to the window, adjust the blinds or shade, move the chair to a slightly different location, and then sit down. During this activity, the physician can shift breathing to the abdomen and prepare to open a new line of discourse with the patient:

> **Doctor:** It's quite obvious how frustrated you are with the way things are going. Let's refocus for a moment on our goals and how things will look for you then.

CONFUSION

Confusion can be helpful in breaking a pattern that locks patient and clinician into repeatedly acting out a script whose negative outcome both can predict. The following caricature illustrates a common script:

> **Patient:** Fix me.
> **Doctor:** Try this.
> **Patient:** That won't work.
> **Doctor:** What do you think will work?
> **Patient:** I don't know. You're the doctor.

When the clinician becomes aware of such a circular pattern, it is helpful to ask "What is the patient anticipating I will say or do next?" If at this point the clinician can do something unpredictable, the result will be temporary confusion, which can be used to shift the patient's trance in a more resourceful direction. The unpredictable action might be the "Columbo technique" (named for the television detective). In this technique, the physician suddenly and dramatically remembers some minor personal problem (e.g., forgetting a spouse's birthday gift), asks the patient's forgiveness for the distraction, and requests the patient's aid. The momentary confusion that ensues (whether or not the patient is able to offer any help) breaks the previous trance and allows the formation of a new one. This temporary role reversal is only one example of the use of unpredictable behavior to induce confusion, interrupting the pattern, and allowing greater rapport and more effective communication.

MINING FOR GOLD

This phrase refers to a technique that shifts the focus of discussion away from distress and toward an exploration of the patient's resources. Useful at any time, this is especially helpful when the tone of meetings with the patient is persistently hopeless, when the patient appears to legitimize the visit by focusing exclusively on somatic complaints, or when the patient's continuing complaints make the clinician feel ineffective or frustrated. In mining for gold, the physician may inquire about things the patient is proud of—past successes, hobbies, travels, relationships, and obstacles overcome. The clinician observes when the patient becomes animated or otherwise shifts out of the negative trance and notes the topic in the chart, returning to this topic briefly in subsequent sessions. Sometimes, the change in the patient's state leads to a change in behavior, emotions, or outlook that had been precluded by the "what's wrong with me" trance. Similarly, the clinician's feeling about the patient may change; renewed interest and curiosity about the patient's personal resources may transform a previously difficult relationship.

ELICITING TARGET STATES

Here the clinician engages the patient in thinking and talking about a future well state, asking the patient to describe what things will be like when the medical problem is resolved or no longer interferes with the patient's life. It is important that the patient be able not only to name the target state ("I want to feel good again" or "I want to be free of pain"), but also to generate visual, auditory, and kinesthetic images of activities associated with that state. This discussion helps physician and patient establish criteria for knowing when the problem is resolved; it also engages the patient in imagining a future well state unrelated to and incompatible with present suffering. This trance shift may be accompanied by positive physiologic changes and increased animation and hope.

CASE ILLUSTRATION (CONTD.)

In the case of the woman with postthoracotomy pain, the physician tried using the technique of eliciting a target state to alter the patient's trance.

Patient: (*grimacing*) I feel trapped. I never imagined it would hurt this bad.

Doctor: How do you imagine it will be when you've completely recovered from your surgery?

Patient: Well, I hope I'll feel better.

Doctor: Well, let's think about what that would be like for you. Once you're feeling better, what do you see yourself doing differently?

Patient: Fly fishing.

Doctor: (smiles; eyebrows raised, voice more animated) You like to fish? (the doctor is a fly fisherman and has shifted automatically into a state of high interest)

Patient: (looks at doctor, smiles) I used to enjoy being out on the river in my waders, fishing for steelhead and Chinook salmon.

The doctor and patient proceeded to discuss various rivers they had fished. The patient had momentarily shifted her mental imagery and her kinesthetic state away from the pain trance toward future health. This created a context in which she could construct a full sensory image of that future well state that was incompatible with the pain behaviors she had displayed. In addition, her image of the doctor, previously associated exclusively with her pain awareness, became, in subsequent visits, associated with images of recovery and hope. The doctor's impression of the patient also changed, so that he looked forward to their meetings instead of dreading them.

MEDICAL APPLICATIONS OF HYPNOSIS

Hypnosis can be an effective therapeutic option for a variety of problems. The neurophysiologic processes by which hypnosis can effect change in such a wide range of complaints are still open to debate. One current theory uses information processing as a heuristic model, with the body, brain, cells, and organs regarded as an information-processing system. In the brain, semantic information (encoded in language) is transduced into molecular information, which uses neurochemical and neurohormonal channels to cause changes in diverse organ systems.

Recent brain imaging studies employing positron emission tomography (PET) and MRI have shown that the hypnotic state is related to a widespread set of cortical areas involving occipital, parietal, precentral, premotor, and ventrolateral prefrontal and anterior cingulate cortices. The antinociceptive effects of hypnosis are correlated with activity in the midcingulate cortex.

In deciding whether to use hypnotic procedures with patients (or to refer them to a hypnotherapist), it is important to consider patients' beliefs about hypnosis, their openness to other therapeutic modalities, and their locus of control. Some religious groups (e.g., Jehovah's Witnesses) forbid use of hypnosis, and some patients may fear that they will surrender control to a powerful "other," who can then control their minds. Brief education by the physician about the nature of hypnosis and its usefulness as a tool to help patients increase control over their symptoms may correct these beliefs. If the patients are not convinced, they are probably not good candidates for hypnosis.

Furthermore, some patients may resist hypnosis because they infer that the physician thinks the problem "is all in their head." For such patients, anything other than a biomedical intervention may be viewed with suspicion. Assuring them that hypnosis is simply part of a comprehensive medical management of their problem may increase their openness.

Locus of control—internal or external—is also a significant factor. Patients with an internal locus of control believe that they can influence many of life's rewards or punishments, and they may be better candidates for hypnosis than those with an external locus of control. This latter group may respond better to biofeedback, which relies on equipment that is external to the patient.

In the following brief descriptions of clinical situations, hypnosis can be considered as an adjunctive or, in some cases, primary treatment.

Relaxation & Stress Management

One of the physiologic effects of therapeutic hypnosis is stimulation of the parasympathetic nervous system. Several stress-related conditions have been attributed to hyperstimulation of the sympathetic nervous system, which is modulated by the parasympathetic nervous system in a dynamic interrelationship. Sympathetic activation can be part of the fight-or-flight response to perceived threats. Given the plethora of real or perceived threats in today's world, stress-related illnesses may be a common presentation of patients' habitual levels of sympathetic arousal (see Chapter 32). Sympathetic responses include tachycardia, muscle tension, adrenaline release, pupil dilation, inhibited intestinal mobility, shortness of breath, and sweating. This autonomic activation is downregulated during hypnosis, and with parasympathetic stimulation the individual becomes relaxed, leading to energy restoration, conservation, and renewal.

Anxiety

Hypnosis can be quite effective as a primary or adjunctive treatment for anxiety. Patients with an internal locus of control will find self-hypnosis an especially satisfying alternative to anxiolytic medication. When introducing this as an alternative treatment, the physician can say:

> **Doctor:** You have a powerful pharmacy in your brain that can produce significant healing effects. Through hypnosis you can learn to mobilize that pharmacy and let it work cooperatively with the other approaches we use.

The clinician can devote 15–20 minutes to inducing a trance, suggesting that the patient imagine being in a relaxing place. If the session is audiotaped, patients can take the tape home for daily practice, learning to self-induce trances and regulate their own levels of autonomic nervous system arousal. The extra time taken for the hypnotic induction can often be compensated by a decrease in time spent on phone calls from anxious patients, since the audiotape allows the patient to access the clinician's voice and suggestions whenever needed.

Pain Management

Because cortical elaboration of nociception is a component of pain, hypnosis can be used to shift the focus of attention away from pain sensations. In some surgical or dental procedures, hypnosis can be used as an adjunct to, or instead of, anesthesia. In addition, patients with chronic pain can be taught to relax the muscles they tense around areas of pain as part of their "guarding" or bracing efforts. This hypnotic relaxation reduces the component of the pain that is due to muscle contraction. Patients with migraine headaches can be taught to dilate blood vessels in their hands and feet through hand- and foot-warming imagery—sitting in front of a campfire, for example. In the early prodromal stage of migraine, this procedure can sometimes reverse the progress of the headache, possibly by increasing peripheral vasodilation and allowing relaxation of blood vessels in the head. Temporomandibular disorders, pain from repetitive strain injuries, and tension headaches have also been treated effectively with hypnosis. Hypnosis has effectively been used for pain relief during labor and childbirth. A recent meta-analysis showed that hypnosis reduces analgesia requirements in labor. Older female patients with osteoarthritis in one study experienced significant increase in their health-related quality of life following a 12-week treatment using guided imagery with relaxation. Recent brain imaging studies have suggested that in hypnosis-induced analgesia prefrontal and anterior cingulate cortices form important structures in a descending pathway that modulates incoming nociceptive input.

Hospice & Palliative Care

Hypnosis has been used adjunctively with other therapies to help patients with chronic and terminal illnesses. Relaxation, overcoming insomnia, relief from pain and dyspnea, and enhancing relationships with relatives and other support persons are some of the benefits of this modality in the hospice setting.

Cancer

There is evidence that hypnosis is effective in alleviating the chronic pain associated with cancer. In addition, hypnosis can control symptoms such as nausea, anticipatory emesis, and learned food aversion; it is also helpful in managing anxiety and other emotions associated with cancer. Hypnosis may also be effective in reducing hot flashes in breast cancer survivors.

Skin Problems

Certain dermatologic conditions, such as warts and alopecia, have been treated successfully with hypnosis. While in trance, patients are given the suggestion to experience tingling or flushing in the affected area. Warts may respond to these suggestions by shrinking in size or—in some cases—disappearing. Burns have also responded to hypnotherapeutic suggestion, both in lessening the degree of the burn and in controlling pain. Other dermatoses for which therapeutic hypnosis may be helpful are acne, atopic dermatitis, herpes simplex, hyperhidrosis, pruritus, psoriasis, and rosacea.

Immune System Function

Hypnosis has been used successfully to treat genital herpes, both in reducing the number of flare-ups and in decreasing the duration of flare-ups. Hypnosis has been shown to decrease blood levels of herpes simplex virus and to increase T-cell effectiveness, natural killer (NK)-cell activity, secretory immunoglobulin A (IgA), and neutrophil adherence. A meta-analysis has shown that hypnosis can reliably alter immune system function. Hypnosis incorporating immune suggestions showed a positive influence on total salivary IgA concentration and neutrophil adherence, along with a modest suppression of intermediate-type hypersensitivity erythema. These effects were mediated through relaxation. Some studies have shown differential delayed skin sensitivity reactions on the right and left arm of subjects depending on which arm was suggested under hypnosis to show no changes.

Respiratory Problems

Patients with asthma have been taught to use self-hypnosis to expand airways and minimize stress-induced attacks. Some patients are able to decrease their bronchodilator use with daily self-hypnosis. Weaning patients off a ventilator in the intensive care unit has been facilitated by the use of hypnosis.

Hypertension

Hypnosis for relaxation can be a useful adjunct to other therapies for hypertension. Daily practice, perhaps using an audiotape made in the clinician's office, can help patients reduce their blood pressure.

Gastrointestinal Problems

Problems such as irritable bowel syndrome (IBS) are amenable to adjunctive treatment with hypnosis. The primary approach is to reduce anxiety, induce relaxation, incorporate abdominal breathing, and suggest warmth in the abdomen and proper functioning in the bowels. Preoperative suggestions have been used successfully to promote an early return of gastrointestinal motility following intra-abdominal surgery, leading to shorter hospital stays.

Sleep Problems

Sleep-onset insomnia—associated with anxiety, obsessive worrying, or sympathetic arousal conditioned to the cue of getting into bed—can be treated with hypnotherapy. By making an audiotaped recording of an induction in which the patient is led into a relaxed state and invited to form positive associations with lying in bed before falling asleep, the clinician can give the patient a new nightly ritual that will enhance relaxation. A relaxing trance can also help the patient return to sleep more quickly after waking up.

Pediatrics

Pediatricians and family physicians skilled in hypnosis find it a useful adjunct in the treatment of children. Children are often amenable to the use of imagination and storytelling as trance induction techniques. Some of the conditions that respond well to primary or adjunctive use of hypnosis include nocturnal enuresis, night terrors, functional abdominal pain, surgical and other office procedures, chronic dyspnea, and symptoms related to cystic fibrosis. Hypnosis was shown to be effective in reducing distress and the duration of an invasive diagnostic test in children with urinary tract abnormalities. In a review of studies on psychological interventions to reduce needle-related procedural pain in children, hypnosis showed the most promise in reducing self-reported pain.

Pregnancy

Hypnosis has been used successfully to reduce symptoms of hyperemesis gravidarum. Habitual aborters have been helped to relieve anticipatory anxiety and lessen the psychogenic risks of spontaneous abortion when organic etiologies have been ruled out.

Preparing for Surgical and Other Difficult Procedures

Patient expectations appear to play a role in the degree of pain and distress felt with surgery and procedures such as colonoscopy. Hypnosis has been used to anesthetize patients who are allergic to anesthetic drugs and to decrease the use of postoperative pain medication. Usually, hypnotic anesthesia requires a deep level of trance, which calls for advanced skill on the part of the hypnotist along with the patient's ability to be hypnotized. Using the naturally occurring trance of patients anticipating surgery, physicians can make simple suggestions to enhance surgical wound healing and reduce postoperative pain. Referring to pain as "discomfort" or an "unusual sensation," the physician can offer a patient a statement such as:

> **Doctor:** No matter what you've been thinking about the time after surgery, you'll be pleasantly surprised at how little discomfort you have.

Presurgical hypnosis can also decrease disorientation and confusion following surgery.

Habit Change

For patients in the preparation/determination or action stage of readiness to stop smoking or to change eating behavior (see Chapter 16), hypnosis can be a useful ally. The ritual pattern of patient behavior around smoking can be viewed as a trance phenomenon. There is an automatic, other-than-conscious sequence of kinesthetic (tactile, visceral, emotional, and postural) awareness and behavior usually set in motion by contextual cues (e.g., finishing a meal, drinking coffee or alcohol, talking on the telephone). Hypnosis can be described to patients in the preparation/determination stage as a useful tool "to help you come out of the smoker's trance and into a more satisfying, health-promoting trance." The clinician can call patients' attention to the automatic behavioral sequence while taking a smoking history (Table 5-1). Asking patients to describe in detail which hand they use to pick up the cigarette pack, take the cigarette out of the pack, hold the lighter or strike the match, and so on will call their attention to the automatic, trance-like nature of their behavior. After inducing a hypnotic trance, the clinician can suggest that patients visualize in slow motion the entire sequence prior to lighting each cigarette. When the previously automatic behavior is raised to the level of awareness, patients are able to break the previous pattern and approach each episode of smoking with increased deliberation. Once patients are in the action stage of cessation, the parasympathetic

Table 5-1. Hypnotic smoking-cessation interview.

The following questions are designed not only to gather information about the patient's smoking behavior and its parameters, but also to raise the patient's awareness about behaviors that are usually automatic and unconscious. The interview presupposes that the patient has already expressed a desire to stop smoking.

- Have you ever quit smoking before? How long were you successful at curtailing your smoking? What allowed you to succeed at not smoking for that long?
- What other habits have you overcome? How have you done that?
- What brand of tobacco have you been using?
- What motivates you to continue smoking?
- Where do you have your first cigarette of the day?
- Where do you have your second cigarette?
- What is the sequence of activities that precede the first cigarette of the day?
- Describe the different situations in which you are likely to smoke.
- Describe the mood or emotional state that usually precedes smoking.
- Describe the urge to smoke in detail.
- Describe how you light a cigarette (if the response is vague, offer the following prompts):
  - Which hand do you use to reach for the pack?
  - Which hand do you use to pull the cigarette out of the pack?
  - Which hand do you use to put it in your mouth?
  - Which hand do you use to light it?
  - Which hand do you use to continue smoking?
- Will you describe in detail all of the reasons that you can think of for not taking a first puff after you have stopped smoking?
- How long will you have to stop before you realize that you are permanently free of smoking?
- How will you tell people that you have stopped smoking?

---

effects of self-hypnosis can be used as an alternative stress-reducing activity.

Hypnosis, when combined with cognitive-behavioral therapy, has been shown to be effective in promoting weight loss.

SELF-HYPNOSIS

With proper training, patients who respond well to hypnotic trances can learn to self-induce hypnosis to achieve both relaxation and specific therapeutic effects. A useful transition to confidence in self-hypnosis is the patient's regular use of a taped hypnotic induction made by the clinician (primary care provider or referral specialist) in the office, thereby extending the clinician's presence into the patient's milieu. As the patient gains experience going into therapeutic trance by listening to the tape, the clinician can teach the patient one of several self-induction protocols, such as the one shown in Table 5-2 (this can also serve as a handout). Some patients are able to develop their skill at self-hypnosis and retain it as a lifelong health resource. One use of a self-induced trance is to enhance one's inner awareness

Table 5-2. Eye roll technique for self-hypnosis.

1. Find a relaxed, quiet place to sit or lie down.
2. Open yourself to a few minutes of inner renewal and refreshment.
3. Use a one-two-three count:
   One: Roll your eyes up to the top of your head.
   Two: Slowly close your eyelids over raised eyes. Inhale deeply.
   Three: Slowly exhale while you relax your eyes.
4. Continue breathing in a relaxed way from your abdomen.
5. Imagine yourself in some pleasant scene or experience for a few minutes.
6. Imagine the sights, sounds, feelings, and smells.
7. While imagining this scene, focus on the desired outcome of this trance (relaxation, pain reduction, and so forth).
8. To alert yourself, use a three-two-one-zero count:
   Three: Tell yourself, "I'm ready to be alert."
   Two: Roll your eyes up under your closed eyelids.
   One: Slowly open your eyes and make a fist.
   Zero: Relax your eyes and your hand. Enjoy reorienting yourself to your surroundings.

Table 5-3. Developing resourceful states with self-hypnosis.

This technique is useful when you anticipate a stressful situation where you would like to access a positive internal resource that is already a part of you. It is founded on the reality that you have already experienced all the inner states you need to be effective in the anticipated situation. These inner states are part of the body's kinesthetic memory and the files containing them can be cross-referenced with your mental representation of the new event. This is a reprogramming technique that allows you to rapidly activate the desired kinesthetic state.

1. Allow yourself to become quiet, breathe from your abdomen, and close your eyes.
2. Build a full sensory image (visual, auditory, kinesthetic) of the stressful situation you expect to encounter. Notice your emotional and physical response.
3. Now break your physical state by changing positions. Become quiet again.
4. Think about the kind of internal resource (attitude, feeling state, level of energy) you would like to have available to you in the stressful situation. Examples would be "confidence," "calmness," or "compassion."
5. Once you have decided on the resource state you want to access, search in your memory for an experience or situation in which you felt that resource to be strong in you. This remembered experience may have nothing to do with the stressful situation you are anticipating and may be from a totally different sphere of your life.
6. Build a full sensory image of the positive experience in which you felt that resource (visual, auditory, kinesthetic). Allow the resourceful feeling to grow in you as you recall that experience.
7. When the resourceful feeling becomes strong in you, **anchor** it by touching together your right thumb and little finger. (An anchor is any stimulus that can serve as a cue for that resource state—it may be a word you say internally, a melody, or a fragrance. The tactile anchor is useful, since it is very portable.)
8. Break your emotional state by changing positions. Now test the anchor you developed by touching your thumb and finger together. Notice what feelings emerge.
9. If you wish to add additional resources to the same anchor to be used in the anticipated situation, repeat steps 4–7 for each additional resource.
10. Now again fantasize the stressful situation. Imagine yourself stepping across a threshold into that scene. As you step across the threshold, activate the anchor and carry the resources you developed with you into the encounter.

or state of mind by accessing somatic memories of positive resource states. This can be useful for either patient or clinician when preparing for a stressful encounter. The method (Table 5-3) is based on the observation that various sensory cues (e.g., music or smell) can trigger associated memories of feeling states. By choosing a desired resource state, constructing a full sensory memory in which that state was felt, then anchoring that feeling state to a tactile cue, the desired state can be reactivated in the new situation. Clinicians might find this especially helpful in shifting toward a positive trance before a patient encounter.

REFERRAL FOR TREATMENT WITH HYPNOSIS

The various medical applications of hypnosis described above require one or more sessions with a trained hypnotherapist. Skilled hypnotherapists spend time with patients prior to hypnosis discussing their understanding and expectations of the hypnotic experience and addressing their anxieties and misconceptions. The aim is to establish rapport and raise positive expectations in the patient's mind. When this preliminary discussion is completed, the clinician proceeds to the induction of a trance, using one of several approaches. (The specifics of these inductions are too numerous and complex to be discussed properly here, and special training is required to use them appropriately and with flexibility to the patient's responses.) Once the patient exhibits signs of a trance, the clinician proceeds to the utilization of that trance for the specific benefit desired. This involves offering suggestions for the patient to imagine changes in somatic sensations, emotions, or future behaviors. The clinician then concludes by alerting and reorienting the patient to the external surroundings. After the procedure, the hypnotherapist can discuss the patient's subjective experiences and answer questions.

As noted earlier, some clinicians become trained in hypnosis (see "Training in Hypnosis," below) so they can integrate this treatment into their medical practices. Others may choose to refer patients to a specialist (psychiatrist, psychologist, clinical social worker, or psychiatric nurse practitioner) trained in hypnosis and familiar with its medical applications. To maximize the therapeutic outcome, it is essential that the referring practitioner communicate with the specialist—before the visit—about the nature of the medical problem, the desired clinical outcome, and the patient's expectations about treatment. It is also important to prepare the patient by explaining the nature of therapeutic hypnosis and by explaining that its intent is to increase the patient's control over both symptoms and their impact.

TRAINING IN HYPNOSIS

Clinicians who are interested in developing their own skills in hypnosis are encouraged to receive formal training from an accredited training program or receive supervision from a licensed health professional with formal training in hypnosis.

SUGGESTED READINGS

Butler LD, Symons BK, Henderson SL, et al. Hypnosis reduces distress and duration of an invasive medical procedure for children. *Pediatrics* 2005;115:e77–e85.

Christensen JF, Levinson W, Grinder M. Applications of neurolinguistic programming to medicine. *J Gen Intern Med* 1990;5:522–527.

Faymonville ME, Boly M, Laureys S. Functional neuroanatomy of the hypnotic state. *J Physiol* 2006;99:463–469.

Gonsalkorale WM, Whorwell PJ. Hypnotherapy in the treatment of irritable bowel syndrome. *Eur J Gastroenterol Hepatol* 2005;17:15–20.

Kupers R, Faymonville ME, Laureys S. The cognitive modulation of pain: hypnosis- and placebo-induced analgesia. *Prog Brain Res* 2005;150:251–269.

Levinson W. Reflections: mining for gold. *J Gen Intern Med* 1993;8:172–173.

Miller GE, Cohen S. Psychological interventions and the immune system: a meta-analytic review and critique. *Health Psychol* 2001;20:47–63.

Pittler MH, Ernst E. Complementary therapies for reducing body weight: a systematic review. *Int J Obes* 2005;29:1030–1038.

Rossi EL. *The Psychobiology of Gene Expression: Neuroscience and Neurogenesis in Hypnosis and the Healing Arts.* New York, NY: Norton, 2002.

Smith CA, Collins CT, Cyna AM, Crowther CA. Complementary and alternative therapies for pain management in labour. *Cochrane Database Systematic Reviews* 2006.

Uman LS, Chambers CT, McGrath PJ, Kisely S. Psychological interventions for needle-related procedural pain and distress in children and adolescents. *Cochrane Database Systematic Reviews* 2006.

WEB SITES

American Psychological Association Web site. http://www.apa.org/divisions/div30/. Accessed September, 2007.

International Society of Hypnosis Web site. http://www.ish-web.org/page.php. Accessed September, 2007.

Society for Clinical and Experimental Hypnosis Web site. http:// www.sceh.us. Accessed September, 2007.

The American Society of Clinical Hypnosis (ASCH) Web site. http://www.asch.net. Accessed September, 2007.

The Milton H. Erickson Foundation Web site. http://www.erickson-foundation.org. Accessed September, 2007.

Practitioner Well-being

6

Anthony L. Suchman, MD, FAACH & Gita Ramamurthy, MD

INTRODUCTION

 CASE ILLUSTRATION

Don, a 38-year-old primary care physician, sighs as he sees Mrs. D.'s name as a last-minute addition to his patient list. It is midafternoon on Friday, and he had blacked out the last hour of the day to attend his son's final softball game of the season. "Of all the days for one of her 'crying headaches,'" Don mutters to himself, "why today?"

Don's skill in handling patients with somatoform problems is respected throughout the health center. Since he assumed responsibility for Mrs. D.'s care, her emergency department visits have fallen by 90%, and she has even taken a part-time job. Don has almost always been able to help her through these spells by sitting with her, holding her hands, and letting her talk.

When he was growing up, Don was always a leader; he was the pride of his hometown, the young man people always thought would "make it out of this place." Now he is back home, as a founding partner in a successful regional health center—and with a waiting list of residents from the university hoping to rotate through his thriving primary care practice.

"Hey, Don!" The greeting comes from Grace, one of Don's partners. Briefcase in hand, she is moving toward the door. "What a great afternoon! My last patient just canceled—I'm going to go home, pour myself a glass of white wine, sit out on the deck, and catch up on some journals. Hope you have a great weekend."

The door opens, the door closes, and frustration, sadness, loneliness, and anger come together as Don watches Grace leave.

Medical practice can be both an enriching source of personal growth and meaning and an unmerciful and depleting taskmaster. It provides us with access to a broad range of human experience—an intimate view of the characters and stories of a thousand novels—and an opportunity to have our very presence matter to others. At the same time, it makes constant demands and surrounds us with perpetual uncertainty; it relentlessly confronts us with our limitations of time, energy, knowledge, and compassion. It is a job that is never done; at best, problems are stabilized until something else goes wrong.

The balance each of us strikes between our own enrichment and depletion is critical to our own physical, emotional, and spiritual health and to our ability to care for others. All too often, however, we lose sight of this balance. We become so outwardly focused, attending to clinical problem solving, that we do not tend to our own renewal. This lack of balance is not surprising; our education has taught us much more about how to care for others than how to care for ourselves. The socialization processes of medical school and residency have cultivated a variety of unrealistic self-expectations and attitudes, especially concerning control and self-sufficiency.

Over time, this imbalance produces a vague but increasing sense of demoralization. The joy of work is lost; patients seem increasingly annoying and adversarial. Work becomes the means to some other end—skiing trips or a vacation house—rather than meaningful in its own right. When the root causes of this dissatisfaction are invisible to us, we blame external sources such as the government, insurance companies, or lawyers. Although there are many legitimate complaints about restrictions and bureaucracy, the most fundamental determinants of satisfaction and well-being are not external but rather are found within.

This chapter discusses important values, attitudes, skills, and healthy work environments, but it must be remembered that simply reading a chapter is not enough to meet the personal challenges that practitioners face. It can, however, help foster practitioners' awareness of important underlying issues that affect their satisfaction and well-being.

BASIC NEEDS OF PRACTITIONERS

The foundation of our well-being is the acknowledgment that we are human, that we have needs and limits, and that to keep on giving we must know and have reliable access to those things that sustain and revitalize us. Unfortunately, the notion that clinicians have needs has been virtually off-limits. An excessively narrow interpretation of the scientific model that guides our work has called on us to be detached and objective observers, leaving no room for our own subjective experience. Moreover, we are exposed early and repeatedly to the ideal of the clinician who is selfless, invulnerable, and omnipotent (the "iron man" model). This ideal is at best unrealistic and at worst dangerous to both ourselves and our patients. Each of us has a variety of needs, both universal and neurotic, that will ultimately assert themselves. The more we are aware of these needs and attend to them consciously and purposefully, the healthier our lives will be.

Among our most fundamental needs are those for human connection, meaning, and self-transcendence—experiencing ourselves as part of something larger than we are. Clinical work is particularly rich with opportunity for human contact and appreciation. Many studies have shown the patient–clinician relationship to be the single most important factor contributing to physician satisfaction (mirroring its central importance to patients). When we are working under excessive pressure or in situations for which we are not adequately prepared, however, clinical work can interfere with the satisfaction of these needs, resulting in depersonalization and alienation from and hostility toward our patients.

Clinical work can also threaten the fulfillment of transpersonal needs through family and community life. Family and career often compete intensely for time and attention, too often to the detriment of the former. Moreover, we sometimes have difficulty shedding the white coat—leaving our professional caretaking role and expressing the spontaneity and vulnerability necessary for intimacy. As tensions build at home, putting more time into work can provide a short-term escape. In the long term, however, avoidance of difficult relationship problems leads to alienation and potentially to the breakdown of crucial personal support systems.

In addition to our universal needs for connection and meaning, we also have very individual neurotic needs—born of pain and conflict—that are intimately related to our medical work. These needs influence both our motivation to go into medicine in the first place and the way we practice. Out of a need to feel loved or appreciated, we often find ourselves in the role of overfunctioning caretakers, and our difficulty saying no quickly leads to overcommitment. Feelings of impotence engendered by childhood experiences of illness—our own or that of a close friend or relative—may be relieved through our work with patients, but the wishful fantasy of controlling disease is constantly challenged by reality. Voyeuristic desires, fear of death, and the fulfillment of parental expectations are other factors, conscious or unconscious, that can motivate our careers.

These darker, neurotic needs are no less legitimate than those less hidden; they, too, are a normal part of life. When these needs operate outside our awareness, however, they can drive us to work excessively, assume unrealistic degrees of responsibility, and otherwise distort our work lives, thereby causing us to suffer. If we invest ourselves in unrealistic solutions that must inevitably fail, we risk chronic anxiety, substance abuse, and even suicide. Through various processes of self-exploration (such as psychotherapy, peer support groups, or mindfulness workshops), we can become more aware of these needs that underlie our work and find healthier ways to satisfy them. We ignore them at our own peril.

PERSONAL PHILOSOPHY

Another important but underrecognized determinant of our well-being is our personal philosophy—the deeply held beliefs and values that address the most fundamental questions of our lives: the meaning and purpose of life, death, joy, and suffering; why things happen the way they do; the nature of our relationship to other people and to the world; and the nature of our goals and responsibilities as human beings. Our personal philosophies define our expectations of ourselves and other people. They guide the way we perceive and respond to our world and help us identify our place in it. They define the framework by which we imbue things in our lives with meaning, joy, or pain and by which we determine what seems right and what seems wrong.

Developing a personal philosophy tends to be a subliminal process—a gradual internalization of attitudes and values from family, culture, education, and life experience. This process makes it possible for us to be entirely unaware of our core beliefs as an ideology; we may take them so completely for granted that they just seem to be part of the way things are. If we do not understand how these beliefs filter our perceptions and shape our behaviors, then we are unable to subject them to critical reflection and to decide which parts work well for us and which parts need to be changed.

The Control Model

An aspect of personal philosophy with special importance to clinical practice is our attitude toward control. Through the influence of Western culture in general and medical culture in particular, we often perceive being in control (of disease, of patients, of the health care team) to be the ideal state (Table 6-1). We use specific intellectual tools for gathering and applying knowledge: *reductionism:* "Sickle cell anemia is attributable to the substitution of a single nucleotide;" *linear causality:* "*A* causes *B*;" and *moving away from the particular toward the general:* "Asthma responds to bronchodilators." All have a distinctly controlling, outcome-oriented focus, that is, to manipulate *A* so as to control *B*. Although this approach has led to important technological advances, it also has important adverse consequences.

The control model creates unrealistic expectations that limit our opportunities to feel successful. Consider, for instance, how our expectations of good control in caring for a diabetic patient allow us to feel successful only when the blood sugar is tightly regulated. The patient's blood sugar, however, is influenced by many factors over which we have no control, the patient's own behavior being foremost among them. We become angry at the patient whose noncompliance stands in the way of our success. If success for us is defined only in terms of controlling disease, we are precluded from feeling successful in many, if not most, situations. Accepting responsibility for outcomes over which we have little or no control is highly stressful and leads us to feel helpless, anxious, and angry.

Our quest for control also creates distance and detachment in the patient–clinician relationship, which, as we have already seen, is an important factor in professional satisfaction. A strong orientation toward control leads to hierarchic relationships. This, coupled with the reductionism and labeling of medical thinking, turns patients into objects, and we find ourselves working more with *things*—organs, diseases, medications, tests—than with people. We, too, become depersonalized in this process, leaving no room for our subjective experience.

The Relational Model

An alternative philosophy that avoids many of these problems emphasizes relatedness rather than control. This model does not reject the insights of reductionism,

but rather builds on them by adding an appreciation of context and relationship. Therefore, although *A* may seem to cause *B*, there are also other mediating factors and bidirectional interactions (*A* and *B* influence each other). For example, the tubercle bacillus causes tuberculosis, but not everyone who is exposed to this bacterium becomes ill; environmental and socioeconomic factors also contribute to the process. The illness, in turn, affects those contextual factors; no portion of the system exists in isolation.

In the relational model, we seek to be with and to understand the patient in a number of dimensions simultaneously—biological, experiential, functional, and spiritual. As we come to understand patients' experiences, we may or may not identify opportunities to recommend strategies or undertake treatments to ameliorate their suffering. We are mindful that patients are ultimately responsible for their own lives; they may or may not accept our suggestions. In some cases, we may have no suggestions or treatment to offer, but we can still find success in offering, in the words of Arthur Kleinman, "empathic witnessing," honoring the patient's need for connection—a healing intervention in its own right.

This relational model helps us avoid unrealistic expectations of ourselves. It offers us the opportunity to feel successful in situations such as untreatable illness or a patient's refusal to accept our good advice that would seem like failures under the control model. The relational model also leads us to more effective action. In contrast to the control model, which attends exclusively to outcomes, this model calls for explicit attention to process, to the quality of communication, and to the values enacted in the way we work together. Paradoxically, it is by letting go of outcomes and focusing more on making the process as good as possible that we achieve the best outcomes. The relational model also gives us more room to look outside ourselves for guidance and solutions—and to admit our own limitations or powerlessness.

Whereas the control model creates barriers between clinicians and patients, the relational model keeps us closer to the experience of both our patients and ourselves,

Table 6-1. A comparison of control- and relationship-based personal philosophies.

Attribute	Control (I-It)*	Relational (I–Thou)*
Phenomenon of interest	Thing-in-itself	Thing-in-context
Epistemologic strategy	Reductionist; linear causality	Emergent; systems model
Clinician's stance	Detached observer	Participant observer
Information deemed relevant	Objective data only	Subjective and objective data
Model for patient–clinician relationship	Hierarchy	Partnership
Focus of attention	Outcome-oriented	Process-oriented

*Terms are from Martin Buber: *I and Thou*. Scribner, 1970.

thereby increasing the opportunities for our work to be meaningful and decreasing the potential for frustration, alienation, and burnout.

SKILLS

There are a number of skills that can make the difference between depletion and thriving in practice.

Time Management

These skills are essential both within the office visit and in arranging work schedules. Negotiating an agenda at the start of each visit focuses attention on the issues that are most important to the patient and the clinician, minimizes time spent on unnecessary tasks, and vastly reduces the emergence of last-minute topics ("Oh, by the way, Doc, I've got this chest pain. . . . ") that lay waste to office schedules. Informing patients at the outset how long their visits will last and reminding them a few minutes before ending allow them to share responsibility for using time effectively. On a more global level, time management skills can help preserve the balance among work, family, community, and recreation that is so important to life satisfaction. Keeping time logs for several days can help us discover whether we are apportioning our time in accordance with our personal goals and priorities. Time logs can also point out time wasters (e.g., unnecessary interruptions) in daily work habits and help us devise more efficient office procedures.

Communication

Given the important contribution of the patient–clinician relationship as a source of meaning, communication and relationship skills become critical tools for well-being. Learning to *be with* the patient requires broadening the goal of the interview from making a diagnosis to understanding the story of the patient's illness as a lived experience. We need to understand the meaning of the illness to the patient—why this disease in this particular patient at this particular time, what its functional effect is, and what role it might be playing in the patient's life. Thus, we need skills for eliciting deeper levels of patients' stories and responding to their emotions. As we become more able to do this, it becomes apparent that there are no longer routine or uninteresting cases—each patient is unique. The patient's personhood enriches our own.

Coaching & Negotiation

Sharing responsibility more effectively and more realistically with patients requires both coaching and negotiation skills. Specifically, we must know how to facilitate patients in articulating their own values, goals, and opinions, including their feedback about their medical care. We must be willing to relinquish our traditional—and burdensome—role of unquestioned authority and adopt instead a more flexible stance, trying to combine synergistically our own knowledge of medicine with patients' knowledge of themselves and the patterns, problems, and balances of their daily lives. We must learn to see patients' increasing capacity for gathering information and making their own decisions not as a threat but as a sign of our success. Knowing how and when to set firm boundaries without being judgmental and how to discuss communication and relationship problems openly can help to resolve impasses with many seemingly difficult patients, making their care less frustrating and more rewarding.

Self-reflection & Self-care

We need to be able to reflect on our own feelings and actions, to acknowledge our vulnerabilities and needs, to seek and courageously follow our sense of calling, and to act in support of our own health. Rather than shutting out as "unprofessional" and "unobjective" feelings such as anger, attraction, or insecurity that must inevitably arise in us, we can learn to use them to gain insights about ourselves and our patients. Through solitary reflection and honest conversation with trusted colleagues (informally or in more organized formats such as Balint groups, workshops, executive coaching, or psychotherapy) we can listen more closely to what our hearts are telling us about the state of our lives. These opportunities to shed the mask of the iron man and disclose our vulnerabilities to each other are also key resources for working amidst uncertainty and coping with mistakes. And finally, we can make choices to limit our work hours, simplifying our material needs to gain more time for whatever it is that truly gives us joy and meaning.

HEALTHY WORK ENVIRONMENTS

Our workplaces have an important effect on our well-being. The local culture of the institutions in which we work—be they hospitals, individual practices, or medical communities—subtly reinforces values through both formal educational processes and everyday policies and practices. The local culture can determine whether we feel able to disclose uncertainty and vulnerability to one another or feel constrained always to maintain the iron man facade; whether we can discuss mistakes and ask for help or be forced to work in perpetual isolation; whether we receive encouragement and respect for setting reasonable limits on our workload so we can be present in our families or feel shamed for being "lazy."

Creating environments that support relationship-centered care is a large topic; a few general principles must suffice for this discussion.

- As clinicians, we tend to treat patients in the same way that we ourselves are treated within our institutions. Core values such as respect, partnership, honesty, and accountability must be explicitly articulated and embodied in institutional policies and procedures. Clinicians and administrators alike may need to learn new communication and relationship skills, and redesign processes for making decisions and maintaining accountability.

- Respecting values and attending to the quality of process must be embraced as the most effective means to high-quality outcomes at the organizational level, just as at the clinical level. This requires a departure from traditional, hierarchic approaches of top-down decision making and control of the work process.

- We can replace the current culture of rugged individualism with a culture of teamwork, accountability, and mutual support. Support groups for all staff, including physicians, may encourage self-awareness, increase sensitivity to patients' concerns, and diminish the isolation and depersonalization that both characterize and accelerate burnout. We can be vigilant to ways in which the local culture reinforces work addiction and inhibits collaboration and work to improve it.

In this time of concern about health care costs and patient safety, clinicians, administrators, patients, and families need to work together in partnership to redesign our medical institutions, making them more respectful and humane, more collaborative in terms of care, and more responsive to the needs of the people they serve and the people who work within them. Clinical outcomes, financial performance, patient satisfaction, and staff satisfaction have all been associated with factors that create healthy work environments for health care providers; institutions thus have a direct stake in maintaining the well-being of their clinicians and staff.

CONCLUSION

Whether the rigors of clinical work become sources of meaning or exhaustion depends on a number of factors. We must be able to know and address deliberately the personal needs that affect our work. The need for connection and meaning is particularly important and when met is sustaining. A more mature perspective of balance, acceptance, and relation must replace the current preoccupation with control. The latter leads only to unrealistic (hence unachievable) expectations and the ongoing specter of inadequacy or failure. We need skills for working with uncertainty, sharing responsibility, and promoting relationship. We must become more attentive to the values expressed subliminally but powerfully in our work environments and begin to make necessary changes so that our environments call forth the best and healthiest of what we have to offer, both as professionals and as human beings. These approaches can help us to appreciate fully the privilege of caring for patients and to realize our best potential for personal fulfillment and growth.

SUGGESTED READINGS

Beach MC, Inui TS. Relationship-centered care. A constructive reframing. *J Gen Intern Med* 2006;21:S3–S8. PMID: 16405707.

Epstein RM. Mindful practice. *JAMA* 1999;282:833–839. PMID: 10478689.

Gabbard GO, Menninger RW. The psychology of postponement in the medical marriage. *JAMA* 1989;261:2378–2381.

Horowitz CR, Suchman AL. What do doctors find meaningful about their work? *Ann Intern Med* 2003;138:772–775. PMID: 12729445.

Novack D, Clark B, Saizow R, et al., eds. *Doc.com: An Interaction Learning Resource for Healthcare Communication.* American Academy on Communication in Healthcare Web site. http://www.aachonline.org. Accessed October, 2007.

Novack DH, Suchman AL, Clark W, et al. Calibrating the physician: personal awareness and effective patient care. *JAMA* 1997;278:502–509. PMID: 9256226.

Quill TE, Williamson PR. Healthy approaches to physician stress. *Arch Intern Med* 1990;150:1857–1861.

Safran DG, Miller W, Beckman H. Organizational dimensions of relationship-centered care. Theory, evidence, and practice. *J Gen Intern Med* 2006;21:S9–S15. PMID: 16405711.

Suchman AL, Matthews DA. What makes the patient-doctor relationship therapeutic? Exploring the connexional dimension of medical care. *Ann Intern Med* 1988;108:125–130. PMID: 3276262.

Suchman AL. Control and relation: two foundational values and their consequences. *J Interprof Care* 2006;20:3–11. PMID: 16581635.

Suchman AL. The influence of healthcare organizations on well-being. *West J Med* 2001:174:43–47. PMID: 11154668.

Vaillant G. Some psychologic vulnerabilities of physicians. *N Engl J Med* 1972;287:372–375.

Wetterneck TB, Linzer M, McMurray JE, et al. Worklife and satisfaction of general internists. *Arch Intern Med* 2002;162:649–656. PMID: 11911718.

Mindful Practice

Ronald Epstein, MD

CASE ILLUSTRATION 1

Jeffrey Borzak, a patient I knew well, seemed to be recovering from coronary artery bypass surgery. On rounds, I sensed that there was something that was wrong, but I could not put my finger on it. In retrospect, his color was not quite right—he was grayish-pale, his blood pressure was too easily controlled, he was even hypotensive on one occasion, and he seemed more depressed than usual. He reported no chest pain or shortness of breath, and had no pedal edema, elevated jugular venous pressure, or other abnormalities on his physical examination. But still I did not feel comfortable, and although there were no "red flags," I ordered an echocardiogram which showed a new area of ischemia. An angiogram showed that one of the grafts had occluded. After angioplasty, Mr. Borzak looked and felt better, and he again required his usual antihypertensive medications.

CASE ILLUSTRATION 2

Elizabeth Grady recently came to be a patient in our practice. The practice, despite having long waits for appointments, was recently reopened to new patients to boost productivity. Mrs. Grady left her previous physician's practice because of a disagreement over seeking care in the emergency room rather than in the office for her out-of-control diabetes. Her blood sugar has never been below 400, and often was in excess of 600 mg/dL. Despite claiming to be on a diet, her weight kept increasing,

and now she weighed nearly 500 lb. At the first visit, an irate sister accompanied her demanding that the patient be hospitalized immediately. On the second visit, Mrs. Grady was so anxious that she could not sit in the examination room; she was pacing in the waiting room until her appointment, and then indicated that she was in a rush to leave even though the appointment was on time. She no-showed for the subsequent appointment, and is now returning for her third appointment.

Excellent patient care requires not only the knowledge and skills to diagnose and treat disease, but also the ability to form therapeutic relationships with patients and their families, recognize and respond to emotionally demanding situations, make decisions under uncertainty, and deal with technical failures and errors. These capabilities require that clinicians have self-awareness to distinguish their values and feelings from those of their patients, recognize faulty reasoning early in the diagnostic thinking process, be attentive to when a technical procedure is not going as it should, recognize the need to gather more data, and be able to incorporate disconfirming data into an evolving assessment of the patient. Often, there is no tool or "instrument" that can help physicians with these situations on a moment-to-moment basis other than their own cognitive and emotional resources and their capacity for reflection and self-awareness. Yet we spend little time during medical training "calibrating" this instrument. For psychotherapists, athletes, and musicians, self-calibration and self-awareness are often important aspects of training. In my view, the clinician who only learns to bring knowledge and technical expertise to patient care is only doing half of his or her job; the other part of developing clinical expertise has to do with cultivating habits of mind that allow the clinician to self-calibrate and reflect continuously during everyday actions. These abilities, in turn, depend on the capacity to be attentive, curious, flexible, and present.

Mindful practice is fundamental to excellent patient care. By "mindful" I mean being attentive, on purpose, to one's own thoughts and feelings during everyday activities (in this case, clinical practice) to be able to practice with greater clarity, insight, and compassion. Mindfulness implies a nonjudgmental stance in which the practitioner can observe not only the patient situation but also his or her own reactions to it before taking action. A mindful practitioner can see a situation from several angles at the same time. Mindful practice implies curiosity rather than premature closure and presence rather than detachment. Mindfulness is especially helpful when dealing with difficult relationships with patients and families, challenging clinical situations, and in recognizing the need for self-care.

In contrast, mindless practice involves some degree of self-deception, often with the illusion of competence. Blind certainty, ignoring of disconfirming data, and arrogance without self-examination or reflection dooms us to "seeing things not as they are, but as we are." Perhaps mindless practice contributes to the common practice of reporting findings that were not actually observed, because "they must be true."

Mindfulness is especially important in the diagnosis and treatment of mental disorders because there are few other anchors to use in judging the severity or pervasiveness of anxiety or depression in a particular patient. However, mindfulness also applies to other cognitive and technical aspects of health care. In this chapter, I will explore several aspects of mindful practice and some ways of recognizing and practicing mindfulness in clinical settings.

MINDFULNESS & CLINICAL CARE

Mindful practice depends on the ability to be aware in the moment. The championship tennis player is being mindful when he or she is not only attentive to the ball, but also to his or her state of balance, expectations for what will happen next, physical sensations such as pain or discomfort, and level of anxiety. All of these factors can affect performance and can be modified by specific attention to them. Like tennis players, physicians' lapses in awareness and concentration can have dire consequences. For physicians, these lapses directly affect the patient's welfare. The result of lapses may include avoidance, overreactions, poor decisions, misjudgments, and miscommunications that affect survival and quality of life for the patient. Thus, physicians have a moral obligation to their patients and themselves to be as aware, present, and observant as possible.

By cultivating the ability to be attentive to the unexpected, mindful practice can improve the quality of care and help prevent errors. Case Illustration 1 presents some observations that led to a change in care resulting in an improved outcome. Being aware in the moment

and receptive to new information—especially that information that is unexpected, unwanted, or upsetting—can help the clinician be more attentive to patients' needs and thus be more likely to meet them. My job in this case would have seemed easier, at least in the short run, if I had ignored my intutions. In that regard, mindfulness involves becoming aware of what we know but don't know that we know. Educators, psychologists, and cognitive scientists have called this "unconscious competence," the "unthought known" or "preattentive processing." Clinicians, whether beginners or experts, often are aware of things before they are named, categorized, or organized into a coherent diagnosis. For example, the unusual gait of a patient walking toward the chair in the examining room may be the first clue to a neurodegenerative disorder.

Conversely, the capacity for inattentiveness and self-deception can be impressive. A patient of mine, hospitalized with a urinary infection, was suspected of having adrenal insufficiency because of hyperpigmented skin. He was later noted to only have hyperpigmented forearms and face; the rest of the body was pale. Yet, the residents and attending physicians continued to evaluate the possibility of adrenal insufficiency in spite of being made aware of the faulty observation. A colleague reported that a patient with two legs was presented on rounds as "BKA (below knee amputation) times 2"; clearly no one had looked. While these examples are dramatic, similar misperceptions are perpetuated with regard to patient personality or psychological states. Consider patients, such as Mrs. Grady (Case Illustration 2), who are labeled "uncooperative," "demanding," or "incompetent"; once so labeled, disconfirming data tend to be ignored. Furthermore, the "difficult patient" is approached as if the difficulty is only the patient's, rather than considering that the physician's expectations and attitudes may also contribute to the difficulties.

Mindfulness also means being attentive to one's own thoughts, feelings, and inner states. Negative thoughts might include pejorative labels ("somatizer"); negative feelings might include anger or disgust; and negative inner states might include boredom or fatigue. Positive feelings also present difficulties. Sexual attraction toward a patient obviously can be problematic, but so can an unusually keen interest in a patient's illness. As a medical student (eons ago!), I was assigned a patient with "hairy-cell leukemia," a disease which was frequently described in leading medical journals at that time. Although she was considered an "exciting" and "fascinating" case, I was disappointed, when meeting her, that she was a sad, weak, pale woman dying of cancer, hardly matching my excitement and that of my colleagues. Awareness of thoughts allows clinicians to follow intuitions and also to be able to identify biases and traps in the process of making clinical decisions. Awareness of feelings is particularly useful in diagnosing mental disorders; clinicians tend to feel "down" when in the presence of a depressed patient. Awareness of fatigue can help clinicians recognize when their cognitive, attentional, or technical capacities are not at their best; the fatigued resident in the emergency room late at night might then get corroboration for an important finding on physical examination (such as the degree of nuchal rigidity in a febrile child) from a trusted colleague.

Mindfulness improves learning. Trainees who are more aware of the difference between what they believe and their actual performance can make adjustments and improvements. Studies show that self-awareness training, for example, improves communication skills. Those without such awareness may believe that they are expert and may be surprised when that notion is challenged by an outside observer or objective test. Other types of professionals—not only medical personnel—also can suffer from the illusion of competence. Among musicians, the well-known adage is that everyone is a "practice-room virtuoso"—referring to a tendency to believe that one plays with technical finesse, an illusion which is often shattered when the performer is put in front of a discerning audience. Clinicians, however, usually practice unobserved, so the opportunities for external validation and learning are much scarcer than for the musician—and the stakes are much higher than a wrong note.

Mindfulness involves cultivating the ability to lower one's own emotional reactivity. Faced with emotionally challenging situations, humans often overreact by blaming (oneself, another clinician, or the patient) or becoming over-involved. Others may underreact by avoiding, minimizing, or distancing. In contrast, a mindful practitioner can observe his or her own reactions, understand their source, and strategize about ways to respond without damaging (and hopefully further building) patient–clinician relationships. In that way, clinicians can respond with empathy based on an understanding of the patient's experience rather than making assumptions about the patient leading to further alienation (see Chapter 2). This same awareness can inform the small ethical decisions that clinicians make during everyday practice.

Finally, mindfulness involves monitoring the clinician's own needs. Self-awareness can directly enhance clinicians' own sense of well-being by helping them feel more in touch and in tune with themselves. Self-awareness can also motivate the clinician to seek needed help and support. Mindful self-care can lead to greater well-being and job satisfaction; clinicians who report greater job satisfaction and well-being tend to express empathy more readily, report making fewer errors, and have patients who report greater satisfaction. The self-reinforcing process of self-care and well-being can contribute to productivity and reduce burnout and attrition (see Chapter 6).

CULTIVATING MINDFULNESS IN ONESELF & TRAINEES

While it is self-evident that self-awareness is a necessary ingredient in developing and maintaining clinical competence, achieving a state of moment-to-moment self-awareness in a chaotic and busy health care environment is not straightforward. For several years, a variety of training venues in medicine, psychology, and other disciplines have offered small group settings for trainees and practitioners to present difficult situations for group discussion, with the intent that the resulting insights then might inform future clinical practice. Four domains that are amenable to these small group sessions might include:

- Clinicians' beliefs and attitudes (health beliefs, beliefs about human behavior and relationships, attitudes toward patient autonomy or psychosocial aspects of care, family, cultural influences, and so on)
- Clinicians' feelings and emotions (joy, fulfillment, vigor, attraction, anger, frustration, conflict, setting boundaries, and so on)
- Challenging clinical situations (difficult decisions, sharing bad news, facing mistakes, apologizing to patients, dying patients, demanding or "difficult" patients, conflict within the health care team, and so on)
- Physician self-care (impairment, balance between home and work, burnout, healthy approaches to stress, finding meaning in work, and so on)

There are a variety of small group formats that are listed in Table 7-1, each with a particular focus but with the common thread of providing both support and insight.

Other educational strategies can enhance the capacity for reflection. Reviewing videotapes of sessions with their patients can be done individually or with a tutor. Learning contracts or agreements can focus learning on areas of deficiency, including becoming more self-aware. We have used peer evaluations of work habits and interpersonal attributes with medical students to foster greater awareness of how students function on the clinical team and interact with their colleagues and patients. Keeping a journal not only promotes reflection on one's actions, but also seems to be therapeutic in itself, offering a venue for self-expression so needed by busy and overwhelmed clinicians.

However, these individual and small group activities may not necessarily translate the insights gained into the moment-to-moment drama of clinical practice. Mindful practice refers not only to reflection on one's actions, but goes one step further by emphasizing habits of mind during actual practice. Mindful practice refers not only to the social and emotional domains of practice, but also the cognitive processes of data gathering and making

Table 7-1. Group learning experiences that promote mindful practice.

Type of Group	Description	Qualifications of Facilitator
Mindfulness-based stress reduction courses	Promote attentive awareness through meditation, yoga and discussion.	Mindfulness training
Support groups	Promote balance between the human and technical aspects of health care by sharing difficult and challenging situations.	Training in psychotherapy or group facilitation
Balint groups	Recognizing that the clinician is a "drug" (a therapeutic agent), groups aim to improve clinician effectiveness by examining thoughts and feelings that may interfere with care.	Training through the International Balint Society
Family of origin groups	By drawing genograms (family trees), participants learn about influences family and culture have on the their values and attitudes.	Family therapy training
Personal awareness groups	Unstructured experience focused on individual needs of participants, these groups examine personal issues that affect a broad array of aspects of being a clinician.	American Academy of Communication in Healthcare offers training courses
Literature in medicine groups	Using published written works or writings of group members, participants explore the human dimensions of health care.	Narrative medicine training
Challenging case conferences	Using videotapes or critical incident reports, participants explore the moment-to-moment actions they took during a clinical encounter.	Facilitation training

decisions and the technical skills employed during physical examinations, surgery, and procedures. Following are some general suggestions on how to enhance mindfulness in practice, for oneself and for trainees:

- *Priming.* Priming refers to creating the expectation for mindfulness. I encourage clinicians to observe what they do during clinical practice to help them be present, curious, and attentive. Sometimes, it is as simple as pausing and taking a breath before entering the patient's room or taking time to look at the patient rather than at the chart or screen. When clinicians report these kinds of techniques for bringing themselves into the present, I then invite them to pay attention to how those techniques enhance their capabilities as clinicians and to think of ways of applying those or similar techniques to other aspects of their practice. When I am with a trainee, I might suggest that they not only pay attention to the patient, but also to their own thoughts and emotions during the clinical encounter. These then can be discussed following the encounter, whether it occurs in hospital or in outpatient settings. Writing narratives about these experiences can help practitioners recognize their own mental states and learn to be aware of how they contribute to creating a coherent patient story while eliciting what often seems like fragmented information from the patient.

- *Availability.* Just as clinicians can make themselves psychologically and physically available to their patients, teachers should carve out time and space in which they are available to observe and discuss students' progress toward greater self-awareness, whether in a small group setting or individually.

- *Asking reflective questions.* Reflective questions explore the inner landscape; no one can answer them but clinicians themselves. They are designed not to elicit facts or answers but rather to foster reflection in the moment. Teachers can ask reflective questions, but more importantly, clinicians themselves can adopt a habit of self-questioning. Examples of reflective questions

Table 7-2. Reflective questions.

- "What am I assuming about this patient that might not be true?"
- "If there were data that I neglected or ignored, what might it be?"
- "What about my prior experience with this patient (or with other patients) is influencing my thinking and reasoning process?"
- "What surprised me about this patient? How did that surprise affect my clinical actions?"
- "What would a trusted colleague say about the way I am managing this patient?"
- "What outcomes am I expecting from this clinical situation? Are those expectations reasonable?"
- "How do I know when I have gathered enough data?"

are shown in Table 7-2. The internal dialogue that they foster can contribute to mindful practice.

- *Active engagement.* When in learning situations, mindful practice can and should be observed directly. Students' reports of what they said and did during a clinical encounter are biased by their own values, expectations, and anxiety; thus presence of a tutor or observer has no substitute. Imagine if in music instruction or tennis lessons, the student simply reported on his or her progress and difficulties, giving a narrative account of how the piece of music or tennis match went. Ludicrous as it sounds, we often do exactly that in medical education.
- *Thinking out loud.* When facing a challenging clinical situation it can be useful to describe one's observations, impressions, or clinical reasoning to a colleague or tutor, or to put them down on paper in the form of a written narrative. Both methods help clinicians hear the story or rationale as if it were told by a third person, allowing them to examine their own thinking processes and emotional reactions, identify what might be missing in their perception of the situation, and correct faulty logic. Both methods can allow for reflection that cannot be accomplished simply by moving forward with problem solving.
- *Practice.* Medicine, like music and tennis, must be practiced; the same is true of mindfulness. "Mantras" for daily practice can be cultivated. Clinicians might use the "it might not be so" mantra when facing a new patient or new diagnosis; the clinician develops a habit of trying to see the situation from another angle that might disprove an emerging hypothesis. "Unexpecting" is a practice of becoming aware of one's own expectations or eliciting those of a learner, and then actively imagining another outcome (the "it might not happen that way" mantra). The goal of using these techniques is not to adopt a different, contrasting perspective; rather their purpose is to

train the mind to consider two or more perspectives at the same time. Most important is a practice of stillness. Even momentary stillness during a busy day can open the mind, allow for new possibilities, and allow greater self-awareness. The stillness may be short—a momentary pause before seeing the next patient, or a "huddle" before commencing a surgical operation. Longer episodes of stillness might include meditation exercises or other contemplative activities. A daily meditation practice can provide a powerful means for learning how to be centered, observant, and attentive. Meditation involves watching one's thoughts, feelings, and bodily sensations (such as breathing) without necessarily trying to change them. By learning to evoke similar states of attentiveness, even briefly, during clinical practice, the clinician can learn to approach new situations with a lowered reactivity and to tolerate ambiguity. Meditation can be an entirely secular activity and need not have religious or spiritual overtones.

- *Praxis.* Clinical skill is not truly learned and known until it is used. Increasing expertise is associated with the development of habits that become second nature. At that point, an expert clinician may not be able to describe easily exactly why he or she is making each decision, because many of the early steps in the decision process may have become automatic or tacit. Just as a habitual approach to history taking or physical examination becomes second nature, mindfulness training should have as its goal developing habits of reflection, self-questioning, and awareness in the moment during clinical practice.
- *Assessment and confirmation.* As is true for any newly acquired skill, some kind of assessment and confirmation of achievement are important for learning and reinforcement. Facilitated self-assessment, assessment by peers, and feedback from supervising clinicians are important to identify markers of and barriers to practicing mindfully. A supervisor might evaluate, for example, the degree to which the learner was able to articulate his or her reactions to a particular patient. Patients and peers can assess presence and attentiveness.

CONCLUSION

Mindful practice is a goal, not a state. Even the most accomplished practitioners cannot claim to be mindful all of the time. Efforts toward becoming more attentive, curious, and present, and to be able to approach familiar situations with a "beginner's mind" can lead clinicians to be better listeners and diagnosticians, and to critique their own technical skills more objectively. Many medical schools and some residency programs offer training in mindfulness and self-awareness, in recognition that these approaches help in the process of professional development, reduce burnout, and improve communication. Resources for mindfulness and self-awareness training are also available through national organizations such as the Center for Mindfulness at the University of Massachusetts (www.umassmed.edu/cfm/index.aspx), the American Academy on Communication in Healthcare (www.aachonline.org) and local organizations such as the Northwest Center for Physician Well Being (www.tfme.org). Research using functional MRI scanning, cognitive testing, and other techniques is only beginning to uncover reasons why mindful practice improves performance and well-being in a variety of professional activities.

SUGGESTED READINGS

Balint E, Norell JS. *Six Minutes for the Patient: Interaction in General Practice Consultation.* London: Tavistock Publications, 1973.

Epstein RM. Just being. *West J Med* 2001;174:63–65.

Epstein RM. Mindful practice. *JAMA* 1999;282:833–839.

Novack DH, Suchman AL, Clark W, et al. Calibrating the physician. Personal awareness and effective patient care. *JAMA* 1997; 278:502–509.

Smith RC, Dorsey AM, Lyles JS, et al. Teaching self-awareness enhances learning about patient-centered interviewing. *Acad Med* 1999;74:1242–1248.

OTHER RESOURCES

Epstein R. Integrating self-reflection and self-awareness. *Web-based Learning Module in Doc.com: An Interactive Learning Resource for Healthcare Communication.* American Academy on Communication in Healthcare Web site. www.aachonline.org. Accessed October, 2007.

WEB SITES

Center for Mindfulness in Medicine, Health Care, and Society. University of Massachusettes Medical School Web site. http://www.umassmed.edu/cfm/index.aspx. Accessed October, 2007.

The Foundation for Medical Excellence Web site. http://www.tfme.org. Accessed October, 2007.

University of Virginia Mindfulness Center Web site. http://www.uvamindfulnesscenter.org. Accessed October, 2007.

SECTION II
Working with Specific Populations

Families

8

Steven R. Hahn, MD & Mitchell D. Feldman, MD, MPhil

INTRODUCTION

Our experience of health, illness, and health care, as patients and as practitioners, occurs in a social context. The "family" is at the heart of that context. Making the patient's social context an explicit part of medical care affects every step of the clinical process, from basic assumptions about who the patient is, to the conceptual framework for the database, theories of causality, and the implementation of treatment. Consider the following vignettes:

1. Despite wondering whether he could have done something more for Joe, his now deceased patient who had gastric cancer, the doctor is gratified and reassured by the family's overwhelming thanks for the "wonderful care" he provided for the past 10 years and in particular during the time preceding the patient's death. The family is grateful for his help in family discussions about end-of-life care.

2. Gina is a 40-year-old woman with diabetes who has extraordinary difficulty following a reasonable diet. Her husband has been unwilling to change his expectations about their meal plans and she has been unable to negotiate a change with him.

3. Mary, 50 years old and previously without complaints, presents with headaches that have been ongoing for 2 months. She's afraid she has a tumor or "something bad." A brief discussion about her family reveals that her 60-year-old husband has been depressed and forgetful for at least 6 months. Two months ago he got lost on his way home from the hardware store. After her doctor listens to her story, she agrees that she too is depressed and very concerned about her husband.

She's upset that he has refused to see a doctor. She accepts her doctor's offer to help her get him evaluated, but she is still worried that her headache is something bad.

4. Eva, who is 27 years old, has multiple somatic complaints and panic disorder. She was raised by her grandmother after her mother died, and when her grandmother died 4 years later, by an aunt 20 years her elder. She and her aunt became very close, "almost like sisters, we did everything together." After completing college she returned to live with her aunt, who had recently begun the first serious relationship of her life. Eva doesn't understand why her aunt needs a boyfriend, and reports that her panic attacks often interrupt her aunt's plans to spend time alone with her fiancé.

In every case, the family context is critical to understanding the situation. In the case of Joe, the doctor has attended to both patient and family and the family is a partner in care and grief. Family function has become a significant barrier to critical self-care for Gina. Mary is having a psychophysiologic reaction to family stress. Eva is a vulnerable young woman whose panic disorders are not only partially a response to her aunt's perceived abandonment but also a high-cost and inadequate "solution."

All health care providers have an intuitive understanding about "the family" and how families work and develop. However, lack of clinically useful tools for making the family an explicit part of care may prevent successful application of this knowledge. Caring for the patient in the context of the family goes beyond involving some families in the management of care. Two case illustrations are presented throughout the chapter that will illustrate the conceptual foundation and basic skills of family assessment and intervention.

THE FAMILY AS THE CONTEXT OF ILLNESS

The family is the primary social context of experience, including that of health and illness. The individual's awareness and perception of health and disease are shaped by the family, as are decisions about whether, how, and from whom to seek help. Use of health care services and acceptance of and adherence to medical treatments are all influenced by the family.

Reciprocal Relationships

There is a reciprocal relationship between healthy family systems and the physical and mental health of its members. Physical symptoms and illness can significantly influence the family's emotional state and behavior, often causing dysfunction in family relationships; and dysfunction in the family system can generate stress and lead to physical illness. Dysfunctional family systems can incorporate a physical illness and symptoms into the family's behavioral patterns, thereby reinforcing the sick role for one or more members and sustaining or exacerbating illness and symptoms. In these "somatizing" families, the presence and persistence of the symptom or illness cannot be understood without examining its meaning in the context of the family.

What Is a Family?

Our understanding of family is based on our experience with our own family and experiences with the families of others. The variety of groups that make up a family is enormous: two-parent nuclear families, single-parent families, foster parents with children from different biological families, families of divorcees blended through remarriage, families with gay or lesbian couples as parents, and married or cohabiting couples without any children. In some cultures, the "family" may be other members of the clan who are not related by blood or marriage. Isolated elderly individuals may think of their home health attendants as family, and for other solitary individuals the only family they may know is their pets.

All of these groups can be experienced as families. They share similarities in the structure of the relationships between their members and the role that the family group plays for the individuals and for the society in which the group exists. So, rather than define the family in terms of its members, we describe it as a *system having certain functional roles*.

The Role of the Family

Family relationships are described more by their roles than by the labels traditionally applied to individuals. For example, in one family an elderly woman may obtain companionship and emotional support from a home health attendant, a friend at the local senior citizen's center, and a daughter, whereas a woman in another family may find these needs met by her marital partner. In one society, the primary education and socialization of children may be accomplished in the household of the child's parent(s) and in community schools. In another, a parent collective or unrelated individuals may accomplish these educational tasks, and play a more prominent, family-like role in children's lives. Hence, for health care practitioners, the patient's family context must be understood as the individuals in the social system who are involved in the roles and tasks that are of central importance to the patient (Table 8-1).

The Family as a System

Families as systems are characterized by:

1. External and internal boundaries
2. An internal hierarchy
3. Self-regulation through feedback
4. Change with time, specifically family life cycle changes

The qualities of these four system characteristics in a particular family help shape the family's internal milieu and functioning.

BOUNDARIES

The family is partially separated from the outside world by a set of behaviors and norms that are embedded in specific cultural systems. Family boundaries are created by norms that determine who interacts with whom, in what way, and around what activities. For example, teaching children "not to talk to strangers" creates a boundary around the family. Different parts of the family system (i.e., subsystems), such as "the parents" and "the

---

Table 8-1. The role of the family: a partial list.

- Reproduction
- Supervision of children
- Food, shelter, and clothing
- Emotional support
- Education: technical, social, and moral
- Religious training
- Health care—nursing
- Financial support
- Entertainment and recreation

children," or each "individual," are separated from one another by boundaries. Internal boundaries work in the same way: children who speak back to a parent may be told that they "don't know their place"; they have crossed a boundary that defines their role. Healthy boundaries balance the individual identity of family subsystems with the openness required for interaction and communication across boundaries.

INTERNAL HIERARCHY

Subsystems of the family relate to one another hierarchically: parents have authority over the children, the older children over the younger children, and so on. A healthy hierarchy is clear and flexible enough to evolve with the needs of the family, and localizes power and control in those who are the most competent. Hierarchies may become dysfunctional for a number of reasons; for example, when they are unable to adapt to change, when the allocation of power or authority is not consistent with the location of expertise or competence in the family, or when the lines of authority are blurred and effective decisions cannot be made.

SELF-REGULATION THROUGH FEEDBACK

Relationships within the boundaries of the family system and its subsystems are regulated by "feedback." All behaviors in the family set a series of actions in motion that in turn influences the original actor.

Feedback maintains the integrity of the family system as a unit, establishes and maintains hierarchies, and regulates the function of boundaries in accordance with the individual family's norms and style. This tendency toward maintaining "homeostasis" is critical. All family systems must learn to balance the desire for stability with the inevitable need to evolve and change.

CHANGE AND THE FAMILY LIFE CYCLE

The family must continually adapt as its members evolve both biologically and socially (Table 8-2). For example, the family with young children must protect them within the boundaries of the family (or that of specific delegates, such as the schools). Adolescents need to achieve a degree of independence and the ability to function without immediate adult supervision. To facilitate this, the family must develop new norms of behavior and relax the boundary between the child and the world and redraw the boundaries between parent and child (e.g., provide more areas of autonomy and privacy). Each stage of the family life cycle presents new challenges, and healthy families are able to modify their hierarchic relationships and boundaries. Families whose boundaries, hierarchies, and self-regulatory feedback are dysfunctional have difficulties at each transition.

HEALTH AND ILLNESS IN FAMILIES: THE "SICK ROLE"

Behavior in social settings can be understood in terms of "roles" that are shaped by shared expectations, rules, and beliefs. All roles have prerequisites, obligations, and benefits or dispensations. One such role is the "sick role," which is temporarily and conditionally granted to individuals when they have an illness perceived to be beyond their control, seek professional help and adhere to treatment, and accept the social stigma associated with being sick. Individuals in the sick role are exempt from many of their usual obligations and entitled to special attention and resources. The sick role therefore has a profound effect on relationships within the family.

The exemption from obligations that is part of the sick role is critical to recovery from illness and adaptation to disability. The obligations and stigmatization of the sick role are important to protect others from abuse. Physicians play a critical role in establishing the legitimacy of the sick role by certifying the prerequisite illness or disability, and attesting to adequate adherence to treatment. Because the sick role has such a profound effect on the family of the sick individual, physicians' obligate role in establishing the sick role makes them a powerful actor in the patient's family system, and makes the family system an intrinsic part of the doctor–patient relationship, whether the physician is aware of these ramifications or not.

The Doctor–Patient–Family Relationship & the Compensatory Alliance

A positive relationship with an active and concerned family can be one of the physician's most powerful tools and rewarding clinical experiences. In these circumstances, working with the family seems quite natural and the complexities of the doctor–patient–family relationship are not apparent. On the other hand, when significant family problems exist, the doctor–patient relationship can become entangled in the family system's dysfunction.

When one or more members have assumed the sick role in response to family problems, the task of providing appropriate care for the patient may be subverted and subsumed by family dysfunction. Some families can achieve internal stability and meet the needs of their members only when one or more individuals are perceived as being sick.

The physician's role in determining that the patient is entitled to the special prerogatives and dispensations of the "sick role" makes the physician a central and powerful member of these family systems. The authority to prescribe changes in role function for the patient further involves the physician in the life of the entire family. In effect, the physician and patient develop an alliance that compensates for the dysfunction and deficit at home. Hahn, Feiner, and Bellin have termed this a *compensatory alliance*.

When the physician is unaware of underlying family dysfunction, the compensatory alliance can become

Table 8-2. The family life cycle.

Life Cycle Stage	Dominant Theme	Transitional Task
The single young adult	Separating from family of origin	Differentiation from family of origin. Developing intimate relationships with peers. Establishing career and financial independence.
Forming a committed relationship	Commitment to a new family	Formation of a committed relationship. Forming and changing relationships with both families of origin.
The family with young children	Adjusting to new family members	Adjusting the relationship to make time and space for children. Negotiating parenting responsibilities. Adjusting relationships with extended families to incorporate parenting and grandparenting.
The family with adolescents	Increasing flexibility of boundaries to allow for children's independence	Adjusting boundaries to allow children to move in and out of the family more freely. Attending to midlife relationship and career issues. Adjusting to aging parent's needs and role.
Launching children	Accepting exits and entries into the system	Adjusting committed relationship to absence of children in the household. Adjusting relationships with children to their independence and adult status. Including new in-laws and becoming grandparents. Adjusting to aging or dying parents' needs and role.
The family later in life	Adjusting to age and new roles	Maintaining functional status, developing new social and familial roles. Supporting central role of middle generation. Integrating the elderly into family life. Dealing with loss of parents, spouse, peers; life review and integration.

Source: Adapted, with permission, from Carter CA, McGoldrick M, eds. *The Family Life Cycle: A Framework for Family Therapy.* New York, NY: Gardner Press, 1980.

dysfunctional and contribute to somatization and non-compliance, and support the ultimately inadequate coping mechanism afforded by the sick role.

PATIENT CARE IN THE CONTEXT OF THE FAMILY: FAMILY ASSESMENT & INTERVENTION FOR PRIMARY CARE

General Considerations

Treating the patient in the context of the family requires a practical method that can be learned and used by health care providers in real world practice and training. The large number of tasks that occupy the provider places limits on the complexity of and time available for family assessment and intervention. A family assessment and intervention method must be focused, time efficient, and consistent with the general scope of care.

All patients should receive a "basic" family assessment that allows the doctor to understand how the family milieu will influence the basic tasks of care, and that identifies family problems requiring intervention (Table 8-3). Basic family assessment consists of two processes: (1) conducting a genogram-based interview and identifying the relevant family life cycle stages and

Table 8-3. Goals of basic family assessment and intervention.

- Understand the pattern of family involvement with the patient's medical problems.
- Communicate with other family members about the management of patient's medical problems.
- Recognize the presence of problem behaviors (e.g., alcohol or drug abuse, somatization, domestic violence, physician experience of the patient as "difficult") and family dysfunction affecting the patient's medical problems or functional status, which require further assessment and intervention.
- Assess the family's behavioral and emotional response to the patient's problems, and provide emotional support to the patient and family.
- Provide counseling to enhance the family's emotional and functional adaptation to the patient's medical problems.
- Perform a preliminary assessment of the doctor–patient–family relationship and recognize a "dysfunctional compensatory alliance" when present or developing.
- Refer the patient or family for further assessment and intervention, or obtain a family systems consultation.
- Understand the triangular relationships and repetitive patterns of interaction among members of the family system, including the development of a "dysfunctional compensatory alliance" in the doctor–patient–family triangle.

---

(2) screening for family problems that are associated with family life cycle stage tasks, or the patient's medical problems. A subset of patients with problems rooted in serious family dysfunction will then require the four-step family intervention described below.

Treating the patient in the context of the family does not necessarily mean bringing the family into the examining room and in adult medicine usually does not. Family assessment and intervention can be accomplished by meeting exclusively with the patient, though meeting with other family members is very often desirable, sometimes necessary, and almost always enhances the care. Using a family systems orientation without meeting directly with other family members requires the ability to explore the life of the family and bring the family into the room through the patient's narrative.

The genogram-based interview, described below, is a powerful technique for accomplishing this goal. However, the task of understanding the patient's family system in this way can be complicated by the fact that patients often give a distorted and incomplete presentation of family life. Such distortion may be conscious, unknowing, or some of both. Therefore, clinicians need to learn to infer what is going on at home—to "see the family over the patient's shoulder"—by imagining how members of the patient's family might be reacting or

behaving in ways that the patient doesn't understand or won't report.

BASIC FAMILY ASSESSMENT: CONDUCTING A GENOGRAM-BASED INTERVIEW, IDENTIFYING FAMILY LIFE CYCLE STAGE ISSUES, & SCREENING FOR PROBLEMS

 CASE ILLUSTRATION 1

Ariana is a 40-year-old Italian-American woman with multiple somatic complaints. She has complained of chronic diarrhea, dyspepsia, and "asthma" but has had a thorough normal gastrointestinal (GI) and pulmonary evaluation. She has made multiple visits to her primary provider and to an urgent care clinic, has been hospitalized two times, and has been seen in several subspecialty clinics. She has made an average of 15 visits per year for the past several years.

Constructing a Genogram

The first step to treating the patient in the context of the family is to create a picture of the family by conducting a "genogram-based interview." A genogram is a graphic representation of the members of a family. It uses the iconography of the genetic pedigree (Figures 8-1 and 8-2) and can be used to record data ranging from family medical history to life events and employment, as well as family issues. The overall objective of the genogram interview is to help the patient tell the family's story.

CONDUCTING A GENOGRAM INTERVIEW

Begin with a blank page, or a designated section of the patient's chart. Place the genogram where the patient can see it and draw a family tree with the patient's help. Note important dates such as marriages, divorces, and deaths, and the general location of individuals in other households. Family systems data can be recorded using lines to enclose household boundaries, double lines between individuals to indicate strong relationships or coalitions, jagged lines to indicate conflict, and triple lines to indicate dysfunctional over involvement.

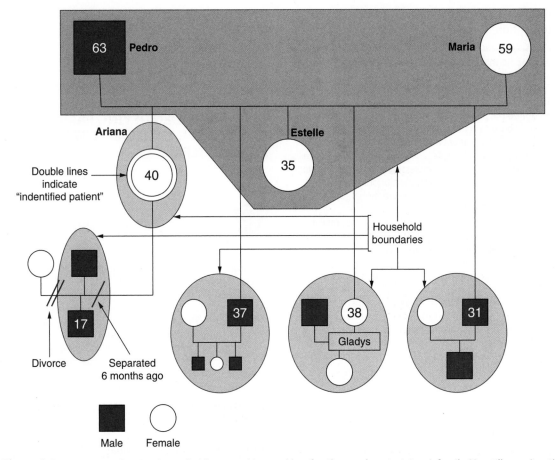

Figure 8-1. Genogram showing household composition and key family members in Ariana's family (Case Illustration 1).

At subsequent visits take a brief look at the genogram to recall the patient's family context, and expand or alter the genogram as the family changes or new issues arise.

FOCUSING THE GENOGRAM

The type of information explored, the number of generations, and the level of detail included in the genogram depend on an initial sense of the importance of family issues. A detailed, comprehensive genogram interview going back more than one generation can be a powerful clinical tool but is too complex for everyday practice. The genogram must be "focused" on the most clinically useful information while providing the foundation for treating the patient in the context of the family. As with most clinical databases, it is harder to know what can safely be excluded than it is to include the entire range of family-oriented data. However, skillful parsimony is acquired with experience, and efficiency is produced by following three principles:

1. Engage patients and encourage active participation—they will take you to the heart of the story.
2. Focus the interview on family life cycle tasks and issues—they are almost always the focal point of stress and dysfunction.
3. Draw and examine the genogram—a picture is worth 1000 words (e.g., picture a single mother, six children, parents and siblings in another country, three different fathers in various places, and a new boyfriend).

Begin with the core members of the family, that is, household members, parents, children, and past and present spouses. Identify the family life cycle stage of the patient's family from the ages, relationships, and household composition of the nucleus of the patient's family. As described below, the family life cycle stage will almost always predict the locus of stress, challenge, or conflict in the patient's family system.

Inquire about the family's responses to any known or presenting problems, and to issues identified using

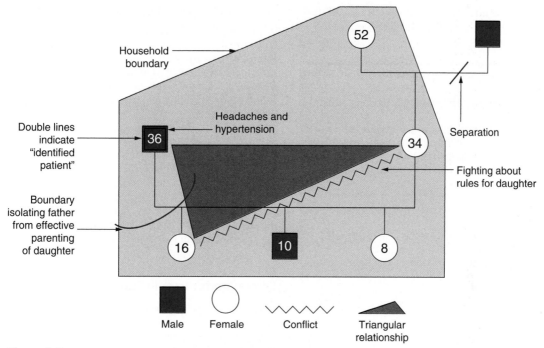

Household boundary

Double lines indicate "identified patient"

Boundary isolating father from effective parenting of daughter

Headaches and hypertension

Separation

Fighting about rules for daughter

52

36

34

16

10

8

Male   Female   Conflict   Triangular relationship

Figure 8-2. Genogram of the family of Case Illustration 2.

the family life cycle screening questions described below. If no significant major problems or dysfunctions are identified, stop the focused genogram interview when you understand the family well enough to take the family into consideration in addressing the patient's medical and other problems. If significant family problems are discovered, continue with the four-step family intervention described below.

Figure 8-1 shows the skeleton of the genogram for Case Illustration 1. The amount of information you gather about each individual and the family should be guided by the evolution of your hypotheses about family function as you go along. When major family issues emerge from the shape of the genogram or the patient's narrative, exploration of family relationships and history can be very focused. If the nature of family issues is initially obscure, but you suspect something important is going on, expand the genogram to include more peripheral family members and examine individual relationships more completely.

In general, it is useful to obtain brief descriptions of family members and important relationships, the history of major life events, immigrations, and comings and goings from the household(s). Record important information on the genogram as the interview progresses to create a picture of the family. Remember, the greatest efficiency in the genogram interview comes from the patient's active participation.

Identifying the Family Life Cycle Stage & Predicting Stress & Conflict

FAMILY LIFE CYCLE STAGE ASSESSMENT

Determining the life cycle stage of the family is the first task of a genogram assessment. The stages of the life cycle are a road map for exploring the important issues in the life of a patient and family.

The family life cycle consists of six stages (Table 8-2). Each stage is grounded in biologically driven and socially and culturally shaped patterns of individual development. The cycle usually "begins" with the separation of the individual from the family of origin (stage 1), followed by the formation of a new family of procreation (stage 2), the raising and "launching" of children into the world (stages 3, 4, and 5), and the family later in life (stage 6). Each of these stages is dominated by a theme and principal task. Each task requires two to four major changes in family structure and function. More often than not, family problems revolve around difficulty with one or more of the developmental tasks of the family's life cycle stage. Of course, the family life cycle is grounded in a specific sociopolitical and cultural context that help determine and shape the themes and tasks of each stage.

THE FAMILY LIFE CYCLE: ROLES AND GENERATIONS

With each stage of the family life cycle individuals acquire new roles: for example, from single adult to

Table 8-4. Presentations and problems associated with family dysfunction that should trigger screening for family dysfunction.

- Noncompliance with self-care regimens
- Alcohol or substance abuse
- Mental disorders, especially psychotic, mood, and anxiety disorders
- Unexplained medical symptoms and somatization
- Physician experienced difficulty in the doctor–patient relationship (i.e., the "difficult patient")
- Health-related habitual behaviors—smoking, eating disorders
- Newly diagnosed, rapidly deteriorating, or frightening illnesses (e.g., HIV infection, cancer, end-stage renal disease, myocardial infarction)
- Disruptions and change in the family system—divorce, separation, death, immigration, or emigration
- Natural and social disaster or trauma—fires, floods, earthquakes, crimes
- Sexually transmitted illness
- Anniversary dates and important holidays
- Domestic violence
- Reproductive health—pregnancy, termination of pregnancy, family planning

husband or wife *and simultaneously* to son or daughter-in-law. Note these roles as you and the patient scan the genogram. A directed open-ended question to screen for problems in each role is an efficient way of exploring the patient's relationships: "What's it like being a grandmother of six? Joe's wife? The daughter of a 95 year old?" If the patient is suitably activated, the whole story may come out after the first inquiry: "Being a grandmother is great, it's being a mother-in-law that I can't stand!"

THE LIFE CYCLE AND PATTERNS OF PARENTING

In probing for life cycle problems be sensitive to the influence of culture, ethnicity, and social class on norms and expected patterns. Pay particular attention to the structure of the parental subsystem: the adaptational strategies of families with one parent, one "working" and one "child care" parent, two working parents, families with extended-family parenting, blended families, and so on have differences that can be anticipated.

CASE ILLUSTRATION 1: DISCUSSION

Ariana (see Figure 8-1) is in the first stage of the family life cycle, an unattached young adult, in her case between families. Her divorce from her husband suggests difficulty forming a new family and moving on to the second stage of the family life cycle. It is noteworthy that the patient's sister Estelle is still at home and having difficulty with the first phase of the life cycle.

Screening for Family Function

After drawing the genogram and determining the life cycle stage of the family, the next step is to screen for family problems (Table 8-4). An activated patient will do the work of screening for you and immediately describe the "real problems." If the patient is reticent or the problem more obscure, the following strategies should aid the exploration.

GLOBAL FAMILY FUNCTION

Begin screening for family problems with open-ended questions about global family function (Table 8-5). The tone and content of the questions should be nonjudgmental, and even normalize the presence of problems, for example, "All families have their ups and downs, how's yours doing these days with all that is going on in

Table 8-5. Family assessment screening questions.

Category	Example
Open-ended assessment of family problems	"How are things going with your family? How is everyone getting along?" "Are you having any problems with (name the key individuals in the genogram)?"
Family problems with the patient's medical problems	"How is your family dealing with your medical problems?" "How is (name the key individuals in the genogram) dealing with it. What is their reaction?"
Problems associated with family dysfunction (see Table 8-4)	"I know you have been feeling quite depressed lately, how has your family reacted to that?" "What has (name the key individuals) said or done about your depression?"
Family life cycle problems	"I see you have a houseful of adolescents. I know that can be quite difficult. How have you been bearing up?"
Problems in the doctor–patient–family relationship: the compensatory alliance	"What does your family think and feel about the suggestions I have made?" "What were you hoping I might say to or do about your family?"

your life?" An effective initial inquiry directs the patient's attention to family issues, in general leaving the patient free rein to respond.

SCREENING FOR FAMILY LIFE CYCLE PROBLEMS

If a question about global function doesn't provide the necessary information, ask a few screening questions about the life cycle tasks that confront the patient's family. For example, the genogram in Figure 8-2 indicates that this family will be dealing with the tasks of "the family with young children" and "the family with adolescents" (see Table 8-2). Six questions, one for each of the three tasks in these two different life cycle stages, can screen for life cycle problems (Table 8-6). However, it is likely that not all of these six questions will have to be asked to identify sources of difficulty, especially if the unique features of any particular family are used to select the initial questions.

SCREENING FOR FAMILY DIFFICULTY WITH THE PATIENT'S MEDICAL PROBLEMS AND SYMPTOMS

The presence of somatization is one of the most important indications for exploring the patient's family, because it is usually driven by the patient's and/or family's need to have the patient occupy the sick role. An effective strategy for exploring the role of symptoms and medical problems in families is to follow the sequence: *symptom—function—family response. Symptom*—"Tell me about your symptom." *Function*—"How does your symptom affect your functioning, your normal activities, and ability to do what is expected?" *Family response*—"If you can't do these things, who does? What does your family do and say?"

Table 8-6. Family life cycle screening questions for families with young children and adolescents.

Stage 3—The family with young children

How are you doing with making time and space in your lives for three children?

How are you and your wife managing with child care responsibilities?

How are you getting along with the children's grandparents, *particularly your mother-in-law,** and your other in-laws?

Stage 4—The family with adolescents

How are you doing with a teenager, *your daughter,* in the house, and setting rules and expectations?

How are you and your wife doing with your work or careers? *Your youngest is going to go to school all day now. Will that change your or your wife's responsibilities or activities?*

What concerns do you have about the health or functioning of your parents or in-laws, *particularly your mother-in-law?*

*Generic questions for this stage of the family life cycle are shown in regular type, questions or elements in italic are modifications specific for the family of the father (see Figure 8-2).

SCREENING WITH RED-FLAG PROBLEMS

Whenever a problem associated with family dysfunction is present, the physician should screen for the family's reaction and response (see Tables 8-4 and 8-5). Many of these problems are emotionally charged and stigmatizing. Nonjudgmental, normalizing, and directive questions are therefore critical. These issues often have immediate clinical and legal implications and raise issues of confidentiality that need to be addressed.

SCREENING FOR PROBLEMS IN THE DOCTOR–PATIENT–FAMILY RELATIONSHIP

Throughout the family assessment consider what role you may be playing in the family system and be alert to the development of dysfunctional alliances with the patient or other family members. Ask the patient or other family members what reactions the family has had to health care providers' suggestions or interventions. It is also useful to determine what the patient wants you to say to other family members. Often these hopes and expectations are implied by patients' words or behavior rather than stated, because patients may not be fully aware of what they want, are too embarrassed to ask for it, or do not feel they have permission to make the request explicit.

 CASE ILLUSTRATION 1 (CONTD.)

In response to an open-ended question about how things are going at home, Ariana immediately identifies as the major problem the stress that Estelle's illness places on her mother and the pressure her mother puts on her (Ariana) to help out. Regarding her family's reaction to her own medical problems, Ariana says her mom has difficulty understanding why she's always so sick. Ariana's sister Gladys has come right out and said that she doesn't think Ariana's problems should be taken seriously. Ariana feels that the pressure of her mother's demands makes it difficult to think about getting involved with anyone. She blames her divorce on her ex-stepson's wildness and her ex-husband's inability to control him. Ariana thinks her mother is depressed about Estelle's illness, and suspects that she resents Estelle's continued dependence but can't admit it to herself or anyone else. Asked what she would like her physician to do in terms of her problems at home, Ariana says that she would like the physician to make her family understand that she really is sick. (Figure 8-3 shows the genogram at this stage of the family assessment.)

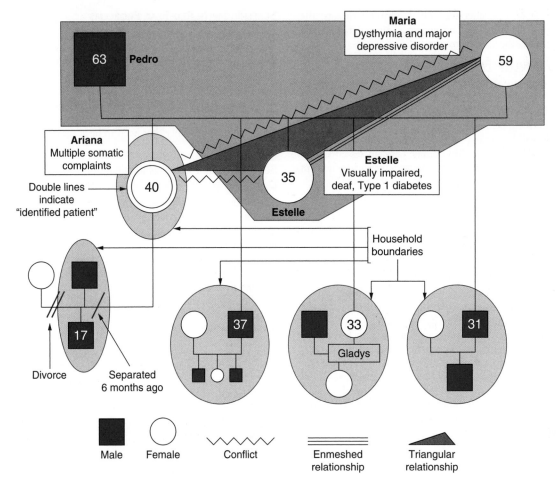

Figure 8-3. Annotated genogram for Ariana in Case Illustration 1.

Treating the Patient in the Context of the Family: Communicating about & Caring for the Patient's Medical Problems

After completing the basic genogram, assessing the family life cycle stage, and screening for problems in family function, the practitioner should be able to provide basic medical care for the patient in the context of the family (Table 8-7). With the majority of families, the interventions described in this step accomplish the basic goals of family assessment and no further intervention is needed (see Table 8-3). A basic family assessment will, by itself, facilitate the following.

ENHANCING THE THERAPEUTIC ALLIANCE

Perhaps the most important consequence of conducting a family systems assessment is to enhance the therapeutic alliance among the patient, provider, and other family members. Patients' perception that their physician cares for them is probably the single most important

variable in the formation of a successful doctor–patient relationship. Few things accomplish this better than talking to patients about the most important people in their lives (see Chapter 2).

COMMUNICATING WITH THE FAMILY

Family assessment enhances communication with the family about the patient's medical problems. This may involve educating them about the patient's condition, discussing self-care regimens and monitoring family involvement with the medical regimen, facilitating the family's role in decision making and advance directives, and helping the family adjust to changes in the patient's functional capacity.

ASSESSMENT AND SUPPORT

Assessing the family's emotional response to the patient's problems and providing needed support are challenging and rewarding family-oriented tasks. It is often difficult for the physician to witness the emotional distress experienced

Table 8-7. Basic family interventions.

- Enhancing the therapeutic alliance by demonstrating interest and concern about the patient's family and life situation
- Communicating with the family about the patient's medical condition
- Providing information about the patient's problems: Discussing prognosis and answering family members' questions about medical problems
- Discussing self-care and enlisting family assistance with medical management
- Facilitating the family's participation in decision making about therapeutic options
- Discussing and mediating the effect of the patient's loss of function on the roles of other family members
- Providing emotional support to the patient and family
- Counseling the family about simple family system problems
- Identifying problems requiring attention from the family
- Preparing for further family assessment, intervention, and referral for further family interventions
- Working in collaboration with family therapists or other mental health specialists

by patient and family in the face of serious medical problems. The temptation to "stick to the facts" and restrict attention to biomedical issues is both strong and understandable, especially in light of the physician's perception that he or she "can do nothing" about the emotional pain. It is important to understand that empathically listening to the family and the patient is a powerful therapeutic intervention in itself—even if it appears to "fix" nothing (see Chapter 2).

It is often possible to make simple family systems interventions by suggesting that families try new behaviors.

CASE ILLUSTRATION 2

A 36-year-old man with hypertension presents to a walk-in clinic with tension headaches that have been going on for 2 weeks. The genogram interview (see Figure 8-2 and Table 8-6) reveals that he is distressed by ongoing conflict between his wife and teenage daughter about rules governing her behavior with peers outside the home. At home, the father remains silent until the fights between mother and daughter become intolerable. Their fights stop only when he complains about the headaches the fights have given him. He has never discussed his own ideas about rules for his daughter's behavior—or of family arguments—or negotiated a common position with his wife.

An appropriate intervention would be to suggest that the patient and his wife discuss the situation before the fights begin and try to develop a plan on which they both agree. If the family has the flexibility to respond to this suggestion, it may help them with the developmental

life cycle challenge. If this intervention fails to help sufficiently, it may be a sign that further family assessment and interventions are required. It is important that suggestions be based on at least as thorough an evaluation as that produced by the preceding steps of this method; premature suggestions based on incomplete assessment are likely to fail.

CAREGIVER COLLABORATION

If the patient or family is receiving treatment from mental health specialists, the physician should actively collaborate, and they should consult with one another when issues come up that are relevant to the other's expertise. Patients may attempt to play one health care provider against the other; for example, they may present somatic symptoms to the mental health specialist and attempt to engage the medical provider in issues being examined in therapy. Patients or family members may complain about the therapist, especially when the family or patient is being challenged to change. Active communication between treating providers is critical if this dynamic arises (commonly referred to as "splitting").

FOCUSING ON THE DYSFUNCTION

Some problems have a clear and potentially devastating effect on the family. Focusing the family's attention on the problems associated with family dysfunction is a crucial clinical task. For example, if a patient or a member of the patient's family has a problem with alcohol abuse or dependence, it is important to assess the family's response, help the family accept the reality of the problem, and support their need to address it. Many families are waiting for just the kind of professional, extrafamiliar attention that the physician can provide. Validating their feelings, and providing information about resources such as Alcoholics Anonymous (AA), may be all that it takes to precipitate action.

On the other hand, the patient's and family's resistance to change may be so strong that basic family assessment is not enough to help them take action. In these cases, it is sometimes preferable to refer the patient to a mental health specialist without further family intervention. However, it is often necessary to proceed to the next level of family intervention to make a successful referral.

CASE ILLUSTRATION 1 (CONTD.)

Ariana greatly appreciated the opportunity to describe the situation at home, especially when the physician expressed sympathy for the burden that Estelle's illness placed on everyone and for the disappointment resulting from Ariana's failed marriage. The physician now had a general feel for Ariana's family. It was clear that Ariana needed to be labeled as "sick" and that every diagnostic test, referral to a specialist, and symptomatic treatment helped create a compensatory alliance establishing the sick role. Ariana, clearly feeling that the physician was on her side after the genogram interview, readily agreed to a family meeting.

FOUR-STEP FAMILY ASSESSMENT & INTERVENTION

If serious family dysfunction is interfering with medical management, the doctor–patient relationship, or the patient's functional status and quality of life, a more intensive, four-step evaluation and intervention is required (Table 8-8). The goals of family assessment and intervention as described here, differ from the structural systems changes that are employed in family therapy. Even if medical providers had the time and training, they could not treat families with commonly employed techniques that require forming alliances with different family members during treatment, because this process can threaten the trust required to deal effectively with the patient's medical problems.

Step 1: Assessing the Family: "Bringing the Pain into the Room"

The previously described basic family assessment is the core and foundation of the first of the four steps of intervention with dysfunctional families (Table 8-8). The difference lies in the need to achieve three goals that go beyond a basic understanding of family functioning. The physician must (1) have a relatively complete

Table 8-8. Family intervention.

Step	Objective	Statement
Analyze, and "bring the pain into the room"	1. Understand the major conflicts in the family system. 2. Understand how the sick role functions in the family system. 3. "Bring the pain into the room," that is, help the patient (and family if present) experience the pain of their problems during the interview.	"Your [family problems] are serious and painful, and you have not been able to resolve them on your own."
Reframe	1. Direct the patient's (and family's) attention to the underlying family problems and away from the sick role establishing somatization, excessive functional impairment, or dysfunctional self-care behavior. 2. Endorse the patient's objectives while separating them from the use of the sick role to obtain them.	"*In addition to* your [symptom/problem] these family problems are equally worthy of attention." "*Even if you were in perfect health* I could understand why you would want your [family problem] resolved in a way that meets your needs."
Empathically witness	1. Provide emotional support and empowerment to the patient. 2. Enhance the therapeutic alliance.	"I am so impressed with how well you are doing despite all your problems."
Refer	1. Provide access to and educate patients about psychotherapeutic intervention. 2. Address resistance to psychotherapeutic treatments.	"You have important questions about how to improve your family situation; therapy is a way of answering those questions."

understanding of the major conflicts or issues in the family; (2) understand how the sick role, if present (and it usually is), is functioning as a coping strategy for the patient and the family; and (3) conduct the interview so that patients can bring the full intensity of their feelings about the family problems out, that is, "bring the pain into the room."

The first step of family assessment and intervention is complete when you can say, with confidence that the patient will agree, "It seems to me that the family problems we are discussing are extremely painful, and that you have been unable to resolve them until now." Bringing the pain of the patient's life "into the room" during the interview is an important part of the process because the shared knowledge will provide the rationale and impetus for the second step of the process, that is, reframing attention to the underlying family problems. The following techniques will help accomplish this first task.

Two features of the way in which family systems work, so called triangles and circles, can help guide exploration of family relationships. First, all dyadic interactions ultimately triangulate. We fully understand the way individuals interact only when we understand the series of triangular relationships they belong to. Second, families that are having difficulty, that are "stuck," engage in a repetitive or "circular" sequence of behaviors that represents the best they can do to cope with their problems. For example, in their study of adolescents with brittle diabetes or poorly controlled asthma, Minuchin and colleagues often observed the following pattern: unresolved marital conflict erupts into an argument between the adolescent's parents; the adolescent, in response to the stress of the fight, becomes acutely ill; the parents stop fighting and focus on caring for their child; the exacerbation of the child's illness resolves; the unresolved marital conflict erupts into another fight, and the process is repeated. From this point of view, it is clear that the outcome of the seemingly dyadic parental conflict cannot be understood without knowing that the child and the illness are "triangulated." It is impossible to understand the behavior of any member of this triangle without examining the interaction with both of the other two.

The triangular relationships among family members are caught up in circular patterns of interactions. The sequence of events that takes place in the adolescent's family may be described in a linear fashion, that is, parents argue, the child is upset and gets sick, the parents stop arguing to help the child, the child gets better. The interruption of the fight, however, also prevents the parents from "finishing" their fight and resolving their problems, thus, the pattern inevitably repeats. Dysfunctional families are often stuck in such a repetitive, self-sustaining pattern.

It is important to understand how the "sick role," created by the patient's symptoms, is embedded in the family system, and how the whole family participates in it. There are no pure victims or villains in such a system: The adolescent is not merely the "victim" of marital discord; the child's sick role and the acute exacerbations of illness have a powerful controlling influence on the inability of the spouses to resolve their conflicts. Looked at from a more positive vantage point, the child's illness is performing the important function of modulating a marital conflict that might otherwise threaten the integrity of the family system more completely. The symptom is the product of and serves the needs of the entire family system. Though the price is high for all involved, and this "solution" is likely to fail in the long run, it is the best that the family can do at the moment to cope with the totality of their problems.

Patient-centered emotion-supporting interviewing techniques can be instrumental in "bringing the pain into the room" during the interview. A "one-two punch" that couples a statement giving permission to express feelings, combined with an open-ended question about an emotionally charged issue, is often effective. For example, you might say to a new grandmother whose single-parent daughter is hoping for child care for her new baby, "setting limits with your children so that you can be a grandparent rather than a nanny can be difficult and even cause a lot of guilt. How's it been for you?"

Conducting a family meeting is a powerful technique for analyzing family systems. The objective of the family meeting is to have the family enact their interactions, and have other members directly report their responses to the patient's sick role symptoms and behavior. If they enact "the pain in the room," so much the better. The physician merely stops the action when it reaches its peak, concludes Step 1 with the statement, "It seems to me that the family problems we are discussing are extremely painful, and that you have been unable to resolve them until now," and moves on to Step 2, "reframing."

 CASE ILLUSTRATION 1 (CONTD.)

During the family interview, the tremendous burden placed on the family by Estelle's visual impairment, deafness, and diabetes became painfully clear as the physician struggled to communicate with her, a process that required writing notes in letters 6 in. high, or having Ariana or her mother slowly and carefully speak so that Estelle could read their lips (Estelle was unable to read anyone else's lips, and the family had tried but failed to learn sign language). It became clear how much the family depended on Ariana and how she stepped ambivalently into the fray whenever Estelle needed attention.

When the subject turned to Ariana's failed marriage and social life, the mother (Maria) expressed some hope, immediately labeled as ridiculous by Ariana, that she (Ariana) would get back together with her ex-husband. Ariana said, "with all this," meaning the problems with Estelle, "how can I find time to get involved with anyone?"

Further discussion revealed that Maria was a worrier and was constantly preoccupied with whichever of her children was having difficulties, especially medical problems. Ariana's medical problems elicited sympathy from her mother, who suggested that since Ariana was no longer married, she should move back into the family house.

Ariana immediately rejected the offer and said that her medical problems were the primary reason she could not move back into the house; she didn't want her mother to see her when she was sick because her mother would worry too much. Ariana added that when she was feeling sick, she needed to stay home by herself, and at these times she didn't even answer the phone or know what was going on in her parents' house.

The physician concluded that Ariana's somatization was embedded in the repetitive pattern of events dominated by her triangular relationship with Estelle and their mother. Ariana's physical symptoms allowed her to remain connected to and receive attention and emotional support from her mother, and simultaneously allowed her to control the family's expectations that she would always be there to help with Estelle. It seemed that Ariana's reason for remaining away from her mother and Estelle was an illness, that is, something beyond her control. The desire to devote more of her life to herself, even though it was closer to the truth, would not be acceptable to either Ariana or the family.

Step 2: Reframing Attention to the Underlying Family Problems

The goal of Step 2 of family intervention, "reframing," is twofold (Table 8-8): (1) focus the patient's and family's attention on the underlying family problems, and away from physical symptoms and sick role-justifying problems; (2) separate the patient's (or family's) objective in using the sick role from the use of the sick role as a tactic to achieve the goal. This is done by recognizing the objective that the patient is pursuing and endorsing it as something that the patient is "entitled to even if [they] are in perfect health."

REFRAMING, "IN ADDITION TO YOUR PAIN ..."

The transition from Step 1 to Step 2 occurs when the interview has "brought the pain into the room," and patients are in touch with their distress, that is, when they agree with the first critical reframing statement, "It seems to me that the family situation you have just described is extremely painful, and that *in addition to* your [problematic symptom or behavior], this family problem is also worthy of attention."

A critical component of the first reframing statement is "*in addition to*" in contrast to either "instead of" or "because of." Even if your understanding, based upon a psychosomatic hypothesis, that family stress is "causing" the somatoform presentation, you must resist saying so. The legitimacy of the sick role and coping strategies that the patient and family currently need to function depends upon there being a "disease beyond one's control" to justify the sick role. If the family intervention begins to have effect, and healthier coping strategies are adopted, then the family will be able to relinquish sick role-based coping. Until that time they must be allowed to retain the sick role strategy. Therefore, the goal of reframing is to establish a *parallel* concern directed at the underlying family problems. Occasionally, a patient or family member will be able to make the connection themselves: "Doctor, do you think that maybe my headache is being caused by all these problems?" In such cases, the psychosomatic hypothesis can be endorsed. The mistake is to make the connection before the patient and family are ready. This will result in the all too familiar, "Doctor, you think it's all in my head. It's not in my head, my pain is real!"

REFRAMING, "EVEN IF YOU WERE THE PICTURE OF PERFECT HEALTH YOU WOULD BE ENTITLED TO ..."

Unless your patient's objectives in occupying the sick role are antisocial, you should be able to identify an essential core of their objective that you can endorse—a new grandmother who doesn't want to be mistaken for a nanny, a father who wants peace in his home and rules for his teenage daughter, a young woman who does not want to become her sister's home health aide, and so on.

The second objective of reframing is to separate the objective from the tactic of occupying the sick role, and to empower the patient and family to adopt other, healthier strategies. This can be done by telling the patient, "*if you were the picture of perfect health, you would be entitled to*—be a grandmother not a nanny, have your daughter follow some agreed upon rules, set limits on your role in taking care of your sister, and so on." This part of the reframing addresses the fundamental function of the sick role, which is to establish entitlement, and uses the authority of the physician to legitimate the desired entitlement on other, healthier grounds.

It was relatively easy to reframe the burden of caring for Estelle as a problem worthy of attention after the painful demonstration of just how difficult it was to just have a conversation with her. It was also easy to reframe Ariana's desire to have some time for herself—a need she was unwilling to claim on her own—as something that would be important for "a woman her age" *even if she was not ill.* Ariana was willing to accept the suggestion that her failure to develop the kind of intimate relationship she desired was also a problem worthy of consideration.

Step 3: Empathic Witnessing: "I Am So Impressed with How Well You Are Doing Despite ... "

The most immediate way to ensure that family intervention has a positive and therapeutic effect is to "empathically witness" the patient's and family's problems and their efforts to cope (Table 8-8). If the interview has succeeded in exposing the family's distress and their best attempts to deal with their problems, the patient and family will recognize that the physician knows the family in a very intimate way. If the physician acknowledges the special nature of this awareness, and responds empathically to the patient and family, the effect can be very therapeutic. The general format for empathic witnessing is to say to the patient (or family) that having heard their story, and seen what they have to cope with, "*I am very impressed with how well you are doing despite all your problems and difficulties.*" It is helpful to remember that even if you cannot praise the patient's behavior or accomplishments, you can usually empathically witness their efforts: "I am impressed that you *want to be* a good mother to your children."

CASE ILLUSTRATION 1 (CONTD.)

The family admitted that the current situation was indeed painful and that they had not been able to solve the problem despite their best efforts. The physician was able to tell Ariana and her mother: "I am so impressed with how well you are both doing despite the tremendous problems you have had to deal with." The physician also remarked on the magnitude of the sacrifice Ariana had made, neglecting her own social life to be available to the family. The physician also commented that it was easy to understand how this area of Ariana's life might be difficult for her to deal with because of her past problems.

Step 4: Referral for Family & Psychotherapy

Referral for therapy is not always indicated. Very often a brief family intervention can empower patients and their families to address their difficulties with new energy, insight, and courage to change. However, when mental health intervention is indicated and proposed, patients and families may not readily accept it (Table 8-8).

Resistance to a mental health referral is common. Referral for therapy may make sense to the provider long before it does to the patient. Framing family problems as "in addition to" will help patients feel comfortable that therapy does not threaten their use of the sick role before they are ready to give it up. Resistance to therapy may be due to fear of dealing directly with painful and powerful emotions. Empathic witnessing and reframing can make this challenge seem more surmountable. Finally, patients may accept the reality of family problems yet not accept the fact that therapy will help: "What's talking going to accomplish?" The process of therapy may indeed seem obscure to patients and it may be useful to restate problems as questions and describe therapy as the process of looking for answers. For example, "you have a serious question to answer. You have to determine how much child care you actually want to provide, and then figure out how to talk to your daughter about it. Therapy can help you find answers to these questions."

Sometimes, patients and their families never get to therapy. Even in that case, the reframing and empathic listening to the patient's family story have a positive effect. *After* performing a family assessment and intervention, the physician may say the following to the patient who has not followed through with referral for therapy and who returns with persistent or recurrent symptoms (as did the father in Case Illustration 2):

CASE ILLUSTRATION 2 (CONCLUSION)

"I am sorry that your headache is still bothering you. Your wife and daughter are still fighting, aren't they? It's too bad that you haven't gotten to the therapist yet. I truly wish that there was more that I could do for you. Now, why don't we check your blood pressure."

The patient—aware that the physician has witnessed the family conflict—knows that the clinician understands the importance of the conflict at home and that this understanding is empathic. Hence, the physician does not have to repeat the assessment and intervention interview, merely recall it for the patient. The physician is in a position to respect the meaning of the patient's symptoms without allowing them to divert the process of care into unnecessary testing, medication, or referrals for more evaluation.

CASE ILLUSTRATION 1 (CONCLUSION)

The physician (1) referred the family for family therapy to explore better approaches to coping with Estelle's medical problems; (2) suggested that Ariana would benefit from individual counseling to explore her difficulties in forming a satisfying intimate relationship; (3) asked Maria's physician to consider the diagnoses of dysthymia and major depression; and (4) recommended that the family try to obtain a home health aide for Estelle to give Maria a break. The family agreed to all four of these suggestions. When Ariana returned for her next visit, she still had numerous symptoms but spoke of them only briefly, allowing the physician to turn the discussion to what was going on at home. Ariana reported that the family had taken no steps toward family therapy and that she was

still considering whether to go to individual therapy. She did report feeling more comfortable setting limits on her mother's expectations of assistance in dealing with Estelle, and reported success in obtaining a home health aide for Estelle. Maria had been placed on an antidepressant, made a few visits to a community mental health center, and was much less symptomatic.

Eight months later, Ariana entered individual therapy and her somatization decreased dramatically and her limit-setting improved. Eventually, she started dating and entered a steady relationship but has not married.

SUGGESTED READINGS

Carter CA, McGoldrick M, eds. *The Family Life Cycle: A Framework for Family Therapy.* New York, NY: Gardner Press, 1980.

Doherty WJ, Baird MA. *Family-Centered Medical Care: A Clinical Case Book.* New York, NY: Guilford Press, 1987.

Doherty WJ, Campbell TL. *Families and Health.* New York, NY: Sage Publications, 1988.

Hahn SR, Feiner JS, Bellin EH. The doctor–patient–family relationship: a compensatory alliance. *Ann Intern Med* 1988; 109:884–889.

Haley J. *Problem Solving Therapy.* San Francisco, CA: Jossey-Bass, 1976.

McGoldrick M, Gerson R. *Genograms in Family Assessment.* New York, NY: Norton, 1985.

Minuchin S. *Families and Family Therapy.* Cambridge, MA: Harvard University Press, 1974.

Children

9

Howard L. Taras, MD

INTRODUCTION

This chapter reviews common childhood behavioral problems and suggests some management guidelines. Pediatric behavioral medicine cannot be easily disassociated from child development because many problematic childhood behaviors have developmental roots.

UNDESIRABLE BEHAVIOR AS A NORMAL PART OF DEVELOPMENT

A child's ability to understand and interact with the environment is constantly evolving. To learn more about the world, a child experiments with ways of interacting with it. Most often, children test the reactions of the people to whom they are closest, their parents. Colloquial phrases such as *"the terrible twos," "she's going through a stage,"* and *"boys will be boys"* indicate that undesirable childhood behaviors are commonly accepted as "normal." But when an undesirable behavior is manifesting in your child, the normalcy can be difficult to accept. And even when the cause is well understood, many parents still need the knowledge and skills to respond to the problem behavior.

EXTRAORDINARY STRESS

Behavioral problems associated with normal childhood development must be distinguished from problems with more complex causes. Aberrant childhood behaviors are often secondary to extraordinary life stresses. This applies to children who witness violence, are members of communities that have experienced a catastrophic event, are exposed to continuous marital discord, have a chronic illness or a chronically ill sibling, or who don't feel wanted. Children living under any condition that seriously threatens healthy and successful transition through a developmental stage are likely to pose serious behavioral problems.

Children, like adults, may appear to be the dysfunctional member of an otherwise healthy family unit even though the problem actually stems from family issues. This is particularly the case with childhood behaviors, because children are dependent on adults in almost every way. Take, for instance, the child who refuses to attend school. Classically, this behavior occurs when one or both parents send subliminal messages to the child to remain home. Although the primary problem is parental anxiety about separation, it is the child who exhibits the apparent symptoms.

INHERENT DISORDERS

In addition to childhood behavioral problems stemming from normal development and extraordinary life stresses, a third general category involves problems caused by disorders inherent to the child. Attention deficit disorders are the most common and well known, but conduct disorders, depression, pervasive developmental disorders, and other psychiatric diagnoses may manifest during childhood. A complete history, observation, and response to treatment help the primary care clinician distinguish these from other causes of behavioral problems.

SCREENING FAMILIES FOR DIFFICULTIES WITH CHILDHOOD BEHAVIORS

Pediatric primary care providers must screen families for difficulties with undesirable childhood behaviors, sort out probable causes for the behaviors, recognize when a mental health referral is appropriate, and manage those problems that are likely to respond to simple environmental changes or to elementary behavioral management techniques.

Practitioner Concern Versus Time Constraints

Many parents do not know where to seek help for behavioral problems such as their baby's night awakenings, their toddler's tantrums, or their fourth grader's class-clown behavior. They do not realize that their child's clinician can assist them. To overcome these barriers, health care providers should take every opportunity to talk about behavioral issues, although time constraints may limit the practitioner's ability to listen to extensive histories. Therefore, clinicians need to screen for behavioral information in ways that are expedient and that leave time to reflect on issues that can be discussed more fully at another time.

Trigger Questions & Questionnaires

One way to elicit information from parents is to ask a preset list of key questions, specific to each age group. Another option is to routinely use formal, standardized questionnaires that are designed so that parents can respond to them by mail in advance of an appointment or in the clinician's waiting room. An excellent source for such screening questions is Jellinek's *Bright Futures in Practice: Mental Health (2002)* (see "Suggested Reading," below). These questionnaires enable parents to take the time to respond thoughtfully to physician inquiries and they include the input of both parents—often exposing differences in parents' opinions. These questionnaires also minimize parents' discomfort with verbalizing certain family problems. They often yield information from a wide range of potential problem areas and do so effectively. Many of these tools are accompanied by a separate set of questions for teachers, which are useful when a problem has been identified.

Table 9-1 lists four behavioral screens that are popular and appropriate for use by primary care clinicians.

Other available questionnaires were reviewed by Simonian (see "Suggested Reading," below). This review is a useful guide for clinicians who wish to identify which tool is most suitable to their needs.

To effectively screen for childhood behavioral problems, practitioners also need to develop their skills of observation and to learn to apply their natural intuitions. Parent–child interaction in the office can be an excellent indicator of problems occurring at home. Incidents in the office that induce parents to discipline their child are opportunities for clinicians to better understand the parent–child relationship and to bring behavioral management issues into discussion. Experienced clinicians have learned to become aware of subtle signs in the office that are indicative of a family's dynamics, such as how a mother holds her baby. A mother who seems uncomfortable feeding her baby, a pattern of noncompliance, or suspicion about the levels of interest mother or father show are all indicative of issues that should register concern with the clinician. Involvement of grandparents and other extended family, references parents make about their own upbringing, and other family characteristics are also worth noting.

Although signs for concern do not always indicate problems, this information is often useful in evaluating a child behavioral issue, although sometimes not until months or years later. Positive impressions that clinicians form about families also provide clinically useful information.

Table 9-1. Behavioral screening tools.

Name	Author/Reference	Characteristic
Achenbach Child Behavior Checklist	Achenbach TM. *Manual for the Child Behavior Checklist/4–18 and 1991 Profile.* Burlington, VT: University of Vermont Department of Psychiatry, 1991.	112 items/ages 2–18
Conners' Parent Rating Scale	Conners CK, Sitarenios G, Parker JDA, et al. The revised Conners' Parent Rating Scale (CPRS-R): factor structure, reliability, and criterion validity. *J Abnorm Child Psychol* 1998;26(4):257–268.	Brief, but only valuable when attention deficit hyperactivity disorder (ADHD) is suspected, less valuable as a general screen
Eyberg Child Behavior Inventory	Eyberg SM. Behavioral Assessment: advancing Methodology in Pediatric Psychology. *J Pediatric Psychology* 1985; June 10(2): 123–139.	36 items/ages 2–16
Pediatric Symptom Checklist	Jellinek MS, Murphy JM, Robinson J, et al. Pediatric symptom checklist: screening school-age children for psychosocial dysfunction. *J Pediatr* 1988;112:201–209.	5 min/35 items for ages 6–12
Behavior Assessment System for Children, Second Edition (BASC-2)	Reynolds CR, Kamphaus RW. *The Behavior Assessment System for Children*, 2nd ed (BASC-2). Circle Pines, MN: AGS, 2005.	Ages 2–22

INTERVIEWING YOUNG CHILDREN

Primary care providers can find themselves in a quandary when they try to elicit information directly from the child. Most children by age 2 1/2–3 years are capable of communicating certain thoughts and feelings to an inquiring health provider. But children do not typically divulge such information to clinicians when questioned directly. Children freely offer their honest opinions on just about any topic, sensitive or banal, but they often do so when it is unsolicited. Parents themselves are often surprised when their children first reveal their feelings about a delicate personal issue to an adult with whom they are not ostensibly very close (a preschool teacher, a friend's mother in their car pool, and so on).

Primary care providers should therefore use tools that help children more freely and predictably disclose what's on their minds. One way is to ask children old enough to understand and comply to draw a picture, for example, to draw "anything they want," "something scary," "their family," or "the worst day at school." The position of the characters in the drawings, facial expressions, and choice of colors can yield important information about what they are thinking and may be indicative of how they are feeling and can be used as a starting point for discussion. Children often find it easier to speak about themselves when the conversation is in the third person, such as "Why would that little girl in the picture want to hit her mommy?"

To avoid alienating parents, you may go through a few such questions when both parent and child are in the room. But many children, and most of those older than age 4 years, respond differently when their parents are in the room. Explain to parents that you would like to interview the child in the same way without them. The general nature of children's responses can be discussed later with parents. Parents should be notified that this will occur. But the interviewer need not feel compelled to reveal children's specific responses to each interview item, particularly if information may be hurtful and not of therapeutic value at that time. Parents and children should know that too.

Other oblique ways of eliciting information from children are to ask open-ended questions using questions that children like to respond to: "Pretend a magical genie in a bottle wanted to grant you three wishes, what would they be?" And "If you could magically turn into any animal you wanted, what would it be?" To their response to the last question, then ask, "Well that's wonderful! And why would you be happy as that animal?"

Sentence completion games are also useful. The clinician begins the first few words of a sentence and asks the child to complete the sentence by making something up. Examples of some are given in Table 9-2, and these (and others like them) can be typed onto colorful

Table 9-2. Samples of "sentence completion" items for interviewing young children.

- I really like it when . . .
- I am ashamed . . .
- I worry a lot about . . .
- My mother . . .
- I hate . . .
- It makes me sad to . . .
- It makes me happy to . . .
- People think that I . . .
- I really hope one day that I . . .

---

cards so that children can choose one at a time and perceive it as a game, not a real interview. Allow the child to be imaginative with responses, and indicate that their responses can be the truth but don't have to be.

Toddlers and school age children are often aware of the clinician's actual intent when these interviewing techniques are used. Despite this, children seem to enjoy going along with this format of questioning and appreciate having an easy way to express themselves. Children respond best when they are comfortable with the clinician. Arranging a number of office visits can help to establish that relationship.

When using drawings, questions in the third person, or questions evoking the child's imagination, it is important not to read too deeply into children's responses. Children have active imaginations: they play around with frightening ideas and with wishful thinking. Sometimes they are merely obsessed with speaking about what they've recently seen on television. To be taken seriously, responses of young children should fit into a general pattern of what the clinician suspects from parent interview and symptoms. One or two worrisome responses should not stand on their own as proof for the etiology to a problem.

BEYOND THE PHYSICIAN–CHILD–PARENT TRIAD

Many toddlers are placed in the care of a day care provider, babysitter, or relative. Virtually, all children older than age 5 spend a large portion of their waking hours in school. Yet despite this, clinicians traditionally rely almost exclusively on parents (and the children themselves) to gather a behavioral history. Some clinicians send questionnaires to school staff to elicit information, or they ask parents about their children's progress at school or day care. It is rare, however, for clinicians to routinely engage in direct telephone contact with child care providers and teachers. Yet these people occupy many, and occasionally most, of children's waking hours. The value of attaining parental permission to speak directly with educational professionals in a child's life cannot be overstated. Teachers and child care providers can provide valuable insight. Many have numerous years of experience with all types of children, and their observations rarely include the emotional biases that sometimes confound a parent's interpretation and recollection of details. Once a behavior plan has been recommended, a relationship with daytime caretakers may extend the plan's implementation to that setting and render it more effective.

NORMAL CHILD DEVELOPMENT

To attribute an undesirable behavior to a developmental stage of childhood, health care providers need to be knowledgeable about stages of normal childhood development (Table 9-3).

Maturational Theory

This theory teaches that behavioral sequences occur by a process of unfolding in all children, that these sequences are regulated by genes, and that detrimental environmental factors could impede this sequence.

Freudian Psychoanalytic Theories

Freud's theories emphasize unconscious and conscious mental processes that children go through. For example, in the anal stage at $1^1/_2$–3 years of age children are

personally focused on elimination and interpersonally focused on "rebellion versus compliance" with parental demands. At this stage, they may fear loss of parental love.

Erikson's Stages of Child Development

Erickson's stages are an expanded version of psychoanalytic theory, and his teachings help clinicians understand children's psychosocial development.

Piagetian Theory

Piaget's staging of children's cognitive development describes, for example, that a child cannot be expected to see a situation from a perspective other than his or her own until school age.

Kohlberg's Theory

Kohlberg's theory of children's moral development describes, for example, how young toddlers understand their actions to be good or bad based on the presence or absence of a resulting punishment or reward.

Each of these theories presents a different view of a single multidimensional entity we call "child development." Each describes child development from another perspective. If one theory illuminates a given child's behavior more than another, then try using it to explain an undesirable behavior and to help guide parents toward a proper response.

Table 9-3. Highlights of child characteristics during stages of development.

Theory	Age 0–2	Age 2–6	Age 6–12
Kohlberg (Development of Moral Judgment)	*Premoral stage* Egocentric, no moral concepts Satisfaction of own needs	*Moral stage* Desires to please others	*Moral stage* Obligation to duty Respect for authority
Piaget (Cognitive Development)	*Sensorimotor/preverbal* Emergence of purposeful activities Learns that objects and people exist even when out of sight	*Preoperational/prelogical* Can deal with one aspect of a problem at a time Learns to use symbols for language, and so on	*Concrete operational/logical* Can deal with multiple aspects of a problem, if not abstract Ability to classify things
Erickson (Psychosocial Development)	*Oral stage (early on)* Initially gaining trust Once gained, seeks independence Uses words like "no" and "me" *Anal stage (2nd year)* Initially learns self-control Then, can develop self-esteem and good will Learns autonomy but struggles with shame and doubt	*Phallic stage* Takes initiative, is curious Becomes more aggressive and competitive Starts to plan ahead Struggles with guilt	*Latency stage* An industrious stage Focused on performance and producing results Struggles with inferiority/inadequacy when meeting some meritable failures

MANAGEMENT & REFERRAL

Primary care providers must often evaluate and manage common child behavior problems in their own offices. In addition, mental health referrals are usually unnecessary since so many undesirable child behaviors are maladaptations or manifestations of normal child development. There are occasions when the need for psychiatric assessment, psychotherapy, or play therapy is apparent from the start. But for most problems that present to primary care practitioners, children respond well to brief, solution-focused strategies. Although no single behavioral management technique works well for all children with similar problems and similar etiologies to their problems, clinicians can quickly learn to tailor their management plans to suit the individual needs of each family. These plans should be based on families' cultural characteristics, size, work schedules, and other factors. A management failure should always first be considered a problem with the behavioral management technique prescribed, not with the child or family.

PREVENTING SUBSTANCE ABUSE, VIOLENCE, & OTHER MALADAPTIVE BEHAVIORS

Primary care clinicians who treat children have the opportunity and responsibility to intervene during these early years to prevent maladaptive behavior. This prevention can take two forms. First, clinicians can work with individual families and patients as they visit the practice for preventive screens and episodic care. Second, clinicians have the power to help modify the environment in which children spend time in their communities, such as schools, playgrounds, and child care centers. This second role of the primary care clinician is an example of "Community-Oriented Primary Care," which is a model that addresses clinicians' role in meeting changing societal needs.

Clinicians can select from several existing preventive theories as they work with children, their families, and communities to thwart the adoption of violence, substance abuse, and self-destructive lifestyles in the children's futures. Two are described here.

Emotional Intelligence

Emotional intelligence is defined as the ability to identify one's own feelings, to identify the feelings of others, and to solve problems that involve emotional issues. The extent to which this "intelligence" is innate versus learned is unknown. Several screening tools for emotional intelligence are used by researchers in this field. But such formal screening is not likely to be useful for practitioners in primary care settings as a routine practice. Although the term "emotional intelligence" is a relatively recent one, the concept of having relative emotional strength or relative weakness, and its impact on one's ability to cope, is not new. Emotional intelligence has been found to be related to having a lower risk for smoking during one's youth. Parents who provide their child with "tools" to handle emotional challenges may be able to increase the emotional ability of their child. By teaching a vocabulary of words that describes emotions, such as "frustrated," "anxious," and "envious," children may become more likely to use them in lieu of acting these behaviors out. Parents are also encouraged to foster an environment in which children will want to describe their feelings. Naturally, this is more easily accepted in theory by parents in your office than at home. Clinicians can ask about specific and recent situations at home that demonstrate the child's personality and point of emotional maturation. By understanding these details, a clinician can offer step-by-step suggestions that are most pertinent to that family's issues and that child's age.

Many classroom programs that are designed to encourage conflict resolution and prevent violence are based on similar theories. Children are taught that anger is an emotion that can be recognized before it is acted upon irrationally. Children discuss and even act out situations that evoke their own anger and those of others. They also learn how to temper these emotions and how to de-escalate a situation. Clinicians have some responsibility to encourage schools and other agencies to make these programs available to children in their neighborhoods.

Developmental Asset Theory

Another preventive theoretical construct is to provide children with a large number of assets in their lives; this will make them less likely to adopt maladaptive behaviors now and in the future. Lists of 40 assets have been developed by the Search Institute (see "Web Sites," below) for various age groups, including preschool and elementary age children. Cumulatively, these assets are purported to foster healthy development. Examples of assets for school-age children are doing service for others in the community or having a supportive relationship with an adult in addition to their parents. For a preschooler, a parent must also have support from people outside the home.

There is still only a limited amount of hard evidence that introduction of these assets prevents untoward behaviors, but promoting these assets is likely harmless and potentially beneficial. Clinicians have opportunity to promote such assets with families in their practices. Moreover, they can help assess the range of opportunities in their communities for children to acquire such assets.

EXAMPLES OF COMMON BEHAVIORAL ISSUES
Infancy: Night Waking

CASE ILLUSTRATION 1

Parents of a 12-week-old girl complain that their daughter rarely sleeps more than a total of 4–5 hours between 8 P.M. and 6 A.M. She may fall asleep at 8 P.M., only to awaken an hour later. She seems to fall asleep during or after short feeds and then remains awake for hours later on. Each night is a struggle of long awakened periods between short spells of sleep. Her parents note that she cries when left alone. She seems content at night when parents walk around with her.

Child development in early infancy is characterized by large fluctuations in temperament and schedules. In the first few weeks of life, infants often sleep as much during the day as at night. In the first 2 months of life, two night awakenings are common, but by 3 months of life most infants are sleeping for 5–6 hours uninterrupted. In this case, the child did not naturally "learn" the difference between night and day, and parents did not train her to do so. But if clinicians ask parents to let their young infants cry themselves to sleep, they set parents up for feelings of inadequacy or guilt. This, in turn, strains the relationship of attachment that parents are forming with their children.

CASE ILLUSTRATION 1 (CONTD.)

On further questioning in this case, the parents reported that their baby falls asleep immediately after daytime feeds and sleeps for 3–5 consecutive hours thereafter. This baby did not adapt to an acceptable or optimal day/night schedule. In this case, their doctor recommended waking the baby up after no more than 2–3 hours of daytime sleep. Parents were to try to occupy their infant's daytime hours by walking around, talking, playing music, and offering other playful activities. It was recommended that nighttime feeds be made minimally stimulating: soften the lights, produce minimal noise, and avoid "fun" interactions at night. Although

sleeping and feeding "on demand" need not always be discouraged, in this case the infant's pattern needlessly disrupted parents' well-being and this justified modification. After 5–6 days of compliance with this schedule, it became easier for parents to keep their daughter awake during the day and the parents settled for a nighttime feed at 11 P.M. before they retired and another feed at 4 A.M.

It is important to note that likely causes for night awakenings change with developmental stages. This same sleep history told by parents of a 9-month-old child would be more likely related to the child's cognitive ability to recognize that parents still "exist" after they leave the room. At that age, if there were no other likely cause, other recommendations would be in order. A nightlight or a transitional object (favorite blanket or teddy bear) could prove to be helpful. The clinician, in this case, should devise a careful behavioral intervention schedule that includes parental reassurance for the child but may also include an allowance for the child to "cry it out" for a couple of nights.

Toddlers: Aggression

CASE ILLUSTRATION 2

The parent of a 3-year-old boy reports that her son throws himself on the floor, throws objects, and screams (usually when he doesn't get his own way). This seems to happen daily. At his child care center, he has begun to bite other children when he is angry, and other parents have begun to complain about him.

Assessment of this behavior begins with elucidating, through history gathering, the extent of the child's aggression and its likely etiology. Angry outbursts are common at 3 years of age, when children often begin to direct their anger at others. Parental response to a given level of aggression differs widely from family to family. Parental expectations of children's behavior, not solely the magnitude of the child's behavior, help define whether a behavior is a problem. Large discrepancies between childhood behaviors and parental thresholds may predict that a child will continue to be problematic in the future. A child who explores the environment very actively may be described as "curious" in one family but as "always climbing the walls" in another. A "difficult and stubborn" child in one family is "persistent—just like his successful grandpa" in another. Perhaps the more positive perspective creates a better self-image for a child and leads to fewer problems later on.

Certain questions may help clinicians assess the etiology of aggressive behavior: Is the child a cruel or unhappy child? Is the child exposed to frequent violent (physical or verbal) outbursts from others at home? Are the incidents that induce these behaviors unpredictable? Is the child cognitively not acting consistently with his or her age? Positive responses to these questions make a normal developmental etiology less likely.

When development is still the most likely cause, there are a number of possibilities to consider. First, children with well-developed cognitive abilities, but with comparatively delayed language abilities, often become frustrated with limited ways of expressing themselves. Second, children at this stage often strive for adult attention and have found aggressive behaviors to be a certain way of getting it. Third, children at this stage need to express their independence, yet some adults have not found enough acceptable ways to allow the child to do this. To ascertain the likely cause(s), clinicians should explore events surrounding these incidents of aggression. Detailed examples of what instigated the last one or two aggressive behaviors are more revealing than letting the parent say, "Oh it happens for just about anything." Always ask parents how they feel when their child acts out. Feeling like "I just don't have time for this" may be a good indication that the child is trying to get attention. If their first reaction is to feel that this is a power struggle, then the child's strivings for independence may be his or her primary incentive. Also ask what parents have done in response to a misbehavior and whether this reaction worked.

CASE ILLUSTRATION 2 (CONTD.)

In this case, the child's degree of aggression was within reason for a child at his developmental stage. His tantrums began as a result of typical frustrations experienced by children his age. Over a period of months as his parent became busier with other family needs, however, he discovered that expressing anger was an excellent way to get adult attention, and the frequency of these behaviors increased. As part of the management plan, his parent was instructed to ignore his anger and put him in his room for a few minutes when he became physically violent with others. Concomitantly, she was to increase time spent doing happier things with him, like playing games, going on walks, and

having him help around the house. At day care, he was given increased individual attention during times he was behaving well. Child care providers were asked to ignore him when he attacked other children and to shower a "noticeable" amount of attention on the attacked child. Within a couple of weeks he stopped biting and seemed happier. Although he still had a terrible temper, these strategies gave his mother the feeling that she had some control over the situation.

Toddlers: Oppositional Behavior

CASE ILLUSTRATION 3

A 3-year-old boy refuses to go to bed on time. He prolongs bedtime rituals by making numerous requests (e.g., for water, use of bathroom, adjusting the door, and so on). He repeatedly leaves his bed. On many nights he finally falls asleep in the living room or his parents' bedroom while spending time with his parents.

CASE ILLUSTRATION 4

A mother solicits your opinion on vitamin supplements to counterbalance her 28-month-old daughter's picky eating habits. She drinks apple juice and eats hot dogs and Honey-Nut Cheerios, and little else. When these foods are not offered, she protests violently and eats nothing.

The behaviors described in these cases are typical for this age group. Toddlers commonly oppose parents for many sorts of issues, including the eating and bedtime cases illustrated here (e.g., getting dressed, putting toys away, wearing seat belt, and so on). A tendency to challenge parents' instructions subsides naturally as children grow older. But they need to be dealt with properly for those months or years they are present. When parents mistake a child's behavior as a personal offense, they react to the behavior in a way that creates additional conflict and heightens oppositional behavior. Therefore, it is important for clinicians to emphasize the developmental component. Children in both illustrative cases have learned to exploit their parents' uncertainty with what exactly is in their child's best interest. In both cases, the clinician should rule out deeper problems by interviewing the parent and, to whatever extent possible, the child. Look for unusual fears, nightmares, and other symptoms that may indicate an unusual etiology to the oppositional behavior. None was found in these two cases.

CASE ILLUSTRATION 3 (CONTD.)

In the first case, the pediatrician recommended to the parents that they explain to the child that from now on after his bedtime ritual he must remain in his bedroom whether he is able to sleep or not. They were to routinely ask their child before leaving his bedroom if he needed anything else. Thereafter, if the child cried, screamed, or tried to carry on a conversation with his parents, they were to ignore him. When he left his bed, they were to physically put him back without talking to him and with expressionless faces. They were to do this even in the middle of the night. They were warned that their child's behavior would likely worsen for one or two nights before improving. In less than a week, this boy resigned himself to making only one unenthusiastic, "face-saving" attempt to stay up before he fell asleep.

Parental persistence must be designed to outlast the child's. It is almost always effective within 2 weeks, and often within 2 nights. If this child shared a room with a sibling, it would have been suggested that the sibling sleep in the parents' room until the index child's behavior became less disruptive.

CASE ILLUSTRATION 4 (CONTD.)

In the second case, the same principles were applied to other behaviors. The child was offered three wholesome meals and one snack at preset times of the day. After telling their daughter once, parents were not to engage in any discussion with

their child about the volume eaten. No other foods in the house were made available to her during this behavioral management period. Between meals this girl was allowed an unlimited quantity of water, but nothing else. After a difficult period of 1 1/2 days (thrown silverware, persistent crying, and so on), she began to nibble at new foods and to enjoy the positive attention for doing so. Although the patient still enjoyed only a limited range of foods, parents were able to expand her repertoire to include broccoli, milk, and pasta.

Parents often worry about harming their child by restricting access to food after a missed meal, so they need to be reassured that this is not harmful and will ultimately improve nutrition. It is all too common for a well-meaning grandparent who resides in the home to "save" the child by sneaking her a cookie between meals (Case Illustration 4) or lying down with the child after a designated bedtime (Case Illustration 3). Such kindly motivated behaviors unwittingly prolong the child's maladaptive behavior, extending the period of inadequate nutrition and sleep. It is imperative that clinicians invite all adult household members to their offices when prescribing a management plan to ensure that all involved endorse both the intent and methods. It is useful to write behavioral management "rules" down on a prescription pad to be taped to the refrigerator door. This helps prevent conflict among adult household members that may arise later. Clinicians should also routinely recommend follow-up visits to their offices once the management plan has been implemented to monitor progress.

Toddlers: Toilet Training

Children must be developmentally ready before toilet training is initiated by parents. First, physiologic sphincter control is necessary. This usually develops between ages 1 and 2 years, and parents often know when their child is beginning to sense a bowel movement because of a characteristic grimace or stance. The ability to follow sequential instructions, the motivation to imitate parents, and the patience to sit on a potty should also be present. It is reasonable to try toilet training at age 2 years if these milestones have been achieved. But disinterest or undue difficulty should alert parents to terminate their attempt and wait 2–3 months before trying again. Some children may not be ready until age 3. Others are ready at 18 months.

Although a number of effective toilet training methods exist, only one method is described here. Place the potty in the bathroom the child typically uses and explain what it is for by drawing parallels with the toilet parents use. The child should be encouraged with praise to sit on the potty for a couple of minutes a day, initially with diaper and pants on and after a few days, without them. The child should accompany the parent to empty soiled diapers into the potty. Parents should avoid commenting on the foul odor of the stool, as some children identify what they've produced as extensions of themselves. Gradually, the child should be asked to sit on the potty more frequently during the day, particularly if there is a time when bowel movements are likely to occur. Encourage the child to let the potty "catch" the stool. Parents should never scold a child for an inability to do this or for any "accidents." Night training, standing at urination, and using a larger toilet are secondary skills that should be introduced only after the child has mastered the basics or if the child expresses interest.

School Age: Primary Nocturnal Enuresis

One workable definition for enuresis is at least one bedwetting incident weekly for a boy older than age 6 or a girl older than age 5. It is considered secondary enuresis if a child had been dry previously for a period greater than 6 months. By this definition, 15% of children have this condition, making it one of the most commonly asked questions of pediatric health care providers. Absence of other urinary tract problems (infection, neurogenic bladder, and so on) can be ruled out with a basic medical examination and history. It is important to recognize that the only problems with primary nocturnal enuresis are the reactions of the child and the parent. Otherwise, it is a self-limiting condition that resolves spontaneously. If a child and his or her parents are not bothered by it, then no treatment is necessary. This is worthwhile to point out to families whenever the option for intervention is offered.

To treat this condition, it is necessary that children themselves, not only their parents, are motivated. Verify that a child is truly motivated and determine the source of motivation by interviewing the child separately. When a child is not genuinely motivated to try something new in order to be dry, clinical efforts should be directed toward other family members. Gauge parental actions and anxieties and if necessary influence them so that their actions and anxieties are not causes of unnecessary stress for their child. Children should never be punished for their enuretic disorder. Even if parents insist that their child help to change wet bed sheets, this task should be carried out with the same attitude as other household responsibilities the child has been expected to take on.

Commercially available alarm devices assist clinicians and parents in instituting "conditioning therapy." This method is of clinically proven use. With this device, an alarm awakens the child with the first few drops of urine. Eventually, this teaches the child to awaken with the sensation of a full bladder. The child is still responsible to get to the bathroom. The alarm is usually effective when used nightly for a couple of months. Setbacks occur after removing the alarm, but these are often corrected more permanently by one further trial period with the device.

Desmopressin (DDAVP), an analogue of antidiuretic hormone, is a pharmacologic therapy of choice. If children respond to this medication they usually do so within 2 weeks. Relapses after withdrawal are not uncommon, however, and this therapy is best offered when the alarm device has failed and for temporary relief (e.g., summer camp). Imipramine has also been shown to be useful in certain circumstances. Sphincter control exercises, fluid restrictions in the evening hours, and urine retention training may be tried, but these methods have shown only limited success.

School Age: Bullying

 CASE ILLUSTRATION 5

During a routine health supervision visit of a 12-year-old girl, your customary questioning of social development reveals that this seventh grade student has been having problems with peers at school. She dislikes school and many of her classmates. Problems began about 3 months ago when another girl knocked an apple out of her hand and onto the cafeteria floor. Your patient tried to swat at the perpetrator (but missed) and was reprimanded by the lunch monitor. Your patient broke into tears at that time and has since been the butt of sneaky jokes among a group of girls and false rumors that have been spread verbally at school and through the occasional e-mail that children write to one another from home in the evenings.

Victims of bullying are likely to internalize bad situations, and it is likely that this child did not reveal much of her distress to her parents at the onset of her problems. Indications that one's child is being bullied may include an increasingly apparent dread of going to school, depressive signs, symptoms of anxiety (e.g., headaches, stomach aches), or changes in academic success. Many children who internalize threats and fears of bullying may believe they are somehow to blame for the behavior of others. Some parents and school staff members view bullying among school age children to be a normal part of growing up. Parents with this attitude need to be educated. Lack of resolution for bullying experiences and situations can result in anxiety disorders, depression, and social withdrawal.

Although some victims of bullying respond with aggression, many more are passive. Sometimes, certain personality characteristics or maladaptive behaviors have made children prone to becoming a victim of bullying. Problems such as having poor social skills, difficulty making friends, or even just being quiet, withdrawn, or shy can be sufficient. Victims are often those who easily become upset or have difficulty standing up for or defending themselves in public. Many feel more comfortable socializing with adults than with age-appropriate peers.

Primary care providers need to assess the level of entrenchment and severity for characteristics that predispose a child to being a victim of bullying behavior. Are there signs that this occurs in more than one environment, including the home? Are improvements recalcitrant to basic interventions? Are there too few positive social interactions with one's own age group? For some, victimization is a sign that the child requires assessment and intervention of a mental health specialist.

 CASE ILLUSTRATION 5 (CONTD.)

The primary care physician made a verbal agreement with the young girl and her parents that they would work together on the problem until there was no bullying at all. The girl would heretofore share her experiences with her parents, despite embarrassment, and parents would take these seriously and keep her from facing these issues alone. Parents would speak with their child's school administration and suggest a plan. Further history taking, in this case, uncovered that this girl is an excellent artist. The parents were encouraged to consciously shower verbal praise for her artistic accomplishments as well as other successes. They were to encourage school staff to do the same. They were also to seek new opportunities for their daughter to exhibit these strengths to herself and to others.

The youngster's parents kept a record of bullying episodes and communicated these with the school principal. Eventually, enrollment in an after-school art class helped this girl develop a couple of new friendships, which lent her a sense of confidence in herself and made her less vulnerable to being bullied.

Primary care physicians must realize that the interventions tendered in this case illustration are often inadequate to turn a situation around and that schools need to play a larger role. An experience with a bullied patient presents an excellent opportunity for a primary care provider to advocate in a local school or district so that bullying is taken seriously and that promising bullying prevention programs are adopted. To be successful, a bullying prevention program requires more than one interested school counselor with a plan or policy. Interventions designed by Olweus have been relatively well-researched and demonstrate encouraging results. School interventions should occur at several levels: school wide interventions (i.e., staff training and development of school wide rules against bullying); classroom-level interventions (i.e., regular classroom meetings and class parent meetings); and individual-level interventions (interacting on a one-to-one level with bullies and victims). School administrators and all school staff must be committed, and each site needs a coordinator responsible for assuring the plan is carried out.

It is no less essential for primary care providers to identify patients who are bullies, as those who are bullied. It is also important to help parents take note of signs that their children may be bullies. Bullies and victims often share problems with friendships, but they manifest these problems in different ways. Parents and clinicians need to be alert to children who are often in trouble at school (but are great at talking themselves out of blame) and who seem to need to control their friends and peers. All too often schools' and parents' only intervention for these bullies has been to punish them. This is typically ineffective because that response alone cannot get to the core of these children's underlying problems. Strict rules, close supervision, and communication with the school are important interventions for parents to adopt. When underlying psychological problems have led to poor conduct, poor peer relationships and emotional upheaval, and when these are not addressed during their youth, it has been found that bullies have a significantly higher chance of engaging in criminal activity later in life. Professional mental health assessment and management are not inappropriate for persistent bullying behavior.

CONCLUSION

With the elicitation of a good history and an understanding of child development, primary care clinicians can develop reasonable hypotheses about childhood behavioral problems. Clinicians who manage childhood behavioral problems become very comfortable with a set of behavioral management protocols that can be applied to many common misbehaviors. Most problems of a serious nature that require psychiatric or psychological intervention become apparent early in the process. It is not only cost-effective to avoid unnecessary referrals; assisting families with behavioral issues that arise with their children in the primary care office improves the relationship that families develop with their primary care clinicians.

SUGGESTED READINGS

Hanna GL, Fischer DJ, Fluent TE. Separation anxiety disorder and school refusal in children and adolescents. *Pediatr Rev* 2006; 27(2):56–62.

Iliffe S, Lenihan P. Integrating primary care and public health: learning from the community-oriented primary care model. *Int J Health Serv* 2003;33(1):85–98.

Jellinek M, Patel BP, Froehle MC, eds. *Bright Futures in Practice: Mental Health—Volume I. Practice Guide.* Arlington, VA: National Center for Education in Maternal and Child Health, 2002.

Law KS, Wong CS, Song LJ. The construct and criterion validity of emotional intelligence and its potential utility for management studies. *J Appl Psychol* 2004;89(3):483–496.

Murphey DA, Lamonda KH, Carney JK, et al. Relationships of a brief measure of youth assets to health-promoting and risk behaviors. *J Adolesc Health* 2004;34(3):184–191.

Roehlkepartain JL, Leffert N. *A Leader's Guide to What Young Children Need to Succeed; Working Together to Build Assets from Birth to Age 11.* Minneapolis, MN: Free Spirit Publishing, Inc., 2000.

Simonian SJ. Screening and identification in pediatric primary care. *Behav Modif* 2006;30(1):114–131.

Taras HL (Ed.-in-Chief), Duncan P, Luckenbill D, et al., eds. *Health, Mental Health and Safety Guidelines for Schools.* Elk Grove Village, IL: American Academy of Pediatrics, 2005. Available at: www.nationalguidelines.org.

PEER-REVIEWED WEB SITES

Cambridge Center for Behavioral Studies Web site. http://www.behavior.org/parentinging.

"Kids Health for Parents" Web site. http://kidshealth.org/parent/emotions/index.html.

"You and Your Family." American Academy of Pediatrics Web site. http://www.aap.org/parents.html.

OTHER WEB SITES

Search Institute Web site. http://www.search-institute.org.

Olweus School Interventions for Bullying Web site. http://www.clemson.edu/olweus.

Adolescents

Lawrence S. Friedman, MD

10

INTRODUCTION

This chapter offers a practical behavioral framework to assist those who provide health care to teenagers. Stages of adolescent development along with behavioral correlates are discussed, and suggestions for effective patient–doctor communication, interviewing, and provision of health services. From a physiologic perspective, adolescence is the interval between the onset of puberty and the cessation of body growth. In psychosocial and behavioral terms, it is the time during which adult body image and sexual identity emerge; independent moral standards, intimate interpersonal relationships, vocational goals, and health behaviors develop; and the separation from parents takes place. Although some of these tasks may begin prior to puberty and evolve into adulthood, they provide the foundation for understanding adolescent behavior.

Health Status & Trends

Most teenagers are healthy. Compared with other age groups, mortality rates for teenagers are low. The majority of health problems in teenagers are behavior related and include unwanted pregnancy; sexually transmitted diseases (STDs); weapon carrying; interpersonal violence; suicidal ideation; alcohol, cigarette, and illicit drug use; and dietary and exercise patterns. Nationally, accidents are the leading cause of death for most populations of teenagers, although homicide (often gang related) leads in some locations. Socioeconomic status and population density, rather than ethnic or racial grouping, define the neighborhoods most at risk for gunshot deaths. Nonetheless, the most common reasons for acute office visits for teenagers are routine or sports physicals, upper respiratory infections, and acne. One of the major challenges to a provider caring for teenagers is eliciting a history that reveals health risk behaviors. Because most adolescent mortality and morbidity are preventable and because many behaviors such as sexual practices, diet, exercise, and substance use that result in adult disease

begin in adolescence, ignoring this age group means missing a major public health opportunity.

In 1992, the American Medical Association published Guidelines for Adolescent Preventive Services (GAPS), the first set of developmentally and behaviorally appropriate comprehensive health care guidelines for adolescents, emphasizing anticipatory, preventive, and patient-centered services. GAPS suggest that promotion of adolescent health and prevention of disease involve a partnership encompassing patients, parents, schools, communities, and health care providers. Although these guidelines have existed for more than a decade, have been well disseminated, and have been shown to be valuable as care standards and as quality measures, there is little evidence that they are being widely implemented.

Adolescent health outcomes—perhaps more than for any other population—are closely linked to cultural, educational, political, and economic policies at the local and national level. Handguns and tobacco are both relevant examples. For example, the availability of handguns is not a problem that the physician can resolve during an office visit, yet making them less available would substantially benefit the health of many teenagers. Many more teenagers would never begin using tobacco if cigarette prices were significantly higher and advertising was eliminated. There is compelling evidence that teenagers who feel connected to parents, school, and community are less likely to participate in health-compromising behavior than teens who feel isolated or disconnected.

STAGES OF DEVELOPMENT

Medical services for teenagers need to be appropriate for each developmental stage. Each of the three recognized developmental stages in adolescence is distinguished by physical, cognitive, and behavioral hallmarks. Not all adolescents fit perfectly into each phase, and they often progress at different rates from one phase to the next. Moreover, rates of physical, cognitive, and behavioral development may not be congruent. For example, a 14-year-old girl who is physically mature may be emotionally and cognitively unable to decide about sexual intimacy and the consequences of pregnancy—or even its possibility.

Early Adolescence (Ages 11–14)

PHYSICAL

Rapid growth causes physical and body-image changes. Many teenagers question whether their growth is "normal," and commonly there is a good deal of somatic preoccupation and anxiety. Gynecomastia, for example (a common transient problem for boys), may cause concern, and prevent participation in physical education class. Because the topic may be too embarrassing for an already self-conscious teenager, clinician-initiated reassurance is essential when the condition is identified during a physical examination. Early or later onset of puberty has widely variable effects. Early puberty may be associated with the increased likelihood of weight concern and excessive dieting and other eating disorders in girls, but it may result in greater self-esteem and athletic prowess in boys. Because self-esteem is linked closely with physical development and peer-group attractiveness, teens who develop later than their peers may have self-esteem problems. Among early adolescents, questions and concerns about menstruation, masturbation, wet dreams, and the size of their breasts (too large or too small) and genitals are common. These questions need to be anticipated and specifically and carefully addressed. Endocrine disorders related to sexual maturation are likely to emerge; early diagnosis and treatment can improve health and self-esteem.

SOCIAL

In adolescence, peer-group involvement increases and family involvement decreases. Friendships are idealized and are mostly same gender. Close peer relationships coupled with curiosity about body development may result in homosexual and other sexual experimentation, anxiety, and fear. Although some heterosexual relationships are initiated, contact with the opposite sex frequently occurs in groups.

COGNITIVE

The transition from concrete to abstract thinking begins. Because experience and emotion play important roles in decision making, improved cognition alone is not enough to prevent many teenagers from making impulsive decisions with little regard for consequences. Increased cognitive ability linked with the search for identity often leads teenagers to test limits both at home and at school. Daydreaming is common.

Middle Adolescence (Ages 15–17)

PHYSICAL

The issues of early adolescence may continue, although most physical development is complete by the end of this phase.

SOCIAL

Independence, identity, and autonomy struggles intensify. Peer groups may become more important than family to some teenagers and result in increasing teen—parent conflict. Experimentation with alcohol, drugs, and sex is common. A sense of invincibility coupled with impulsiveness leads to relatively high rates of automobile accidents and interpersonal violence. Suicide, impulsively linked to failed love relationships, or poor self-esteem because of difficulty finding peer-group acceptance may also occur during this phase. Despite adhering to peer-group norms regarding music, dress, and appearance (including body piercing, clothes, hair color, and makeup), the expression of individuality is common. Many teenagers find identity and support in school, sports, community, or church activities. For teenagers whose support systems or community resources are inadequate, gangs may supplement personal strength and provide a sense of identity. Teenagers from alienated and disenfranchised ethnic groups are at particular risk for gang activity. In spite of slowly improving cultural acceptance, gay, lesbian, and transgendered teenagers may feel increased isolation, alienation, and bullying. This may lead to depression, sexual promiscuity, or suicide.

COGNITIVE

Improved reasoning and abstraction allow for closer interpersonal relationships and empathy in this group. Evaluation of future academic and vocational plans becomes important. Poor school performance may heighten anxiety and concern about vocational choices and lead to "escape" in drugs and alcohol. Practical guidance that identifies strengths and builds self-esteem can help avoid frustration and failure.

Late Adolescence (Ages 18–24)

PHYSICAL

Body growth is usually no longer a concern. The quest to become comfortable with one's physical appearance often continues throughout adulthood.

SOCIAL

If the adolescent's development has occurred within the context of a supportive family, community, school, and peer environment, individual identity formation and separation will be complete. In reality, however, at least some developmental issues usually remain unresolved into adulthood. Late adolescents typically spend more time developing monogamous interpersonal relationships and less time seeking peer-group support. Ideally, decision making, based on an individualized value system, is modulated by limit setting and compromise.

COGNITIVE

Vocational goals should now be set in practical terms, and there should be realistic expectations about education and work.

ADOLESCENTS & THE MEDICAL INTERVIEW

A general health assessment should include a review of systems and an evaluation of health-related behavior. This should include risk factors for accidents, STDs, including human immunodeficiency virus (HIV), pregnancy, interpersonal violence (including past physical or sexual abuse), nutrition, substance use, exercise, learning, and mental health problems. Guidance about promoting healthful behaviors and preventing disease should be integrated into the discussion. From the patient's perspective, the clinician's inquiries and assessment of some behaviors may be viewed as embarrassing, intrusive, or trivial. It is therefore helpful to explain, prior to questioning, that (1) the same questions are asked of all patients and that (2) the encounter goal is patient self-awareness and health education. During the interview it is important to reinforce and praise healthy decisions, such as sexual abstinence.

Confidentiality

Certain ground rules are important. Ensure the adolescent that, unless homicide or suicide is threatened or ongoing abuse is reported, all conversations are confidential, and the information will not be shared with parents, teachers, or other authorities without permission. Discussions about sex and drugs should always occur in private unless otherwise requested by the patient. If the patient is accompanied by a parent, solicit parental concerns, and then ask the adult to leave the room and conduct the interview in private. It is also helpful to let the parent know (if present) about the confidential nature of the patient–clinician conversation.

Although most teenagers want to receive health information and discuss personal behavior, these discussions must generally be initiated by the physician. Many teenagers are not accustomed to interacting in such participatory, nonjudgmental conversations with adults. The willingness of a teenager to share personal or intimate information depends on the perceived receptiveness of the provider. Teenagers need to feel that

they have permission to share personal, behavior-related information. For example, it is usually not difficult for patients and clinicians to discuss routine chronic medical conditions such as diabetes or asthma. Control of these conditions in some teenagers, however, may be related to dietary indiscretions and cigarette use, than to insulin or inhaler use. Such health-compromising behaviors must be identified before they can be dealt with; comments, facial expressions, or body language indicating disapproval can undermine the patient's willingness to disclose confidential behavior (Table 10-1).

Legal Issues

Many practitioners worry about the legality of evaluating and treating teenagers without parental consent. Because laws vary by state, it is essential to become familiar with the applicable local statutes. Many states permit the diagnosis and treatment of teenagers with sex-, drug-, and alcohol-related problems without parental notification or consent. States do vary at the age about which teens can receive such services without parental permission. Likewise, most states permit medical care if a condition is potentially life threatening. Documentation of the rationale leading to the decision to proceed without parental permission, in a potential "life-threatening" situation, is essential.

Interview Organization

A comprehensive health-risk assessment should cover issues dealing with home, education, activities, drug use, sexual practices, and suicidal ideation (HEADSS).

Table 10-1. Interview suggestions.

1. Ensure doctor–patient confidentiality. Don't inquire about health-related behaviors in front of parents.
2. Use the HEADSS format to organize the interview.
3. Assess the patient's cognitive and developmental level through interactive dialogue.
4. Initiate discussions about behavior and offer anticipatory guidance that is culturally and developmentally appropriate.
5. Listen actively to patients' opinions and perspective.
6. Be familiar with and refer to local resources for cases of domestic violence, runaways, and substance abuse.
7. Include patients in discussing and making all diagnostic and therapeutic decisions.
8. Review the behavioral stages of development with parents. Emphasize the importance of instilling confidence and building self-esteem in their children.
9. Reinforce good behavior. Congratulate teenagers who do not use drugs and who are not sexually active.
10. Address all teenagers with respect, and be nonjudgmental about their behaviors and traits.

Using the HEADSS format helps with organization and standardization. Assessing cognitive ability using interactive dialogue needs to be done in the first few minutes of the interview. The following interview goals and questions facilitate communication.

HOME

1. **Goal**—Determine household structure, family structure and function, conflict-resolution skills, the possibility of domestic violence, and presence of chronic illness in the family (see Chapter 8).

2. **Questions**—"Who lives where you live?" If only one parent is at home, the interviewer should inquire about the other parent's whereabouts, visitation pattern, reasons for leaving (especially domestic violence and substance abuse), and whether the teen moves back and forth between parents. Teenagers caught between divorced parents or those who feel neglected may "act out" and get into trouble to gain parental attention, sometimes in the hope that their problems will reunite separated parents. For single-parent families, the patient can be asked, "Does your mom or dad date? How do you get along with the people he or she dates?" Questions about domestic violence should include "What happens when people argue in your house?" and "Does anyone get hurt during arguments? How about you?" and "What if someone has been drinking or using drugs and they argue?" and "Have you ever seen your mother hit by anyone?" "Are there guns in your house" if there are, ask if they are always locked and who has a key. Educate parents and patients about accidental gunshots. Ask about siblings, including their health and whereabouts. Somatization may be learned by observing a family member who receives attention for a chronic medical condition.

EDUCATION

1. **Goal**—Identify attention deficit hyperactivity disorder (ADHD) and other learning disabilities, school performance, cognitive ability, and vocational potential.

2. **Questions**—"What grade are you in?" "What type of grades do you get?" "How do they compare with your grades last year?" Falling grades may indicate family, mental health, or substance-abuse problems. "Have you ever been told you had a learning problem?" "Can you see the blackboard?" Most teenagers respond that everything in school is okay. Specific questions about courses and content need to be asked, including the student's favorite and worst subjects and his or her career aspirations. Generally, teenagers who perform well in school are less likely to participate in multiple health risk behaviors. The teen should be asked about attendance, and truancy or other school troubles. Teenagers with chemical dependency may enjoy going to school because, although they may rarely attend class, school is where they visit friends and purchase or sell drugs. Students who get all "A's" should be asked about school-related stress and what would happen if they didn't receive high grades. Depression and even suicide can be related to unrealistic grade expectations by teenagers and their parents.

ACTIVITIES

1. **Goal**—Evaluate the patient's social interactions, interests, and self-esteem.

2. **Questions**—"What do you do for fun?" "Are you involved in school, community, or religious activities, such as youth groups, clubs, or sports?" Self-esteem is often related to successful participation in these activities. Teenagers actively involved in "productive" activities are less likely to participate in delinquent behavior. The clinician should ask about gang or fraternity/sorority membership, either of which can be a source of inappropriate peer pressure. Gangs may provide the strongest sense of family or community available to some teenagers.

Questions should be asked about dietary habits, including the frequency and amount of "junk" food, who cooks, and dieting or self-induced vomiting (see Chapter 20). It is also important to inquire about patients' physical activities, and to educate and to make recommendations about regular exercise, protective headgear, and seatbelts.

DRUGS

1. **Goal**—Evaluate the patient's current habits, patterns of use, and the genetic or environmental risk factors (Table 10-2). Distinguish between those who drink because of social, cultural, and peer pressure, those who are genetically predisposed, and those who drink or use illicit drugs because of comorbid mental health problems.

2. **Questions**—It is less threatening to begin by asking, "Are you aware of alcohol or drug use at your school?"

Table 10-2. Substance-abuse risk factors for adolescents.

1. Family history of use
2. Low self-esteem and body image
3. Depression or thought disorder
4. Antisocial personality traits
5. Peer and cultural pressures

and "Do any of your friends drink or use drugs?" followed by "Have you ever tried alcohol or drugs?" The physician should inquire specifically about cigarettes, alcohol, marijuana, recreational "pills" (e.g., ecstasy, ketamine), cocaine, lysergic acid diethylamide (LSD), crystal methamphetamine, anabolic steroids, and heroin. The quantity, frequency, circumstances, and family patterns of use are important. To learn about family drinking, ask specific questions about each parent and both maternal and paternal grandparents, including whether anyone in the family attends Alcoholics Anonymous (AA) or other self-help groups. When parents do not recognize or admit to a problem, a child may not identify them as alcoholics. The teenager should be asked to describe the parent's pattern of alcohol use. "Have you ever seen your mother or father drunk?" If the answer is yes, "When and how frequently?" The CRAFFT questions (Table 10-3) have been validated as a useful brief screening test for teenagers suspected of substance abuse. Two or more YES answers on the CRAFFT indicate a significant problem.

Recognition of a parental problem is also essential. Even the best treatment program will fail if a teenager is discharged back into the home of an actively using parent. The willingness of parents to change either their own drinking or family behavior patterns is one of the best predictors of adolescent treatment success.

Among many teenagers, the use of drugs and alcohol is often not considered abnormal or dangerous. Only about 5–10% of teenage drinkers or drug users develop substance-abuse problems as adults. Because serious physical consequences, other than accidents, usually do not occur until later in life, there is little negative association with alcohol or drug use. Abused, neglected, disabled, or chronically ill teenagers may consider drugs or alcohol one of the few things that, at least temporarily,

make them feel good and accepted by peers. If legal involvement, school problems, or family conflict are present, it is important to assess the role of alcohol and drugs. Even if use seems minimal, it should be pointed out that problems are best solved sober.

Referral to a substance-abuse expert is indicated when use significantly interferes with school, family, or social functioning. Anticipatory guidance should address age-appropriate concerns. Advising teenagers to stop smoking cigarettes because of the possibility of future lung cancer and heart disease is usually meaningless. Talking about wrinkled skin, bad breath, and yellow teeth is much more relevant to body-image concerns and far more likely to prevent or stop cigarette use. Similarly, the association between alcohol and date rape is more important to teenage girls than are other future consequences.

SEX

1. **Goal**—Determine the level of the patient's sexual involvement and sexuality, use of birth control, protection against STDs, and any history of abuse.

2. **Questions**—An opening question such as "Have you ever been sexually involved with anyone?" is preferable to "Are you sexually active?" The word *active* is notoriously misinterpreted. Questions need to be open-ended and should not assume heterosexual orientation. Assumptions about boyfriends or girlfriends inhibit discussion or questions about homosexual partners or feelings. Because teenagers frequently practice serial monogamy, the sequential number of different partners and their ages should be determined. A 15-year-old teenager with a peer-group partner is at less risk for STDs, especially HIV, than is one with a substantially older partner. For the sexually involved, discuss birth control techniques and condoms. One of the most common reasons for not using a condom is the belief that birth control pills provide adequate protection against STDs. When appropriate, physicians should reinforce sexual abstinence with congratulations and support.

Sexual abuse is unfortunately common. A history of such should be sought by asking, "Have you ever been touched sexually when you did not want to be?" Obtaining this history may be pivotal in helping a teenager who has developed abuse-related behavioral problems, such as sexual promiscuity, depression, substance abuse, delinquency, and an eating or somatization disorder.

Although in decline over the past decade, teenage pregnancy is still at epidemic proportions. Risk factors are complex but include ignorance, lack of access to family-planning services, cultural acceptance, and poor self-esteem.

Table 10-3. CRAFFT* questions.

1. Have you ever ridden in a CAR driven by someone (including yourself) who was "high" or had been using alcohol or drugs?
2. Do you ever use alcohol/drugs to RELAX, feel better about yourself, or fit in?
3. Do you ever use alcohol/drugs while you are by yourself, ALONE?
4. Do your family or FRIENDS ever tell you that you should cut down on drinking or drug use?
5. Do you ever FORGET things you did while using alcohol or drugs?
6. Have you gotten into TROUBLE while you were using alcohol or drugs?

*Two or more YES answers indicate a significant problem.

SUICIDE

1. **Goal**—Identify serious mental health problems and distinguish them from normal adolescent affect and moodiness. Primary risk factors are listed in Table 10-4.

   Distinguishing significant psychiatric illness from normal fluctuations in a teenager's affect is challenging. In spite of the general perception to the contrary, most teenagers are not maladjusted, and the rates of mental health problems are no higher than in adults. Few teenagers announce that they are feeling depressed or are in emotional turmoil. Depression may be reflected in sexual promiscuity, drug and alcohol abuse, or in the commission of violent and delinquent acts. Chronic somatic complaints such as headache, abdominal pain, or chest pain without an identifiable biological explanation may also indicate depression secondary to abuse.

2. **Questions**—Physicians should identify vegetative signs of depression, such as sleep disturbance, decreased appetite, hopelessness, lethargy, continuous thoughts about suicide, hallucinations, or illogical thoughts. It should also be noted that many of these symptoms may also be caused by substance abuse. Evaluation of lethargy should be done from the patient's perspective. Energy may be low relative to the parents' desires or expectations—but sufficient for the teenager. There may be insufficient energy to clean, help with household chores, or complete homework but plenty of energy available to play sports, go on a date, party with friends, travel miles and wait for hours to obtain concert tickets.

Table 10-4. Risk factors for major depression and suicide.

1. Prior episode of serious depression or suicide
2. Family history of suicide or mental health problems
3. History of victimization
4. Substance abuse or dependency
5. Gay or lesbian sexual identity
6. Availability of handguns (increases rate of success)
7. Recent loss of significant friends or family
8. Extreme family, school, or social stress

This case illustrates several important adolescent issues. First, teenagers may concretely interpret questions. When Lauren was asked by the nurse if she was taking any medication, she answered honestly. A combination of clinical judgment at the time of interview related to Lauren's inattentiveness, knowledge that teenagers may interpret concretely, and that they may not make the connection between behavior and health consequences are all important to this case. Second, teenagers seek peer conformance. Medication compliance problems may relate to avoiding peer awareness of medications and therefore being labeled as different. Taking medication at school, camp, or at the house of a friend may all make a teenager feel different. Lastly, instructions about medications should be given in terms of what is important to the patient. Lauren may have known that medication was beneficial for school performance but may not have realized that it would improve concentration with other tasks that required focus and attention.

Case Illustration 1

Lauren is a 15 year old admitted to the hospital with an arm fracture requiring surgical repair. The fracture occurred during cheerleading practice while climbing a pyramid of other cheerleaders. She reported being distracted while climbing, lost concentration, and fell to the ground. During the admission history the patient was talkative and easily distracted. Although she did not report taking any medications to the admitting nurse, when asked "are you supposed to be taking" any medications, Lauren reported that she should be taking medication for ADHD (see Chapter 24). She had not taken medication for the last several days because she was staying with a friend and did not want her friend to know that she took medication.

Case Illustration 2

Two days after sustaining minor injuries in a traffic accident, Jeff, a 16-year-old teenager, comes to the physician's office complaining of left shoulder pain. He is accompanied by his mother, who is concerned because Jeff was also recently arrested for driving under the influence of alcohol. There is no history of medical or behavioral problems, although, on questioning, his mother describes a 12-month history of moodiness and falling school grades. Using the HEADsS format assessment, the physician assesses Jeff's health risks:

Home: Jeff lives at home with his biological mother and father. The parents are first-generation immigrants who both work full time. There are few arguments at home, and Jeff describes both parents as stoic, religious, and unemotional.

Education: Although he was an above-average student until last year, Jeff's education is now being adversely affected by his truancy and lack of interest.

Activity: Although Jeff previously played several sports at school, watching television is now his favorite activity.

Drugs: Jeff admits to using drugs frequently. He drinks alcohol at least twice a week and smokes marijuana daily. Since this use is no more frequent than that of his friends, he does not consider it excessive.

Sex: Jeff has no steady sexual partners, but has had several short-term relationships.

Suicide: Jeff denies being suicidal or depressed. When asked about significant losses, however, he becomes tearful and talks hesitantly about his older brother, a construction worker, who died accidentally 2 years ago. Since the burial, his brother was never talked about at home.

The connection between increased substance use, declining grades, and the brother's death seems obvious. Because the substance use began insidiously, and significant trouble did not occur until more than a year after his brother's death, neither Jeff nor his parents associated the events. Furthermore, this is a family that seemingly does not share emotions, and Jeff never learned how to discuss his feelings. In this case, simply learning about his drug use, home situation, school performance, and activities was not enough. The facts all confirmed his substance abuse but did not explain it. With a teenager who previously has been without significant behavioral problems, it is crucial to search for personal or family events, including losses, that underlie and precipitate behavior change.

Both Jeff and his parents must be made aware of the connection between the substance use and the brother's death. It is imperative that Jeff acknowledge his drug problem and be referred to a practitioner experienced in treating adolescents with substance-abuse problems (see Chapter 21). Although Jeff should respond to psychotherapy that addresses his grief and loss, psychotherapy may not be effective if mind-altering substances are being used concomitantly.

SPECIFIC AT-RISK POPULATIONS

Homeless & Runaway Teenagers

There is a heterogeneous group of between 500,000 and 2 million homeless teenagers in the United States. Some are homeless because their families are, some live on the streets for brief periods of time, and others find shelter with friends or relatives. Those who leave home, do not return, and no longer depend on parents for financial support or shelter constitute a significant proportion and may be more precisely called *throwaways*. Before they leave home, these teenagers have usually had repeated contacts with social service agencies and have histories of severe parental conflict and high rates of physical and sexual abuse. Family abandonment because of sexual orientation is not uncommon. The social network designed to protect them has failed, and their experience of neglect, abuse, and abandonment results in a distrust of adults and institutions.

Leaving home and living on the streets may initially be a liberating experience. Once on the street, multiple substance use is common, often becoming a short-term pleasant escape from an otherwise dismal existence. Survival often depends on trading sex for drugs, food, or shelter. Other survival techniques, such as selling drugs and theft, create risks for interpersonal violence and victimization. Poor self-esteem, depression, and suicidal ideation are common in this group. Usually—within weeks or months—the liberating experience of independence becomes one of desperation and hopelessness.

The initial medical evaluation may seem overwhelming. Many of these patients qualify for emancipated-minor legal status and may be eligible for Medicaid or other entitlements. Distrust of adults, the inability to navigate a complicated health system, and reluctance to disclose personal information may, however, keep them from receiving benefits and proper health care. It is important for the clinician to prioritize such a patient's health issues and be familiar with community referral sources. Shelter, food, safety, social support, substance abuse and mental health counseling, and medical evaluation are all usually necessary. Developing a trusting working relationship is essential and may require several visits. Keeping medical appointments and complying with referrals may be complicated by a reversed sleep–wake cycle. As with other teenagers, questions about sex and drugs are best kept in a medical context; it should be made clear that they are asked only because of their health implications. Rather than asking whether a teenager has been a "prostitute," asking, "Have you ever had sex in order to obtain drugs, food, or a place to sleep?" is nonjudgmental and will be readily understood. Questions about sexual orientation may be confusing to a teenager with a history of sexual abuse and survival sex and may provoke anxiety and shame. These issues are best raised after a stable living situation and support system have been established.

Chronic Disease & Disability

At least 2 million teenagers in the United States have chronic disabilities or diseases. Although this is a diverse group, its members share some similar behavioral issues.

Unlike other teenagers whose identity and self-esteem are molded by the acceptance of a peer group, chronically ill or disabled teenagers have limited ability to conform and often have poor self-esteem. Too frequently this leads to depression, family conflict, and social isolation.

Like those of other teenagers—usually revolve around physical, social, and sexual development. Frank discussions, including realistic assessments of their hopes and expectations, need to be initiated by the physician. It is crucial to identify and encourage the interests and skills that may realistically be expected to strengthen self-esteem. Predictors of successful coping include friendships with healthy as well as ill or disabled peers, parents who are not overly protective, involvement with family activities, and appropriate household responsibilities.

Chronically ill teenagers are often "noncompliant" with medical regimens. Adolescence is no less a time of experimentation, self-discovery, and testing of limits for the chronically ill teen than for other teens, and chronically ill teenagers—like others are often noncompliant. Issues about compliance are often issues about control and of testing of limits. The struggle for independence conflicts with the limitations of the disability itself as well the relationship with parents and health care providers. Table 10-5 lists some suggestions for ways of improving compliance.

Gay & Lesbian Youth

Gay and lesbian teenagers are at risk for social isolation, depression, STDs, substance abuse, and interpersonal violence. The relationships they develop with a health

Table 10-5. Strategies for improving compliance.

1. Have patients participate in all therapeutic and diagnostic decisions.
2. Discuss developmentally appropriate consequences of noncompliance. For instance, the renal or neurologic complications of poor diabetes control will not seem very important to a 14-year-old teenager. Emphasize the positive instead—such as how proper glucose control will allow continued participation in sports and other peer activities.
3. Parents need guidance on how to balance protectiveness with their teenager's need to make independent decisions. Role-playing in specific scenarios may be helpful.
4. When possible, communicate directly with the patient without using the parent as a conduit. Let patients know that their opinions and questions are important.
5. Refer patients and parents to local peer support groups such as diabetes, asthma, and epilepsy societies. Support groups exist for almost all chronic illnesses and can usually be found through local telephone directories or agencies such as United Way.

Table 10-6. Recommendations for addressing needs of gay or lesbian youth.

1. Assess the patient's level of comfort and self-acceptance.
2. Evaluate and discuss external stressors, such as parents, school, and the patient's social and religious environment. Refer the patient (and parents, if necessary) to mental health experts if the stressors are severe and interfere with daily activities.
3. Reassure the patient that from a medical perspective, homosexuality is a normal variant like left-handedness.
4. Refer patients to local gay youth groups for peer support; most cities and colleges provide resources for lesbian and gay youth, and telephone directories usually list local resources. Refer parents to local parent support groups, especially the local chapter of Parents and Friends of Lesbian and Gay Youth (P-FLAG).

care provider may help them cope with the negative stereotyping they receive from other parts of society. A nonjudgmental and supportive attitude by the clinician helps lessen the weight of such cultural negativity.

Although some teenagers may volunteer information about their homosexual concerns or ideation, many do not unless they are specifically asked or given permission to do so. Some teens may have feelings of anxiety, shame, and guilt about same-sex experiences. Such experiences are common, especially among young adolescents who may not yet have firm sexual identity. Such experiences do not necessarily reflect future sexual orientation. The risk of HIV infection increases when gay teenage boys have older partners, who themselves may have had multiple partners. Table 10-6 lists some suggestions for working with gay and lesbian youth.

SUGGESTED READINGS

Centers for Disease Control and Prevention: Youth Risk Behavior Surveillance—United States, 2005. *Morb Mortal Wkly Rep* 2006; 55(SS-5):1–108.

Elster AB, Kuznets NJ, eds. *AMA Guidelines for Adolescent Preventive Services (GAPS)*. Philadelphia, PA: Williams & Wilkins, 1994.

Knight JR, Sherrit L, Shrier LA, et al. Validity of the CRAFFT substance abuse screening test among general adolescent clinic patients. *Arch Pediatr Adolesc Med* 2002;156:607–614.

Kulig J and the Committee on Substance Abuse. Tobacco, alcohol and other drugs: the role of the pediatrician in prevention, indentification and management. *Pediatrics* 2005;115:816–821.

WEB SITES

Position Papers on Adolescent Health. American Academy of Pediatrics Web site. www.pediatrics.org. Accessed September, 2007.

Official Position Papers on Multiple Relevant Topics. Society for Adolescent Medicine Web site. www.adolescenthealth.org. Accessed September, 2007.

Older Patients

11

Clifford M. Singer, MD, Jay Luxenberg, MD, & Elizabeth Eckstrom, MD

INTRODUCTION

We are an aging society. By the year 2020, one in five Americans will be over the age of 65, compared to a little over one in eight today. The oldest of the old, those over 85, comprise an increasing proportion of the elderly, and present special challenges to health care providers. The clinical care of older adults relies on knowledge of normal aging and the common diseases of old age. This chapter focuses on these aspects of mental health and illness.

NORMAL PSYCHOLOGICAL AGING

Although chronic and degenerative diseases impact quality of life, most older adults are active, engaged, and pleasure seeking. They remain curious and continue to learn throughout their lives. Temperament (i.e., energy, intensity, reactivity) remains stable through adult life, whereas personality (learned behavior patterns) undergoes refinement and change over time in most healthy adults. Predictable changes in intellect occur in most people as they age. Although judgment, knowledge, and verbal skills increase through the lifespan, mental functions relying on memory and processing speed are adversely affected by aging.

Successful adaptation to old age is difficult to define and variably expressed. Signs of successful aging include acceptance of change, affectionate relationships with family and friends, and a positive view of one's life story. Another indicator might be the ability to find new sources of self-esteem independent of raising children, career, physical strength, or beauty. Factors that promote successful adaptation are luck (good genes, avoiding injury) and health behaviors that include proper diet, adequate sleep, plenty of physical activity, and stress management. Having enough money for basic needs, and strong kinship and extended family bonds add extra protection from disease and despair, as do spirituality, having friends and confidants, and feeling valued by society. Opportunities to be productive and assist younger generations can provide a sense of connection to one's community and a feeling of completeness.

Patients and families will often ask for advice on staying engaged and active. Many communities have senior centers, agencies, or programs that organize discussion groups, lectures, hobby groups, book groups, adult education classes, and volunteer activities. Similar programs or groups can be created, even in the smallest communities, by forming book or knitting groups, foster grandparent services, or peer support programs. The local Area Agency on Aging may have information for specific resources and volunteer opportunities in your community.

Social conditions that contribute to demoralization in old age include highly mobile and rapidly changing communities, youth-oriented aesthetics, the deaths of friends and family members, and forced retirement. Physical conditions that limit function, such as urinary incontinence, chronic pain, gait and mobility problems, and hearing and vision loss also contribute to demoralization. Declining hygiene, poor nutrition, falls, alcohol abuse, social withdrawal, chaotic finances, and denial of severe health problems are clues that an older person is failing at home because of diminishing physical, emotional, or intellectual function. Recognizing these problems can be difficult. Health care practitioners may not detect problems if older patients are reclusive, try to look their best in the office, or avoid discussion of problems they face functioning at home. Often it is family members, friends, neighbors, and others who first recognize a person's functional decline. Their impressions can be very helpful to the clinician, but sometimes family need to be specifically asked to investigate the well-being of the patient. In extreme cases, Adult Protective Services or a local Council on Aging may be asked to investigate patients' safety in their own environment. The challenge is to obtain the needed information while abiding by HIPAA (Health Insurance Portability and Accountability Act) regulations, and obtaining the information while retaining the confidence of the patient. If time permits, a home visit by the physician, nurse, or other clinician may be especially revealing.

Older adults experience obstacles to obtaining medical care. Financial barriers to mental health care are compounded by the lesser coverage for mental compared to physical illness under the Medicare insurance program. Elderly patients may also deliberately avoid seeking help, particularly for emotional and cognitive problems. Some seniors do not view emotional distress as something to discuss with physicians. They suffer silently or disguise their distress with physical symptoms or irritability and withdrawal from family, friends, or caregivers. Unfortunately, the prejudicial attitudes of physicians and mental health providers about mental and emotional problems in old age play into this silence and contribute to the under recognition and treatment of these disorders. Clinicians may be reluctant to prescribe treatment for problems viewed as inevitable parts of aging or they may simply consider treatment to be futile.

Providing medical care to elderly patients requires an understanding of normal changes in mental and emotional functioning in old age, and skill in determining when intervention is needed. Addressing the concerns of family and caregivers, accessing community services, and advising patients about end-of-life and long-term care options all require sensitivity and skill. Diagnosing mental disorders in older people is challenging as multiple clinical syndromes—including both mental and medical—often overlap. While it is challenging to care for the vulnerable elderly, we provide some case discussions that illustrate how clinicians can effectively treat this population.

Case Examples

CASE ILLUSTRATION 1

Martha is an 87-year-old woman who never married and who lives alone in her own home, as she has for 48 years. Her doctor is a family physician who has been asked to see Martha by her niece Joanne, a current patient. Martha's sister (Joanne's mother) died not long ago and was the only person with whom Martha had significant contact in recent years.

Joanne tells the doctor that she recently went to see her aunt and was appalled by her living conditions. Martha had more than 20 cats, many of whom appeared sick. The house reeked of cat urine and the entire first floor was full of trash and newspapers. Cat food, soda pop, cookies, canned spaghetti, and candy bars were the only food in the house. Although the house had gas, electricity, and running water, there was no phone service. Unpaid bills, bank statements, a social security check, and some cash were stuffed into a coffee can in the kitchen sink.

The following week, Joanne brings her aunt to the doctor's office. Martha is a thin, disheveled, and

foul-smelling woman with poor dentition. She shakes the doctor's hand and comments pleasantly on how nicely she has been treated by the office staff. She has not seen a physician in 30 years and has no physical complaints. She cooperates with the physical examination that reveals she is 5 ft 4 in. tall and weighs 82 lb. Her blood pressure is 180/98. The remainder of the neurologic and physical examination is unremarkable. Her blood work is normal except for a hematocrit of 30 and an albumin of 3.0.

The doctor asks Martha how she is managing at home. This seems to irritate her, and as he is about to proceed with a mental status examination, she politely but firmly states that the interview is complete, that she feels fine, and she has no need for his services. She dresses herself and says she will be sitting outside in the waiting room. When she is out of earshot, Joanne says, "See what I mean? Even when she was young she was off and now she's totally unreasonable. Can you help me get her into a nursing home?"

The doctor must now consider what other information is needed to determine whether Martha has a mental disorder and how different diagnoses would affect his approach to the situation. Some important issues need to be addressed: Can Martha safely remain in her home? What else does the doctor need to know about her cognitive function? What is Joanne's role?

CASE ILLUSTRATION 2

Mr. and Mrs. J. have been patients in this internal medicine practice for several years. Mr. J., a retired engineer, is 89 years old. Mrs. J., also 89, is a retired teacher who until recently had volunteered as a church secretary. In their retirement they have been very active, particularly in church-related activities. The couple has two daughters living in the area, but one is in ill health, and the other, a single mother, has a demanding job and children to care for. Neither of the daughters is in a position to care for their father, who has been diagnosed with Alzheimer disease.

Now, 3 years later, he has almost caused a fire by leaving a glue gun burning in the garage and has had to give up woodworking, his favorite activity. Mrs. J. is also concerned because her husband has wandered away from the house several times, and on one occasion had to be brought home by the police. His personality changes have been particularly difficult. At church several months ago, Mr. J. began swearing loudly during the service and his wife had to take him home. Mrs. J. has been too embarrassed to return. Nights are also difficult in that Mr. J. gets up and wanders. Sometimes at night he doesn't recognize his wife and demands she leave his house.

Today Mrs. J. brings her husband in for an evaluation. During the appointment she begins to cry, saying she cannot go on much longer. She believes God is punishing her for being a bad wife and she feels guilty because she has been losing her temper with her husband. The physician discovers that Mrs. J. has lost 15 lbs and is suffering severe sleep deprivation.

What interventions might help Mr. J. become more manageable? What services could help Mrs. J. gain respite from the burden of caring for her husband? Does Mrs. J. need treatment herself?

CASE ILLUSTRATION 3

Mr. L. is a 79-year-old man whose wife of 45 years died unexpectedly 2 months ago. The marriage was not an easy one: Mr. L. drank heavily, had numerous affairs, and was verbally abusive to his wife. Since his retirement at age 65, however, their relationship improved and Mr. L. treated his wife with more respect and affection.

Mr. L.'s daughter, Eleanor, calls her parents' long-time physician to say she thinks her father is becoming "senile." He seems to be at a complete loss since his wife died. He has not paid any bills, and the only food in his refrigerator is what neighbors and Eleanor bring. He hasn't changed his clothes or bathed for at least a week. One of the neighbors called Eleanor last week to say her father was wandering around the yard at night. Even more alarming to Eleanor, she has found him talking to his deceased wife as if she was there.

Eleanor makes an appointment for her father. When they come in for the office visit the doctor is taken aback by Mr. L.'s haggard appearance. Although he seems distracted on mental status examination, Mr. L. proves to be oriented to year and month but not the date or day of the week. His thinking and speech are very slow. Everything he is asked reminds him of his wife and makes him tearful. Mr. L. complains of insomnia and asks for sleep medication.

What is happening to Mr. L.? Is he developing dementia or mental illness? Is this just normal bereavement? What assessment and interventions should the physician consider?

THE CLINICAL ENCOUNTER

Considerations for Communicating with Elderly Patients

THE CLINICAL SETTING

Clinicians should adapt their office setting to facilitate communication and rapport with older patients whenever possible. Larger, wheelchair accessible rooms close to the front door will make it easier for slowly mobile patients to get to the examination room. Minimizing distracting noise and providing soft lighting can make it easier for older patients to concentrate on the medical encounter. Educating staff to sit next to patients when gathering data, to make sure that their own face is illuminated by the light source, and to ask about patient comfort with transfers can enhance safety and ease anxiety during the visit.

PATIENT INTERVIEW

Clinicians should inquire early in the interview whether they are being heard and understood. Projecting one's voice and speaking distinctly are helpful for many older persons, but clinicians should not assume this is necessary and shout at all patients just because they are very old. Speaking slower facilitates communication much better than speaking louder. Assistive devices such as portable amplification, for example, PocketTalker, can be invaluable in obtaining useful information. Active listening methods, such as maintaining eye contact, nodding, and paraphrasing the patient's questions and statements should be used (see Chapter 1). Attention to the light source is important, being certain not to sit or stand with your back to the window or light fixture so patients will be able to see your face. Shorter more frequent visits for patients with many symptoms or greater need to talk will reduce the physician's frustration, improve communication, and better meet the patient's emotional needs for contact with the physician. One of the true pleasures of caring for elderly patients is hearing their life stories, but time constraints may mandate that this occur over several visits.

FAMILY AND CAREGIVER INTERVIEW

Most frail elderly patients should be accompanied by a family member or caregiver so that the clinician can obtain a complete view of the problem. Patients with dementia may not be aware of their memory impairment and can actively deny they have any problem. They may also have limited insight into functional decline in their own activities of daily living (ADL), depressive symptoms, or paranoid thinking. Delusional thoughts may seem perfectly logical until the family or caregiver is consulted (sometimes, of course, the patient is correct—abuse and exploitation must be ruled out). Family consultation must be pursued with sensitivity to the patient's feelings, and may need to occur outside the examination room (with permission from the patient) to avoid alienating the patient. It is during these separate interviews that clinicians can obtain more candid reports of impaired ADLs, psychiatric symptoms, and memory problems.

Assessment

HISTORY

When assessing older adults, clinicians should pay special attention to past episodes of symptoms similar to the chief complaint, recent changes in function, time course of symptoms, modifying factors, and all prescribed and over-the-counter medications. Vitamins, food supplements, and homeopathic remedies are used by a significant percentage of older patients and need to be surveyed as well. Alcohol use should be evaluated. A useful acronym we have developed for a geriatric review of systems (MOMS AND DADS) is presented in Table 11-1.

PHYSICAL ASSESSMENT

General appearance, weight and nutritional status, hygiene, vital signs, and physical and neurologic examinations help determine whether the patient is medically stable, well cared for, or taking care of himself or herself adequately. Evidence of abuse, such as suspicious bruises or injuries, or evidence of medical neglect

Table 11-1. The "MOMS AND DADS" geriatric neuropsychiatry review of symptoms.*

M	Mobility	Gait and balance, recent falls, use of walking aides
O	Output	Bowel function, urine output, bladder continence
M	Memory	Emphasis on recent memory function
S	Senses	Changes in hearing and vision
A	Aches	Pain survey
N	Neuro	Neuro symptoms such as dizziness or weakness
D	Delusions	Psychotic symptoms, paranoia, hallucinations
D	Depression	Dysphoria, anxiety, fearfulness, irritability, hopelessness
A	Appetite	Food and fluid intake
D	Dermis	Changes in skin color, integrity, dental problems
S	Sleep	Problems initiating or maintaining sleep, daytime alertness, abnormal nocturnal activity

*This offers a helpful supplement to the standard organ-system-based review of systems.

should prompt an adult protective services referral through the local Area Agency on Aging.

MENTAL AND COGNITIVE STATUS EXAMINATIONS

An assessment of orientation, recent memory, problem-solving ability, judgment, insight, initiative, mood and affect, and the presence of suspiciousness, paranoia, or unusual beliefs is essential for ruling out dementia, depression, or delusional disorders (see Chapter 27 for tools to assess cognition). Use of a standardized mood rating scale, such as the Geriatric Depression Scale (GDS), can dramatically improve detection of depression in primary care settings. The GDS is self-administered, although a clinician can read the "yes-no" questions to a patient. The shorter, 15-question version has good validity and is time efficient. Cognition rating scales should be used routinely to screen for memory and cognitive impairment. The Folstein Mini-Mental State Exam (MMSE) is the most widely used, but many others are available. For example, the Mini-Cog, which consists of a three-word recall and clock-draw test, is an extremely time-efficient way to do a preliminary screen for cognitive impairment. Although an initial screening for depression and dementia can be done quickly with these brief, validated instruments, diagnosis and referral (as necessary) will usually require an extra office visit for additional mental status assessment, neurologic examination, and family interview. Executive functions, judgment, and insight are the most subtle and complex aspects of mental function to assess (see Chapter 27), but health care behavior and decision-making ability provide the clinician with clues about these functions. The latter, however, must be interpreted in light of the patient's cultural and religious values.

FUNCTIONAL ASSESSMENT

One thing that sets the evaluation of older adults apart from assessment of younger patients is the importance of performing functional assessment. The ability to do activities of daily living, such as bathing, dressing, grooming, eating, transferring, and toileting can be affected by medical illness and mental disorders. Instrumental activities of daily living (IADLs), such as telephone use, money and medication management, shopping, cooking, driving, and transportation are impacted by even mild dementia. Status of ADL and IADL function needs to be assessed to determine a person's safety at home. Improvements in ADL and IADL status will demonstrate response to medical treatments and allow patients to remain at home and independent for as long as possible.

SOCIAL SYSTEM ASSESSMENT

When frail patients are dependent on caregivers, the caregiver's capacity and coping become the clinician's concern. Caregiving is often associated with depression and health problems. The clinician should tactfully probe for indicators of stress, feelings of burden, and breakdown in the caregiver's ability to provide care (there are a number of tools available to assess caregiver burden, such as the American Medical Association's *Caregiver Self-Assessment Questionnaire*, available on their web site). The potential for abuse should also be assessed, keeping in mind that hostile remarks and impatience are risk factors for physical aggression and neglect. Many states require physicians to report suspected abuse, and all communities are required by federal law to have Area Agencies on Aging that provide adult protective services.

ENVIRONMENTAL ASSESSMENT

Community nursing and senior care agencies can assist health care providers by making home assessments and evaluating patients' safety in their own environment. These services are often covered as a Medicare benefit, especially if the patient is homebound. Fall risk, fire safety, medication management, and hygiene concerns are among the many things that can be evaluated. Removing loose throw rugs, keeping the path to the bathroom lit at night, adding bars next to the toilet, and other simple interventions can markedly increase safety and prolong independent living.

DIAGNOSIS

Major Mental Disorders of Old Age

DEPRESSION

Major depression is common in older adults (2–4% of community-residing elderly), but the prevalence is much higher in the chronically ill. Major depression in geriatric patients manifests in all the usual ways seen in younger adults (see Chapter 22), but nonspecific and atypical symptoms are common and may dominate the clinical presentation. Although depressed mood and hopelessness have diagnostic value, less specific symptoms may be prominent and give valuable clues to the underlying diagnosis. Anhedonia, anxiety, fearfulness, irritability, cognitive impairment, apathy, dependency, and numerous somatic complaints should prompt the consideration of depression even when the patient denies feeling depressed. Instruments such as the GDS can increase detection of depression and are also helpful for determining the severity of depression in primary care settings. The prognosis for depression in old age is fairly good, at least for acute symptoms, and patients need to be told this to counter the hopelessness they feel. However, partial remissions and relapses are common, especially in patients with previous episodes of depression. Other negative predictors include persistent health problems that compromise function or comfort and ongoing psychosocial stressors. Antidepressant medication and psychosocial support are known to improve

outcomes and reduce the risk of relapse in older adults. Cognitive impairment associated with depression may improve with remission of the mood disorder, but is predictive of an underlying neurodegenerative dementia. Such patients need close follow-up to catch the dementia early and ensure safety at home.

Many older people look and act depressed but do not feel sad or meet the diagnostic criteria for major depression. These minor depressions or so-called "masked depressions" often occur in the context of chronic medical illness, weight loss, and functional decline, creating the clinical syndrome of "failure to thrive." Apathy may be prominent. Some of these patients experience a slow recovery from an acute physical illness, with poor oral intake and little motivation to regain strength. Standard treatments for depression can be targeted to improve initiative and motivation, appetite, and pain tolerance in failing patients when there are many or unclear underlying causes of the syndrome. Psychostimulants such as methylphenidate or D-amphetamine may be helpful as short-term adjunctive treatments. The apathy syndrome, however, may be due to underlying vascular or degenerative disease and be very resistant to improvement.

Occasionally, bipolar affective disorder is diagnosed in older patients, either as a primary mania or hypomania developing for the first time or previous illness that went undiagnosed. Secondary mania from stroke, epilepsy, neurodegenerative diseases, and medical conditions is also seen. Mood is frequently dysphoric and irritable (prompting a misdiagnosis of "agitated depression" in some patients), although classic euphoria is also seen. Impulsivity, talkativeness, and intense, labile affect are clues to the correct diagnosis. Hyperactivity, reduced sleep, paranoia, and hypersexuality are very suggestive of the diagnosis but are not always present. Rapid cycling—with several episodes of depression and mania every year—is common in elderly bipolar patients. Treatment must include mood stabilizers such as divalproex and atypical antipsychotic drugs, rather than antidepressants.

ANXIETY DISORDERS

Elderly patients have the highest per capita use of antianxiety medications. These figures are probably higher than necessary, since many of the anxious elderly are actually suffering from depression as their primary illness. Apart from depression, the differential diagnosis of anxiety in the elderly includes transient apprehension and fear, adjustments to life changes, phobic avoidant behaviors, obsessive-compulsive disorder, panic disorder, posttraumatic stress, and generalized anxiety disorder (see Chapter 23). Secondary anxiety disorders are also very common; medications, chronic obstructive pulmonary disease, and endocrinopathies are often implicated.

DELUSIONAL DISORDERS

Delusional thinking arises from a number of disturbances in old age. A primary delusional disorder of unknown etiology, previously known as paranoia, is typically seen in elderly women who live alone. Although these patients describe persecutory delusions of an intense nature, highly suggestive of schizophrenia, they do not have other manifestations of this disease, such as hallucinations, loose associations, disorganized behavior, and functional decline. Elders who do exhibit these cardinal symptoms of schizophrenia have usually had the disease for many years, although it can develop in late life. Paranoia and delusions can also be the presenting symptoms of dementia, depression, mania, and alcohol abuse.

DEMENTIA

The prevalence of dementia increases with age, approaching 20% at age 80 and 50% by age 90. The diagnosis of dementia is made when intellectual impairment is severe enough to affect independent functioning. Alzheimer disease (AD) is the most common cause of dementia in the elderly, and can be diagnosed with fairly good accuracy by using formal diagnostic criteria (see Chapter 27). The presence of progressive decline in recent memory, normal motor function (without weakness, ataxia, or parkinsonism), and deficits in at least one other higher cortical function (language, praxis, visual-spatial, calculations, and executive functions), is highly supportive of the diagnosis. Mild cognitive impairment (MCI) is diagnosed when memory is impaired but other cognitive functions remain intact. MCI gradually progresses to AD in most individuals, but the diagnosis of AD is delayed until dementia is actually present; that is, in addition to memory, independent function is also impaired. Medical treatment of AD includes long-term maintenance on acetylcholinesterase inhibitors and memantine (for modest improvement in symptoms and slowing of functional decline), treatment of neuropsychiatric symptoms when necessary, and attention to comfort (especially pain), continence, and caregiver distress. Although high dose α-tocopherol (vitamin E 800–2000 IU/day) has been used based on evidence that it slows disease progression, recent evidence of excess cardiovascular death has discouraged its use for AD. Prescribing atypical antipsychotic medications to treat agitation and psychosis in patients with dementia is complicated by clinical trial evidence of higher mortality risk (60–70% higher vs. placebo) and a Food and Drug Administration (FDA) warning against their use in this population. A recently published multicenter trial funded by the National Institute on Aging, indicates that the efficacy of these drugs is often limited by rapid discontinuation because of side effects. Nevertheless, the atypical antipsychotics remain in widespread clinical use, partly because of the high risk of the symptoms these drugs are used to

treat, and also a relative lack of evidence for safety and efficacy of alternative medications. If used in this population, these medications should be dosed very conservatively, and patients should be closely monitored for oversedation.

Another common dementia of old age is Dementia with Lewy Bodies (DLB). This is diagnosed when a patient manifests a progressive dementia, parkinsonism (especially bradykinesia and rigidity without tremor), daily fluctuations in mental status similar to delirium, and visual hallucinations. Sleep disturbance is common, especially daytime sleepiness and excessive motor activity during REM (rapid eye movement) sleep. DLB accounts for 5–10% of cases of old age dementia, and may occur mixed with AD. Treatment of DLB involves trials of acetylcholinesterase inhibitors and psychotropic medications for targeted neuropsychiatric symptoms. Older antipsychotic medications such as haloperidol must be rigorously avoided. Most clinicians will prescribe low doses of quetiapine (12.5–100 mg a day in divided doses) for delusions and hallucinations that do not respond to acetylcholinesterase inhibitors. For neuropsychiatric symptoms that persist after cholinesterase treatment within package insert dosing guidelines, there is some evidence that higher doses can be tolerated with improved efficacy. Parkinsonism can respond modestly to L-dopa, but care must be taken to balance the doses against worsening neuropsychiatric symptoms.

Vascular dementia is another common cause of intellectual and functional decline in old age, accounting for about 5% of dementia cases and contributing to worsening dementia in many more patients as a comorbid condition with AD. Large cortical strokes produce a stepwise decline with noticeable points of change associated with strokes (multi-infarct dementia). Small vessel disease producing lacunar infarcts in subcortical structures is associated with hypertension and diabetes. Also known as Binswanger's dementia, this condition produces a more gradually progressive dementia that looks similar to AD, but with more obvious gait impairment, incontinence, parkinsonism, and affect lability. Executive functions and cognitive processing speed are usually affected more than memory. Circulatory problems in the absence of stroke (i.e., congestive heart failure, hyperviscosity states, and so forth) can also produce cognitive impairment. Patients with vascular dementia can potentially benefit from a trial of cholinesterase treatment.

DELIRIUM

Delirium is characterized by the acute (within hours) or subacute (within days) development of disorientation and confusion. Inability to focus and sustain attention are key to the diagnosis. Hallucinations, fearful or paranoid perceptions, fluctuating awareness, and alterations in the sleep–wake cycle are other frequent symptoms.

In patients with mild delirium, the decreased level of alertness may not be obvious. Patients will often have psychomotor slowing, listlessness, and apathy. These patients may be misdiagnosed as depressed or demented, although there frequently is an underlying dementia. Delirium is often the first symptom of medical illness in frail elderly people. The most common causes of delirium in older patients are infections (usually urinary tract and pulmonary), medications, metabolic abnormalities, alcohol or sedative intoxication and withdrawal, stroke, seizures, and heart failure. In patients with dementia, problems such as pain, fecal impaction, and urinary retention can cause rapid changes in mental status and behavior that look like superimposed delirium.

Many, if not most, older adults have at least mild delirium when hospitalized for an acute illness or surgery. In this setting, delirium increases fall rates, hospital stays, and risk of poor outcomes. Adequate pain control and correction of metabolic problems or infections will help shorten the time course of the delirium. Agitation, paranoia, and sleeplessness may require separate pharmacologic management (see Chapter 27). Low doses of haloperidol (0.25–1 mg IV, IM, or PO) given every few hours as needed up to 2–3 mg daily is the treatment of choice in most instances. Younger patients, patients in withdrawal from alcohol or other substances, or those with primary mental illness may need higher doses, or alternate therapies.

SUBSTANCE ABUSE AND POLYPHARMACY

Often overlooked, substance abuse is very common in the elderly; alcohol abuse is the third most common mental disorder in elderly males. Unexplained falls, ataxia, confusion, malnutrition, burns, head trauma, and depression should prompt questions about surreptitious alcohol abuse. Sedative-hypnotic medications; over-the-counter remedies for constipation, sleeplessness, and pain; and numerous vitamins and supplements are also overused. Seeing multiple physicians and practitioners and patronizing several pharmacies are clues to the clinician that prescription abuse is likely (see Chapter 21).

Because of their greater number of chronic medical conditions, older patients generally take more prescription medications than younger patients. Although often necessary, polypharmacy increases the risk of adverse drug reactions, a leading cause of confusion, depression, falls, and functional decline. An ongoing effort to evaluate the current need for everything being taken is prudent.

SOMATIZATION

Geriatric patients are not immune to somatic perceptions for which there are no known physical causes. Of course, older patients often manifest illness in vague and nonspecific ways, so an open mind is necessary when thinking through mysterious symptoms. Nevertheless, the clinician should avoid unnecessary interventions while continuously supporting the needs of the patient to be heard and understood. Although regularly scheduled appointments with brief, focused examinations that allow the "laying on of the hands" continue to be the most effective interventions, major depression and anxiety disorders commonly underlie hypochondriasis. Antidepressants and psychotherapy may improve function and a sense of well-being in somatically focused patients (see Chapter 25).

TREATMENT

Caring for Elderly Patients

HELPING OLD PEOPLE STAY AT HOME

The focus of treatment planning with the frail elderly patient is always the provision of comfort and the maintenance of independent functioning. Although there are clearly times when safety becomes the paramount issue, as in the case of the elderly driver who is becoming a hazard behind the wheel, independence is usually the shared goal of patient and clinician. To achieve this in the face of aging and progressive disease, treatment planning must include utilization of community care resources, skillful medical management, and rehabilitation therapies.

COMMUNITY CARE OPTIONS FOR THE FRAIL ELDERLY

Clinicians should become familiar with the services available in their community that provide case management, in-home assistance, and emotional support to elderly patients and caregivers. Local and county agencies providing services for seniors, private case management firms, local chapters of the Alzheimer's Association, and home health care agencies will be resources to you and your patients in arranging the services necessary to keep your patients at home longer than would otherwise be safe. In rural areas without these resources, family, neighbors, and lay networks of helpers can sometimes fill in the gaps and keep frail elders cared for at home. The Family Caregiver Alliance web site (www.caregiver.org) provides information on local resources supporting caregivers in every state.

Patients with round-the-clock care needs will eventually exhaust many family caregivers. Some patients with dementia-associated agitation, delusions, and misperceptions can be combative and make caregiving frustrating and occasionally dangerous. Caregivers, family, and paid professionals all face depression and health risks beyond their peers. There comes a time when placement in a long-term care facility becomes necessary for both the patient's as well as the family's well-being. Physicians, nurses, and other practitioners play important roles in assisting patients and families through this transition. Clinicians can help them anticipate the need to leave home for supervised living settings, familiarize them with different long-term care options in the community, and also help families with feelings of guilt experienced when they have to make the decision on the patient's behalf. This role requires clinicians to know what the patient's care needs are and what type of facility can safely meet those needs. People who need assistance only with housekeeping and cooking will do fine in retirement homes and residential care facilities. Residential care facilities may be able to administer medications and provide assistance with ADLs for additional cost. A few states allow people to provide care for up to five frail elders in a private home. These "adult foster homes" or "care homes" provide a home-like alternative to residential care facilities. Additional care needs may be met by an independent or assisted living facility. Assisted living or "independent living" facilities may provide some nursing supervision and occasionally may even have a medical director. However, the amount of nursing and medical involvement varies greatly based on state regulations and the management philosophy of the owners. These facilities are very popular with patients and families and are increasingly seen as alternatives to skilled nursing facilities because they are less expensive and much less "hospital like" than nursing homes. Many assisted living facilities allow patients to "age in place" and even allow them to receive hospice-level care at the end of life without having to move to a skilled nursing facility. However, it is important to inform patients and families that these facilities cannot generally provide the same level of nursing assessment and care that skilled nursing facilities provide. Many patients with complex care needs will still need nursing homes, but there are now many other options for less frail patients.

MEDICAL TREATMENT PLANNING

The motto of the British Geriatrics Society, "Adding Life to Years," is useful to keep in mind when treating elderly patients. Comfort and increased activity become the goals of treatment. Providing adequate pain relief, physical therapy, and treatment of depression are all integrated into comprehensive treatment plans.

Immunizations, blood pressure management, smoking cessation, weight loss, exercise, and proper nutrition should continue to be a focus of preventive care in the elderly. It is also important to explore the expectations of both the patient and the caregiver and to discuss end-of-life treatment decisions. If possible, this discussion should take place before an acute medical condition forces interventions that may be invasive, futile, or unwanted. These "advance directives" should extend beyond cardiopulmonary resuscitation and include the patient's goals of care. If the decision is to forego these interventions, the clinician should provide assurances

that the comfort of the patient will be maintained (see Chapter 37).

Given the high prevalence of mental disorders in old age, it is not surprising that the elderly are prescribed psychotropic medications at a higher rate than younger adults. Special care must be taken to start most medications at a lower dose in older patients (generally half the usual starting dose in young-old patients, i.e., 65–80 years, and a third the usual dose in old-old patients, i.e., over age 80). In the case of benzodiazepines, antipsychotics, and mood stabilizers, the effective treatment dose will also usually be one-half to one-third the dose used in younger patients. However, in the case of antidepressants, the eventual effective doses are frequently at the same levels used in young adults.

FUNCTIONAL REHABILITATION

Functional rehabilitation of elderly patients with mental disorders following stroke, fracture, or medical illness ideally involves a multidisciplinary team approach. Mental disorders, such as depression, can by themselves induce substantial physical disability through increased time in bed. The goal is to treat the mental disorder and primary disability, while preventing secondary disabilities such as immobility and incontinence, and complications such as skin breakdown and infection. The composition of the team varies widely and may include rehabilitation professionals such as physical, occupational, and speech therapists. The rehabilitation plan, like the medical plan, must have realistic goals that are individualized to the patient. This plan must be frequently re-evaluated and revised as the progress of patients toward reaching their goals is reassessed. Older patients lose function rapidly when hospitalized and bedridden for even a few days, and a brief period of strengthening rehabilitation may be needed for those who lose the ability to ambulate or transfer independently while in hospital.

CASE DISCUSSIONS

 CASE ILLUSTRATION 1

Despite her niece's concerns, Martha may only be an eccentric person, and not one with a neurodegenerative condition or mental illness. The so-called "Senior Squalor Syndrome" or Diogenes Syndrome, however, is often due to underlying dementia, depression, paranoid disorder, schizophrenia, or alcoholism. Occasionally, fear of losing autonomy and being forced from the home will lead seniors to cover-up their physical incapacity to keep up at home. Knowing whether this represents a change in personality and a recent decline in function inconsistent with past habits will allow the clinician to

determine whether this is just an eccentric lifestyle preference in an otherwise healthy person or a pathologic condition of old age. A mental status examination and functional assessment would be helpful. Knowing she is paranoid or has memory and self-care deficits will alter the clinician's approach to eliciting her cooperation. Documenting specific ADL and IADL deficits in the patient's abilities and safety hazards in the home (fire, food safety, fall risk, ability to summon emergency services) are key to determining whether intervention is necessary. Martha has apparently been paying electricity and water bills, which indicates some preservation of cognitive function. Perhaps she could remain home safely if she received help with housekeeping, shopping, and nutrition. Phone service would also be helpful, assuming she could afford a phone and be able and willing to use it.

Several things will determine the success of the physician's efforts to intervene. First, because Martha seems to be sensitive and defensive, the doctor needs to approach her thoughtfully, emphasizing the shared goal of her staying healthy and independent. Second, Martha's financial status may limit her options. She needs a social worker or case manager to help sort out her finances and arrange necessary community services. Treating the dementia, depression, or psychosis may have a large impact on function.

The local humane society or animal protection league needs to take some of the cats away. The remaining ones need veterinary care and neutering. Because the cats are important to Martha, if she did have to leave the home, placement in a facility that allows her to have a cat or two would be important for her well-being.

Joanne is Martha's only living relative, and if Martha is found to have impaired decision-making capacity, Joanne will need to assume a formal role as power of attorney, guardian, or conservator. Her ability to represent Martha's interests will need ongoing assessment by the clinician and the court.

CASE ILLUSTRATION 2

Like many caregivers, Mrs. J. is overwhelmed by the problems she faces and needs to use more support services. Options available in most areas include caregiver support groups, respite care, day programs, and housekeeping and home health services. Learning how to manage the behavioral symptoms of her husband's dementia will decrease her feelings of helplessness. Involvement with the local chapter of the Alzheimer's Association should

be strongly recommended. If agitation and delusions become severe, the newer antipsychotic medications can be very effective. Antidepressants and anticonvulsants can be effective with agitation as well. Sleep medication for Mr. J. may give both the patient and caregiver some rest.

Mrs. J. may be depressed. She is also at risk for other caregiver stress-related health problems. Treatment for the depression and counseling focused on grief and anger management would be very helpful. Even with treatment of the depression, Mrs. J. may no longer be able to effectively care for her husband in their home, and a discussion with the family about Mr. J. moving to a dementia care facility will help prepare them for what may be necessary in the future.

CASE ILLUSTRATION 3

The major diagnostic considerations in Mr. L.'s case are bereavement, major depression, dementia, and alcoholism—which can all coexist. His symptoms are consistent with bereavement: disorganization, dishevelment, talking to the deceased, and poor sleep. Although medications to aid sleep may be helpful, benzodiazepines are a risky choice for him given his past alcoholism, advanced age, and cognitive impairment. Antidepressant medication might be indicated if the severe symptoms of dysphoria persist. Grief counseling and in-home support services could both be helpful. Although making major life decisions should be avoided during a period of acute grief, a move to a residential care or assisted living facility might provide a balance of privacy, socialization, independence, and support for daily activities.

CONTINUING EDUCATION RESOURCES

The American Geriatric Society (770 Lexington Avenue, Suite 300, New York, NY 10021), The Gerontological Society of America (1275 K Street NW, Suite 350, Washington, DC 20005-4006), the American Association of Geriatric Psychiatry (PO Box 376A, Greenbelt, MD 20768), and the American Medical Director's Association (10480 Patuyent Parkway, Suite 760, Columbia, MD 21094) publish outstanding journals, have useful web sites, and sponsor educational conferences for physicians and other health care providers.

SUGGESTED READINGS

Blazer DG, Steffens DC, Busse EW, et al., eds. *Textbook of Geriatric Psychiatry*, 2nd ed. Washington, DC: American Psychiatric Publishing, Inc., 2004.

D'Ath P, Katona P, Mullan E, et al. Screening, detection and management of depression in elderly primary care attenders. I: The acceptability and performance of the 15 item Geriatric Depression Scale (GDS15) and the development of short versions. *Fam Pract* 1994;11:260–266.

Folstein MF, Folstein SE, McHugh PR, et al. "Mini-Mental State": a practical method for grading the cognitive state of patients for the clinician. *J Psychiatr Res* 1975;12:189–198.

Jacobson SA, Pies RW, Katz IR. *Clinical Manual of Geriatric Psychopharmacology*, 2nd ed. Washington, DC: American Psychiatric Publishing, Inc., 2007.

Niven D. *The 100 Simple Secrets of the Best Half of Life*. San Francisco, CA: Harper, 2005.

WEB SITES

American Association of Geriatric Psychiatry Web site. www.aagponline.org. Accessed October, 2007.

American Geriatric Society Web site. www.americangeriatrics.org. Accessed October, 2007.

American Medical Director's Association Web site. www.amda.com. Accessed October, 2007.

British Society of Gerontology Web site. www.britishgerontology.org. Accessed October, 2007.

Canadian Geriatric Society Web site. www.canadiangeriatrics.com. Accessed October, 2007.

Family Caregiver Alliance Web site. www.caregiver.org. Accessed October, 2007.

Gerontology Society of America Web site. www.geron.org. Accessed October, 2007.

International Psychogeriatric Association Web site. www.ipa-online. org. Accessed October, 2007.

National Institute of Aging Web site. www.nia.nih.gov. Accessed October, 2007.

Cross-cultural Communication

12

Thomas Denberg, MD, PhD & Mitchell D. Feldman, MD, MPhil

INTRODUCTION

Effective clinician–patient communication involves verbal and nonverbal sharing of information across cultural and linguistic boundaries. In the medical arena, these boundaries are populated on the one side by clinicians who represent the esoteric world of biomedicine, and on the other side by patients and families who often lack familiarity with biomedical concepts and procedures and may have their own strongly held beliefs about illness—what it means, how it should be diagnosed, and how it should be treated. The goals of effective cross-cultural communication (or "cultural competency," as it is sometimes called) are threefold: (1) to understand illness from the perspective of the *patient*; (2) to assist patients in understanding diseases and treatments from the perspective of *biomedicine*; and (3) to help patients and their families navigate, express themselves, and feel comfortable within large, complex, and often impersonal health care organizations. These activities require some awareness of the wider context of patients' lives, and of how the worlds of biomedicine and the lay public interact and, at times, conflict and misunderstand each other.

Cross-cultural communication skills are best developed through practice, reflection, and reading about and interacting with diverse patient populations. Knowing a few facts about the illness beliefs of an immigrant group or ethnic minority is not enough. It is important to develop ways of perceiving and interpreting what *individual* patients say and do in the context of their previous experiences with illness, structural positions within society, and membership within particular ethnic and religious communities. True cultural awareness also involves understanding how biomedicine is itself a cultural system, and how it is likely to be perceived and (mis)understood by patients.

As the dominant form of health care in the United States, biomedicine is practiced by highly specialized professionals and relies on detailed, scientific information about the human body and the use of pharmaceutical and surgical interventions to prevent or treat anatomic and physiologic disorders and their associated symptoms. It has a definite body of knowledge, set of practices, strengths, non-evidence-based biases, and inherent limitations. Each of its many specialties and subspecialties has unique conventions, systems of knowledge, and ways of making sense of people and events. To patients of all backgrounds, much about biomedicine is obscure; difficulties agreeing with and accepting medical explanations and recommendations are commonplace. Therefore, the perspective that orients the discussion in this chapter is that although cross-cultural communication is especially important and challenging for immigrant and minority patients, it has relevance to *all* patients.

CULTURE & SOCIAL LOCATION

Culture

Culture refers to beliefs, values, rituals, customs, institutions, social roles, and relationships that are shared among identifiable groups of people. Typically, one's own culture is taken for granted; it feels entirely natural, consisting of those assumptions and routines that make the world what it is "supposed" to be. Unconscious learning and modeling play important roles in the acquisition of cultural assumptions and routines. Within the family, one of the most influential cultural systems, there is generally a clear-cut division of labor, regular routines such as meal and work times, explanations (or myths) about family origins, and strategies for fulfilling common goals and passing down shared values. It is also within the family that beliefs are first developed about the causes of illness, acceptable ways of expressing symptoms, and strategies for diagnosing illness and restoring health. Individuals, of course, are also shaped by, and participate in, cultures related to work, school, worship, political affiliation, social clubs, and so on, each of which may also have important—and sometimes contradictory or inconsistent—influences on beliefs about and responses to illness.

Cultures are neither pure nor static, but constantly intermix and evolve. Particularly in the United States—a highly mobile, diverse, and media-saturated society—millions of people move in and out of multiple domains, borrowing and adapting ideas and customs from other groups. Because cultural change over time and across generations is considerable, it should not be *assumed* that particular patients have certain beliefs or engage in certain behaviors solely on the basis of their last name, physical appearance, or national origin. Inferences—always open to revision—should be based on detailed knowledge of patient attributes that go beyond race and ethnicity alone.

THE RELATIONSHIP OF CULTURE TO RACE, ETHNICITY, AND NATIONAL ORIGIN

In some cultural competency training, various racial, ethnic, and national groups are said to possess distinctive cultural traits with which the clinician should become familiar in order to render more effective care. Commonly cited examples include beliefs in "fallen fontanelle" and "evil eye" among Latinos and "high blood/low blood" among African Americans, as well as values such as "individualism" among North Americans and "family centeredness" among Asians. Although these generalizations may illustrate a wide spectrum of cultural influences on illness and healing, this approach is too simplistic. It implies that race, ethnicity, and national origin are the most important determinants of an individual's understanding of and response to illness, and ignores the tremendous heterogeneity among individuals *within* each of these groups.

Take the case of the United States, in which the primary racial/ethnic categories include African American, white, Asian, American Indian, Pacific Islander, and Latino. Some people may self-identify using these terms, and the labels are often important politically, but there are significant differences among people within each of these categories in terms of age, place of birth, religion, social class, level of education, and so on. Conceptualizing differences in health beliefs and behaviors on the overarching levels of race and ethnicity may promote stereotyping and does little to advance more effective medical care. In general, assumptions about cultural beliefs and practices should be based on more specific identification of group membership, such as recent immigrants; particular U.S. subpopulations such as the homeless, southern rural African Americans, or inhabitants of particular city neighborhoods.

Social Location

As we move beyond ideas of culture determined solely by race and ethnicity, knowledge of patients will be enhanced by awareness of their *social location*. Social location specifies one's position in society relative to others and is based on an amalgam of characteristics that include not only race and ethnicity, but also gender, age, immigration status, language(s) spoken, neighborhood of residence, length of time and number of generations in the United States, educational attainment, income, occupation, religion, and prior experiences with racism. Gender and age are two fundamental variables that influence how patients give meaning to illness and express themselves in relation to it. Men and women, and people over the age of 50 and under 20, although from the same city or region, will generally belong to distinctive subcultures: they may share certain core beliefs, values, and customs, but not others. Another fundamental influence on disease risk, health behaviors, and familiarity with biomedicine is degree of acculturation. One's neighborhood of residence, with its quality of housing and schools, population density, associated level of crime, and access to public transportation, also dramatically shapes one's understanding of the world and strategies for dealing with adversity. Religion, spirituality, and membership in a community of like-minded believers also have significant bearings on attitudes toward health and illness. Historical experiences of racism can engender feelings of helplessness, anger, and distrust that may, in turn, significantly affect attitudes toward medical providers as well as interpretations of illness. Finally, the elements of social class—education, income, and occupation—have a profound influence on beliefs about illness and opportunities and strategies for restoring health.

The attributes of social location are more complete, specific, and clinically relevant than race and ethnicity alone. In this way, a clinician will not simply note that a patient is Latino, or even Mexican American, and then attempt to remember "typical" cultural traits that apply to members of this group. Instead, they will observe that the U.S.-born patient is 20 years old, unemployed, has completed high school, speaks little Spanish, and lives with her Mexican-born, primarily Spanish-speaking, rural-origin parents in a mixed race, working-class neighborhood. Each of these characteristics, alone and in combination, provides important clues about *this* patient—clues that help in interpreting the patient's statements and symptoms and that facilitate patient education and tailored treatment.

Obviously, the more experience practitioners have with patients from a specific, narrowly defined population or community, the more they will become aware of the health problems and themes important to that group as a whole. The ability to communicate effectively with patients from such groups can be enhanced by spending time in the local community—in senior citizen centers, at cultural and sporting events, churches, and schools—as well as by reading relevant neighborhood newsletters, ethnographies, social histories, census reports, novels, and biographies. Although such activities and materials do not constitute the normal corpus of medical duties or references, they can sensitize the clinician to the issues that are important to patients—in their own terms and from their own points of view. Detailed knowledge of a specific population can also help the clinician understand not only the literal sense of a patient's words, but also other kinds of meanings contained in what the patient says (or chooses not to say), and in what the patient does (or chooses not to do), such as adhere to prescribed treatments.

IMMIGRANTS & ETHNIC MINORITIES

Recent immigrants bring a number of unique issues and challenges to medical cross-cultural communication. Relocating to a new country often results in dramatic alterations in social status, occupation, and daily routines; isolation from previous friendships and networks of social support; and the upending of traditional roles as older individuals rely on those who are younger to support the family, locate housing, and interpret local events. Anomie (a sense of purposelessness) and alienation (lack of feelings of belonging) can contribute to anxiety, depression, and a decreased ability to cope with the new stresses of daily life. Refugee experiences of war and natural catastrophe exacerbate these problems. The astute clinician will be aware that many individuals somatize this distress.

Recent immigrants are more likely to hold beliefs and practices that to "Western"-trained physicians may seem colorful or strange. These illness beliefs and behaviors are often cited in discussions of cultural competence but are generally most applicable to elderly and/or recently arrived immigrants. Processes of globalization, including the growth of tourism, the opening of commercial markets, and the spread of popular culture from the United States and Europe, have familiarized large numbers of third-world immigrants with life in industrially advanced, capitalist societies. In addition, a substantial proportion of first- and second-generation residents quickly assimilate into U.S. society, often because of a keen desire to "fit in" or "become American." Even among individuals who speak English poorly, are poorly assimilated, or actively resist assimilation, many will have had a significant amount of experience with biomedicine in their countries of origin. Although they may not have previously encountered the technological and organizational complexity that characterize biomedicine in the United States, they may be familiar with its reductionistic, scientific foundation, status as a profession, and its conventions for diagnosing and treating illness. It is difficult, if not impossible, to accurately gauge a patient's level of sophistication about biomedicine and "Western" disease categories through visual inspection or knowledge of the patient's race and ethnicity alone; the clinician should avoid assumptions and instead learn by observing and asking questions to the patient.

BIOMEDICINE AS A CULTURAL SYSTEM

Focusing on "culture" primarily in relation to immigrant or minority patients may convey the notion that biomedicine is itself without culture. In fact, while biomedicine is informed by scientific knowledge (a "culture" with its own values and beliefs) it is also shaped by the politics of government funding, insurance reimbursement, rivalries among specialties, as well as by competing ideologies of profit versus altruism, changing fashions and trends, best guesses, and regional biases. Biomedicine comprises many cultural worlds and languages—primary care, cardiology, surgery; the hospital, the clinic; nursing, physicians, pharmacists; and so on—that for many patients are strange, potentially threatening, and difficult to understand. Awareness of how different kinds of patients are likely to experience and interpret biomedicine is essential to enhancing cross-cultural communication. It is equally important for clinicians to be aware of their own roles in perpetuating the culture of biomedicine, and to realize the extent to which they are both the products and practitioners of this cultural system. Table 12-1 lists several characteristics that have been associated with biomedicine and its practitioners.

Tensions and misunderstandings between practitioner and patient are often strongly rooted in many of the attributes listed under (A) in Table 12-1. Often most problematic from the perspective of patients is biomedicine's tendency to sharply differentiate body from mind and to emphasize organic pathophysiology over the psychosocial ramifications and origins of illness. Nonetheless, many of biomedicine's major successes have been achieved despite—or often because of—such tendencies. These are the characteristics that set biomedicine apart from other systems of healing. They are also quite resistant to change. The clinician's goal should be to act as a cultural broker, making these features of biomedicine more accessible and understandable to the patient while at the same time exploring and attending to the psychosocial dimensions of illness from the patient's perspective.

Individual practitioners vary greatly in the degree to which they conform to the attributes of professionalism listed under (B) in Table 12-1 (see Chapter 39). Although common, none is a *predictable* feature of biomedicine in the same way as those listed under (A). A central problem, however, is that many patients have difficulty understanding or sympathizing with the attributes in either category, compounding communication difficulties and leading some to hold many of the negative impressions listed under (C) in Table 12-1. This is especially true when patients desire a more personal and less professional relationship with their physicians, or when social distance compounds the patient's feelings of powerlessness. The culturally competent

Table 12-1. Characteristics of biomedicine and its practitioners.

(A) Biomedicine *as a system of healing rests upon and esteems the following:*

- Empiric science
- Written knowledge as opposed to oral tradition
- Rigorous and lengthy training
- Technological sophistication and innovation
- Action orientation and interventionism ("doing something rather than nothing")
- Materialism (disease in the individual, physical body rather than in the family, social group, mind, or spirit)
- Differentiating among acute illness, chronic illness, and prevention
- Reductionism (pathophysiology is molecular and anatomic; symptoms are expressions of underlying disease rather than diseases themselves)
- High levels of bureaucratic organization and subspecialization
- Efficiency
- Cost containment
- "Defensiveness" or avoiding malpractice
- The prolongation of life

(B) *Many* **clinicians** *value these traits:*

- Hard work
- Self-sacrifice
- Self-reliance and autonomy
- Strong career orientation
- Status consciousness
- Respect for authority and hierarchy
- Hygiene
- Punctuality
- The physician as the expert
- Deliberateness
- Articulateness
- A clear separation between personal and work lives
- Conservatism in dress and expressions of emotion
- Quality judged by one's colleagues

(C) *Common attributions that* **patients** *have about biomedicine and its practitioners:*

Negative	Positive
Arrogant	Highly competent
Elite	Honest
Judgmental	Careful
Remote and inaccessible	Thorough
Narrow minded	Methodical
Difficult to comprehend	Caring
Money hungry	Accurate
Rushed	Reliable
Dogmatic	Responsible
Rigid	Impartial
Uninterested in the patient as a person	Putting the patient's welfare first and foremost

clinician will understand these common features and negative patient perceptions of biomedicine, recognizing when they contribute to misunderstandings and impair a patient's ability to feel at ease, communicate, and benefit from a biomedical approach.

COMMUNICATION

Communication involves the exchange, processing, and interpretation of messages—both verbal and nonverbal. In this complex process, there are myriad opportunities for miscommunication: messages can be incomplete, confusing, and contradictory; language barriers as well as emotional and physical distractions can interfere with the receipt and relaying of information; and unspoken assumptions can influence the meaning one person attributes to another's statements or actions. Much of this takes place outside of conscious awareness. With this in mind, this section reviews three fundamental aspects of communication to which the clinician should direct particular attention: (1) attempting to understand the illness from the *patient's* perspective; (2) ensuring that the patient understands, as much as possible and at an appropriate level, *biomedical* explanations of the illness and its treatment; and (3) guiding patients through the *ritualized* clinical encounter and the health care bureaucracy in ways that increase their familiarity and comfort with it.

The Patient

Barriers to health care affecting both immigrants and disadvantaged minority groups—such as lack of insurance and other financial resources, physical distance, and low literacy—often make biomedical treatment an option of last resort. Clinical consultations for such patients will frequently be more time consuming and require increased patience by the clinician. Extra effort may sometimes be needed to teach such patients to be assertive, ask questions, and raise concerns. Clinicians who treat large numbers of such patients will benefit the most from reading about and becoming personally familiar with them outside of medical settings.

EXPLANATORY MODELS

Explanatory models refer to theories of disease causation, prognosis, typical symptoms, and appropriate treatment. Eliciting patients' explanatory models of disease offers unparalleled insight into their sense of self and relationships with significant others while yielding clues about how they are likely to interpret, resist, or accept biomedical explanations and treatments. Knowledge of the patient's perspective also facilitates the ability to ease patient fear and anxiety. Understanding the patient's *explanatory model* of illness is especially important when treating potentially debilitating chronic conditions, where nonadherence is a common concern and where the psychosocial dimensions of illness loom large.

Typically, the most important component of a patient's explanatory model is the idea of illness *causation* (see Table 12-2). To elicit this belief the clinician can ask, "What do you think caused your problem?" and then listen carefully to the answer as it is likely to reveal crucial feelings related to moral failings, discord with significant others, financial and practical challenges in daily life, and whether there is a sense of hope for the future. The clinician should not expect patients

Table 12-2. Questions to elicit a patient's explanatory model of illness.

- What do you think caused your problem?
- What do you think you have?
- What is the name you give to this condition?
- Why do some people get this illness but not others?
- What do you think needs to be done to relieve this problem?

to answer questions about causation with simple and mechanistic explanations. Additional probing may also be required. For example, the clinician could follow up with questions such as "What do you think you have? What is the name you give to this condition?" "Why do some people get this illness and not others?" "Who or what is responsible (or to blame) for this problem?" and "Do you ever think that you did (or didn't do) something to bring this on yourself, or that someone else did (or didn't do) something?" Additional questions can allow patients to elaborate on their explanatory model: "What do you think should be done to treat you?" "Do you think a complete cure is possible?" "How long will the problem last?" "What do you think needs to be done to relieve this problem?" The advantage of such questions is that they are open-ended, are applicable to every patient, and can help to correct or refine initial clinical assumptions or preconceptions. They are also powerful in their ability to provide clues about what the patient may find difficult to understand or accept when it comes to explaining the illness in *biomedical* terms.

Some patients, especially recent immigrants, may be reticent about sharing their explanatory models of illness out of concern that their beliefs will be viewed as ignorant or superstitious. Alternatively, such patients may feel that they have come to hear the doctor's expert opinion, and that their own perspective is of little consequence. It is sometimes prudent to allow patients' explanatory models to emerge slowly, through gentle probing, over the course of several visits. Inference combined with direct questioning (e.g., "other patients believe X, what do you think about this?") and background knowledge of the patient's social location will often be necessary to form a coherent picture.

Fatalism

Members of some groups, including many immigrants, may seem to be fatalistic in their attitudes toward illness. They may be passive about seeking treatment, persist in unhealthful behaviors, or accept misfortune because they believe it is preordained. It is important not to assume that this style of explaining and dealing with illness is indelibly rooted in the culture or religion of the patient's racial or ethnic group. In fact, fatalism is widespread and is common among people who have little control over the circumstances of their lives. It also emerges out of a kind of valid logic that observes that serious illness can befall even those who have no bad habits and live a "clean" or "virtuous" life. Fatalism does not usually imply a lack of interest in preventing or treating disease. Rather, it can be viewed as an idiom for describing a person's perceived powerlessness in the world, lack of hope, and even distrust. The doctor can approach this problem by acknowledging the real challenges the patient faces, and by clearly articulating the practical steps the patient can take to resolve or manage the illness.

CASE ILLUSTRATION 1

A 56-year-old African American woman who completed a grade-school education declines colon cancer screening. On questioning, she believes that cancer is a "death sentence" and cannot be cured. Cancer terrifies her and she therefore sees no point in learning she might have it. The clinician explains that from a medical perspective cancer takes many years to develop, and that in people over 50 it can happen in a few individuals out of a hundred. She then tells the patient that the purpose of colon cancer screening—a relatively safe procedure performed thousands of times every year—is not to find a big cancer (which would be extremely unusual) but to save lives by finding a few areas (polyps) where cancer could develop and then snip them out. She provides the patient with an illustrated brochure to look over and consider.

In addition to the patient's beliefs about cancer, the clinician suspects that she distrusts the idea of doctors doing something to her that she, herself, has not requested or previously thought about. Over the course of several appointments, the clinician gently revisits the issue. A year later, the patient agrees. Trust—developed through a continuing relationship, manifest concern on the part of the clinician, and openness in explaining the purpose of medical tests—was a key factor in the patient's decision. Had the patient continued to decline screening, however, the clinician appropriately would have respected her decision , without overt negative judgment.

THE PASSIVE PATIENT

Some immigrants and older patients may be exceptionally reserved or deferential in clinical interactions, often preferring to avoid direct eye contact. The clinician should not assume that such patients are shy, uninterested, unintelligent, or uneducated simply because they avoid eye contact, agree with everything the doctor says, express a great deal of uncertainty about instructions, or are not forthcoming with information. In these circumstances, the clinician should speak clearly without reverting to an overly simplistic, commanding, frustrated, or patronizing tone of voice. Further clinic visits and gentle elicitation of questions and concerns may be necessary before the patient begins to interact more openly. The patient's behavior may reflect not only cultural norms toward those in authority, but uncertainty, fear, the expression of trust through passivity, or a desire to attain a better impression of the clinician before revealing intimate details.

CASE ILLUSTRATION 2

An older patient, originally a schoolteacher from the Philippines, is hospitalized for community-acquired pneumonia. The hospitalization is uneventful and on the day of discharge, the medical team enters his room to review his discharge instructions. When asked for his input about preferred follow-up or his understanding of the ongoing treatment, he averts his eyes, speaks quietly, and seems unable to comprehend the discharge plan. He repeatedly asks for instructions about the various forms. The team leaves the room uncertain of his understanding. Later that morning, the pharmacist on the team returns to review his discharge medications with him. She sits down and speaks softly and respectfully. Eventually, he opens up and it becomes apparent that he understood the prior conversation completely and speaks articulately about his concerns, although he continues to avoid eye contact.

INTERPRETERS

Trained medical interpreters can greatly facilitate patient–clinician communication and improve quality of care. Unfortunately, perhaps because of economic constraints and clinicians' beliefs in their own ability to simply "get by," well-trained interpreters are underused in many medical settings, with negative consequences for patient care. For example, although clinicians with some ability in conversational Spanish may assume they understand a Puerto Rican patient's use of the term "ataque de nervios" (literally a "nervous attack"), the patient is actually referring to a culturally specific syndrome with identifiable precipitants and clear symptoms that has little to do with a "nervous breakdown."

Although family members often act as de-facto interpreters, this can also introduce problems. For example, a relative who "already knows" what is wrong with the patient may not wish to bother the physician with the full details of the patient's complaints, thereby omitting important symptoms. Children and adolescents are inappropriate interpreters for many reasons, including an often incomplete mastery of English, insufficient knowledge of the subtleties of translation, and issues of relationship and status.

Trained medical interpreters can provide more than literal paraphrasing: they can interpret patient's illness labels and idioms for the practitioner, and translate biomedical concepts and instructions into the patient's vernacular. Interpreters should be treated as full members of the health care team. Prior to the interaction, the clinician may want to meet briefly with the interpreter to review the goals for that discussion (e.g., addressing the patient's understanding of and compliance with a particular medication). In addition, the clinician should periodically stop the interview to seek clarification from the interpreter: "The patient has mentioned 'nerves' a few times. I was assuming that she felt nervous, but now I'm not so sure. Could you explain to me what she means?."

When using an interpreter, it is important to consider the physical arrangement of the participants. The clinician should always face and speak to the patient directly. The interpreter can sit next to the physician (though some patients may find this arrangement threatening), or the patient and interpreter can sit side by side. Some clinicians prefer the traditional triangular arrangement so that all parties have equal space and symbolic power, but the easy flow of conversation may be compromised as patient and provider often cannot resist the impulse to direct their attention toward the interpreter instead of toward each other.

The Clinician

Understanding illness from the patient's perspective—traditionally regarded as the essence of cultural competence—must be balanced by the equally important task of knowing how to communicate *biomedical* explanations about the disease and its treatment to the patient (i.e., serving as interpreter of biomedical culture for patients). The desire for such information is usually one of the patient's primary motivations for visiting a doctor. The clinician should offer explanations in terms the patient can understand and then gently test this understanding.

NAMING AND EXPLAINING THE DISEASE IN NEUTRAL TERMS

Naming a disease helps to transform a patient's inchoate fears into something that can be perceived and addressed directly. Speaking about disease in neutral and mechanistic ways can also dispel feelings of shame

and ideas about etiology that are rooted in personal weakness and social failure. Patients will often seize upon, and benefit from, explanations that appropriately relieve them of personal responsibility for their misfortune. Giving a specific name to a disease and explaining it in neutral terms should be regarded as one of the primary goals of communication. Reaching this point, of course, may depend upon an initial period of testing and observation.

 CASE ILLUSTRATION 3

A 65-year-old immigrant and former physician is diagnosed with cancer. The clinician is able to elicit the patient's belief that cancer often occurs in people with "repressed personalities." Believing that he brought his disease upon himself because of such a character flaw, he feels a lack of hope and is less inclined to treat the disease. He benefits from an impersonal biomedical interpretation of cancer that focuses on damaged cellular DNA leading to unchecked cellular proliferation, and treatment aimed at destroying aberrant cells.

MEDICALIZATION

Although reductionistic disease labels and explanations are often helpful, they may contribute to the medicalization of conditions whose etiologies reside in adverse environmental (e.g., polluted air and water) or social circumstances (e.g., racism, intimate partner violence, sexual abuse, and work-related stress). In other words, defining illness entirely in terms of how it adversely affects the body can direct attention away from other, more fundamental causes. It is important to remain mindful of, and at times acknowledge, the broader context that gives rise to the illness. This is often very difficult for physicians to do, in part because they are not trained to recognize these links and are limited in their ability to resolve problems such as poverty, unemployment, poor housing, or lack of education and opportunity. For example, declaring that a patient's asthma is made worse by living near a factory from which, for economic reasons, the patient cannot easily move away may imply that nothing can be done about the problem. Nonetheless, awareness of such constraints can help the clinician to better understand and sympathize with the patient and tailor therapies that are realistic and appropriate. In addition, it is extremely common for patients of all backgrounds to believe that illness is caused by breaches in the moral order, social discord, and the failure of one's self or significant others to fulfill expected roles. Purely mechanistic biomedical explanations cannot simply replace these types of beliefs, which tend to be deeply rooted and resistant to change. Educating the patient about disease terms and pathophysiology should complement but not supersede the importance of understanding and acknowledging these other aspects of the patient's explanatory model.

"BLAMING THE VICTIM"

When it is possible to trace the etiology of disease to potentially destructive personal behaviors, such as "risky" sex, smoking, alcoholism, and drug abuse, or the worsening of disease to medical nonadherence, two pitfalls should be avoided. One is emphasizing personal culpability at the expense of helping the patient to understand the nature of the disease itself. Without adequate education, patients may have a difficult time perceiving the relationship between their behavior and the outcomes these generate, and will therefore see less reason to make changes. Although it is important to stress that certain habits are harmful and should be altered or discontinued, this should be done in a straightforward and nonjudgmental manner. The second pitfall is failing to acknowledge the personal situations and social contexts that contribute to or sustain these behaviors. Low self-esteem, depression, chronic pain, social isolation, lack of "legitimate" employment, and a strong desire to experience a sense of social belonging can contribute to many varieties of harmful and risky practices. To the extent possible, clinicians should attempt to determine the factors that perpetuate or encourage harmful behaviors and discuss these with their patients in an open and frank manner. Doing so will demonstrate empathy and concern, and help patients understand how their behavior (arising as it might for understandable reasons) should nonetheless be modified, and how this might be achieved (see Chapter 16).

COMMUNICATING BAD NEWS

Naming the disease is a cornerstone of communication in the biomedical model. However, a more flexible approach to informing patients of their diagnosis is often appropriate, particularly when the diagnosis is cancer or a terminal illness. Knowledge of a patient's social location and explanatory models of illness (including cancer), as well as in-depth questioning of the patient and family, will provide the best understanding of cultural differences and preferences. Chapter 3 offers a more complete discussion of this topic.

PSYCHIATRIC DIAGNOSES

For patients of many backgrounds, profound stigma is often attached to behavioral and psychiatric diagnoses. Labels such as "depression," referrals to psychiatrists, or prescriptions for "mind-altering" medications may be strongly resisted, interpreted as insulting by some, and

may severely compromise the practitioner–patient relationship. For such patients, somatization is often the most "legitimate" way of expressing distress. If there is any doubt regarding the patient's perception of psychiatric labels and referrals, the clinician should carefully explore the meanings that patients and their families attribute to them.

 CASE ILLUSTRATION 4

A Mexican immigrant, working-class mother is taken aback by the pediatrician's diagnosis of "attention deficit disorder" in her child and concomitant referral to a child psychiatrist and prescription for stimulant medication. She believes these recommendations imply that her child is "crazy" and, by extension, that she, first and foremost, as well as the family as a whole, have somehow failed. Her anguish is compounded by the extreme importance she attributes to her role as a mother and homemaker. Furthermore, she holds that psychiatric medicines are "too powerful" for her child who, like all children, is "sensitive and vulnerable." She would have benefited from a discussion that elicited these beliefs in advance, followed by an approach that acknowledged her fears, reaffirmed her maternal skills and concern, and attempted gently to address her beliefs and values.

PATIENT INTERPRETATIONS OF ACUTE ILLNESS, CHRONIC ILLNESS, AND PREVENTIVE MEDICINE

Many patients do not clearly differentiate acute from chronic illness, nor do they make distinctions among curing, managing, and preventing disease. Commonly, they assume that symptoms or diseases are self-limiting or curable with a single course of therapy. This can frustrate the clinician's ability to provide education and can contribute to poor adherence. If in doubt, the clinician should determine whether patients believe a cure is possible (*not* generally the case with chronic illness) or whether patients believe the absence of current symptoms implies the absence of future disease (suggesting poor understanding of preventive medicine). Gently correcting patients' misconceptions should be viewed as an ongoing process that takes time and bears repetition.

PATIENTS WITH POOR ENGLISH LITERACY

It is estimated that up to 21% of American adults are functionally illiterate and many more are only marginally literate, limiting their ability to understand medical information and engage in meaningful discussions with their providers. Feelings of embarrassment may lead patients to conceal this problem. Strategies for managing such patients include speaking slowly, using simple terms, targeting written materials to at most a fifth-grade reading level, and using clear pictures and diagrams whenever possible. Instruments such as the Test of Functional Health Literacy in Adults (TOFHLA) can provide rapid estimates of the ability to read and comprehend common medical and lay terms. Such tools can assist clinicians in tailoring both written and spoken information, and are probably more accurate at assessing the patient's reading and numerical skills and ability to function effectively in health care settings than subjective clinician impression alone.

REVIEWING MEDICATIONS

Failure to discuss medications is one of the most frequent lacunae in practitioner–patient communication. Misunderstandings and fears about medications are extremely common and are major contributors to nonadherence. Pharmaceuticals, however, are generally the most tangible and therapeutically important products that result from the clinical encounter. Special care should therefore be given to explaining their purpose, mechanism of action, and common side effects. Eliciting patient concerns and questions to uncover erroneous beliefs is also important. This is particularly likely to benefit patients who are reticent or unable to express these concerns on their own.

Sometimes it may be helpful for clinicians to personalize information by acknowledging common challenges they face in educating and treating patients.

 CASE ILLUSTRATION 5

A patient has been diagnosed with hypertension. After explaining the benefits and risks of treating hypertension with medication, the physician tries to help the patient see the clinical challenge from her perspective. She explains, "As doctors, we often have difficulty helping patients understand why they should take medicines even when they have no unpleasant symptoms. Understandably, patients often hate to take medicines, especially if they feel perfectly fine. Yet medicines are important for preventing very serious problems down the road."

This kind of approach may help some patients to understand and sympathize with the challenges faced by the clinician, promoting a sense that the two are allies in achieving a common objective.

CONTROVERSIAL AND ALTERNATIVE TREATMENTS

Sometimes there is medical uncertainty about the value of a medical test or intervention (e.g., prostate-specific antigen [PSA] screening). Sometimes there may be more than one treatment option, none of which is clearly superior in terms of prevention, cure, or control of symptoms, but each of which differs significantly in terms of cost or in the likelihood of various adverse effects on quality of life (e.g., worry over a PSA value of 5). In these instances, before taking action the clinician should attempt to gauge both the patient's desire for information as well as preferences for decision making. Studies have shown that most patients wish to be "maximally" informed about their diseases as well as medical treatments and evaluations, but there is wide variability in their desire to assume or share responsibility for making actual treatment decisions. Only through probing is it possible to determine how much information patients want in order to feel comfortable and whether they want to share in the decision-making process. Providing too much information or attempting to make the patient accept responsibility for a medical decision can be counterproductive, but so can an approach that is overly paternalistic. One strategy is for the provider to state that there is a choice and perhaps some medical controversy or uncertainty; briefly mention the pros and cons of each option; elicit patient outcome preferences; and then wait for the patient to ask for more details, voice concerns, or express a preference for the provider to make the ultimate decision.

ASSESSING PATIENT UNDERSTANDING

To ensure that biomedical explanations are correctly understood, the clinician should ask patients close- and open-ended questions about their disease process and ask them to repeat instructions. For example, "Tell me what you understand about the cause of your diabetes and what you think will happen if we cannot adequately control your blood sugar. How often should you check your blood sugar? What should you do if you feel light-headed and sweaty?" Such checks will help to reinforce knowledge and understanding and identify areas that benefit from further counseling.

The Clinician as Cultural Broker and Institutional Guide

As described above, cross-cultural communication is enhanced by attention to patients' social location because it allows provisional inferences to be made about how patients, as *individuals*, are likely to interpret and respond to their illness. Initial clinical impressions are then modified by eliciting patients' explanatory models of illness. This information helps to tailor communication regarding the *biomedical* perspective. Finally, communication is further enhanced by understanding how patients perceive key features of the clinical process and by guiding them through its ritual and bureaucratic aspects.

CLINICAL RITUALS

Repetitive and predictable patterns and rules circumscribe patient–clinician interactions. In the ambulatory setting, for example, the nurse measures the patient's blood pressure and then brings the patient to see the physician, who directs the proceedings according to a predefined format of greeting the patient, asking questions in a certain order, examining the patient, and offering explanations and recommendations. The patient is given a specific place to sit and generally knows that the consultation will last a fixed amount of time. In the hospital, the medical team rounds in the morning and obtains a standard template of subjective and objective information. The basic format of these rituals is fairly simple and can be readily learned by patients and by the new initiates into the profession.

Such ritual aspects of medicine can both facilitate and impede effective communication. For example, consistency minimizes confusion about what is acceptable and unacceptable and about what will happen. Ritual offers a sense of security when patients are undressed or are sharing personal information. The ground rules and scripts of ritual are translatable from one setting to another and operate even if practitioner and patient have never met. They allow the involved actors to focus greater attention on the *content* of their exchanges and, in themselves, these rituals can be comforting and even therapeutic.

On the other hand, rituals can impair communication if patients and practitioners differ in their expectations about how they are supposed to work, or if rituals become inflexible, blind routines that leave little room for digression, variation, and opportunities for patients to express themselves freely and in fully emotional ways. This frequently happens when the clinician is pressed for time and wants the patient to provide the "facts" as tersely as possible, or when the patient yields all spontaneity of self-expression to the perceived all-knowingness and authority of the doctor. Ritual should not become so fixed that its participants become inflexible. Awareness of these pitfalls and the ability to make spontaneous adjustments to unspoken aspects of ritual can do much to enhance communication with the patient. Brief, unexpected, or even surprising disruptions to ritual—such as a joke, a doctor's personal reflection, allowing the patient to shed a tear or relate a piece of medical history during the physical examination, or briefly and politely answering a patient's personal question about the doctor or his family—can, when judiciously applied and without breaking the overall structure of the encounter, foster more effective communication and enhance the therapeutic relationship.

For almost all patients, illness is not simply an individual malady, but a social disruption that both affects and requires the involvement of significant others. The paradigmatic private, dyadic nature of biomedicine's doctor–patient relationship can also impair communication when working with patients for whom the involvement of family members is very important. When desired by the patient, and to the extent possible, allowances and arrangements should be made to incorporate the family into diagnostic and treatment plans (see Chapter 8).

INSTITUTIONAL GUIDE

The provider should be sensitive to immigrants and other vulnerable patients who have a poor understanding of how the health care system works. Providing education about where to report for laboratory work and procedures, when results will be returned and what will be done with these, the roles of various office staff, the hours of operation, rules pertaining to the presence of children, and so on will increase efficiency, improve patient use of resources, and also likely increase patient trust by helping to demystify what seems to be a complex and threatening bureaucracy. Of note, some patients may not wish to fill out forms because of fears of deportation; it is important to be explicit about the purpose and confidentiality of medical information.

"COMPLEMENTARY" & "ALTERNATIVE" HEALERS

Despite its depth of knowledge and undeniable efficacy in many areas, biomedicine is for many patients simply *one* healing option among many others, some of which are employed simultaneously and without apparent contradiction.

If the patient wishes to discuss or solicit the provider's opinion about other healing modalities, the clinician—unless there are concrete reasons to the contrary—should be willing to acknowledge the beneficial role that nonbiomedical approaches may have for the patient. If there are potential adverse interactions or side effects of "alternative" therapies, or if there is concern that potentially beneficial biomedical therapies might be thwarted by other types of healers, the clinician should express these concerns but should always respect the fact that patients are the ultimate arbiters regarding the healing modalities for which they are best suited (see Chapter 30).

RACE/ETHNICITY & GENETICS

By virtue of their race or ethnicity, patients are sometimes said to be "at risk" for certain diseases. Examples include diabetes mellitus among Native Americans, breast cancer among Ashkenazi Jews, and prostate cancer among African Americans. Particular forms of treatment are also believed to be more (or less) effective among certain racial/ethnic groups compared with others. For example, among African Americans compared with whites, it is said that the combination of isosorbide dinitrate and hydralazine is more effective for treating heart failure, angiotensin-converting enzyme (ACE) inhibitors are less effective for essential hypertension, and a therapeutic response to selective serotonin reuptake inhibitor (SSRI) antidepressants takes place at lower doses. Each of these examples is highly controversial, reflecting long-standing, often heated disputes about whether race and ethnicity are primarily social constructs or, instead, meaningful and valid surrogates for biological difference. It is beyond the scope of this chapter to summarize the elements of this debate. We believe, however, that in communicating with patients it is important for clinicians to avoid oversimplifying the relationship between race/ethnicity and genetics. Although knowledge of race or ethnicity might prompt genetic testing or detailed family history taking in particular instances, the issues are simply too complex and the evidence too uncertain in a relatively small number of conditions for clinicians to make unqualified assertions to patients that they are "at risk" for a particular illness or unlikely to respond to therapies solely on the basis of their racial/ethnic background. In very real ways, believing that one is "at risk" can unnecessarily increase stress, fear, and feelings of stigma, uncertainty, and worthlessness. When discussing with patients the possible relevance of race and ethnicity, clinicians should openly acknowledge that experts do not always agree and they should quantify and convey individual risk through a consideration of as many relevant variables as possible.

CONCLUSION

Cross-cultural communication can be learned and enhanced through reflection and practice with a variety of patients from different cultures. Biomedicine has its own distinct culture and practices that may be difficult for many patients to comprehend and access. Cultural stereotypes are rarely useful in clinical encounters; instead clinicians should attempt to understand the social location of their patients as reflected in their race and ethnicity, gender, age, immigration status, literacy level, occupation, and other characteristics. As their skills develop, clinicians will find enormous gratification in caring for patients who are in some way different from themselves.

SUGGESTED READINGS

Doak CC, Doak LG, Root JH. *Teaching Patients With Low Literacy Skills.* Philadelphia, PA: J.B. Lippincott, 1985.

Fadiman A. *The Spirit Catches You and You Fall Down.* New York, NY: Farrar, Strauss & Giroux, 1998.

Helman C. *Culture, Health, and Illness,* 2nd ed. Oxford: Butterworth-Heinemann, 1992.

Kaiser Permanente National Diversity Council. *A Provider's Handbook on Culturally Competent Care.* (Available for Latino, African American, Asian/Pacific-Islander, and Eastern European populations.)

Kleinman A. *Patients and Healers in the Context of Culture.* Berkeley, CA: University of California Press, 1980.

Weigmann K. Racial medicine: here to stay? The success of the International HapMap Project and other initiatives may help to overcome racial profiling in medicine, but old habits die hard. *EMBO Rep* 2006;7(3):246–249.

WEB SITE

Cross-cultural Resources in Clinical Practice Web site. http://medicine.ucsf.edu/resources/guidelines/culture.html.

Women

Diane S. Morse, MD, Judith Walsh, MD, MPH, & Martina Jelley, MD

INTRODUCTION

There are developmental transitions adults attain, conceived as stages of the family life cycle. In this chapter, we describe behavioral issues for adolescents, young adults, middle age and older women using this framework. We discuss expected behavioral issues normally occurring as part of the life cycle, as well as problematic ones requiring medical surveillance or intervention.

ADOLESCENCE: A TIME OF POWER IN THE MIDST OF INSECURITY

The task of adolescence is to find one's own beliefs, moving from childhood to adulthood physically and in relationships. A number of events can occur during this time that will require the sensitive attention of the primary care physician, but numerous studies have suggested that confidentiality must be maintained for the physician to be trusted and helpful to an adolescent.

Approach to the Gynecologic Examination

Many women fear a pelvic examination, especially when they are undergoing it for the first time. Little research has been done on what strategies are best in performing a pelvic examination, but several techniques have been found to be helpful in clinical practice.

Before performing the examination, clinicians should ask women if they have ever had a pelvic examination. In addition, they should take a complete sexual history, and specifically inquire about a history of sexual abuse or sexual dysfunction such as dyspareunia, vaginismus, and disorders of sexual desire. Problems with sexual desire can sometimes be related to underlying conditions such as hypothyroidism or depression. During the pelvic examination, potential causes of dyspareunia and vaginismus such as vaginal lesions, infection, and dryness or atrophy can be ruled out.

It is useful for the clinician to describe exactly what is being done before and during the examination; providing more information about the reproductive organs may also be helpful. When the examiner is male, it is appropriate for a nurse or chaperone to be present.

Other techniques include appropriate draping, using a warm speculum, using the narrowest speculum that will allow adequate visualization of the cervix, being as gentle as possible and encouraging the patient to use relaxation techniques including deep breathing and mental imagery. Deep breathing is suggested when the patient feels uncomfortable, and mental imagery (encouraging the patient to form and talk about a mental image) can be used to help further relax the pelvic muscles, and may be particularly useful for young women and for those who have been victims of sexual abuse. In addition, elevating the head will facilitate eye contact and may make it easier for some women to relax. In situations where a patient has suffered extreme abuse; anxiety, posttraumatic stress disorder (PTSD), or even dissociation may occur and a onetime dose of a benzodiazepine may be required.

Research has shown that the experience of the first pelvic examination strongly influences attitudes about subsequent examinations; therefore, it is important for clinicians to make the first pelvic examination as positive an experience as possible. In a study describing experiences of the first pelvic examination, a negative evaluation of the examination was associated with pain, embarrassment, and having insufficient knowledge about the examination and what the doctor was doing. Spending time at the first examination providing knowledge and encouraging realistic expectations of the examination may be useful in shaping attitudes about subsequent examinations.

If a gynecologic examination is being done on an adolescent in the context of reproductive health care or to screen for sexually transmitted infections, it is important to be aware of the legal requirements of confidentiality in the United States. The details of this may vary from state to state, however up-to-date information regarding this issue is available on the Alan Guttmacher Institute web site: http://www.guttmacher.org.

Adolescents should be encouraged to involve their parents or care providers in medical decisions as much as possible, and providers should be aware of mandatory reporting laws in the case of nonconsensual sexual activity, sex with an older adult, or other abuse. Attempts by the parent or the adolescent to involve the physician in lying or keeping secrets should be resisted by encouraging the parties to talk to each other and adhering to confidentiality.

Chronic Pelvic Pain & Vulvodynia

Another condition that can affect women starting in teen or early adult years is chronic pelvic pain (CPP), which is defined as noncyclical pain of at least 6 months duration that occurs in the pelvis, abdominal wall, lower back or buttocks, and is serious enough to cause disability or lead to medical care. CPP can be severe and debilitating and accounts for 20% of the hysterectomies performed in the United States. Women diagnosed with CPP are more likely to experience depression, anxiety, somatoform disorders, sexual dysfunction, and substance abuse, though these conditions may be a cause or effect of the CPP. A history of sexual or physical abuse, often during childhood, but including intimate partner violence, has been identified in over 50% of patients. Medically unexplained symptoms (MUS) and other functional symptoms, specifically irritable bowel syndrome (IBS) and fibromyalgia, are frequently associated with CPP (see Chapter 26).

The possible causes of CPP are many and include endometriosis, pelvic inflammatory disease, and interstitial cystitis, although no underlying physical cause can be found in more than half of patients. Scientific evidence to guide treatment of the patients with no clear underlying physical source is limited. Tricyclic antidepressants have been shown to be somewhat effective in the treatment of other chronic pain syndromes and are commonly used despite lack of supportive data. Medroxyprogesterone acetate can reduce pain especially in those with pelvic congestion syndrome. Cognitive behavioral therapy (CBT) and counseling are effective for reducing pain and improving mood. A multidisciplinary approach utilizing techniques effective for other types of chronic pain may be useful in addressing the issue of CPP. It is important for the primary care provider to consider the possibility of prior or ongoing abuse or sexual trauma, and adjust interviewing strategies accordingly.

Vulvodynia is vulvar discomfort occurring in the absence of relevant visible infections, inflammatory, neoplastic findings, or a neurologic disorder, again typically requiring gynecology involvement. The pain is usually described as burning and may be provoked by sexual or nonsexual contact or be unprovoked. The pain is more common in women older than 30, menopausal, and Hispanic women. Women with vulvodynia report a substantial negative impact on quality of life. Comorbidities associated with vulvar pain are low back pain, IBS, migraine, and fibromyalgia. It is thought that vulvodynia is a neuropathic pain and pharmacotherapy has been based on this premise. Tricyclic antidepressants and gabapentin have been used although there have been no controlled trials. For the primary care provider, counseling the patient about the disorder and its course, giving emotional support, and facilitating appropriate subspecialist involvement are recommended.

SCREENING & DETECTION OF EATING DISORDERS

Issues Around Food & Eating Disorders

Eating disorders are common and challenging in young women, and the primary care physician plays an important role in their detection (see Chapter 21). The primary care physician also manages the medical complications, determines the need for hospitalization, and coordinates care. In addition, for patients with milder forms of disordered eating who may not be seeing a mental health specialist regularly, the primary care physician may have responsibility for ongoing care, including exacerbations that may mandate coordination with mental health and/or nutritional support. Two groups at high risk for eating disorders are female athletes and females with diabetes.

Binge eating disorder is defined as eating in a discrete period of time, an amount of food that is significantly larger than most people would eat under similar circumstances for at least 2 days per week for 6 months. The binges must have at least three of the following criteria: (a) eating much more rapidly than normal, (b) eating until uncomfortably full, (c) eating large amounts of food when not feeling physically hungry, (d) eating alone because of embarrassment, and (e) feeling disgusted, depressed, or very guilty after overeating. The estimated population prevalence is 2–3% and it is more common in females. Binge eating has been strongly associated with obesity; in one study 25–30% of adults presenting for weight loss treatment qualified for a diagnosis of binge eating disorder, although all the measures were self-report. While many obese patients report binge eating, not all have binge eating disorder. As expected, obesity-related complications are likely to exist, and binge eating disorder may be more common in weight cycling patients. Evidence is limited, but preliminary studies suggest that selective serotonin reuptake inhibitors (SSRIs), antiepileptics, and appetite suppressants may be useful in treatment.

Screening for Eating Disorders

Because many women will not seek care for an eating disorder, the clinician must remain alert for clues, such as amenorrhea, concern about weight loss by a family member, abdominal bloating, and cold intolerance. Questions that are useful in ascertaining eating habits include: "Are you trying to lose weight?" "What did you eat yesterday?" and "Do you ever binge eat (eat more than you want) or use laxatives, diuretics, or diet pills?" Two questions have been shown to be useful in screening for bulimia nervosa in the primary care setting: "Do you ever eat in secret?" and "How satisfied are you with your eating habits?" Another screening tool, the SCOFF Questionnaire, may prove to be useful in screening for eating disorders. The questions include the following: (1) Do you make yourself Sick because you feel uncomfortably full? (2) Do you worry you have lost Control over how much you eat? (3) Have you recently lost more than One stone (14 lb) in a 3-month period? (4) Do you believe yourself to be Fat when others say you are too thin? (5) Would you say Food dominates your life? A "yes" answer to any question is worth one point and a score of two is highly predictive of anorexia nervosa or bulimia nervosa; however, this test has not yet been validated prospectively in a broader population.

Clinicians should remain alert for the possibility of binge eating disorder in obese patients. Questions such as, "Do you ever binge eat? Do you often eat alone? and Do you ever feel guilty or depressed after overeating?" may be useful in detecting this disorder.

Treatment of Eating Disorders: A Framework

The various treatments for eating disorders are described in full in Chapter 20. A theoretical framework for treating patients with eating disorders based on the self-determination theory of behavior change is described below (see Chapter 16). A patient may not be willing to accept full multidisciplinary treatment for an "eating disorder," unless she is intrinsically motivated to do so. The first step in this process may be assessment of her knowledge and education by a primary care provider. She may then agree to work with one member of the treatment team, for example, a nutritionist, without acknowledging that seriously disordered eating is present. Similarly, counseling for developmental or family issues, or treatment for depression, may be acceptable, again without acknowledgment of the presence of an eating disorder or clear interest in changing the behavior. Family counseling may be helpful in limiting pressure from the family. Since the family is extrinsic to her, pressure may be less likely to result in changed behavior than to generate resistance from the patient. A counselor trained in treating adolescents may be able to help the patient navigate some of the peer issues involved in the behavior. Whether or not referral to a nutritionist or psychologist

is accepted, periodic medical visits to follow the presenting symptom(s), for example, amenorrhea, low heart rate, or loss of weight, allow the primary care clinician to monitor the severity of symptoms (particularly cardiac status or other indications for hospitalization) while gently informing a patient of the medical risks of her condition. Evidence of associated medical risks, such as osteopenia, dental erosion in the case of bulimia, or concerns about fertility (particularly when the patient has low weight or is estrogen deficient) may encourage a patient to acknowledge the diagnosis and begin full treatment. Danger signs such as bradycardia and electrolyte disturbances may mandate involuntary hospitalization, which the primary care provider often must initiate.

In summary, the primary care practitioner should be equipped to detect an eating disorder, and then must work as a member of a multidisciplinary team, including a mental health professional and a nutritionist, to ensure that the patient gains weight as appropriate, modifies her eating habits, and receives appropriate psychological and/or medical therapies.

YOUNG ADULTHOOD: LEAVING HOME & PUTTING IT ALL TOGETHER

In this phase of life, one begins to accept financial and emotional self-responsibility, to differentiate from the family of origin, and to develop intimate relationships with peers.

Healthy Behaviors & Health Care Maintenance

Safety in relation to sexuality, substance use, contraception, motor vehicles, and preventive care are ultimately the patient's responsibility, but the physician can play an important role in establishing lifelong healthy habits and collaboration in this realm. The physician who uses gender neutral and nonjudgmental styles of history taking and is alert to patient cues will be more likely to be told about challenges for the patient that may have long-term modifiable consequences such as gender identity issues, substance abuse, unsafe sex, intimate partner violence, eating disorders, and depression. Engaging with patients in partnership works best, allowing them to identify pros and cons of their choices, and reinforcing their ability to make changes if needed. Intrinsic motivation to change and patient belief in ability to make a change are positively associated with successful changes in behavior and maintenance of those changes.

Role of Culture

Identity also includes a patient's determination of her cultural role; if she is African American, a first-generation South Asian immigrant, or a child of fundamentalist

Christians, she will need to establish herself in her family unit and this can impact on her health and illness behavior (see Chapter 12). If, perhaps, she feels great pressure to succeed as an engineer, but prefers to be an artist, this can cause stress-related symptoms and bring her to the health care system. Somatoform behavior and MUS are common across all cultures and may be reinforced in preference to the expression of emotions in some families, masking a mental health disorder.

For women, unique issues regarding culture can relate to appearance and behavior as well. African American women, for example, may feel pressure from the dominant culture regarding slender body weight, but conflict may arise if their internal, sex partner or family value system is concordant with a larger body habitus. Some Asian women are encouraged verbally and through custom to be subservient to men, though this can be manifested to varying degrees, and may or may not result in conflict. Social support may be lacking as they become more acculturated in the United States. Immigrants engaged in a cultural transition process may experience criticism from their older relatives as they assimilate to the new culture, and from their younger relatives as they maintain connection to the culture of origin. Immigrants or people of color may experience pressure to succeed academically and professionally beyond the level of previous generations, or to support others in that process, to the exclusion of their own needs. Also, traditional cultures may promote respect for elders and traditional gender roles, often a family-strengthening behavior, but reinforce secrecy around family violence and abuse. All of these issues may affect women uniquely, in the traditional role in the family and physicians should be alert for clues that problems are occurring. In Ethiopian immigrant families, for example, many non-English speaking women have experienced clitorectomy, a procedure unknown in the United States.

Pregnancy & Infertility: Psychosocial Issues

INFERTILITY

Psychosocial stress is common in individuals struggling with infertility, and may influence the outcomes of infertility treatment as well as the couple's desires about whether or not to continue treatment. Some studies have shown that the prevalence of psychiatric disorders is higher in infertility patients than in a primary care population. Psychosocial stress has also been shown to be stronger in the partner with the infertility problem than in the other partner.

When asking infertility patients about stress, it is important to assess the impact of the infertility on their relationships with their partner, their sexual health, and their social lives. Helpful questions can include: "Do you find that you only make love during the fertile times of your cycle?" "Do you and your partner agree about your plans for infertility treatment?" "Do you feel blamed of at fault for the infertility?" "Do you feel uncomfortable around pregnant women or small children?"

Generally, stress levels tend to increase as treatment becomes more complex. In addition, the psychosocial stress of infertility is a major contributor to many individuals stopping fertility treatments. Some studies have suggested that increased stress may be inversely correlated with the likelihood of subsequent pregnancy.

If psychosocial stress can negatively impact infertility patients, can psychological interventions make a difference? Psychotherapy has been shown to be useful in reducing the associated anxiety and depression, and may be associated with an increase in pregnancy rates. CBT is generally used for patients with infertility and has been associated with an improvement in symptoms. Most cognitive behavioral programs use multiple sessions and often include the partners.

Patients with preexisting anxiety or depression can have worsening symptoms during infertility treatment. Women at high risk for depression or anxiety during infertility treatment include those with a history of psychiatric illness, pregnancy loss, longer duration of infertility and medical diagnoses associated with poorer prognosis for fertility treatment. In addition, many patients discontinue psychotropic medications in anticipation of becoming pregnant, which can worsen symptoms. Women with significant symptoms of anxiety and/or depression should discuss the risks and benefits of psychiatric medications given recent evidence suggesting that SSRIs are associated with increased risk of fetal cardiac defects.

DEPRESSION IN PREGNANCY

Prevalence of major depression during pregnancy has been estimated to be between 3 and 5%. Women with a history of depression are at highest risk. Other risk factors include family history of depression and either discontinuing or decreasing antidepressant medications. The symptoms of depression in pregnancy are the same as in the general population. It is recommended to screen for depression in pregnant women with a standard screening instrument such as the PHQ-9.

TREATMENT OF DEPRESSION IN PREGNANCY

If the person is not suicidal and has mild depression, starting with psychotherapy is recommended. Psychotherapy for depression has been shown to be equally effective as antidepressant medications. Often the focus of psychotherapy in this setting is on the transition to motherhood and the acquisition of the requisite skills.

The decision about prescription of psychotropic medications is complex: the risk of medication exposure to the fetus must be balanced against the risk of untreated depression for the mother, other children in the home and, ultimately, the infant. Decisions about medication include factors such as the severity of the depression, the number of prior depressive episodes, and history of response to medications. Women with major depression who discontinue medications during pregnancy are at a high risk of relapse; the risk is lower in women with milder forms of depression.

The SSRIs and serotonin norepinephrine reuptake inhibitors (SNRIs) are very effective for the treatment of depression during pregnancy and until recently, observational studies had suggested that they were generally safe. Recent studies have suggested that women exposed to paroxetine during pregnancy have an increased risk of fetal cardiovascular malformations. Some other studies have suggested an increased risk of neonatal behavioral issues among women taking SSRIs and SNRIs. These results have appropriately led to more caution in prescribing these drugs. Less evidence is currently available on pregnancy outcomes and bupropion, which is commonly prescribed for depression and smoking cessation, and so it is generally not considered a drug of first choice in pregnancy. Overall, fluoxetine and sertraline are the most studied and have relatively good safety records, and hence, may be the preferred drugs for treatment of depression in pregnant women.

In summary, psychotherapy is recommended as initial treatment in all pregnant women with mild to moderate symptoms of depression. For women with moderate to severe depression, psychotropic medications should be considered and the risks of fetal exposure balanced against the risks of untreated depression.

Postpartum Depression

During the postpartum period, women can experience mood changes, including postpartum blues, postpartum depression, panic disorder, and postpartum psychosis. Although these women are often seen by their obstetricians, primary care clinicians may be seeing these patients and should remain alert for symptoms suggestive of mood disorders.

Postpartum blues are common, occurring within a few days of delivery in 40–80% of women. Postpartum blues often include mood swings, irritability, sadness, and crying spells. The symptoms are generally transient, peaking at about 10 days and resolving within about 10 days. Women with postpartum blues are at an increased risk of developing postpartum depression.

Postpartum depression has been estimated to occur in about 6% of women. The diagnostic criteria are the same as those of major depressive disorder, but the symptoms occur within a month of birth. The biggest risk factor for postpartum depression is a personal history of depression.

Other risk factors include lack of social support, history of miscarriage or other pregnancy loss, not breast-feeding, and family psychiatric history. Some of the symptoms of postpartum depression such as fatigue, sleeping problems, and decreased sexual drive are common symptoms of the immediate postpartum period, making the disorder more difficult to detect. Feeling overwhelmed or guilty, being unable to care for or bond to the baby, or not sleeping even when the baby is sleeping, should all alert the clinician to the possibility of the diagnosis.

The Edinburgh Postnatal Depression Scale has been validated and used in multiple settings to screen for postpartum depression. Other scales such as the Beck Depression Inventory can also be useful in screening for postpartum depression. Clinicians should ask about mood, appetite, sleep, and being overwhelmed during postpartum visits. Women who express thoughts about harming the baby should receive immediate evaluation by a mental health professional. Pediatricians should also remain alert for postpartum depression as they often see the mother most frequently. When evaluating a woman for possible postpartum depression, thyroid disorders should be ruled out as both hypothyroidism and hyperthyroidism are more common in the postpartum period.

Postpartum psychosis is rare, and is associated with an increased risk of infanticide and suicide. Common symptoms include extreme disorganization of thought, bizarre behavior, delusions, and hallucinations. Postpartum psychosis is often a manifestation of bipolar disorder. Women with suspected postpartum psychosis should be emergently evaluated and treated by a psychiatrist.

Treatment of Postpartum Depression

Women with mild to moderate symptoms should be initially treated with nonpharmacologic measures. Promotion of adequate sleep can be very beneficial, as can psychotherapy. CBT, group therapy, and interpersonal therapy have all been shown to be beneficial. Family therapy can also be beneficial.

Few studies have focused on the role of pharmacotherapy specifically in postpartum depression. Antidepressant drugs are generally initiated in the same fashion as in the usual treatment of major depression. An important consideration for postpartum depression is whether or not the woman is breast-feeding.

The SSRIs are the drug of first choice for major depression, given their safety profile and relative low risk of side effects. Although there are limited data about their use in breast-feeding women, there are only few reports of adverse effects. In particular, sertraline and paroxetine seem to be excreted in very low levels into breast milk and therefore, may be better SSRI choices.

As with major depression, it is generally recommended that treatment continue for at least 6 months after full remission. A slow taper of medications is also recommended to avoid the risk of withdrawal and to enable intervention if symptoms recur.

Irritable Bowel Syndrome

Young adult women may present to their physicians with IBS, as it is the most common gastrointestinal disorder seen in primary care. It is characterized by chronic abdominal pain and altered bowel habits in the absence of an organic cause. IBS is estimated to occur in 10–15% of the population with a female predominance of 2:1. Only 15% seek medical care for their condition yet the volume of patients is large and burden to society in health care costs and missed work is significant.

The pathophysiology of IBS remains unknown. It is thought to be a disorder of gastrointestinal motility, dysregulation of the nervous system, and increased visceral sensitivity. Psychosocial stressors have been shown to precipitate and exacerbate symptoms but are not thought to be a cause of the underlying condition. Women who have a history of physical or sexual abuse are more likely than controls to suffer from IBS and other functional bowel disease. Patients with a history of abuse have poorer health outcomes as manifested by an increase in pain, physician visits, and surgical procedures than patients without an abuse history. Although women seeking treatment for IBS are more likely to suffer from depression, anxiety, panic disorder, somatization, or other mental illness, those who do not seek treatment for the symptoms have the same incidence of these problems as the general population. Hence, it is unclear whether psychiatric stressors exacerbate the disease or contribute to the underlying etiology, perhaps varying in different individuals. Other conditions related to IBS include sleep disturbance, depression, and fibromyalgia. Interestingly, health-related quality of life appears to be more related to extraintestinal symptoms rather than traditionally elicited gastrointestinal symptoms in patients with IBS.

Effective treatment for IBS involves an integrated behavioral and pharmacologic stepwise approach individualized to the patient's main symptom. Treatment for mild disease can involve only education, bulking laxatives, and antispasmodics. The tricyclic antidepressants are effective in some patients but can exacerbate constipation. A few studies have shown modest benefit with SSRIs, specifically paroxetine and fluoxetine. Newer treatments include tegaserod and alosetron. CBT has been shown to be helpful in several studies although results are somewhat mixed and effects were short-term in some studies. In the largest trial testing CBT in women, CBT was significantly more effective than education alone. Certain subgroups of IBS sufferers may be especially responsive to CBT. Simple educational interventions designed to help patients learn more about their bodies and IBS can be helpful in reducing anxiety and improving health-related quality of life. However, similar to other disorders overlapping with a history of childhood or adult abuse or sexual trauma, psychiatric comorbidities, or somatization disorder, sensitive communication strategies are crucial.

Premenstrual Syndrome & Premenstrual Dysphoric Disorder

Another condition frequently effecting young adult menstruating women is premenstrual syndrome (PMS), characterized by cyclic occurrences of a variety of somatic, affective, and behavioral symptoms. As many as 150 symptoms have been attributed to PMS but the most common are fatigue, irritability, bloating, anxiety or tension, breast tenderness, mood lability, depression, and food cravings. Symptoms typically occur 7–10 days prior to menses and usually resolve within a few days after the onset. Estimates of the number of women who have PMS are as high as 80%, but those have included all women who have any premenstrual mood or physical symptom. The more severe form of PMS is premenstrual dysphoric disorder (PMDD, also known as late luteal phase dysphoric disorder) and occurs in only 3–8% of women. These women experience symptoms that impair work, school, relationships, or some other aspect of daily living. The diagnostic criteria for PMDD, as classified by the DSM-IV-TR, specifically exclude premenstrual exacerbation of a known underlying psychiatric disorder. Therefore, it is important to evaluate and treat any underlying psychiatric disorder if it is present in this group of patients. The DSM-IV-TR criteria for PMDD require documentation of physical and behavioral symptoms (using diaries) being present for most of the preceding year. Five or more symptoms must have been present during the week prior to menses, resolving within a few days after menses starts. The five symptoms must be one of: (1) sadness, hopelessness, or being self-critical; (2) tension or anxiety; (3) labile mood interspersed with frequent tearfulness; (4) persistent irritability or anger; and (5) increased relational conflicts. Additional emotional symptoms may include: decrease in usual activities, social withdrawal, difficulty concentrating, fatigue, lethargy, changed appetite, possibly associated with binge eating or craving specific foods, hypersomnia or insomnia, or feeling overwhelmed. Physical symptoms can include breast tenderness or swelling, headaches, musculoskeletal pain, feeling bloated, or weight gain.

Because of varied symptoms and overlap with other conditions, a prospective daily symptom scale for PMS can be an important tool in diagnosis. Several calendars have been widely used and validated, including the Calendar of Premenstrual Experiences (COPE), which includes a 4-point Likert scale for each of the 10 most commonly reported physical symptoms and 12 most common behavioral symptoms rated daily throughout the menstrual cycle. A total score on this inventory of less than 40 during days 3–9 of the cycle combined with a score greater than 42 during the last 7 days of the cycle has been shown to be an excellent predictor or women who meet inclusion criteria for PMDD. The timing of the onset of symptoms around the time of ovulation and a symptom-free period are crucial to the diagnosis. The calendar can also be therapeutic to the patient.

Treatment for PMS is approached in a stepwise fashion. For less severe cases, a set of behavioral changes is recommended before pharmacotherapy is begun. Encouraging the patient to exercise regularly, limit salt and caffeine intake, and keep a regular sleep schedule may be beneficial. These recommendations arise from retrospective studies of risk factors for PMS. Calcium at a dosage of 1200 mg daily and vitamin D supplementation are related to lower incidence of PMS symptoms and should be recommended for all women due to other beneficial effects. As mentioned earlier, the prospective daily symptom scale may be therapeutic as it can help the patient identify symptoms and how they relate to the menstrual cycle. This allows her to be proactive in anticipating, managing, and avoiding symptoms. Since stress has been shown to increase symptoms, relaxation exercises, counseling, coping strategies, and psychotherapy may be effective. There is some evidence from controlled trials that women with PMS benefit from individual cognitive therapy or coping skills training.

Most patients with PMDD require pharmacologic therapy for significant improvement. The SSRIs are considered first-line therapy and have been proven effective in multiple studies, for both behavioral and physical symptoms. Fluoxetine is the most studied and is Food and Drug Administration (FDA)-approved for this use, and shows response rates from 60 to 75%. Doses from 20 to 60 mg have been used with the higher doses being no more effective but causing more side effects. Other SSRIs with efficacy are sertraline, paroxetine, and citalopram. More recent studies have shown that SSRIs can be administered continuously through the month, intermittently from ovulation to the onset of menstruation, or semi-intermittently with increased doses in the late luteal phase. The benzodiazepine alprazolam (0.25 mg tid) can be used in the luteal phase to reduce symptoms, but the effect is smaller than with the SSRIs. Patients who do not respond to SSRIs or anxiolytics are candidates for ovulation suppression agents, such as gonadotropin-releasing hormone (GnRH) analogues. Because these agents cause a "chemical menopause," several types of steroid "add-back" regimens have been developed. A meta-analysis of studies using GnRH analogues (e.g., leuprolide) concluded that this treatment is effective for premenstrual symptoms and the add-back therapy reduces side effects without reducing efficacy.

Although oral contraceptives prevent ovulation, hence theoretically improving PMS symptoms, most studies have not shown significant improvement. However, recently, two studies using low-dose estrogen and the progestin, drospirenone, given for 24 days with a 4-day pill-free interval, displayed significant improvement over placebo in mood, physical, and behavioral symptoms. Continuous oral contraceptives have been proposed to improve PMS symptoms by eliminating hormonal fluctuations, but no clinical trials have been published. Other treatments showing some benefit are vitamin B_6 supplementation and spironolactone.

THE MIDDLE YEARS: FAMILY & TRANSITIONS

Women with children negotiate a myriad of changes in themselves, their children, their families of origin, and their committed relationships. In the childbearing years, they need to incorporate the child into a primary relationship. This is mapped upon changes in emotional and physical self, career, and the rest of the family on all sides. This is perhaps, the most profound example of multitasking. As children age, the parent(s) must accommodate varying tasks in the children's lives, helping them with their transitions, as the parents, sometimes paradoxically, achieve their own. Simultaneously, as their parents, parents-in-law, and other older relatives age, women are the most likely ones to care for all these relatives. Expected physiologic changes or unexpected illness further impact women in these years. It is imperative that primary care providers anticipate these developmental processes and incorporate them into their approach to these patients. For women who do not have children, many of the same developmental processes occur, as they have to do with maturation as well.

Menopause: Managing Symptoms

Personal, cultural, and family attitudes can have a large effect on the emotional and functional impact of menopausal symptoms. A biopsychosocial approach, which includes inquiring about the impact of these developmental processes, and whether symptoms can be managed without medication is crucial. Since publication of the results of the Women's Health Initiative, which showed increased risk of breast cancer and cardiovascular disease associated with use of estrogen/progestin, many women and their physicians are reluctant to use hormone therapy for treatment of menopausal symptoms. Use of systemic estrogen, and progesterone if the woman has a uterus, is a personal decision that many choose after trials of other therapies and assessment of the risks and benefits. The primary care provider can help women patients sort through the multitude of options to make their own best decisions. Comorbidities such as family history of breast cancer, use of cigarettes, cardiac risk factors, and personal or family history of thromboembolic disease may impact on this decision.

The average age of menopause in the United States is 51. More than 50% of postmenopausal women experience "hot flashes," a manifestation of vasomotor instability associated with the abrupt withdrawal of estrogen. Hot flashes, also known as hot flushes, are sensations of feeling warm, frequently associated with perspiration, palpitations, and anxiety. When they occur at night, they can be manifested by night sweats, frequent awakening and consequently, sleep disturbance.

Another important menopausal symptom is urogenital atrophy. The loss of estrogen causes thinning of the vaginal epithelium and may lead to vaginal irritation, dyspareunia, and increased risk of vaginal infections. When the urethra is affected, urinary frequency, incontinence, and bladder irritation or infection can also occur.

Treatment of Vasomotor Instability

Determining the efficacy of treatments for vasomotor instability is challenging, as about 30% of women will respond to placebo (Table 13-1). However, estrogen has been shown to be most effective in reducing the frequency of hot flashes, associated with an 80% reduction in hot flash frequency.

Nonestrogen therapies that have been used for vasomotor symptoms include SSRIs, SNRIs, high-dose progestins, clonidine, gabapentin, and several complementary therapies.

At least 10 trials have evaluated antidepressants (SSRIs and SNRIs) in the treatment of postmenopausal hot flashes. Several of the early trials were on women with breast cancer, although several more recent trials also included women without breast cancer. Drugs that have been found to be effective include venlafaxine

Table 13-1. Alternatives for treatment of hot flashes.

Treatment	% Reduction in Hot flashes
Estrogen	80%
SSRIs/SNRIs	60%
Megace	0–50%
Clonidine	40%
Phytoestrogens	30–40%
Placebo	20–30%

(a SNRI) and paroxetine (a SSRI), generally associated with about 60% reduction in hot flash frequency.

High-dose progestins (megestrol acetate or Megace) have been associated with about a 50–60% reduction in hot flashes, although prolonged therapy can be associated with weight gain.

Clonidine has been studied in at least 10 trials and has been associated with about a 40% reduction in hot flashes. Clonidine is usually given transdermally for this indication, although can be given orally. Side effects such as dry mouth and dizziness often limit its use. Gabapentin has also been associated with a reduction in hot flash frequency. In one study, a dose of 600 mg a day was associated with a reduction in hot flash frequency of about 30–45%.

Several complementary and alternative therapies have been used for treating hot flashes, although the trials are often small, short in duration, and lack a placebo arm. In addition, the dose of the supplements often varies among studies. Isoflavones are contained in soy products and red clover, and have been frequently used for the treatment of menopausal symptoms; however, studies have yielded mixed results. Recent meta-analyses have not shown a significant effect of either red clover or soy isoflavones. Several herbal remedies have been promoted for hot flash reduction. Although evidence is limited, black cohosh may be associated with reduction in hot flashes. In another study, vitamin E was associated with reduction in hot flashes that was statistically, but not clinically, significant. Herbal remedies that have been used but do not have proven efficacy include wild yams, natural progesterone cream, ginseng, dong quai, and evening primrose oil.

Many women go through menopause without medications, using behavioral strategies such as exercise, hydration, wearing layered loosely fitting clothes, and short daytime naps to compensate for hot flash-interrupted sleep. It is important for primary care providers to establish a collaborative relationship with patients, allowing them to discuss issues that may compound menopausal symptoms. Normalizing these sometimes stressful transitions may help a woman to accept a trial of watchful waiting or even psychotherapy to address the stress of these changes. Discussion of menopausal symptoms may not necessarily be a request for medications, but should trigger discussions about the variety of available management strategies.

Treatment of Urogenital Atrophy

Oral estrogen therapy is quite effective for urogenital atrophy, although it is currently being used less frequently because of the above-noted issues. The mainstays of treatment are currently vaginal moisturizers and vaginal estrogen therapy.

Regular use of vaginal moisturizers and use of lubricants during intercourse can be beneficial. Topical estrogen can be quite helpful and results in higher concentrations than can be found when administered systemically, causing a minimum effect on serum estradiol levels. Estrogen cream (conjugated or synthetic) can be given in a low dose (e.g., 0.3 mg of conjugated estrogen or 0.5 mg of synthetic estrogen) every night for 3 weeks and twice a week thereafter. An alternative mode of administration is an estrogen ring inserted into the vagina (Estring), which secretes a small amount of estrogen into the vagina daily.

Maintaining Sexual Function

It is important for physicians to inquire about sexual function; a national study of 1749 women and 1410 men aged 18–59 years found a prevalence of sexual dysfunction for women of 43%. Sexual function in women is both emotional and physical. As some women age, they experience a liberation from the responsibilities of young children, relationship struggles, and financial concerns that allows them to enjoy sex more than they ever have. This may also be due, in part, to a relative rise in testosterone, as estrogen levels decrease, that improves sexual function in some women. Others experience physiologic changes described above that diminish sexual function, such as urogenital atrophy or sleeplessness from hot flashes. Expectations may be different between a male and female in a couple, especially if a male is able to treat erectile dysfunction medically. Besides lubrication, women can be advised to try a slower pace of sexual activity, as it is normal for reaction time to diminish with age in both genders. If estrogen is used to treat vasomotor symptoms of menopause, the relative drop in testosterone can diminish sexual drive or function in some women and that subgroup of patients may benefit from the addition of small amounts of testosterone. An internist or family physician may defer prescription of these medications to a gynecologist or endocrinologist, but should be familiar with the physiology and be able to make recommendations accordingly.

WOMEN IN LATER LIFE: SHIFTING ROLES & OPPORTUNITIES

Women in their later years are achieving the tasks of shifting generational roles and changes in couple and family functioning. Challenges may include: loss of spouse, family members, and friends, along with physiologic aging and financial concerns. Opportunities exist, however, for life review and integration, along with time for new friendships and activities. Additionally, a woman may enjoy being appreciated for her wisdom, without many of the burdensome responsibilities of younger years. A primary care provider should be prepared to assist in these challenges and supportive of the opportunities.

Osteoporosis & Falls

Both osteoporosis and falls are more common in older women than men. More than half of all women will develop osteoporosis by age 80. Fractures are 2.2 times higher in women over 65 than men. Women appear to recover more slowly from these injuries, which may contribute to increased medical costs for falls in women. Hence, prevention of falls is an important issue for older women and has several behavioral components. Interventions shown to reduce falls include: muscle strengthening and balance retraining, multidisciplinary health and environmental risk factor screening and intervention programs, group exercise with tai chi, home hazard assessment, and withdrawal of psychotropic medications.

Fear of falling can significantly impact an older woman's life by inhibiting activities, leading to a loss of independence. In one survey, 80% of women answered that they would rather be dead than experience the loss of independence and quality of life that results from a bad hip fracture and subsequent admission to a nursing home. Clinicians caring for older women should address this fear and consider interventions. Some of the same activities that reduce incidence of falls can reduce fear of falling. These include tai chi and strength training.

Urinary Incontinence

Although urinary incontinence affects men, prevalence is higher in women, increasing with age, with up to 50% of elderly women reporting some incontinence. Daily incontinence occurs in 21% of community-dwelling women aged 85 or older. Many women do not tell their health care provider about their situation and just try to live with it. The psychological morbidity from this "hidden" problem can be high. Problems may include social withdrawal, depression, and sexual dysfunction. Urinary incontinence can significantly affect the quality of life of older women, but this is quite variable. The clinician can uncover these problems with thorough history taking.

Several behavioral treatments have been found helpful in urinary incontinence. For stress incontinence, avoiding overfilling of the bladder and regular muscle contraction (Kegel) exercises are beneficial. In urge incontinence, bladder retraining in cognitively intact women can decrease episodes of incontinence by 50%. Biofeedback has also proven to be effective for some women and was shown in one study to be more effective than traditional pharmacotherapy. In cognitively impaired women, prompted voiding by a caregiver can reduce incontinent episodes.

A wide array of medical treatments exists for the treatment of urinary incontinence. The primary care physician should be well versed in these treatments but should also be aware that they can be used in conjunction with behavioral treatments.

Cognitive Dysfunction

Cognitive dysfunction, including mild cognitive impairment and the dementias, is a major issue facing older women, with up to 10% of people over 65 and 50% of those over 85 having Alzheimer's dementia. Women appear to be at higher risk of developing dementia and, because of women's longer life span, there are many more older women suffering dementia than men. Prevention of dementia would be optimal in reducing the burden of this disease and many of the prevention strategies involve behavioral approaches. Risk factors for dementia include hyperlipidemia, diabetes, hypertension, low levels of physical activity, low levels of mental activity, and poor social network. Older women should be encouraged to adopt a "brain-healthy" diet, which includes a decrease in overall fat and an increase in foods high in monounsaturated fats and antioxidants (fruits, vegetables, nuts, and cold-water fish). They should also maintain a healthy weight, get regular physical activity, participate in social activities, and exercise the mind (learn new things, read, play games, crossword puzzles, and so forth).

The role estrogen plays in cognitive dysfunction in women has been a hot topic of study over the last several years. A biological basis exists for the relationship of cognition and estrogen. For this reason, it has been hypothesized that hormone replacement therapy (HRT) after menopause would help decrease the risk of cognitive dysfunction and dementia. Several prospective population cohort studies found fewer declines in cognitive function in women taking HRT. Earlier small clinical trials have shown some cognitive improvement in women taking HRT, but the more recent and much larger Women's Health Initiative actually showed an increase in cognitive decline in some groups taking HRT, both estrogen-alone and estrogen-progestin groups. As this study started several years after menopause for most of the participants, no conclusions regarding early postmenopausal therapy can be made. Using current evidence, HRT should not be prescribed for the sole purpose of preserving cognition.

SUMMARY

There are a number of behavioral issues in the care of women by the primary care provider and these should be integrated into preventive care and management of medical issues from a biopsychosocial perspective. Although the developmental stages women experience include challenges, there are also opportunities for fulfillment both for the patients and those who care for them.

SUGGESTED READINGS

Alan Guttmacher Institute: *Sex and America's Teenagers.* New York, NY: Alan Guttmacher Institute, 1994.

American College of Obstetrics and Gynecology: ACOG Practice Bulletin No. 51. Chronic pelvic pain. *Obstet Gynecol* 2004; 103:589–605.

American Psychiatric Association. *Diagnostic and Statistical Manual of Mental Disorders,* 4th ed. Washington, DC: American Psychiatric Association, 1994.

Basson R. Women's sexual dysfunction: revised and expanded definitions. *CMAJ* 2005;172:1327–1333.

Carter B, McGoldrick M. *The Changing Life Cycle: A Framework for Family Therapy.* Needham Heights, MA: Allyn and Bacon, 1989.

Chatzisarantis NLD, Hagger MS, Biddle SJH, et al. The cognitive processes by which perceived locus of causality predicts participation in physical activity. *J Health Psychol* 2002;7: 685–699.

Domar AD, Broome A, Zuttermeister PC, et al. The prevalence and predictability of depression in infertile women. *Fertil Steril* 1992;58(6):1158–1163.

Grady D. Postmenopausal hormones-therapy for symptoms only. *N Engl J Med* 2003;348(19):1835–1837.

Grady-Weliky TA. Premenstrual dysphoric disorder. *N Engl J Med* 2003;348:433–438.

Hendrick V, Altshuler L. Management of major depression during pregnancy. *Am J Psychiatry* 2002;159(10):1667–1673.

Holroyd-Leduc JM, Straus SM. Management of urinary incontinence in women: scientific review. *JAMA* 2004;291: 986–995.

Leserman J, Zolnoun D, Meltzer-Brody S, et al. Identification of diagnostic subtypes of chronic pelvic pain and how subtypes differ in health status and trauma history. *Am J Obstet Gynecol* 2006;195:554–560.

Morgan JF, Reid F, Lacey JH. The SCOFF questionnaire: assessment of a new screening tool for eating disorders. *BMJ* 1999;319(7223):1467–1468.

Murray L, Carothers AD. The validation of the Edinburgh Postnatal Depression Scale on a community sample. *Br J Psychiatry* 1990;157:288–290.

Nelson HD, Vesco KK, Haney E, et al. Nonhormonal therapies for menopausal hot flashes: systematic review and meta-analysis. *JAMA* 2006;295(17):2057–2071.

Steiner M, Pearlstein T, Cohen LS, et al. Expert guidelines for the treatment of severe PMS, PMDD, and comorbidities: the role of SSRIs. *J Womens Health* (Larchmt) 2006;15: 57–69.

Walsh JME, Wheat ME, Freund K. Detection, evaluation and treatment of eating disorders: the role of the primary care physician. *J Gen Intern Med* 2000;15(8): 577–590.

Wisner WL, Parry BL, Piontek CM. Clinical practice. Postpartum depression. *N Engl J Med* 2002;347(3):194–199.

Lesbian, Gay, Bisexual, & Transgender (LGBT) Patients

14

Donald W. Brady, MD FAACH, Jason Schneider, MD, & Jocelyn C. White, MD, FACP

INTRODUCTION

Lesbian, gay, bisexual, and transgender (LGBT) people have become more openly accepted into the framework of society. Likewise, the medical literature has expanded its discussion of the health needs of LGBT people, though often addressing the issues from a strictly sexual behavior perspective (e.g., "men who have sex with men"). Specific knowledge and skills are essential for the health care provider to be able to ascertain the sexual orientation of patients; communicate acceptance and understanding of LGBT health issues; screen for conditions amenable to behavioral medicine; and provide information and resources specific to the needs of LGBT patients. Providers can use these skills to provide access to competent medical care for LGBT patients.

Lesbians and gay men make up anywhere from 1 to 10% of the general population—depending on the source quoted and the sampling method used in the study. In most studies, self-identified bisexuals are a small fraction of the lesbian or gay population. Whatever the exact percentage, however, in absolute terms, LGBT persons constitute a significant group of patients with unique medical, psychological, and social needs. Many primary care providers care for LGBT patients without being aware of the patients' sexual orientation or gender identity and are therefore unable to recognize or acknowledge their unique needs.

DEFINITIONS & CONCEPTS

Sexual Orientation, Sexual Behavior, & Identity

Sexual orientation refers to sexual attraction to another person, including fantasies and the desire for sex, affection, and love. Sexual orientation is distinct from and not necessarily predictive of sexual behavior or activities. Being gay, lesbian, or bisexual assumes awareness of this sexual attraction to people of the same gender or both genders, respectively, and development of an identity based on this awareness. This identity is formed by emotions, psychological responses, societal expectations, individual choices, and cultural influences. Most lesbians and gay men prefer the terms *lesbian* and *gay*, because such terms incorporate emotions, behavior, and a cultural system, as well as sexual orientation. Compared to the term *homosexual*, often interpreted as more clinical and sometimes pejorative, *gay* and *lesbian* are viewed as nonjudgmental.

Sexual orientation, sexual behavior, and identity are interrelated but function independently. Most self-identified lesbians and gay men are sexually active with a partner of their own gender. However, despite this identity, some lesbians and gay men are celibate or have sexual partners of the opposite gender. In fact, most lesbians have had at least one sexual experience with a man, but would not self-identify as bisexual. On the other hand, some men and women who identify as bisexual enter into and codify long-term relationships with a partner of the opposite gender while maintaining sexual relationships with partners of the same gender. Because of the variable relationship between orientation, behavior, and identity, physicians must remain sensitive, open-minded, and nonjudgmental (see "Doctor–Patient Interactions," below).

Race and ethnicity have a strong influence on sexual identity and behavior. "Down low," a popular term coined in African American hip-hop culture, refers to nondisclosure of same-sex sexual behavior among men who identify as heterosexual. Sexual behavior in conflict with sexual identity is not unique to African American men. Men and women from racial and ethnic minority communities are less likely to identify as gay, lesbian, or bisexual because of the complex interactions of homophobia (see "Homophobia and Transphobia," below), religious institutions and influences, and cultural norms. As an example, the concept of *machismo* or masculinity is highly valued in Latino culture. A gay male Latino identity runs counter to this norm.

Gender Identity, Gender Expression, & Gender Roles

Gender identity refers to the deep-seated beliefs, emotions, and thoughts that create the self-perception of being male or female. A person is considered transgender when gender identity conflicts with physical sexual characteristics or manifestations. Gender expression is the behavioral manifestation of gender identity. Toddlers and school-age children often engage in sex-discordant gender expression normally. In transgender individuals, this conflict between sex and gender is pervasive and long-lasting. Although the current edition of the Diagnostic and Statistical Manual defines transgender as a "gender identity disorder," most transgender individuals do not view themselves as manifestations of a pathologic state.

The gender expression and roles that transgender people exhibit vary widely, influenced by personal preference and access to health care resources. Some transgender men and women may only desire an outward physical appearance (e.g., hair style, cosmetics, clothing) consistent with their identity. Others may seek cosmetic and/or full sex reassignment surgery. Many transgender individuals interact with the health care system actively in transition from one gender to another.

The spectrum of gender identity is distinct from sexual orientation and identity. A transgender person can have either same-gender sexual attraction, opposite-gender sexual attraction, or both. Regardless of the gender of sexual partners, transgender individuals do not necessarily identify as gay, lesbian, or bisexual.

Homophobia & Transphobia

Homophobia is defined as an irrational fear of or prejudice against gay men, lesbians, and bisexuals. Transphobia is a more recent term reflecting a similar fear or prejudice against transgender individuals. In daily life, LGBT individuals experience homophobia and transphobia as interpersonal, workplace, societal, or political bias. In other words, homophobia and transphobia reflect prejudice or hatred based solely on perceptions of sexual orientation and gender identity. LGBT people often find it difficult to act in accordance with their identity for fear of bias, discrimination, or violence.

The stigma that accompanies attitudes of homophobia and transphobia contributes to chronic stress and negative health outcomes for LGBT persons. Societal discrimination both creates a disparity in social support and resources and limits access to appropriate health care resources. Internalized homophobia (i.e., self-hatred) and self-concealment can create adverse mental health outcomes. Conversely, disclosure of LGBT identity often leads to better psychological adjustment. However, if self-disclosure by an LGBT individual is not supported, it can lead to its own stressor and risk behaviors (see "Coming Out," below).

Provider Bias

LGBT patients frequently report detrimental experiences with health care providers. In a survey of its members, the Gay and Lesbian Medical Association reported that greater than 50% of respondents were aware of substandard care delivery because of a patient's sexual orientation. In a 1998 survey of nursing students, 8–12% of those responding "despised" gays and lesbians. Several studies document negative reactions after patients self-disclose their identity to a provider.

Each negative experience with a health care provider decreases the likelihood that LGBT patients will continue to seek health care. Providers must work to overcome judgmental attitudes and biases toward LGBT patients. The *Code of Ethics* of the American Medical Association states that professional obligation limits a physician's prerogative to choose whether to enter into a relationship with a patient, in that "physicians cannot refuse to care for patients based on race, gender, [or] sexual orientation . . . " Health care providers must recognize that patients of all orientations and identities are likely to be encountered in the daily practice of medicine (see "Doctor–Patient Interactions," below).

DOCTOR–PATIENT INTERACTIONS

The doctor–patient relationship is the key to providing competent and respectful care to LGBT patients. Without a good provider–patient relationship, patients may avoid medical care and providers who are uncomfortable working with LGBT patients, or who fail to recognize the sexual orientation of a patient, will not provide quality care. Patients who do not obtain competent primary care services, including screening and health-risk and psychosocial counseling, are likely to have a lower health status than their heterosexual counterparts. Providers can develop a good relationship with LGBT patients by showing an understanding of their health needs and communicating a nonjudgmental attitude.

 CASE ILLUSTRATION 1

Robert, a middle-aged high school teacher, comes to the doctor's office. This is his first visit, and he hasn't completed the intake history form. After the introductions, the physician looks at the form and prepares to take a social history.

Overcoming Barriers to Communication

Many LGBT persons are reluctant to share their sexual orientation with health care providers for fear of negative judgments and homophobic responses. Some fail to share this information even when asked directly. Unpleasant experiences with health care providers have made LGBT people more likely to avoid health care and routine screening. Even sympathetic health care providers are often uncomfortable with the interaction. They may lack experience with LGBT health issues or feel unsure as to what language to use to elicit information respectfully from these patients. When both patient and provider are uncomfortable, important information is not shared.

THE SEXUAL HISTORY

Gathering information about a patient's sexual orientation or sexual practices is often a challenge for health care providers. Asking about orientation only while taking a sexual history and not at other times can limit the opportunity to learn important details about the patient. The initial focus should be on sexual behavior, not identity, as many people with same-sex partners do not identify as gay or lesbian. In addition, the most commonly used questions set up barriers between the provider and patient and can lead to inaccurate or incomplete information: "What form of birth control do you use?" "Are you married, single, widowed, or divorced?" "When was the last time you had intercourse?" When LGBT individuals hear these questions, they may not know how to answer because these questions are based on the assumption that the patient is heterosexual. Because the options given do not necessarily pertain to them, the patient must either provide false information or awkwardly stop and explain. Needing to give such explanations can make obtaining an already challenging sexual history even more difficult for both parties. To avoid this awkwardness, patients may play along with the assumption of heterosexuality, which may negatively impact their health care.

THE SOCIAL HISTORY

This may be a more comfortable part of the interview in which to raise issues of sexual orientation. By asking questions that do not have heterosexual assumptions, the provider can increase the opportunities for, and comfort level in, discussing these issues. Providers learn about the patient's family structure, any stressors the patient might have, and personal and community resources on which patients would be likely to draw.

SENSITIVE COMMUNICATION

Sensitive questions make no assumptions about sexual orientation and are easily phrased: "Are you single, partnered, married, widowed, or divorced?" "Who is in your immediate family?" "Over your lifetime, have your sexual partners been men, women, or both?" "If you become ill, is there someone important whom I should involve in your care?" "How do you feel about my documenting your sexual orientation on the chart?" "What percentage of the time do you use safer sex?" Transgender individuals very early in a transition to another gender may have an appearance that is discordant from the intended gender. Others may have not yet changed the assigned sex or name on legal documents or the medical record. It is perfectly acceptable to inquire about the preferred use of personal pronouns: "What name do you prefer? Would you prefer I address you as he or she?"

Because LGBT people come in all shapes, sizes, ages, and colors, providers need to use questions such as these with all men and women, not just those they suspect of being LGBT.

In the initial visit with the patient, it is important to discuss explicitly the documentation of sexual orientation in the chart. Many LGBT persons keep their sexual orientation hidden for legal, employment, or child-custody reasons. When an LGBT patient does not want sexual orientation documented, a coded entry can be used. The code serves to remind providers of the patient's sexual orientation for medical purposes but will prevent inadvertent breaches of confidentiality.

 CASE ILLUSTRATION 1 (CONTD.)

The doctor starts the social history:

Doctor: *Are you single, partnered, married, widowed, or divorced?*

Robert: *I'm divorced, with a 20-year-old son, and I'm partnered now. His name is Tim.*

Doctor: *How long have you been together? How's the relationship?*

Robert: *Six years, and there's some tension now.*

Further questioning reveals that Tim is younger than Robert—and openly gay. Robert is uncomfortable being that open; he is afraid of a scandal at school and the loss of his job. As the history taking continues, the physician asks how Robert feels about having the fact that he is gay documented in the chart. After some discussion, the two decide on a coded entry of the information. At the end of the visit, Robert thanks the doctor for being so understanding; the doctor is also happy with the visit because he has been able to screen the patient appropriately and provide him with his first physical examination in 6 years.

Enhancing the Relationship

Providers who show a nonjudgmental attitude are much more likely to develop trusting relationships with gay and lesbian patients. Providers can improve the relationship in several simple ways: offering to include a partner in the discussions, ensuring that an LGBT patient's partner is treated as a spouse in the office and the hospital, including partners in discussions of next-of-kin policies and advance directives, and using office and hospital forms with words that do not assume a heterosexual family structure.

LESBIAN, GAY, BISEXUAL, AND TRANSGENDER PROVIDERS

Lesbian, gay, bisexual, and transgender patients often prefer working with LGBT health care providers because of the presumed absence of homophobia in the relationship. LGBT providers, however, train in the same settings as their heterosexual counterparts and, thus, may have learned communication skills without recognizing heterosexual bias. Gradually, more information is emerging about lesbian and gay health issues (though not as much about bisexual or transgender issues) and new language habits for bias-free communication is being disseminated.

Lesbian and gay providers may find themselves in a situation in which the question of whether to disclose their own sexual orientation to their patients arises. The question the providers should ask themselves is whether disclosure of sexual orientation is in the best interest of the patient. In many cases, such disclosure may be beneficial. When a patient clearly needs to understand that there will be no overt homophobia in the interaction before agreeing to remain in care, it may be reassuring to know that the provider is LGBT. As patient–provider relationships develop, patients often want more personal information about the provider. LGBT providers must weigh for themselves the therapeutic benefit to the patient, the patient's need for information, and their own level of comfort in self-disclosure. Although many LGBT physicians have reported ostracism, harassment, and professional discrimination from colleagues, teachers, administrators, and health plans, others report being open about their sexual orientation without experiencing any negative consequences.

COMING OUT

The process of discovering one's sexual orientation and/or gender identity and revealing it to others is known as *coming out* and can occur at any age. Stage theories for coming out have been well described and have been summarized as a four-step process:

1. Awareness of homosexual and/or transgender feelings
2. Testing and exploration
3. Identity acceptance
4. Identity integration and self-disclosure

Recent research suggests that there may be different sequences of coming out for younger and older individuals, with individuals who come out in adolescence often identifying and disclosing themselves as homosexual prior to any consensual sexual experiences. The process of coming out involves a shift in core identity that can be associated with significant emotional distress, especially if family and peers respond negatively. Prevailing social attitudes also influence the experience. Most often, individuals come out to other people in person, but some may choose to come out initially through virtual arenas, a process with its own potentially complicating factors, including issues of privacy or unintended disclosure to other individuals. Societal and internalized homophobia often causes lesbians, gay men, and bisexual individuals to perform a fatiguing "cost–benefit" analysis for each situation in which they consider coming out. This process can be even more taxing for transgender persons as each situation may involve issues of both orientation and gender identity. Data show that women who have children before coming out are slower in reaching developmental milestones in this process than either women without children or women who have children after coming out. If the costs of self-disclosure are repeatedly high, an individual may ultimately become socially isolated or revert to denying their LGBT identity. On the other hand, disclosing at work and working for more gay-supportive organizations correlates with higher job satisfaction and lower anxiety at work.

ADOLESCENTS

Lesbian, gay, bisexual, and transgender adolescents are particularly vulnerable to the emotional distress of coming out, and this distress can make adolescent development even more difficult (see Chapter 10). Adolescents who self-identify as homosexual prior to consensual sexual experiences may have a more rapid progression through the coming out stages, have fewer or no heterosexual encounters, and may engage in less risky sexual experiences. Cultural factors, such as race and ethnicity, do not seem to hamper the formation of identity but may delay identity integration. Parental acceptance of the adolescent during the coming out process may be the primary determinant of healthy self-esteem. Primary care providers need to screen for signs of sexual-orientation confusion in their adolescent patients. These signs may include depression, diminished school performance, alcohol and substance abuse, acting out, and suicidal ideation. Providers noting these signs need to consider sexual-orientation confusion in the differential diagnosis, along with depression and substance abuse. Providers also need to be willing to discuss sexual orientation with their adolescent patients, as their attempts to discuss same-sex attractions and homosexual orientations may be the patients' first disclosure of these feelings. If providers meet such reaching out with reticence, dismay, or contempt, then adolescents may be less likely to share their feelings with others and either revert to denial or engage in more covert, risky behaviors.

OLDER ADULTS

Coming out can occur at any age. Because there are varying degrees of disclosure, older individuals may be "out" to themselves and a partner or close friends but no one else beyond that trusted circle. Older gay, lesbian, or bisexual individuals are vulnerable to social isolation, and primary care providers are often among the primary support resources for older individuals. Older homosexual individuals are more likely to engage in same-sex sexual experiences prior to self-identifying as gay or lesbian than adolescents, and thus may be at greater risk for adverse health consequences because of risky sexual behavior. In exploring the social support network for their older patients, primary care providers need to be alert to the possibility of a lesbian or gay identity and the needs this engenders.

RELATIONSHIPS

Community

Many LGBT individuals experience support and nurturing from their biological families after coming out to them. For others, the support network of LGBT individuals may not include their biologic family, as many families do not accept the sexual orientation or gender identity of the individual. In either situation, partners, friends, and community organizations can serve as an extended family. Primary care providers should be aware of a few useful resources to which they can direct patients (some resources are listed at the end of this chapter). LGBT people in rural or suburban geographic areas may have difficulty in accessing community-based support networks available in urban environments. In a study focused on men who have sex with men (MSM), those outside concentrated urban areas were less likely to identify as gay, be in a long-term relationship, be involved in a gay community, and were more likely to be out to a smaller number of people. In rural areas, a caring, open-minded physician may be an especially important source of support for LGBT patients.

Partners

Like most heterosexuals, the majority of LGBT people express a desire to find a partner and develop a relationship. And like heterosexuals, LGBT people can form and maintain long-lasting relationships. LGBT couples have commitment ceremonies and get married (in some localities), own homes together, share finances, and raise children. Physicians should be aware of local, state, and federal laws that allow LGBT individuals to codify their relationships with partners and children, ensure health care and retirement benefits, document advance directives, and secure inheritance rights.

Because of potential isolation from family, coworkers, and religious organizations, the relationship with a partner can be particularly important to a LGBT individual's well-being. As a result, discord in the relationship may be even more stressful than it might be for a heterosexual couple. In times of relationship stress, an individual may have limited resources for help in coping. Primary care providers should screen for such stressors and be able to provide appropriate referrals for individual and couples therapy.

Parenthood

Parenthood plays a role in the lives of many LGBT people, and the decision to become parents is usually deliberate and carefully made. LGBT individuals or couples may have children from previous heterosexual relationships or through adoption, artificial insemination, in vitro fertilization and surrogacy, heterosexual intercourse, or by serving as foster parents. Dual gay and lesbian couples raising children together is becoming more common.

Studies of the attitudes of gay and lesbian couples toward parenting find more similarities than differences compared to heterosexual couples. Children of gay or lesbian parents are no more likely to be gay or lesbian or to have gender identity confusion than the general population. Current evidence indicates that children of gays or lesbians develop normally and fare better in relationships where parents share responsibilities equally and have a low level of interpersonal conflict. Though they may face additional stigma in the school or community, children of gay or lesbian parents, like all children, are resilient and cope well with this challenge. Many professional medical associations, including the American Academy of Pediatrics and American Medical Association, have policies supporting same-sex coparent adoption.

Loss

GRIEF

Grieving the loss of a partner may be more difficult for a lesbian or gay man if a support system is not available. Gay men and lesbians have been particularly affected by the deaths of partners and many friends from AIDS. When a partner dies, the survivor, in effect, loses a spouse. This fact often goes unrecognized in the survivor's own social network. Frequently, the family of the deceased partner excludes the survivor or will not allow him or her to take part as a spouse in the funeral. A close-knit network of surviving friends is often neglected when a grieving family takes over funeral plans.

Occasionally, parents and family of the deceased are shocked and embarrassed to learn of the individual's sexual orientation or gender identity. In such cases, the family may feel intense guilt or the need to hide their grief, unable to share it with their support network because of embarrassment. Family members of gay or lesbian individuals can find information and support for this and other issues by contacting Parents and Friends of Lesbians and Gays, a national organization with local chapters (see the list of resources at the end of this chapter).

Primary care providers can assist surviving partners and friends in the grieving process in several ways. Providers can assist the survivor in talking about the loss and expressing his or her feelings, identify and interpret normal grieving behavior and timelines, provide ongoing support throughout the grief process, encourage the survivor to develop new relationships and support structures, and help the survivor adapt to new roles and patterns of living. In some cases, the health care provider may be the only individual in whom the survivor can confide.

ADVANCE DIRECTIVES

The durable power of attorney for health care is particularly important for lesbians and gay men. Because many are unable to marry legally, LGBT individuals need to execute these documents to appoint their partners as surrogate health decision makers. Without such a document, the next of kin is considered the surrogate decision maker. Completing this document is the best way to avoid tragic decision-making conflicts between a partner and the estranged family members of seriously ill patients in time of crisis. As with all patients, a discussion of advance directives should be included in the preventive medicine check-up (see Chapter 37).

CLINICAL ISSUES

The American Psychiatric Association removed homosexuality from its list of mental disorders in 1973. Psychiatric and behavioral interventions, like reparative therapy, used to "cure" patients of homosexuality have proven neither effective nor necessary. Nonetheless, primary care providers must be aware of the unique psychosocial issues that face many LGBT people.

Depression & Suicide

Multiple studies indicate a higher prevalence of depression among both gay men and lesbians. Higher rates of suicidal behavior are also evident compared to the general population, though the prevalence is equivalent between gay men and lesbians. Lesbians are four times more likely to report suicidal ideation than heterosexual women, and gay men are six times more likely to attempt suicide than heterosexual males.

Adolescents are particularly vulnerable to depression and suicide. One report suggests that approximately one-third of gay or lesbian adolescents will attempt suicide. Much of the literature on this topic, however, comes from surveys of self-reported behavior subject to report bias. Whatever the exact prevalence of suicidality, gay, lesbian, and transgender youth face additional risk of suicide related to coming out early, rejection by family members, rejection by religious institutions, interpersonal violence, and additional levels of marginalization (e.g., homelessness, racial and ethnic minority status).

Smoking

LGBT populations have a 1.6 times higher prevalence of smoking compared to heterosexual populations. The Women's Health Initiative survey data documented a 10–14.4% prevalence among lesbian respondents, compared to 7.2% among heterosexual counterparts. The Urban Men's Health Study data indicate a 31.4% prevalence of smoking among MSM. Theories supporting the increased rates of smoking among these groups include higher levels of stress secondary to homophobia and discrimination, bars as a frequent social focus, potentially higher rates of associated drug and alcohol use, and targeted advertising by cigarette manufacturers. As with any group of patients, asking about tobacco product use is a vital part of the social history for LGBT individuals.

Substance Abuse

Inquiring about drug and alcohol use is also important for LGBT patients (see Chapter 21). A provider should specifically explore the type of substances, the frequency and quantity, and whether patients use them during or preceding sexual activity. Many substances have a disinhibiting effect on the user and may make individuals more likely to engage in unsafe sex practices. In a multivariate analysis of drug use among men who have sex with men, amyl nitrate ("poppers"), crystal methamphetamine ("crystal meth"), cocaine, and heavy alcohol use were all associated with unprotected anal intercourse, independent of partner-specific variables. Similar to many other populations, crystal meth, with its highly addictive potential, has had a profound impact on many gay men. There is a strong association between crystal meth use and prolonged, unprotected sexual activity. Although drug and alcohol use is an important issue for the entire LGBT population, there is controversy about its extent. Based on more recent literature, alcohol use among gay men is probably the same as or slightly more prevalent than among heterosexual men. Drug use is more common among gay men compared to their heterosexual counterparts. According to a comparison of a population-based sample of lesbians in the San Francisco Bay area with a control group, alcohol use appears to be no more prevalent among lesbians than among heterosexual women. There are no population-based studies of drug use among lesbians compared with heterosexual women.

Domestic Violence

Contrary to some popular beliefs, battery of LGBT persons by their partners exists. The exact prevalence of battery in same-sex relationships is not known, but recent literature suggests the rate of same-sex domestic violence (SSDV) to be at least equal to that of opposite-sex domestic violence (OSDV). Unfortunately, gender-role stereotyping both in the likelihood of the perpetrator inducing injury (men more capable than women) and the seriousness of the violence (women are more likely to sustain serious injury) exists and likely influences the recognition of SSDV, the consequences to the perpetrator, and empathy for the victim. Lesbians perceive that interpersonal power imbalances contribute to battery. They also report that many women's shelters are not responsive to their specific needs. Gay men may find it even more difficult to obtain services related to battery.

Minority stress (e.g., internalized homophobia, discrimination) negatively influences SSDV perpetration and victimization among LGBT persons. There is likely a similar, if not greater, effect among transgender individuals. Primary care providers should screen their gay and lesbian patients—and all patients—for the possibility of domestic violence and be able to give referrals to lesbian- and gay-sensitive resources, including shelters and counselors (see Chapter 35).

Hate Crimes

Also known as bias crimes, these are words or actions directed at an individual because of membership in a minority group. The U.S. Department of Justice reports that LGBT individuals may be the most victimized group in the nation and that the incidence of hate crimes against LGBT persons is rising. Many studies report crimes ranging from verbal abuse and threats of violence to property damage, physical violence, and murder. The number of hate crimes reported by LGBT persons is increasing every year. Lesbians at universities, for example, report being victims of sexual assault twice as often as heterosexual women. Youths who report same-sex or both-sex romantic attractions are more likely to be both victims and witnesses of violence.

Perpetrators of hate crimes often include family members and community authorities. Many gay and lesbian adolescents leave home because of an abusive family member, and homeless LGBT youths are of increasing social concern. LGBT survivors of hate crimes display more symptoms of depression, anger, anxiety, and posttraumatic stress than other recent crime victims. When patients present with symptoms of depression or anxiety, providers should consider violence, including hate crimes, as a possible correlate.

EDUCATION, REFERRALS, & RESOURCES

Patient Education

This is a cornerstone of primary care. Providers who care for LGBT patients must know how to advise patients in health issues, refer them to appropriate educational and community resources, and provide appropriate reference materials to hand out at visits.

Instruction

Instruction in preventing the spread of HIV and other sexually transmitted diseases should be clear and specific to individual sexual practices. Physicians should be able to educate LGBT patients about risks and screening for cancer. They should be able to counsel patients, or refer them for counseling, about issues such as safer sex, parenting, coming out, violence, substance use, and depression.

Referrals

Referrals should include other providers and community-based resources sensitive to the needs of LGBT people. Specialists of particular importance to delivering appropriate, multidisciplinary care include gynecologists, urologists, general or colorectal surgeons, plastic surgeons, and endocrinologists. Local resources with which to be familiar include bookstores, youth groups, senior groups and retirement centers, community centers, supportive religious organizations, substance abuse treatment programs, and support groups. LGBT-oriented periodicals from a nearby urban area may have resources listed for surrounding suburban and rural regions.

Provider Education

Health care providers can obtain additional information about specific health issues and communicating LGBT patients through textbooks, review articles, teaching videos, and workshops at both national and regional medical conferences. See below for details on individual resources.

General Background

- Gay and Lesbian Medical Association <<www.glma.org>>
  - Resources for providers and patients
  - Provider referral network
- The GLBT Health Access Project <<www.glbthealth.org>>
  - Community standards of practice for provision of quality health care services for LGBT clients
  - Educational posters
- National Coalition for LGBT Health <<www.lgbthealth.net>>
- National Association of Gay and Lesbian Community Centers <<www.lgbtcenters.org>>
  - Directory (for centers throughout the United States which will have additional referrals for local LGBT-sensitive services—e.g., counseling services, support groups, health educators, and legal resources)
- GLBT National Help Center <<www.glnh.org>>
  - National nonprofit organization offering toll-free peer counseling, information, and local resources, including local switchboard numbers and gay-related links: 888-THE-GNLH (843-4564)
  - GLBT National Youth Talkline
  - Youth peer counseling, information, and local resources, through age 25: 800-246-PRIDE (7743)
- Substance Abuse Mental Health Services Administration/National Clearinghouse for Alcohol and Drug Information <<ncadistore.samhsa.gov/catalog/results.aspx?h=audiences&topic=31>>
  - Substance abuse resource guide: lesbian, gay, bisexual, and transgender populations
  - Guidelines for care of LGBT patients

5. General lesbian health
   - The Lesbian Health Research Center at UCSF <<www.lesbianhealthinfo.org>>
   - Mautner Project, the National Lesbian Health Organization <<www.mautnerproject.org>>
   - Lesbian Health Fact Sheet <<www.4woman.gov/owh/pub/factsheets/Lesbian.htm>>

6. General gay men's health
   - GayHealth.com <<www.gayhealth.com>>
   - The Institute for Gay Men's Health
     - A project of Gay Men's Health Crisis and AIDS Project Los Angeles <<www.gmhc.org/programs/institute.html>>

7. General bisexual health
   - Bisexual Resource Center Health Resources <<www.biresource.org/health>>

8. General information: National LGBT Rights
   - Human Rights Campaign <<www.hrc.org>>
     - National organization working for LGBT equal rights on federal government level
   - Lambda Legal <<www.lambdalegal.org>>
     - National LGBT legal and policy organization protecting civil rights of LGBT and people living with HIV
     - Legal helpdesk: 212-809-8585
   - National Center for Lesbian Rights <<www.nclrights.org>>
     - Hotline: 415-392-6257
   - National Gay and Lesbian Task Force <<www.ngltf.org>>
     - National organization supporting LGBT advocacy efforts at state and federal levels

9. PFLAG (Parents, Families, and Friends of Lesbians and Gays)
   <<www.pflag.org>>
   - Promotes the health and well-being of gay, lesbian, bisexual, and transgender persons, their families and friends

10. Media/brochures (for waiting room)
    - American Cancer Society
      - Cancer facts for gay and bisexual men
      - Cancer facts for lesbians and bisexual women
      - Tobacco and the LGBT community
      - Place order for free brochures by phone: 800-ACS-2345
    - American College Health Association <<http://www.acha.org/info_resources/his_brochures.cfm>>
      - Man to man: three steps to health for gay, bisexual, or any men who have sex with men
      - Woman to woman: three steps to health for lesbian, bisexual, or any women who have sex with women

11. Transgender health
    - International Foundation for Gender Education <<www.ifge.org>>
    - Transgender Forum's Community Center <<www.transgender.org>>
    - Transgender Law Center
      - Recommendations for Transgender Health Care <<www.transgenderlaw.org/resources/tlchealth.htm>>

12. Youth
    - National gay, lesbian, bisexual, transgender youth hotline: 800-347-TEEN
    - Youth Guardian Services: on-line support <<www.youth-guard.org>>
    - Youth Resource: a project of Advocates for Youth <<www.youthresource.com>>

- National Youth Advocacy Coalition <<www.nyacyouth.org>>
13. Elders
    - SAGE: Services and Advocacy for Gay, Lesbian, Bisexual, and Transgender Elders <<www.sageusa.org>>
14. Intimate partner violence
    - Community United Against Violence <<www.cuav.org>>
    - National domestic violence hotline
      - Local referrals, including LGBT-sensitive: 800-799-SAFE (7233) (24 hours in English and Spanish)
      - TDD: 800-787-3224
    - Network for battered lesbians and bisexual women hotline
      - *info@thenetworklared.org*
      - 617-742-4911

SUGGESTED READINGS

Floyd FJ, Bakeman R. Coming-out across the life course: implications of age and historical context. Arch Sex Behav 2006;35(3): 287–296.

Mills TC, Stall R, Pollack L, et al. Health-related characteristics of men who have sex with men: a comparison of those living in "gay ghettos" with those living elsewhere. *Am J Public Health* 2001;91(6):980–983.

O'Hanlan K, Cabaj RP, Schotz B, et al. A review of the medical consequences of homophobia with suggestions for resolution. *J Gay Lesbian Med Assoc* 1997;1:25–39.

Ryan H, Wortley PM, Easton A, et al. Smoking among lesbians, gays, and bisexuals. *Am J Prev Med* 2001;21(2):142–149.

Solarz AL, ed. *Lesbian Health: Current Assessment and Directions for the Future.* Washington, DC: National Academy Press, 1999.

Stall R, Mills TC, Williamson J, et al. Association of co-occurring psychosocial health problems and increased vulnerability to HIV/AIDS among urban men who have sex with men. *Am J Public Health* 2003;93(6): 939–942.

Vulnerable Patients

15

Dean Schillinger, MD, Teresa Villela, MD, & George Saba, PhD

OBJECTIVES

- Describe the elements of building a therapeutic alliance, eliciting the patient's narrative, and assessing the patient's vulnerabilities and strengths.
- Explore critical components of the therapeutic alliance: building trust, conveying empathy, and collaboration.
- Describe the relevance of the therapeutic alliance to the effective care of vulnerable patients.
- List the benefits of eliciting the patient's narrative.
- Review common psychosocial vulnerabilities and illustrate how identifying them can help create a patient-centered clinical encounter.

INTRODUCTION

CASE ILLUSTRATION 1

Ms. Sviridov is a 67-year-old woman with chronic arthritis pain, hypertension, prior stroke, diastolic dysfunction, and diabetes. Despite a sizable, guideline-based medication regimen and frequent visits to both a primary care physician and a cardiologist, she has recalcitrant heart failure, requiring multiple hospital admissions. An extensive cardiac workup has been unrevealing.

Ms. Sviridov's new primary care physician asks about her life. She describes an active singing career and a rich family life in the past, and the importance of her church. She acknowledges that profound depression and concern over the welfare of her drug-abusing son, however, now interfere with caring for herself.

Ms. Sviridov's physician suggests he make a home visit. Exploring her initial refusal, he learns that her son deals drugs from her apartment. Eventually, with the support of her physician and adult

protective services, she is able to demand that her son leave. She receives support and assistance from home-health services and her church group. Her conditions stabilize and she is not rehospitalized.

Social characteristics—living in poverty, having a low level of education and limited literacy skills, being from a minority background, having no health insurance, speaking little English, among other factors—make individuals vulnerable to contracting illness and to facing overwhelming obstacles in the care of that illness. Vulnerable populations tend to experience these health risks in clusters, making both individuals and communities more susceptible to declines in health. For example, it is not uncommon for an individual living in poverty to have limited literacy skills and no health insurance; to simultaneously have diabetes, heart disease, or depression; and to smoke or to live in a community with limited access to high quality grocers and safe outdoor space for physical activity.

Clinicians must learn to successfully engage those most at risk by virtue of this clustering. Unfortunately, vulnerable patients experience a triple jeopardy when it comes to health care: they are more likely to be ill; more likely to have difficulty accessing care, and when they do, the care they receive is more likely to be suboptimal. This reflects the mismatch between the psychosocial vulnerabilities that they bring to the clinical encounter and the knowledge, attitudes, skills, and beliefs of the clinicians caring for them as well as the priorities and policies of the health systems in which they receive care. In this chapter, we focus on the centrality of strong provider–patient relationships to all efforts to improve the health of vulnerable patients. Three essential strategies are recommended to promote a context for effective care for vulnerable patients: building a therapeutic alliance, eliciting the patient's story or "narrative," and assessing for the patient's psychosocial vulnerabilities and strengths. Clinicians can use a combination of these approaches to create more productive and effective interactions and relationships with vulnerable patients (Figure 15-1).

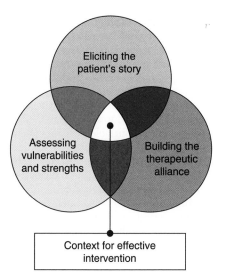

Figure 15-1. Creating a context for effective intervention in the clinical care of vulnerable patients.

VULNERABILITY & THERAPEUTIC ALLIANCE

Psychosocial vulnerabilities can affect health and health care, either alone or in concert (see Figure 15-2). The first path is a direct one, a situation in which the vulnerability in and of itself leads to poor health. Concrete examples of this mechanism might be intravenous drug abuse and skin abscesses or intimate partner violence and head trauma. A second path is an indirect one, where the vulnerability attenuates the benefits of medical treatment on coexisting medical conditions; that is, the vulnerability presents a barrier to optimal acute,

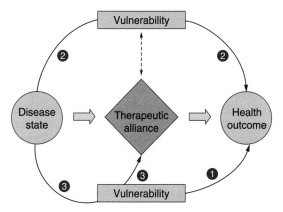

Figure 15-2. Pathways by which psychosocial vulnerabilities affect health and health care in the clinical encounter (see text for details).

chronic, and/or preventive care, thereby accelerating disease course. Examples of this include the effects of depression on nonadherence to medications among patients with heart disease; or inability to pay for medications and poor diabetes control. The third mechanism, also an indirect one, is mediated entirely through the therapeutic alliance. In this path, the vulnerability affects components of the relationship or therapeutic alliance with the provider (such as open disclosure, mutual trust, caring, and engagement), thereby limiting the benefits of a collaborative relationship on care. Examples of this include a patient with an undisclosed illness that is inconsistent with a prescribed treatment plan; a physician whose belief systems regarding addiction impedes true engagement with a patient with a substance use disorder; or a patient with depression that impedes follow-through with a prescribed treatment plan, thereby leading to mutual frustration and blame (Saba et al., 2006).

What is the Therapeutic Alliance?

In the field of medicine, a therapeutic alliance exists when patient and provider develop mutual trusting, caring, and respectful bonds that allow collaboration in care and treatment (Balint, 1957, Bordin, 1979, Bordin, 1994). "Patient-centered" and "relationship-centered" care models build on the notion of the therapeutic alliance, and research reveals that patients reporting greater trust, increased satisfaction, and more collaborative relationships with clinicians had increased adherence to medication and treatment regimens and better health outcomes (Kaplan, 1989, Kaplan, 1995, Stewart, 2000).

Key dimensions of the Therapeutic Alliance include:

- **Mutual trust**—Patients need to trust in their clinicians' integrity and competence, and clinicians need to trust that patients enter the relationship trying to do their best.
- **Empathy**—Demonstrating empathy, or recognizing and understanding the beliefs and emotions of another without injecting one's own, allows the clinician to connect emotionally with the patient without pity or over identification.
- **Respect**—Expressing respect for patients and treating them with dignity are important and require creating a context in which communication can occur as equals.
- **Collaboration**—Collaboration requires a meaningful partnership in which clinician and patient perceive that they are working together toward a common goal and committed to resolving conflicts that inevitably emerge about treatment goals.
- **Broadening the alliance**—The therapeutic alliance must be broadened beyond the one-to-one relationship between clinician and patient to include other

important people (e.g., family; consulting clinicians) (McDaniel, 1990, Pinsof, 1994). Health systems can foster or erode the therapeutic alliance based on the policies they promote (Wagner, 1998, Schillinger, 2004).

Therapeutic Alliance & Vulnerable Patients

 CASE ILLUSTRATION 2

Mr. Jackson is a 52-year-old man with Type 2 diabetes, hypertension, and end-stage renal disease. He receives care intermittently at a public clinic. He was recently referred for dialysis but missed his appointment for evaluation. He was a construction worker and now is unemployed; he lives alone and is episodically homeless. He is African American and has two sons living in the area.

He was admitted to the Family Medicine Service of a county hospital and found to be in diabetic ketoacidosis. During the admission, the inpatient team rediscusses his need for dialysis. His initial meeting with the Renal Team ends with him becoming angry and refusing dialysis. The resident assigned to his care urges him to reconsider, and he becomes withdrawn. She attempts to arrange dialysis again, and the Renal Team, citing his history of alcohol use, his intermittent homelessness, and his lack of follow-through, declares him a "poor candidate" for dialysis.

The resident meets with Mr. Jackson to better understand his thinking. Initially he remains distant; as she expresses her concern for helping him receive the best care, he is able to express his anger at the medical system over the years. He feels he has not been given information about his illness in a manner that he understands, he is unable to implement the many self-care suggestions given his living situation, and feels that doctors have only been interested in him if they can "learn medicine" by experimenting on him. The resident expresses her concern and regret for how he has been previously treated and offers to do her best to help him now. He is able to talk about his experience with diabetes, his fear about dying, and his desire to change. She expresses her appreciation for his willingness to be forthright and offers to become his primary care physician. She also offers to advocate for him with the Renal Team to initiate dialysis both in and out of the hospital.

A growing body of evidence suggests that it is precisely with vulnerable patients that the therapeutic alliance can have its most profound benefits. Through a therapeutic alliance, clinicians offer a professional relationship aimed at helping patients feel comfortable to be as open and honest as is necessary to receive the best care. Clinicians are permitted access to the interior of patients' lives that few other people are allowed. Using this privileged position, they can help build an alliance which empowers patients and reduces barriers to their care.

Empowerment—Vulnerable patients often experience human relationships as broken or disrupted (e.g., due to violence, immigration, mental illness, homelessness, illness). Through the therapeutic alliance, clinicians can offer a reliable, dependable, and continuous presence which is supportive, accepting, and nonjudgmental. They can provide safety, thus allowing patients to tell the stories of their lives and illness and disclose their vulnerabilities. By examining the patients' strengths and resources, clinicians can provide a sense of dignity and hope. Through validating their experiences, clinicians can help patients feel less marginalized. In supporting patients as competent and strong, clinicians can help empower them to become actively involved in their care.

Access to care and related resources—Vulnerable patients often face limited access to health care and social services. In part, they may be unaware of what is available and may not have the facility to negotiate complex, bureaucratic systems. Clinicians are in a position to remedy both of these barriers. Through the therapeutic alliance, clinicians can help patients feel safe enough to reveal concerns or problems beyond the presenting problem, which they might not otherwise have done. For example, a patient seeking care for her diabetes may disclose that she lives with an abusive partner, drinks alcohol regularly, or is only sporadically housed. The clinician has the ability to collaborate on treatment plans and to facilitate entry into the various health and social systems that can help address vulnerabilities. The therapeutic alliance can help patients feel assured that clinicians will not abuse the disclosure of information (e.g., leading to rejection or legal action) but will help them access resources critical for their health.

What Can Happen When the Therapeutic Alliance is Absent?

The absence of a therapeutic alliance can result in serious consequences for the health of vulnerable patients.

Trust—Clinicians often enter into relationships with patients assuming they share the same goals and will trust each other to do their best to attain them. However, many patients enter into the relationship with a degree of mistrust. This may result from personal experiences with institutions in which they have felt betrayed or unwelcome or may be rooted in broader, historical experiences of their community. Clinicians should not automatically assume that they have patients' immediate, total trust; rather, they should earn it by demonstrating trustworthiness.

Clinicians can indicate their trustworthiness by:

- *Being transparent*: Vulnerable patients often experience external intrusions into their lives and little privacy; they may not understand why clinicians ask about personal information. Explaining the context of questions that may not seem immediately pertinent to the patient's concern may dispel patient's concerns about hidden agendas (e.g., "I am asking about who you live with, not to pry, but to see who might be available to care for you following your operation."). Similarly, vulnerable patients may believe clinicians are interested in ordering particular laboratory tests, imaging studies or procedures in order to learn at the expense of the patient or to increase financial resources. On the other hand, patients may fear that they are being denied particular treatments to save the health care system money. Explaining why one is recommending a particular diagnostic course or treatment regimen can build trust (e.g., "I want you to get the treadmill test, because I think it is the best way we have to know how best to help you and to decide the best treatments.").

- *Following through*: Vulnerable patients are accustomed to hearing that something will occur (e.g., appointment scheduled; prescription ordered; referral to social service made) and then learning, for whatever reason, that it did not happen. By taking the extra time to follow-through on promises, clinicians can show patients that they can be counted on to make ensure the best care ("I told you I would call when I found out how to help you find housing; here's what I've learned." "My homework after your last appointment was to find out about Spanish-speaking support groups for patients with diabetes; there is one not to far from your home.").

- *Addressing concerns*: Vulnerable patients may experience clinicians as rushed, interested in their own agendas, and nonresponsive to those of the patient. By taking the time to ask and answer questions and focus on what the patient needs, clinicians can indicate that they are interested in helping the patient and can be trusted to care ("While there are many things that I want to talk to you about, what are you most concerned about?" ("I know that I am more worried about your high blood pressure than you are. I also know you are more concerned that you cannot work because your elbow is so painful. Let's work on both today.").

Caring—Poor and minority patients frequently receive care in teaching hospitals and community health centers where the turnover of providers is high. Patients may question provider's motivation and commitment, fearing that they are educational fodder for trainees who will go on to care for the privileged. When clinicians do not offer certain treatments, patients may be suspicious about the clinicians' willingness to expend resources for them. When clinicians persuasively argue for unwanted treatments, they may fear being used as experimental "guinea pigs." Rather than risk raising concerns or disagreements with a clinician whose motives they question, patients may choose not to follow-through on recommended treatment or simply not return for care.

Respect—Perceived disrespect and discrimination due to race or socioeconomic status has been associated with lower satisfaction with the health care system and worse health outcomes among patients with chronic illness (Piette et al., 2006). Significant proportions of African Americans, Latinos, and Asians and those with lower educational attainment have reported that they were treated with disrespect, were treated unfairly, or received worse care because of their position in society (Blanchard and Lurie, 2004). These perceptions influenced whether patients followed recommended advice or delayed needed care for chronic illness. Communicating respect is essential to convincing vulnerable patients that clinicians are willing to enter into a relationship based on equality and dignity.

Mutual agreement and collaboration—In the absence of a trusting relationship, true collaboration may be difficult to achieve. Fear of being punished or treated unfairly for speaking truthfully can lead patients to withhold their beliefs and values about a suggested treatment or to refuse to follow-through on a recommendation. Clinicians, in turn, feel frustrated and mistrustful when they wonder if they are being misled or if patients really care about their health.

Shared decision making is often promoted as a model for mutual agreement and collaboration. However, research with diverse populations suggests that clinicians and patients, seemingly engaged in the cardinal behaviors of shared decision making, may still not perceive that a collaborative partnership exists between them (Saba et al., 2006). Indeed, being treated with respect and dignity may be more important than engaging in shared decision making—and may itself lead to positive outcomes (i.e., higher satisfaction, adherence, receipt of optimal preventive care) (Beach, 2005).

BUILDING A THERAPEUTIC ALLIANCE WITH VULNERABLE PATIENTS

There are no simple, protocol-like statements or behaviors that we can employ to make another human being feel that they are cared about or respected. However, if we consciously strive to transmit a sense of trust, caring, and respect, along with a desire to enter into true partnership, we increase the likelihood of forming productive relationships with patients. Some guidelines to consider in this process include the following:

- **Demonstrate commitment to the relationship.** We need to state clearly our desire to be available to our patients within the scope of our practice (e.g., "I will be your regular doctor. Here is my telephone number with a voice mail; I check it daily and will get back to you as soon as possible."); be clear with what we expect ourselves to do for the patient between visits (e.g., "I will check into support groups and tell you at our next appointment."); and follow-through on what we have promised.

- **Allow for the humanity of the patient and the clinician to emerge.** The humanity of the health care worker and the patient should be expressed and elicited. This may include the sharing of beliefs, values, and feelings as they relate to the clinical issues facing them (e.g., express concern about suffering, *"I am sorry you have to deal with this pain"*; self-disclosure to identify a shared history or common interests with the patient, *"As a parent, I can't imagine how incredibly strong you had to be to escape with your children."*).

- **Elicit patients' stories or health "narratives."** This interviewing approach can provide critical insights into a patient's illness model, allow for expression of the patient's humanity, and uncover important psychosocial vulnerabilities (see "Eliciting the Patient's Story or 'Narrative,'" below).

- **Search actively for patients' strengths and resources.** We commonly focus on what is wrong or dysfunctional in the patient's life. Just as vital as the search for deficits, is the identification and validation of the strengths and resilience each patient has (e.g., *"You have been through a lot of suffering in your life, how have you been able to survive?" "Who gives you the strength to deal with difficult things?"*). Reflecting on how the patient has used these resources in previously difficult times can provide a positive starting point for healing (e.g., *"You have talked about turning to God when dealing with other major crises in your life; have you thought of doing that now?"*). The power for healing does not rest solely with the clinician, but must involve an empowered patient and their family (e.g., *"Your sister gave you strength to leave an abusive relationship; can she help now in dealing with your diabetes?"*).

- **Express caring overtly.** We need to clearly state that we care about our patients as people, and not assume they know. When hearing patients describe difficult or painful experiences, we can acknowledge their perspective (e.g., *"I can't imagine how difficult your life has been"*; *"What you have lived through sounds so frightening"*; *"I know you're afraid of going through these tests and treatments; is there anything I can do to make it less scary?"*). A number of nonverbal behaviors and verbal statements can also overtly express that we care: (a) body language (e.g., *sitting in proximity; a focused, unhurried posture*); (b) active listening and reframing (e.g., *"It sounds to me that you felt betrayed by the people you trusted most; am I right about that?"*) ; (c) support (e.g., *"I know you are trying very hard to live on your own now; I think you are doing great, and I want to do whatever I can to support you."*) ; and (d) validation (e.g., *"You are right to feel that you do not deserve to be abused."*) . Caring can also be communicated a number of indirect ways, such as making an unexpected phone call to follow-up with a patient in crisis (e.g., *"I know you had your colonoscopy yesterday, and I wanted to see how you are doing."*) . Not all patients (nor all clinicians) are comfortable with touch. Some patients may even believe clinicians are afraid to touch them. Respectful physical contact during painful or uplifting moments can help cement a mutual human connection.

- **Create a context for conflict to emerge and get addressed.** We need to convince patients that when they have beliefs, opinions, or ideas different from ours, we will welcome discussing them. We must allay any fears patients have that voicing disagreement will incur displeasure or even punishment from the provider. A corollary to this is that patients need to understand that they can change their minds about treatment plans and decisions at anytime. Patients need repeated reassurance and reminders that disagreement will not cost them the provider's regard and care (e.g., *"I will not be angry or upset if you disagree; it would be very helpful to know how you really feel, because together we can figure out the best thing to do."*) . Building a therapeutic alliance doesn't require us to deny our educated viewpoint but to adopt nonthreatening ways of communicating differences with our patients.

- **Clarify boundaries.** Vulnerable patients may often experience considerable intrusion into their personal lives by government institutions or social service agencies. They may be required to disclose more information than others, and then find it shared across agencies without their knowledge or permission. We should clarify why we are inquiring about certain information (e.g., *"I want to ask more specifically about your family because they seem important in your care, and I want to understand how they help you."*) and what is confidential or required to be shared (e.g., *"I will keep whatever you tell me confidential unless I think you may harm yourself or someone else; then I must tell others to protect you from any harm."*) .

We should also clarify our own boundaries; it is not uncommon for a relationship between a clinician and a patient to evolve into one of unhealthy dependence or unrealistic expectations. For example, as we learn more about the hardships our patients face and their difficulty navigating the system, we may feel tempted to reach out to them differently than we would for non-vulnerable patients. We may be inclined to give them a pager number or even our home phone because we want to improve access; we might lend them money or give them a ride. While these behaviors might not, in and of themselves, prove problematic, they do represent a crossing of boundaries that are commonly set with patients and signal us to reflect upon and to consider potential consequences. We can avoid creating problematic relationships by remaining mindful of the role we play in the therapeutic relationship and by regularly reflecting on our interactions. Communicating with colleagues about our patient challenges (including boundaries) can provide a critical and supportive perspective as we strive to make appropriate decisions in building the therapeutic relationship.

- **Address the therapeutic alliance directly**. When caring for a patient who is doing poorly clinically but receiving optimal "medical" management, we should consider if the therapeutic alliance needs attention. We can directly state our desire to have a strong relationship and a real sense of partnership. We can ask if the patient would want any changes in the relationship, reassuring them that speaking honestly is not only acceptable, but essential to working together.

ELICITING THE PATIENT'S STORY OR "NARRATIVE"

What is the Patient's Perspective?

Many factors (individual, familial, societal, spiritual, cultural) shape a person's concepts and experiences of health and illness. These inform an individual's sense of responsibility as a patient; expectations of health care providers and family members and the meaning of healing and recovery. Personal concepts of health determine what preventive and self-care behaviors are considered appropriate, which symptoms seem worrisome, and when to seek help from health care professionals. These explanatory models encompass the meaning of the illness, the presumed cause, its proposed trajectory, the degree of hope of cure, and how treatment should be conducted (Kleinman, 1988).

The same factors that influence how a person thinks about health and illness obviously affect other aspects of their life, and eliciting information about these influences can unveil perspectives important to health care. For example, how an individual makes decisions about health care may resemble how they make decisions about parenting or work; the process for how a family decided to immigrate to the United States may be very similar to how they will approach a difficult treatment decision; one's explanation of life difficulties and the narrative of how one has prevailed over them may illustrate how one will face challenging health problems as

well. Illness may be framed hopefully or pessimistically; patients may identify themselves as efficacious or as victims; they may prefer being independent or isolated or they may find strength in support from others.

Importance of Eliciting the Patient's Perspective

A patient's perspective, a complex mixture of very personal beliefs, values, and assumptions reflecting multiple influences, can determine how patients develop a relationship with their clinician, and whether they feel understood and respected or misunderstood and discounted. Clinicians, in turn, have their own individual perspectives on health and illness, and ascribe specific meaning to their role as healers. Assuming a shared understanding and not exploring the differences may in fact lead to greater distance and misunderstanding. Eliciting patients' perspectives allows for accurate empathy and can uncover interests or experiences common to both patient and clinician, thereby reducing the social distance that often impedes the development of a therapeutic alliance.

Eliciting the patient's story can also improve patient trust, satisfaction, and adherence. In a meta-analysis of the effect of physician communication on health, Stewart found that effective communication within the history-taking section of the visit consistently correlated with improved health outcomes, including emotional health, symptom resolution, function, physiologic measures (e.g., blood pressure and blood glucose), and pain control (Stewart, 2000). In his studies of patient trust, Thom found that physician's receptive communication behaviors such as "letting the whole story be told" was associated with patient trust, satisfaction, and adherence (Thom, 2004). Clinicians benefit from understanding their patient's stories too. It enriches and brings meaning to interactions and allows providers to be more effective and engaged.

Furthermore, sometimes the way people frame their illnesses can cause suffering. Within the context of a strong therapeutic alliance it is possible, as part of the healing process, to recast some narratives. A patient who feels incompetent, for example, might grow, through learning to control his illness, to feel capable and empowered in realms beyond the medical.

ASSESSING & ACKNOWLEDGING PSYCHOSOCIAL VULNERABILITIES

Much of clinical training and guideline development focuses on pathophysiology, disease, diagnosis, and treatment. Seasoned clinicians, however, are acutely aware of the gap between the outcomes that are expected (e.g., from reading textbooks or following guidelines) and the outcomes that are actually achieved

---

BOX 15-1. GENERATING A DIFFERENTIAL DIAGNOSIS OF PSYCHOSOCIAL VULNERABILITIES.

Violence
Uninsured
Literacy and/or Language barriers
Neglect
Economic hardship
Race/ethnic discordance, discrimination
Addiction
Brain disorders (e.g., depression, dementia, personality disorder)

Immigrant
Legal status
Isolation/Informal caregiving burden
Transportation problems
Illness model
Eyes and Ears (vision and hearing problems)
Shelter

---

in practice. While there are many reasons for the observed variation in quality and health outcomes, one of the most important and frequently least appreciated factors, is the patient's social context. A wide range of psychosocial vulnerabilities can impinge on a patient's ability to carry out the treatment plan and interfere with the therapeutic alliance (see Box 15-1).

When faced with a patient who is doing poorly from a clinical standpoint, many clinicians do not reflect on the psychosocial factors that may be influencing the patient's course. They may simply throw up their arms and attribute a patient's clinical decline to his or her social milieu in a global or at times derogatory fashion, referring to such a patient as "nonadherent," a "difficult patient," or a "social nightmare," without digging deeper. Such clinicians often believe that addressing psychosocial problems is "not my job," stating, "I can't fix his social problems." Still others may not have the communication skills to uncover underlying psychosocial problems, or to address them and integrate this knowledge into treatment plans to forge a more genuine, engaged therapeutic alliance.

Screening for psychosocial vulnerabilities is central to caring for patients in any setting and at many points during the process of care, particularly when treatments appear to be failing. Some vulnerabilities will be apparent from the first encounter, while others may be hidden. For some problems, it is not until a collaborative relationship has been established that a patient might feel comfortable enough to disclose sensitive information. Similarly, patients may perceive a problem to be irrelevant to their health and neglect to discuss it. When assessing for areas of vulnerability, the clinician should be nonjudgmental, allowing the patient to respond at his or her own pace. Using open-ended questions and responding to patient cues may enable a patient to reveal the important nonclinical factors that may be impeding their progress (see Table 15-1).

It is important to raise four important *caveats* about assessing for psychosocial vulnerability. The first is that

in the pursuit of identifying vulnerability, the clinician should be reminded of the importance of simultaneously identifying and acknowledging an individual's *strengths, resilience,* and range of *resources,* such as one's belief in a higher power or support from a religious community; or the love and support provided by a spouse, friend, or pet. Reviewing and reflecting patients' past experiences of overcoming difficulty and helping them identify patterns of success is critical to building self-efficacy and developing a therapeutic alliance in the face of vulnerability.

Secondly, vulnerability is *context-dependent.* For example, in countries with universal health care coverage, lack of insurance simply does not contribute to vulnerability. Conversely, absence of interpretation services may exacerbate the effects of limited English proficiency when compared to settings with medical interpretation; presence of a methadone treatment program or a mobile treatment van in one's clinic may mitigate the untoward health effects of heroin addiction and housing instability, respectively. As such, the effects of vulnerability on health care can be influenced by altering the context in which caregiving takes place, which most frequently means adapting the clinical

Table 15-1. Common pitfalls in assessing for vulnerability.

- Failing to recognize the contribution of psychosocial vulnerabilities to the patient's illness.
- Failing to acknowledge vulnerability and to explore how vulnerability may be affecting care.
- Failing to address specific vulnerabilities.
- Failing to integrate knowledge of vulnerability into treatment plans.
- Failing to recognize the shame and stigma associated with vulnerabilities.
- Neglecting to identify and acknowledge strengths, resilience, and range of resources.

---

encounter. This suggests that when caring for vulnerable populations, clinicians and systems should also perform *self-assessments*, and carefully explore the ways in which the caregiving context can be adapted to best attenuate (or even eliminate) the health effects of vulnerability.

Thirdly, in the process of assessment, the clinician should be sensitive to the concerns of patients with respect to shame and stigma (Lazare, 1987). It is clear that a number of factors listed in Box 15-1 may elicit feelings of shame, such as having limited literacy, being marginally housed, having mental illness, or being addicted.

Fourthly, after identifying vulnerability, the clinician should not forget the important step of exploring with the patient, in a supportive and nonjudgmental manner, how the vulnerability may be affecting both health and care and how to mitigate them. Only by doing so can the clinicians develop a more effective treatment plan while simultaneously enhancing the therapeutic alliance.

UNIQUE ASPECTS TO BUILDING THE THERAPEUTIC ALLIANCE WITH VULNERABLE PATIENTS

There are a number of additional strategies that may be especially useful in developing and sustaining a therapeutic alliance with socially vulnerable patients. These include *showing* patients in concrete ways that you care (i.e., "going the extra mile"); *advocating* for patients with the myriad bureaucracies that they struggle with; *connecting* them to appropriate community resources (e.g., immigration lawyer, domestic violence counselor, exercise groups); *networking* with others, including family, friends, public health, and community resources, so as to encourage them to support the patient's efforts to achieve health; engaging in *self-disclosure* to narrow social distance and encourage the sharing of personal stories.

Building a therapeutic alliance with vulnerable patients comes with both special rewards and challenges. Working with the underserved allows a clinician to apply his or her skills to assist those who are most in need, fulfilling one of the basic humanitarian ideals in Medicine. Developing a therapeutic bond with patients that do not represent the "typical patient," or that many consider too difficult to manage, can be rewarding in and of itself, often involving a process of shared discovery and reflection.

It is not uncommon, however, for unseasoned clinicians to be overwhelmed by the many challenges inherent to caring for vulnerable patients. Developing patterns of codependency, such as repeatedly "rescuing" patients from the decisions that are in their control, may be a prelude to clinician "burnout." Clinicians should be aware of signs of "burnout," such as exhibiting their anger and frustration at patients or staff, or developing an overly passive style of patient engagement.

Clinicians who have been able to sustain therapeutic relationships with vulnerable patients and maintain fulfilling careers in the care of vulnerable populations tend to (a) elicit patients' agendas so as to establish an understanding of patient expectations, (b) set realistic goals for what they can accomplish and share these goals with their patients, (c) limit what they aim to accomplish in any given encounter and see their work with patients as evolving over a long period of time, (d) continually clarify boundaries, (e) maintain a sense of curiosity and discovery about the patients' clinical and personal profile, (f) acknowledge that many of the problems experienced by vulnerable patients are structural/societal in nature, and not always a result of patient choice, (g) engage in public health-related or social advocacy efforts to affect structural determinants of health, (h) seek the advice and support of colleagues who share common ideals and practices.

CONCLUSION

A strong therapeutic alliance creates a trusting context for patient care. Building a therapeutic alliance, eliciting the patient's narrative and assessing for vulnerabilities and strengths are critical to creating this context. Fostering the therapeutic alliance requires developing trust, conveying empathy, and collaborating about treatment goals. Depending on the skills, attitudes, and orientation of clinicians and the systems in which they work, the clinical encounter can increase social distance and exacerbate the effects of vulnerability on health, or it can lead to productive engagement with patients to mitigate or even eliminate the effects of vulnerability on health. While it may be especially challenging to develop and sustain a therapeutic alliance with those who are socially vulnerable, the benefits to patient and clinician can be profound.

KEY CONCEPTS

Vulnerable patients often experience fragmentation and disconnection in their lives and in their health care.

- The therapeutic alliance is an important means to reduce the effects of vulnerability on health outcomes.
- Eliciting the patient's story or perspective is an effective means to uncover health beliefs, develop shared meaning, enable empathy, and enhance the therapeutic alliance. It also serves to uncover patient vulnerabilities and reveal patients' resilience.
- By identifying vulnerabilities and acknowledging to the patient and to other clinicians involved in the patient's care how such factors might influence the effectiveness of treatment, clinicians will be better equipped to develop effective treatment plans.

CORE COMPETENCY

Eliciting the Patient's Perspective

- Let patients know that hearing their perspective is important to you.
- Explain that you think discussing family, coping styles, and their personal story is important to an individual patient's health.
- Take the time necessary, and use the time well.
  - Set a climate of interest, concern, and calm.
- Use an inquiry style that fosters more, not less, information.
  - Maintain a high degree of curiosity, be aware of patient's verbal or emotional cues.
  - Follow-up on cues—such as *"it seemed that talking about that brought up some feelings for you. Why is that?"*
- Use open-ended questions and reflective statements.
- Discover the patient's explanatory model.
  - Ask the Kleinman questions:
  What do you call the problem? What do you think has caused the problem? Why do you think it started when it did? What do you think the sickness does? How does it work? How severe is the sickness? Will it have a short or long course? What kind of treatment do you think you should receive? What are the most important results you hope to receive from this treatment? What are the chief problems the sickness has caused you? What do you fear most about the sickness? (Kleinman, 1988)
- Consider the interpersonal context of patients' general health care framework.
- Focus on the meaning of what patients are saying.
- Avoid using technical, medical jargon.
- Do not try to gather the entire perspective in one appointment, but try to gain some insight every time.

DISCUSSION QUESTIONS

1. Discuss clinical experiences you have had with vulnerable patients in which the presence or absence of strategies such as building a therapeutic alliance, eliciting patients' narratives, and assessing for vulnerabilities and strengths influenced the process and perhaps the outcome of their health care.

2. Consider what structural and health policy changes would need to be made to better incorporate the strategies of building a therapeutic alliance, eliciting patients' narratives, and assessing for vulnerabilities and strengths into the day-to-day clinical care of vulnerable patients.

3. What are some of the most surprising or fascinating nonmedical pieces of information you learned about the last patient you cared for and how did it influence either the treatment plan or your relationship with the patient and his or her family?

4. Discuss how personal beliefs, values, and assumptions about vulnerable patients affects your ability to create a context for effective care using strategies such as building a therapeutic alliance, eliciting patients' narratives, and assessing for vulnerabilities and strengths.

SUGGESTED READINGS

Balint M. *The Doctor, His Patient and the Illness*. New York, NY: International University Press, 1957.

Beach MC, Sugarman J, Johnson RL, et al. Do patients treated with dignity report higher satisfaction, adherence, and receipt of preventive care? *Ann Fam Med* 2005;3:331–338.

Blanchard J, Lurie N. R-E-S-P-E-C-T: patient reports of disrespect in the health care setting and its impact on care. *J Fam Pract* 2004;53:721–730.

Bordin ES. The generalizability of the psychoanalytic concept of the working alliance. *Psychotherapy theory, research and practice* 1979;16:252–260.

Bordin ES. Theory and research on the therapeutic working alliance: new directions. In: Horvath AO, Greenberg LS, eds. *The Working Alliance: Theory, Research and Practice*. New York, NY: Wiley, 1994, p. 1337.

Freedheim DK. *History of Psychotherapy: A Century of Change*. Washington, DC: American Psychological Association, 1992.

Kaplan SH, Gandek B, Greenfield S, et al. Patient and visit characteristics related to physicians' participatory decision-making style. Results from the Medical Outcomes Study. *Med Care* 1995;33:1176–1187.

Kaplan SH, Greenfield S, Ware JE Jr. Assessing the effects of physician-patient interactions on the outcomes of chronic disease. *Med Care* 1989;27(Suppl):S110–S127.

Kleinman A. *The Illness Narratives: Suffering, Healing and the Human Condition*. New York, NY: Basic Books, 1988.

Lazare A. Shame and humiliation in the medical encounter. *Arch Intern Med* 1987;147:1653–1658.

McDaniel S, Campbell T, Seaburn DB. *Family-Oriented Primary Care*. New York, NY: Springer-Verlag, 1990.

Piette JD, Bibbins-Domingo K, Schillinger D. Health care discrimination, processes of care, and diabetes patients' health status. *Patient Educ Couns* 2006;60:41–48.

Pinsof W. An integrative systems perspective on the therapeutic alliance: theoretical, clinical and research implications. In: Horvath AO, Greenberg LS, eds. *The Working Alliance: Theory, Research and Practice*. New York, NY: Wiley, 1994, pp. 173–195.

Saba GW, Wong S, Schillinger D, et al. Shared decision-making and perceived collaboration in primary care. *Ann Fam Med* 2006;4:54–62.

Schillinger D. Improving chronic disease care for populations with limited health literacy. In: Nielsen-Bohlman LEA, ed. *Health Literacy: A Prescription to End Confusion*. Washington, DC:

Institute of Medicine, National Academy Press, 2004, pp. 267–284.

Stewart M, Brown JB, Donner A, et al. The impact of patient-centered care on outcomes. *J Fam Pract* 2000;49:796–804.

Thom DH, Hall MA, Pawlson LG. Measuring patients' trust in physicians when assessing quality of care. *Health Aff (Millwood)* 2004;23:124–132.

Wagner EH. Chronic disease management: what will it take to improve care for chronic illness? *Eff Clin Pract* 1998;1:2–4.

RESOURCES

American Academy on Communication in Healthcare. Web site. http://www.aachonline.org. Accessed September, 2007.

Lipkin M Jr, Putnam SM, Lazare A, eds. *The Medical Interview: Clinical Care, Education, and Research.* New York, NY: Springer, 1995.

Young RK, ed. *A Piece of My Mind: A New Collection of Essays from JAMA, the Journal of the American Medical Association.* Chicago, IL: AMA Press, 2000.

SECTION III
Health-related Behavior

Behavior Change

16

Daniel O'Connell, PhD

INTRODUCTION

Despite advances in medical technology and evidence-based guidelines, most efforts to improve health require some change in behavior on the part of patients. These changes in behavior might involve reduction or elimination of destructive behaviors (e.g., smoking and alcohol dependence), promotion of healthier lifestyles (e.g., regular exercise, safer sex), and adherence to medical regimens intended to treat acute or chronic illness (e.g., taking medications, dietary restrictions checking blood glucose). Most clinicians, however, feel more confident in their diagnostic and treatment skills than they do in their ability to ensure that patients will make necessary lifestyle changes or closely adhere to medical regimens.

In this chapter, I will describe and integrate three of the most researched approaches to behavior change: the Stages of Change Model of James Prochaska and Carlo DiClemente, the Motivational Interviewing Model of William Miller and Stephen Rollnick, and the Self-efficacy Model of Albert Bandura. My goal is to outline a practical approach to influencing patients that respects the complexity of human behavior while breaking clinician interventions into manageable steps.

SUMMARY OF BEHAVIOR CHANGE MODELS

Stages of Change

The Stages of Change Model introduced the idea that people move through a succession of six relatively distinguishable stages in making changes in behavior.

1. *Precontemplation stage:* There is little thought about the problem or its solution.
2. *Contemplation stage:* The problem and the potential methods, costs, and benefits involved in trying to address it are explored and evaluated.
3. *Preparation/Determination stage:* Choosing and committing to a specific course of action and timetable around which to commit energies to change.
4. *Action stage:* New behaviors are initiated and problem behaviors are replaced (e.g., following a diet and exercise program on a consistent basis).
5. *Maintenance stage:* Successful changers begin to incorporate Action stage behaviors into a "new normal" way of living.
6. *Relapse stage:* There is a return to an earlier stage after an initial period of successful change.

The change process starts in the Precontemplation stage during which people have a problem but are not thinking much about the problem or its solution. Problem awareness typically begins in response to some "bad news" that can arise in myriad forms, for example, physical symptoms, clothes that don't fit, workplace prohibition on smoking, doctor reports problem with routine blood pressure or lab test. The disturbing data prompt entry into the Contemplation stage where they begin to think more about the problem and begin weighing the pros and cons of trying to address it. They may make halfhearted efforts of change, but lack the commitment needed to sustain them. In the Preparation/Determination stage they become more committed to a specific plan as they prepare to take action. In the Action stage people are "doing it"; engaging in changed behavior on a regular basis (e.g., walking a mile five times a week, closely following a diet plan). The daily effort of behavior change is hard to sustain. Changers learn that they must stay conscious of their specific intentions and muster sufficient resolve to overcome moment-to-moment temptations to slip back into old behaviors. To achieve long-term success individuals must move into the Maintenance stage where they incorporate their Action stage behaviors into their lifestyle, although perhaps with reduced frequency and intensity (e.g., attending fewer Alcoholics Anonymous [AA] meetings, or allowing previously forbidden foods back into their diet in a controlled manner). Maintainers are thinking of the long-term success (e.g., staying sober, keeping weight off). This is different from Action stage thinking about behavior change as an extraordinary but mercifully a temporary effort (e.g., the dieter's fallacy of temporary draconian dietary changes until a goal weight is achieved with the expectation that the diet can then be abandoned and weight will not increase). For any single attempt at behavior change it is as common for people to relapse back to an earlier stage as it is to move on to the next stage. For example, an individual may profess a commitment to a course of action (Preparation) but lose enthusiasm and stall before they really get started. Or, they may have started to take action on a daily basis (Action) but then are overcome by obstacles and so fail to sustain it. Finally, they may have had initial success, but through a series of slips that were not corrected, could not maintain the new behavior and now find themselves relapsed into former problem behavior patterns. Some relapsers may now be feeling discouraged and stuck, while others are still committed to change and are already regrouping for another try (see Table 16-1 for a summary of these stages).

Motivational Interviewing

Miller and Rollnick's Motivational Interviewing Model challenged the existing assumption that people change primarily when they are pressured from outside. Deci and Ryan's Intrinsic Motivation research lent support to this insight. They realized that many attempts to influence patients were limited to "pushing" types of interactions in which the clinician lectured, explained, exhorted, criticized, inspired, or threatened the patient with dire consequences if change did not occur. They saw little support in the research for the effectiveness of such a heavy-handed, coercive or even an inspirational approach. The theory of reactance posits that individuals are strongly motivated to maintain a sense of autonomy and to resist coercion by others. Reactance creates its own logic. People who might otherwise have admitted their concern over a problem may instead feel compelled to defend their behavior when criticized. Miller and Rollnick demonstrated that the most effective way to influence patients' behavior is to build on their own self-motivation to change. This is accomplished through an interview style that emphasizes empathy, curiosity, self-determination, and acceptance on the clinician's part. The clinician is advised to expect and explore the patient's ambivalence about change and roll with resistance rather than pushing back with arguments. They encouraged "pulling behaviors" such as asking questions, eliciting values, clarifying and supporting patients' autonomy, "Of course these are your decisions to make." Concern not control, and curiosity rather than command, is a hallmark of Motivational Interviewing.

> **Doctor:** I am concerned that you will continue to worry about another heart attack unless you can change some of the continuing risks we have been discussing. What do you think about that?

Social Learning Theory

Albert Bandura is a leading figure in the development of Social Learning Theory which describes how people learn social behaviors, evaluate the desirability of behaviors, and influence and are influenced by others to adopt behaviors and beliefs. A wide body of research has looked at many types of social influence. Examples include modeling (motivating by example), lecturing/explaining, and social reinforcement (e.g., praise). This

Table 16-1. Stages of change and patient characteristics.

Stage	Patient Characteristic
Precontemplation	The problem exists, but the patient minimizes or denies it.
Contemplation	The patient is thinking about the problem and the costs and benefits of continuing with the problem or trying to change.
Preparation	The patient commits to a time and plan for resolving the problem.
Action	The patient makes daily efforts to overcome the problem.
Maintenance	The patient has overcome the problem and remains vigilant to prevent backsliding.
Relapse	The patient has gone back to the problem behavior on a regular basis after a period of successful resolution.

research has helped explain how these interactions impact individuals' rational as well as emotional self-assessments about both the importance and desirability of a change and the confidence in their capacity to behave differently. They showed that motivation to try new behavior comes from an interaction of two forces: a **conviction** that the behavior is necessary/valuable and the **self-efficacy/confidence** that he or she could successfully carry it out.

Conviction and confidence are continuous rather than dichotomous dimensions (more or less rather than all or none). Questions that assess conviction and confidence in the medical interview are as simple as:

> **Doctor:** How convinced are you that cigarette smoking is really hurting you?

> **Doctor:** How confident are you that you could quit smoking if you really wanted to? What gets in the way of your feeling more confident that you could quit?

Clinicians should be looking for things that boost the conviction of the insufficiently convinced and/or increase the confidence of the individual who feels change is overwhelming in some way. Motivational Interviewing advises the clinician to approach these tasks through empathic conversation rather than lecturing/advising. The Stages of Change Model shows how the content of the message and recommendations made should be matched to the patient's stage of change.

Influence Versus Control

Research indicates that clinicians can influence patients' behavior but they cannot control it. Fewer than 20% of patients report that they are ready to take action on a health behavior change in the next 30 days (e.g., quit smoking or start a weight-loss program). Therefore, much of the clinician's work involves increasing patients' readiness to take action by helping them to contemplate, choose, and then commit themselves to a specific plan.

Clinicians are not burdened with the sole responsibility for promoting healthier behaviors. Friends, family, media, employers, laws and law enforcement, commercial enterprises, and self-help groups all attempt to generate motivation and provide resources for behavior change. Linking up with these other sources of interest and motivation increases the clinician's influence and reduces the burden.

The Ideal Clinician Demeanor: Empathy & Curiosity

Research has consistently demonstrated the power of an empathic and involved supporter in promoting growth and change (see Chapter 2). But empathy and curiosity may not come easily to the busy clinician who is frustrated by the patient's inability or unwillingness to act upon obvious health improvement recommendations and treatment plans. The clinician needs to raise behavioral issues without provoking defensiveness or rationalizations which can neutralize his or her impact. The most productive clinician demeanor is one of respectful curiosity that focuses the patient on identifying motivations and overcoming specific obstacles to change.

Here is how that might be done.

> **Doctor:** I'm curious about what happened with the exercise program that you seemed ready to commit yourself to at your last visit? (Pause for the count of three to signal the importance of the patient's response.)

> **Doctor:** I can hear that you have not found diets to be effective for you in the past. If you give me a more detail about how you have dieted in the past, then perhaps we could figure out together why you weren't able to lose more weight.

Since behavior change requires an active patient outside of medical visits, we need the patient to be an active participant during the discussion as well. Here are some follow-up questions that utilize the "pulling" approach of empathy and curiosity in discussion of behavior change.

> **Doctor:** What do you think is the biggest thing you must do or overcome in order to get an exercise program started? (Pause) How convinced are you that losing weight is important for you now?

> **Doctor:** How would you make that decision?

> **Doctor:** Remind me of why you originally felt this change would be helpful for you?

> **Doctor:** It sounds to you like that's a lot to take on right now, yet I know how upsetting it has been to you to watch your weight increasing and the hemoglobin A1-C scores continuing to rise.

> **Doctor:** If in a few years I were to learn that you succeeded in quitting smoking, what do you think would be the reason you would tell me that finally convinced you to quit?

Many clinicians report that, once they let go of the illusion of "pushing" as their main responsibility and strategy, these kinds of conversations are more enjoyable. It helps to know that research supports the clinician in a less controlling and therefore frustrating approach to influencing behavior change. The clinician can discharge his or her appropriate advisory responsibility quite simply and then devote what time remains available in the discussion to exploring the patient's intrinsic motivation and urgency.

Doctor: The research tells us that quitting smoking is probably the best thing you could do for your health. But where are you in your own thinking about quitting?

Clinicians accept the theory of reactance and the natural resistance to coercion and criticism and do not try to force change on patients because of their own sense of urgency. A clinician who is concerned about the pregnancy of a teenager who smokes cigarettes and drinks alcohol will have no more influence over this behavior than the strength of the clinician–patient relationship and the ability of the clinician to prompt genuine self-re-evaluation allows. When patients feel shame or embarrassment they are as likely to become defensive and avoidant of a topic and the clinician as they are to be spurred into action. To the pregnant teenager the clinician might better say, "I imagine that learning you are pregnant is a big piece of news all by itself. On top of that, here I am telling you that things like alcohol and cigarette smoking could really hurt your developing baby. What do you think about all that?" Rather than attempting to take control over decisions that are in the patient's realm of responsibility, the clinician can increase the patient's involvement by asking questions that emphasize her self-determination. For example the doctor might say, "There are many things that we like to go over in a prenatal visit, but let's start with your questions first, OK?" A 3-second pause with eye contact is a good way to signal your genuine intention that the patient is expected to be an active participant in all aspects of her care.

Ambivalence

An important contribution of the Motivational Interviewing Model is its emphasis on understanding and exploring ambivalence. People almost always feel two ways about behavior change. They see discomfort and disruption of their familiar routines in the short term balanced against the hope of desirable outcomes in the longer term. Trying to lose weight certainly fits this model. "On the one hand doctor, I'd love to lose some weight, but on the other hand I hate being on a diet and don't see where I would get the time to exercise regularly." Addictive behavior highlights the difficulty of trading short-term pleasure in hope of longer-term benefit. Smoking cigarettes brings smokers immediate pleasure and not smoking brings them immediate discomfort. It is typically when the smoker sees how all the various costs will mount up eventually that he seriously considers quitting.

The effective clinician asks about and empathizes with this ambivalence by inviting the patient to talk about the resulting stalemate and its effects. This is better done through surfacing and reflecting on the patient's mixed feelings about the change rather than through rhetorical questions (e.g., "Don't you think

that . . . ?") that encourage a "correct" rather than a genuinely felt response. Here is an example of exploring ambivalence:

Doctor: It sounds like you're weighing the time and effort of regular exercise against the upset you feel with yourself for not doing more to reduce your risk of another heart attack? How do you imagine you will ultimately decide what to do?"

The clinician can translate his or her sense of urgency into an expression of concern that the patient's goals may not be met unless the ambivalent impasse is resolved. Using the language of "I am concerned." emphasizes the desire to be helpful over the tone of judgment that people so easily hear and resent.

Doctor: I am just concerned that you will feel progressively weaker unless you can get yourself out of the house for some activity every day. But what do you think?

Doctor: I am just concerned that without restarting the home stretching and conditioning program, you will continue to feel limited by this back pain and perhaps end up choosing the surgery that you told me initially you wanted to avoid." (Pause for response.)

Apply the Model to Yourself First

Most clinicians will recognize that they have also been contemplating, or even promising to change some behavior for years without consistent success (e.g., regular exercise or getting sufficient sleep). This awareness can help them to appreciate the time span, false starts, progress, and relapses that are normal in the process of change. Since clinicians have been able to exert enormous discipline over portions of their lives, they are sometimes surprised to recognize the paralyzing affect of the ambivalence ("Don't you think that I would love to . . . but can't you see it is hard for me to because . . ."). The result can be more accurate empathy and therefore a more finely tuned intuition about what might be most helpful to say or propose next in a conversation with the patient.

What Makes a Successful Encounter?

Clinicians may fear that they will be shirking their duty to advise and appear too permissive if they don't press patients to take action immediately to change potentially harmful behaviors. They may react with frustration and hopelessness with a patient who appears resistant. It is natural to imagine that more force will be needed to overcome more resistance or conversely to be too passive if you believe that change is impossible for some people or with some problems. Eschewing criticism and confrontation is not the same as avoiding a careful focus on health behavior change process. One of the most valuable contributions of these models has been to better understand the natural history of behavior change and how to use the most effective approaches to accomplish the work of each stage.

Change is a process not an event. The clinician's task at any time is to promote movement through the stages leading up to the patient's taking consistent action and then translating the new behavior into a lifestyle that resists relapse. The patient remains in control; the clinician thoughtfully applies his or her influence as the opportunities arise.

INTEGRATING THE THREE APPROACHES

Determining the Current State of Change Organizes the Clinician's Approach

Assessing stage of change starts most naturally with a statement bridging to the clinician's reasons for pursuing the behavioral issue. Let's use a discussion of smoking cessation with a hospitalized chronic obstructive pulmonary disease patient (COPD) patient as an example.

Doctor: Let me ask you about a few behaviors that usually worsen COPD and create the kind of crisis that led to your admission. For instance, how do you think your smoking might be affecting this?

Doctor: I imagine it was pretty scary to feel that you couldn't get a breath. How much effort would you be willing to put in at this point to avoid another breathing crisis like that one. (Pause for response.)

Doctor: I'm wondering if you are ready to talk about how we could help you quit smoking.

The self-efficacy construct offers a very helpful diagnostic and planning metric for the clinician. The clinician can ask the patient to rate himself from 1 to 10 on how convinced he is that his smoking is a problem (Or stated differently, how convinced is he that quitting smoking would be helpful right now.) If the patient is barely convinced that the change is valuable at this time (e.g., "I don't see how that would really help."), then exploring his understanding of the impact of smoking on his COPD will be the place to start. If the patient is already convinced that the change would be very valuable (e.g., "I know that smoking is killing me, but I have never been able to quit."), then clinician's time is best spent enhancing confidence that it can be achieved.

Doctor: Tell me a little more about what part of quitting smoking has been the most difficult for you and I will see what ideas we might have that could help with that.

Here are more examples of questions to assess conviction and confidence as part of understanding the patient's current stage of change and deciding where best to spend additional effort in the interview:

Doctor: How convinced are you that cigarette smoking is really damaging your health?

Doctor: How confident are you that you could quit in the near future? (Pause) What affects your confidence the most?

Doctor: So in order to help you feel more confident that you could quit, we would need to find some way to reduce that initial craving? Tell me what you already know about things that can help with craving and I will fill in the blanks.

This same style of question can be adapted to a wide range of health problems and health behavior changes. For example:

Doctor: How convinced are you that stretching and strengthening exercises will reduce your back pain?

Doctor: What are you doing now to control your weight?

Doctor: Is this something that you are ready to make a commitment to do in the near future?

Doctor: Has there ever been a time when you have lost a good deal of weight? ... Tell me more about how you lost it and then how you think you relapsed into regaining it.

Doctor: Being in the hospital allows patients time to plan for the lifestyle changes that will be essential for their recovery. What ideas do you have already about changes that will be important for you to make after discharge?" (Pull before push, ask before tell.)

Research suggests that it is best to focus on specific rather than general targets. Consider the list of behavior changes that would be advised for an inpatient following a heart attack: exercise, diet, medication adherence, cardiac rehab and regular follow-up, smoking cessation, alcohol moderation, and stress reduction. These are each separate behaviors to the patient. He may have previously quit smoking, but done little to change diet and exercise. Some patients, in the face of a new diagnosis of a medical problem will want to commit themselves immediately to a broad range of lifestyle changes. Yet even with this enormous surge of motivation many will not succed unless they work through each of the stages and build a commitment to a sustainable strategy and then apply their intended strategy on a consistent basis.

Once the clinician has established the patient's current stage of change for a specific behavior, the next step is to focus on brief interventions that identify and target specific obstacles to movement to the next stage (Table 16-2). Each conversation is in furtherance of this goal, yet the patient is the one who dictates how much movement is possible in any period.

Table 16-2. Stages of change and clinician strategies.

Stage of Change	Patient Characteristic	Clinician Strategy
Precontemplation	Denies problem and its importance. Is reluctant to discuss problem. Problem is identified by others. Shows reactance when pressured. High risk of argument.	Ask permission to discuss problem. Inquire about patient's thoughts. Gently point out discrepancies. Express concern. Ask patient to think, talk, or read about situation between visits.
Contemplation	Shows openness to talk, read, and think about problem. Weighs pros and cons. Dabbles in action. Can be obsessive about problem and can prolong stage.	Elicit patient's perspective first. Help identify pros and cons of change. Ask what would promote commitment. Suggest trials.
Preparation/Determination	Understands that change is needed. Begins to form commitment to specific goals, methods, and timetables. Can picture overcoming obstacles. May procrastinate about setting start date for change.	Summarize patient's reasons for change. Negotiate a start date to begin some or all change activities. Encourage patient to announce publicly. Arrange a follow-up contact at or shortly after start date.
Action	Follows a plan of regular activity to change problem. Can describe plan in detail (unlike dabbling in action of contemplator). Shows commitment in facing obstacles. Resists slips. Is particularly vulnerable to abandoning effort impulsively.	Show interest in specifics of plan. Discuss difference between slip and relapse. Help anticipate how to handle a slip. Support and re-emphasize pros of changing. Help to modify action plan if aspects are not working well. Arrange follow-up contact for support.
Maintenance	Has accomplished change or improvement through focused action. Has varying levels of awareness regarding importance of long-term vigilance. May already be losing ground through slips or wavering commitment. Has feelings about how much the change has actually improved life. May be developing lifestyle that precludes relapse into former problem.	Show support and admiration. Inquire about feelings and expectations and how well they were met. Ask about slips, any signs of wavering commitment. Help create plan for intensifying activity should slips occur. Support lifestyle and personal redefinition that reduce risk of relapse. Reflect on the long-term—and possibly permanent—nature of this stage as opposed to the more immediate gratification of initial success.
Relapse	Consistent return to problem behavior after period of resolution. Begins as slips that are not effectively resisted. May have cycled back to precontemplation, contemplation, or determination stages. Lessening time spent in this stage is a key to making greater progress toward fully integrated, successful, long-term change.	Frame relapse as a learning opportunity in preparation for next Action stage. Ask about specifics of change and relapse. Remind patient that contemplation work is still valid (reasons for changing). Use "when," rather than "if," in describing next change attempt. Normalize relapse as the common experience on the path to successful long-term change.

We now look at each stage and identify its main characteristics and strategies to promote movement to the next stage.

Helping the Precontemplator Start to Contemplate

In the Precontemplation stage patients typically minimize or deny the importance of a problem behavior. This topic was not on their agenda. Much of the resistance to discussion can be understood from reactance theory if the patient reacts to feeling criticized, embarrassed, and pressured.

It is useful for clinicians to differentiate the true, unaware Precontemplator from the mistrustful Contemplator's reluctance to discuss uncomfortable issues due to shame, demoralization, or a lack of trust in the clinician (e.g., the obese patient who frets constantly about her weight, yet dreads the issue arising in the doctor's office). Some patients are only too well aware of the problem and its costs, but feel overwhelmed and powerless to succeed in its resolution. The clinician's interview style will greatly influence these patients' willingness to discuss the problem. For example, drug and alcohol addiction are often described as diseases of denial. How can someone appear oblivious to the damage this behavior is causing? Closer examination often reveals that abusing or addicted individuals may spend considerable effort trying to unsuccessfully manage their addictive behavior. Sensitive questioning increases the likelihood that the precontemplator will be willing to contemplate the problem and potential solutions. Resist your urge to "push" information at the precontemplator and instead build his or her involvement by "pulling" ideas from him or her.

> **Doctor:** Tell me a little about how you think your weight might be a factor here?

> **Doctor:** Many of my patients tell me that they feel hopeless about their weight. How are you thinking about your weight at this point?

> **Doctor:** The research has made it clear that losing 10% of your current weight is likely to provide some valuable benefits in terms of your diabetes, hypertension, and joint pain. Were you aware of that? (Pause for response.)

The clinician wants the precontemplator to start contemplating the problem and its solution during the visit and later on his or her own. Once the patient becomes engaged in the contemplation or preparation stages for weight loss, for example, then the myriad of books, diets, and experts will probably be a much better source of ongoing information than the doctor himself or herself. That frees the doctor up to focus his or her brief moments with the patient where he or she can have the most impact, namely, the collaborative identification of the patient's current understanding of the obstacles and motivations and seeing the pathway to change.

> **Doctor:** Let's start thinking about the pros and cons of making a change. Then you can investigate the strategies/diets/programs that best fit your needs and, when you're ready, get started. Make sense?

> **Doctor:** Fortunately, there are excellent books that accurately describe the nutritional issues and offer very effective weight-loss plans for you to think about. Do you have a favorite already or could I suggest one or two?

 CASE ILLUSTRATION 1

Jack is 50 years old and is being seen by his internist. The appointment was encouraged by Jack's wife Clara, ostensibly for follow-up of treatment for persistent high blood pressure. The actual reason, as she explained confidentially to the nurse, is her concern about her husband's drinking and his failure to follow the clinician's latest recommendations for blood pressure control. During his time alone with the doctor, Jack does not mention any problems with alcohol or any difficulty following the recommended regimen. When the doctor presses Jack for more details about the amount of alcohol he is consuming, Jack becomes evasive and irritated. The physician backs off and ends the visit with only a change in antihypertensive medication—and a feeling of frustration.

Defensiveness can often be defused if clinicians ask the precontemplator for permission to talk about the problem and makes a bridging statement to introduce the topic. For instance:

> **Doctor:** Would it be all right if we talk a little more about things that can elevate blood pressure and cause other problems? First I'd like to get an idea of what you think might be contributing to some of the symptoms you mentioned today?

The clinician explores the patient's degree of awareness as a way to move the conversation further into contemplation. For example, over the course of a brief exchange, the clinician might ask questions such as:

> **Doctor:** What concerns do you have about your alcohol use? (Pause) Is there anything about it that worries you? (Pause) What is your wife most worried

about? What has happened to make this such a concern to her? (Pause) How important is her concern to you?

Depending on the specific problem there may be well worked out sets of screening questions that fit in nicely here (e.g., CAGE or MAST questions for alcohol, brief screening inventories for depression or anxiety, or the SOAPES screening questionnaire to assess the risk of abuse or dependency when prescribing opiates for pain).

Doctor: I have a brief questionnaire that can be helpful in determining how much depression or anxiety may be contributing to the problem. Why don't you take a moment to complete it now and we will score it together and see what it suggests to us.

When offering the clinician's perspective or providing data the **Provide-Elicit-Provide-Elicit** approach helps to keep the patient actively involved. Instead of giving extended lectures or explanations, the clinician gives a piece of information and then quickly elicits (pulls) the patient's reaction. For example:

Doctor: High blood pressure can be dangerous for many reasons. What do you already know about the risks of sustained high blood pressure?

Asking patients to contemplate the possible connections between their physical symptoms or medical condition and the behaviors that may be contributing to them is among the most helpful ways to get precontemplators thinking.

As much as possible, the physician's agenda should be linked to concerns the patient has already expressed. If a female patient asks for birth control, the clinician can use her concern about pregnancy as a basis for asking how else she had been protecting herself when having sex. This may lead naturally to a discussion about using condoms with new partners, an issue that was not on her agenda for this visit.

Many patients seem unaware of the interaction between their emotional and physical health. Sixty to eighty percent of patients with depression or anxiety present with medical symptoms rather than emotional concerns. Often the clinician first works up all the "legitimate" medical causes of symptoms before inquiring about emotional involvement. An alternative is to ask early on in the visit about psychosocial contributors to the somatic symptoms since these factors may suggest behavior changes or treatments that are necessary for symptom relief. For example:

Doctor: Tell me about anything that is going on in your life that could be affecting the frequency or the intensity of those headaches. (Pause)

Conversely, when the patient brings up the stresses in his or her life, the clinician can be listening for linkage to physical symptoms or the ability to adhere to a challenging medical regimen.

Doctor: With all that is going on in your life, I imagine it can be difficult to keep on top of your diabetes self-care regimen. What have you noticed?

Discrepancies between the patient's present behavior and his or her expressed goal of feeling better can be pointed out empathically. Physicians can also express their concern that the patient may not achieve the desired improvement without addressing the behavior that contributes to it.

Doctor: I'm concerned that you'll always worry about another heart attack unless you know that you've changed your lifestyle to lower the risks.

Doctor: I'm concerned that none of these medicines will be able to relieve your stomach discomfort as long as your diet contains so many things that can irritate it.

Much of the actual work of contemplation is done between visits. Clinicians can ask the patient to think about, keep track of, and read about the problem and potential solutions—or talk to someone else about them—before the next appointment. The clinician notes the patient's response and mentions it at the next visit to affirm its importance.

Doctor: Many of my patients feel they are eating very little and still gaining weight. I wonder if it be helpful for you to sit down with our nutritionist and let the two of you map out exactly how many calories you are taking in and where they're coming from?

Doctor: Sounds like you and your wife disagree about how much and how often you are drinking. You could resolve that by noting on the calendar each day how much alcohol you had to drink. Then it would be more clear to the two of you how much of an issue there actually is. How does that sound to you?

Doctor: What would you look at to tell you whether your drinking was causing trouble in your life?

Doctor: I am curious. Why do you think that I place so much emphasis on finding alternatives to narcotics for dealing with your back pain? (Pause) When you have a moment this handout might clarify for you the criteria we are required to use when deciding when it is safe and legal to prescribe narcotics on a long-term basis.

For the precontemplator, most of the motivation of statements are being made by others and can feel like coercion or criticism. We want the patient to begin reflecting on the situations without feeling pressured by others.

Doctor: If the narcotics were helping you to live better with your back condition, what would you be doing differently in your daily life that would tell us they were working?

The precontemplator is often initially spurred to contemplation by forces acting upon him rather than by his own choosing. Perhaps his wife threatens to leave him, or his boss threatens to fire him if he continues to drink/drug. Perhaps the clinician gives unexpected news about cholesterol, hemoglobin A1-C, blood pressure, or makes an upsetting diagnosis. The sensitive interviewer uses this moment to "induct" the patient further into the Contemplation stage.

Doctor: Now that you have that data, what goes through your mind? (Pause) How aware are you of the relationship between these elevated hemoglobin A1-Cs and the increased likelihood of complications from your diabetes? (Pause) Remind me of what you already know about the keys to improved diabetes management. (Pause) How would you rate yourself on each of those?

When the patient increasingly thinks on his own about the problem and how it might be solved, then he has moved into the Contemplation stage of change and the clinician's efforts shift to firming up commitment to a plan of action.

Helping Contemplators Prepare to Commit Themselves to a Course of Action

In the Contemplation stage the patient demonstrates some of the following characteristics:

- The patient is open to thinking about and discussing the problem with little prompting and may even raise the problem himself or herself.
- The patient appears interested, may ask for additional information, and weighs the pros and cons of changing or not changing the problem behavior.
- Unless the patient feels pushed to make a specific commitment to take action, there is less risk of resistance.
- The Contemplation stage can be prolonged or obsessive as the patient searches for more convincing data and looks for an ideal time and situation in which to initiate change.
- Patients may be dabbling in action without a clear and firm commitment. They may, for example, decline an occasional dessert, and go for a walk on the weekend. Contemplators may learn they can

reduce immediate guilt or anxiety by making a vague promise to change in the future or overestimating the value of intermittent behavior change.

- Contemplators may be thinking about obstacles from too limited a framework, for example, doubting that they have sufficient willpower, or thinking that they are genetically prone to obesity and therefore overlooking practical ways to reduce or burn calories.

Contemplation builds the foundation for later successful resolution of the problem. Patients must anticipate costs and obstacles, identify their motivations, reassess how easy or difficult the behavior change might be, and feel that they are making informed and independent decisions, rather than being coerced by others. Although some people claim that they impulsively threw away their cigarettes, or that they quit drinking suddenly and never once looked back, research suggests that even these people were quietly doing contemplation work in the years and months leading up to the presumably impulsive action.

 CASE ILLUSTRATION 2

Joanna is 44 years old and has been smoking a pack of cigarettes a day since she was 17. When prompted by her primary care provider she is very willing to discuss the pros and cons of smoking. Joanna tells her doctor that she is being pressured by her children about secondary smoke and that she agrees with their position. She thinks that the habit is both expensive and stupid. On the other hand, she believes that smoking is one of the few things that relax her throughout the day at work and at home. One of her friends quit smoking and gained 25 lb; this possibility is frightening to Joanna, who is already concerned about her weight. Her doctor asks what she knows about ways to reduce the craving for nicotine that also help prevent weight gain. Johanna says she has tried nicotine gum in the past, but wants to know more about other smoking cessation aides and medications. By the end of the discussion Johanna has promised her doctor to think more seriously about trying to quit, but makes no commitments to a specific approach or quit date. Johanna is in contemplation about smoking cessation.

The clinician's goal with the Contemplation stage is to help patients resolve their ambivalence sufficiently to enable them to commit to a plan and timetable for taking action. In order to accomplish this, the clinician elicits the patient's perspective before offering advice, asking questions that encourage self-reflection and self-motivational statements. This works in the inpatient as well as outpatient settings. For example, the hospitalist can assess the patient's stage of change quickly and then initiate a focused 2-minute conversation linking smoking cessation with discharge goals.

> **Hospitalist:** As we move closer to discharge, what are your thoughts about your cigarette smoking and why quitting would be particularly helpful for you now?

> **Hospitalist:** Being in a hospital gives people a chance to think and talk with loved ones about life changes they need to make in order to recover and stay healthy. Let's make a list of the two or three behavior changes that would be most beneficial to you.

Patients can be helped to identify the pros and cons of change and to examine the current pleasures and ultimate consequences of a problem behavior. It is axiomatic that people engage in unhealthful behavior because they desire the pleasures such acts bring. Many patients already believe that they would be better off if they ate differently, exercised more, drank less, stopped or cut down on drug use, lost weight, reduced stress, and so on. Contemplators often become stuck in ambivalence because they fear the change process will be psychologically or physically unpleasant, costly, and likely to fail. This is often where the clinician is tempted to pounce with ideas and encouragement that unfortunately often oversimplify the issue in a "just do it" admonition. While encouragement is a wonderful part of the doctor–patient interaction, it loses some power if it comes across in a generalized or pat way. Linked with a moment more of respectful exploration, encouragement focuses the contemplator on how to succeed.

> **Doctor:** There is no doubt that increasing the strength and flexibility in your back muscles, reduces your risk of re-injury and even more disability. What has been the biggest obstacle to doing the back strengthening exercises at home? (Pause) What ideas have you had for how to work around that? (Pause) Is there more we could be doing to help?

Patients often claim that because of insufficient willpower they are powerless to stop smoking, quit drug or alcohol abuse, or change some other behavior. Clinicians often feel stuck when the conversation moves into the "willpower" realm. Reframe willpower as an energy that rises and falls in relation to how convinced the patients are that change is valuable and the size of the step that they are asking themselves to take.

> **Doctor:** If you were to become convinced that your life depended on your not smoking for 3 months, do you think you could resist temptation that long? (Pause) Where would the willpower to do it come from?

> **Doctor:** You may be asking yourself to take too big a step at one time. Let's think about an amount and type of physical activity that you would be able to fit into your week right now.

> **Doctor:** Willpower can be thought of like money. It goes a lot further when we spend it wisely. Let's think about taking smaller steps that initially cost less willpower.

Similarly, patients can be asked what they think would bring about a commitment to change the behavior in some future period.

> **Doctor:** If I were to meet you years from now and find that you had completely stopped using marijuana, what do you think you would tell me was the reason you finally quit? (Pause for response.) How do you imagine you would have accomplished this?

In order to promote movement from prolonged contemplation to a specific action, clinicians can encourage patients to think about an upcoming time in which taking action to resolve or improve the problem situation would make most sense.

> **Doctor:** I understand this is a bad time to get started, but I wonder if you can anticipate another upcoming period that seems more promising.

Since self-efficacy is related to the size of the step to be taken, suggestions for limited trials of smaller steps can build the patient's confidence and willingness to commit to some more concerted action. Questions in the form, "Would you be willing to try . . . ?" frame these changes as both thought experiments as well as real suggestions for steps to think about between visits.

> **Doctor:** Would you be willing to cut down from 20 to 15 cigarettes a day and make a note of how hard or easy this is for you? That way you will learn more about what will work best when you try to quit completely.

Patients in the Contemplation stage usually need to evaluate not only the pros and cons of the problem, but also the advantages and disadvantages of different means of overcoming the problem. The clinician can sometimes be most helpful by assisting the patient in contemplating the many ways that change can be accomplished in order to increase their readiness to commit to a plan of action.

> **Doctor:** There are a number of over-the-counter and prescription medications that reduce the craving caused by nicotine withdrawal when you first stop smoking. Tell me what you already know about these and I can help us think about which would be most effective for you to consider.

Sometimes the clinician is asking the contemplator to take a smaller step now in order to make behavior change easier in the future.

Doctor: Would you be willing to always carry a condom with you so that it's available the next time you have the opportunity for sex?

Doctor: Would you be willing to check with your health plan now about your options for getting alcohol treatment in the evening? That way, if you should decide to start treatment, you wouldn't miss work and no one there would need to know about the problem.

The clinician can briefly summarize the issues to facilitate contemplation at resolution to the ambivalence.

Doctor: It sounds as though you realize that losing weight will be best for you in the long term, and now you're also trying to choose the best approach and timetable for taking action.

The clinician can also delegate the contemplation work to another resource.

Doctor: There is so much valuable information about diet changes for diabetes and weight control that I suggest we give you a chance to sit down with our nutritionist and think this through. Should we arrange that next?

Doctor: It sounds to me that stresses at home are a big part of your depression. I am concerned that we don't have enough time here to give the situation the careful consideration it deserves. What do you think about sitting down with a counselor and giving yourself the time to understand this better and decide what to do?

Motivation to move from what may have become prolonged contemplation to a commitment to a specific course of action may come from many quarters; salient information arriving at an opportune moment, threats or pressure from people or circumstances (e.g., the alcoholic husband whose wife threatens divorce, the smoker who learns she is pregnant), an inspiring model, an opportunity for social support from others undergoing similar changes (e.g., workmates deciding to join a weight-loss program together) , or an opportunity for a fresh start, such as a job transfer or move or a new health plan that covers behavioral health better. Like many things that move quickly when they get "unstuck" by a jolt or force from outside, the patient with a new diagnosis of heart disease may be energized to move rapidly through contemplation, and seek out behavior recommendations that were previously ignored or resisted. Such changes lead to the Preparation/Determination stage.

Encouraging Preparation/Determination to Take Action

In the Preparation/Determination stage the patient experiences a mounting sense of urgency and commitment to change.

- The patient talks about having made the decision to change, in contrast with the contemplator's wish for change.
- The patient chooses a specific goal: "I am going to stop smoking completely." "I will exercise three times a week." "I want to get my blood sugars under X."
- The patient mentions a specific time to begin the activity: "Next month. . . ." "After my surgery. . . ." "When the kids start school in September. . . ."
- The patient has chosen a specific course of action, such as joining a commercial weight-loss program or Alcoholics or Narcotics Anonymous (AA, NA), or is asking for a referral so the health plan will cover a behavior treatment.
- The patient anticipates and is ready to pay the costs of change, including out-of-pocket expenses, the time required for the change, physical discomfort, self-consciousness, and risk of failure.
- The patient considers the potential reactions of important people who may resist or be threatened by the change. A spouse or partner who smokes or drinks or is overweight, for example, may react negatively to the patient's plans to overcome the problem, perhaps anticipating pressure to face their own problems. In other cases, spouses, partners, and friends may resist the patient's decision to change because of some anticipated personal inconvenience (e.g., the spouse who must watch the children while his wife goes to an aerobics class or support group, or live with a change in diet as the spouse shifts the family's meals in healthy directions). The Preparation/Determination stage involves consolidating conviction and confidence in order to commit to take action. Below is an example of a teenager who has crossed the threshold into commitment to change.

 CASE ILLUSTRATION 3

Mike is a 15-year-old boy who has been doing poorly in school for several years. Although he had previously been diagnosed with attention deficit hyperactivity disorder (ADHD), his parents, teachers, and pediatrician have been unable to convince him that he should take a medication that could help. Now he has asked for an appointment with his pediatrician to discuss the situation. During the

visit, Mike confesses that he is increasingly frustrated by his problem behavior and poor school performance as he starts to think about college someday. Further questioning by the physician reveals that one of Mike's friends admitted to being treated with medication for ADHD. Mike noticed and envied his friend's success; he asks the physician to prescribe "Whatever it will take to help me." Mike's parents are invited into the examining room, and all agree on a plan that will begin with a trial of stimulant medicine. The effects of the medication will be reassessed in a month, based on questionnaires filled out by Mike and his parents and teachers. Mike is in Preparation/Determination stage of change ready to take action.

In this stage, it is appropriate for the clinician to encourage the patient to make a firm commitment to a specific plan and set a date to start action on the problem. Summarizing what has been said up to now can mark this transition.

Doctor: So you're planning to start Weight Watchers at work next month with the goal of losing 35 lbs this year?

Doctor: You've committed yourself to getting 30 minutes of aerobic exercise four times a week.

Doctor: You want to try on your own first, but you are willing to join a support group if you don't have success?

These commitments can be noted in the chart in the patient's presence, and the patient can be told that the clinician is looking forward to hearing about what happens next.

Patients are supported by reassurance that initiating action to change problem behavior is always the right thing to do. Even when the attempt is not fully successful, the experience will yield helpful information about how to succeed eventually. It is important not to appear so enthusiastic and hopeful that patients who are unsuccessful want to avoid you. Because public commitments are more likely to be kept than private ones, patients should be encouraged to tell others about their plan and ask for specific support when needed.

Follow-up is helpful, whether by scheduling an appointment, or requesting a note or phone message soon after the proposed start date. Some people will move back and forth between Determination/Preparation and Contemplation stages a few more times before actually moving into Action stage. We have all stood on the edge of the water believing we were ready to jump in, only to talk ourselves out of it. The clinician's role is to help these patients develop their commitment to a specific course of action. They can do this by focusing the limited time available in a medical encounter on exactly which obstacles are causing the delay in launching the action plan.

Action

In this stage, patients engage in a consistent course of action intended to achieve the goals they have set in the earlier stages. The clinician may not always fully agree with the patient's initial action plan. For example, a patient's diet and exercise regimen may be too limited to produce the desirable weight loss. Yet it is easier to make adjustments to a plan in Action than to overcome the inertia of getting a plan started in the first place. The clinician can genuinely support any plan that will provide the patient with some useful information, and help move them in a direction of change. Some characteristics of the Action stage include the following:

- The patient is attending a weight-reduction group, has started going to AA, has recently quit or cut down on smoking and may be wearing a nicotine patch, or has begun exercising regularly, or recording daily glucometer readings.
- The patient may be focusing on "one day at a time" or trying to look past the initial discomfort by focusing on the long-term benefits.
- The patient recognizes and deals with the obstacles that arise, making adjustments when necessary to adhere to the overall plan.

Unlike in the Contemplation stage, Action stage behavior is more than experimental dabbling in change to see what it might be like. There is now greater determination to succeed. Of course, it remains to be seen whether the action plan can be maintained and if it will show sufficient results to keep the patient motivated. By reminding the patient of his or her motivations for change, the patient can withstand discomforts and obstacles that would shake a less well-developed commitment.

The Action stage is a time of maximum focus and effort. The patient is experiencing most of the discomfort and not yet realizing much of the desired benefit. The greatest risk is that second thoughts may undermine the patient in a moment of weakness. The action plan may then be abandoned precipitously or allow exceptions (slips) that ultimately dilute and unravel the strength of the original commitment. Successful changers have usually anticipated these risks and have an intention and plan to address them.

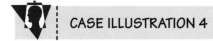

CASE ILLUSTRATION 4

Martha is a 45-year-old diabetic patient. Over the past few years, her doctor has encouraged her to lose weight and exercise regularly, without much success. Martha comes in today and proudly reports that she has joined a weight-loss group that is held at her work site. Two colleagues have also joined, and they have all been attending faithfully and following the dietary recommendations for the past 3 weeks. The doctor encourages Martha to talk about her efforts. She is eager to talk; she reports feeling a sense of pride and satisfaction. She admits that although she had been disgusted with herself for getting so heavy, she never before felt ready and able to tackle the problem. When her friends suggested that they join the group together she understood that this was the situation she had been hoping for, one that could provide support in making a difficult change.

Martha also admits to some anxiety. Since many people now know that she is trying to lose weight she does not want to fail publicly. Although she has been tempted to cheat on the diet, she has resisted the urge. She admits to the doctor that she had felt somewhat discouraged when she did not lose as much weight as she had hoped the previous week and wonders aloud what might have been the cause.

While checking the weight-loss program's recommendations, Martha's doctor warmly reinforces the effort at change. The doctor may offer additional helpful suggestions to reduce the risk of relapse and orient Martha more firmly toward long-term maintenance. The doctor's warm, curious, and engaged demeanor has reverberations beyond the visit. Martha can use the pleasant memory of the encounter to further internalize the value of the effort toward change. While the doctor will have little control over Martha's weight-loss success, she is pleased to have efficiently used what influence she does have to encourage Martha's efforts. Martha leaves feeling that an important person is rooting for her success.

Strategies for the Action Stage

In this stage, the clinician and patient anticipate what might be needed to maintain the initial behavior changes. This involves problem-solving obstacles that are already emerging as well as planning ahead for how slips will be checked before a full-blown relapse can set in.

As in the above example, a moment of warm inquiry about the specifics of the patient's program reinforces the clinician's interest and provides encouragement for the patient.

Clinicians can also ask about any obstacles the patient has encountered (obstacles and second thoughts are to be expected) and offer help in thinking through potential solutions. For example, one clinician suggested that her patients write out the pros of making the change and post them prominently as an aid to maintaining motivation.

Patients can be asked for permission to consult with other professionals involved in the program. A brief contact with a chemical-dependency counselor, diabetic educator, smoking-cessation group leader, psychotherapist, and so on demonstrates that the physician values and supports the patient's efforts during the most vulnerable period of active change and helps resolve any mixed messages the patient may be getting.

Asking about slips that have occurred and the patient's plan for quick recovery can be helpful in this stage (e.g., smoking a cigarette, having a drink, missing an exercise session or AA meeting, or having seconds at a meal). A slip need not become a fall into relapse if patients have anticipated the possibility and prepared how they will think about the slip and react once it is recognised, e.g., throw out the rest of the cigarette pack; pour out the remainder of the bottle; add another exercise session or AA meeting; eat a smaller-than-usual portion at the next meal; and reaffirm the commitment to conquer this problem.

Some type of follow-up (e.g., a note or call, an appointment) can be helpful to get a progress update and to show support for the patient. Making a note on the chart will remind the physician and office staff to inquire about the change effort at the next patient contact. One of the potential problems that arise in the transition of care from the hospitalist to the outpatient is the discontinuity when the patient is discharged and returns to usual care. Since time in the hospital is often triggered by a "crisis" where there is momentarily greater willingness to consider behavior change (either lifestyle change or greater adherence to outpatient medical regimens), it behooves the hospitalist to give the patient some written follow-up plan that includes summarizing what they have discussed and committed themselves to in terms of behavior change and to include the details of the plan in the discharge summary to the outpatient clinician.

Doctor: Well Mr. Smith, it sounds as if you are ready to commit yourself now to quit smoking and continue to use the nicotine patches that we started while you were in the hospital. I will be rooting for your success and will let your regular doctor know our plan.

The Action stage is a time of concerted effort to behave differently. The behaviors feel new or unfamiliar and therefore somewhat vulnerable. It will require longer-term commitment, vigilance, and activity to make continued progress toward a goal (e.g., weight loss, firmer sobriety, lower hemoglobin A1-C) and to prevent backsliding into relapse. This sustained vigilance and continued activity characterizes the Maintenance stage. For people who must control their weight, for instance, this stage may last a lifetime. In one study, former smokers reported some temptation to smoke 18 months after quitting. Problem drinkers may continue in AA for many years before they feel safe with their sobriety. Clinicians should be concerned about patients who have made good progress in initially changing their behavior but cannot describe their long-term maintenance plans. Helping patients anticipate and find satisfying answers to the questions addressed in the next section is an important way in which clinicians can promote long-term success.

Maintenance

The Maintenance stage is the period where initial success from the Action stage is transformed into the new "normal," a part of the patient's lifestyle.

- The patient has achieved a period of success—as he or she has defined it—in overcoming the problem. For example, the patient may have cut down or stopped drinking, reduced to the goal weight, or gone without cigarettes for several months. He or she may be managing time and commitments better so that stress is no longer overwhelming or may have gained consistent control over a short temper, or accomplished other desired outcomes.
- Some patients assume a positive identity as people who have overcome a problem and whose lives have gone in a new direction. Patients who begin an exercise and diet program to lose weight, for example, may become avid hikers whose leisure time is now devoted to rigorous outdoor adventures and who stay in shape in order to enjoy them. These people have made an identity change in which the former sedentary lifestyle has no place.

In order to maintain behavioral improvements, the patient must be able to handle both predictable (e.g., working through the "deprived feeling" that often accompanies dieting or substance-abuse recovery) and unpredictable challenges (e.g., not reverting to smoking during a period of unexpected personal stress). Successful maintenance requires dealing appropriately with the temptations and frustrations that inevitably arise in the months and years following successful action.

Some patients may feel disappointed that success in dealing with one problem has not brought about hoped-for changes in other areas. For example, while 10% weight loss may produce improvements in blood sugar and cholesterol control, it may not lead to a hoped-for degree of slenderness and attractiveness. Abstinence from crack cocaine may not be enough to improve all relationship, job, and financial problems. Chronic disease management adherence may postpone but not eliminate increasing disability. Patients who reduce their workaholic schedules so as to spend more time with their families may find they've traded more admiration at home for less at work. Adherence to psychiatric medication may control target symptoms but bring troublesome side effects.

Maintenance often involves a tapering off from the intensity of effort that marked the Action stage. Attendance at support-group meetings, for example, may have become less frequent. The patient may be wondering whether it is now safe to quit the group or treatment program or to end a specific diet. It is hard to know when one is "out of the woods" and the problem resolved. Successful maintenance requires both accurate self-appraisal and ongoing vigilance for lapses into the problem behavior. "I'll have just one glass of wine when I'm out with friends." "I'll only have a cigarette if I'm feeling really tense." These seductive thoughts must be resisted if successful maintenance is to continue. It may be necessary to renew the more intense effort of the Action stage to do so (e.g., rejoining Weight Watchers, returning to 12 Step Support Group, going back to psychotherapy and/or psychiatric medication).

 CASE ILLUSTRATION 5

At 55 years of age, Bill is doing very well overall, seeing his internist periodically for health maintenance. Bill had been a very heavy drinker for 20 years. Five years ago a citation for driving under the influence of alcohol and the threat of divorce by his second wife pushed him into an alcohol treatment program. He achieved abstinence while attending the formal, court-mandated, 2-year outpatient treatment program. Since that time he has continued in AA, attending at least two meetings a week and occasional weekend conferences and workshops. Bill also sponsors a younger man in the AA group. In his conversations with his doctor, Bill describes himself as a recovering alcoholic. During his last appointment with his doctor he describes a great deal of distress over problems his son is experiencing—for which he holds himself partly responsible. The doctor thinks antidepressant medicine might be helpful, particularly in light of Bill's disturbed

sleep and preoccupied demeanor. Bill questions the internist closely about the risk of addiction and explains his reluctance to use "another crutch" to control his moods.

Bill's doctor recognizes that because Bill is in maintenance for his alcohol problem he is extremely vigilant about anything he sees as a threat to his sobriety. The doctor asks respectfully how Bill believes antidepressant medication might undermine his sobriety or stimulate a new addiction. Bill says that he is basically afraid of becoming dependent on the medication. The physician then explains that antidepressant medications are not addictive and that individual psychotherapy is also an effective treatment, and advises Bill to think about the recommendation, to speak with other AA members and confidants about the two alternatives, and to give him a call when he is ready to discuss it further.

Strategies for the Maintenance Stage

Inquiring about how well the patient is maintaining the changed behavior and what improvements or disappointments he or she is noticing is an important first step in supporting maintenance.

Doctor: What have you been doing to keep your weight down? (Pause) How have you noticed your lifestyle changing as a result?

Doctor: How have your support-group meetings been going? (Pause) How would you decide if you needed to attend them more regularly again?

Doctor: How have you been doing with your exercise program? What are your goals at this point?

Doctor: Patients sometimes have second thoughts about continuing medications after they have been feeling better for a while, particularly if there are some unpleasant side effects. What have you noticed in that regard?

Doctor: Living well with a chronic illness is a great accomplishment. I am impressed with how well you manage your arthritis and are able to live a very active life.

Patients can be asked about slips that have already occurred and how they responded. Patients should be prepared for the likelihood of a slip and have a plan for how to deal with it at once. They may protest that the clinician is being too pessimistic. Explaining that such preparation is a way that patients can protect their investment in all they have accomplished and can provide a more positive rationale for anticipating and planning for how they will respond to slips.

Ask how convinced they are now that the change is beneficial and how confident they are that they will maintain the improvement over the next time period. Anticipate threats to maintenance by asking patients to describe situations in which the risk of a slip or relapse is high—such as going to a party or experiencing emotions such as anger, sadness, or exuberance—and how prepared they feel to handle these high-risk situations without a slip.

Each of these recommendations shows interest, support, and curiosity and suggests that anticipation and vigilance are the keys to successful maintenance. The busy clinician may not be taking a leading role in the change (e.g., counselors, diabetic educators, and support-group members may be much more actively involved), but his or her empathic curiosity and focused advice can still be very supportive.

Clinicians should be alert for any signs of waning enthusiasm and express empathic curiosity about the cause. Are they discouraged or disappointed, or merely forgetting the problem or risk that existed previously now that so much time has passed? They may feel that others do not recognize and appreciate the effort that they have made to change. A sincere compliment from a clinician accompanied by a message that "I am rooting for you" creates a memory that can be recalled during moments of discouragement.

Relapse

Unfortunately, clinicians know from both research and experience that many patients' attempts to lose weight, stop alcohol or drug abuse, to reduce stress, alter their diets, and even to floss their teeth daily end in relapse. The false starts, failed promises, and pounds promptly regained tend to obscure the fact that persistent effort often does eventually result in a more successful resolution of the problem. Although any single effort to change may get derailed before the patient achieves successful long-term maintenance, repeated efforts tend to yield the desired result eventually. It is worth noting that more than 45 million Americans have now quit smoking, many on their third or fourth serious try. Since relapse is so common, the effective clinician should have a comfortable way of helping people learn from previous experience and rebuild their commitment to tackle the problem again.

Relapse begins with "slips." These are brief episodes of problem behavior after a period of self-defined success in having overcome the problem. A slip might involve engaging in an undesirable behavior such as smoking, or not engaging in a desirable behavior such as exercising. In the Relapse stage, the patient has reverted to consistent problem behavior, the "old normal."

- The patient may now talk or act like a person in an earlier stage of change. For example, he or she may have entered a period of resistance and avoidance that is characteristic of the Precontemplation stage. "It's impossible. I give up." Alternatively, the patient may be contemplating change again, possibly even preparing to begin a course of action again in the near future. "I'm going to try again in the Spring."

- The reasons offered for the relapse provide clues to the problems that the patient must address for success in future.

The time the patient spends in the Relapse stage before initiating the next Action stage of change accounts for much of the observed slowness in achieving final success for many health-behavior problems. We know that to have had any period of successful action the patient must have contemplated the problem, committed himself or herself to a course of action, been able to achieve some initial success, all of which potentially provide a useful springboard to the next attempt to change.

 CASE ILLUSTRATION 6

Barbara is a 28-year-old woman who is being seen 2 months after the birth of her second child for renewal of her birth control prescription. Her physician is delighted to see Barbara again. As the interview evolves, Barbara sheepishly reveals that she is back to smoking a pack of cigarettes a day. The clinician is both disappointed and surprised, since Barbara had been quite proud of the fact that she stopped smoking during the pregnancy. The doctor takes a deep breath and calmly asks Barbara how this happened so quickly. Barbara talks about how frazzled she has felt taking care of both her baby and her 3-year-old son with her husband away so much for work. She explains how, at first, she found it relaxing to smoke a cigarette or two after dinner after the kids have been put to bed. She had not pictured herself going back to smoking a pack a day again. Soon, however, she was smoking with a friend who stopped in to visit. Now she has begun looking forward to a cigarette whenever she has a break from the immediate demands of her family. She tells her doctor that although she tries not to smoke when the baby is up, even this control is starting to erode.

Barbara has relapsed. The doctor's first challenge is to manage her own frustration and not leave Barbara feeling judged and ashamed. She reminds Barbara of her previous success in caring for her (then) 2-year-old

child and dealing with the mood swings and physical discomforts of pregnancy without smoking. She supports Barbara's commitment not to smoke around the baby. Next, the doctor asks where Barbara is now in her thinking about continuing to smoke versus quitting. This tells her Barbara's current stage of change (the relapser settles into one of the earlier stages) and allows her to apply the strategies we have discussed previously in order to encourage Barbara's movement toward another attempt at smoking cessation.

If addressed empathically, patients in the Relapse stage are usually willing to talk about the problem behavior without denial or argument. They had already concluded at least once that change was needed and can typically recount the costs of continuing the problem behavior. From self-efficacy theory we recognize that relapse undermines confidence more than conviction. Patients may come to the wrong conclusion, for example, "I guess I don't have the willpower," unless helped to analyze and learn something specific and helpful from the relapse. A next attempt at change can be discussed as inevitable—when rather than if.

Doctor: It sounds like you have more than enough willpower when your intention to never use drugs is clear. The problem may have come about when you began to think you could use them in a controlled manner. That made for endless decisions rather than the single clear decision that launched you to successful sobriety originally. What do you think?

Doctor: It sounds like all your original reasons for changing are just as valid today. You also know that you have the willpower to stick with your exercise plan if you sign up for scheduled classes at the Y. What this relapse may have taught you is that you need to have a backup exercise plan to use when other important commitments interfere with your primary plan. What do you think?

CONCLUSION

One aspect of using these behavior change models is the hopefulness it generates for both clinician and patient. While clinicians are usually convinced that behavior change would be helpful, they often lack confidence in their ability to influence patients' behavior in brief medical interviews. The goal of this chapter has been to map out pragmatic approaches that can be utilized in even the briefest encounters in order to have a positive influence on the patient's behavior. Assessing patients' Stage of Change leads to focused examination room or hospital room conversations to promote movement toward behavior change. Motivational Interviewing teaches the demeanor of empathic and respectful curiosity that acknowledges patients' autonomy while exploring the ambivalence that marks all difficult choices. The clinician learns to pull from the patient self-motivational thoughts and feelings rather than push at the patient with lectures, threats, and inspiration. Finally, Social Learning Theory teaches that behavior changes when both conviction and confidence cross a threshold that tips toward action. At each stage of change the clinician must understand what is affecting the patients' conviction that the problem requires attention as well as his or her confidence that success is possible. This enables the clinician to focus on areas where his or her involvement is most likely to catalyze change.

SUGGESTED READINGS

Miller WR, Rollnick S, eds. *Motivational Interviewing: Preparing People for Change*. New York, NY: Guilford Press, 2002.

Prochaska JO, Norcross JC, DiClemente CC. *Changing for Good*. New York, NY: Guilford Press, 1994.

Rollnick S, Mason P, Butler C. *Health Behavior Change: A Guide for Practitioners*. London: Churchill Livingstone, 1999.

Rollnick S. Readiness, importance and confidence: critical conditions of change in treatment. In: Miller WR, Heather N, eds. *Treating Addictive Behavior*, 2nd ed. New York, NY: Plenum Press, 1998.

WEB SITES

The *Motivational Interviewing Page* Web site. http://www.motivationalinterview.org/. Accessed October, 2007.

Patient Adherence

Summer L. Williams, MA, Kelly B. Haskard, PhD, & M. Robin DiMatteo, PhD

INTRODUCTION

When patients fail to follow treatment recommendations made by their physicians, problems in clinical care can result. **Nonadherence** (also called **noncompliance**) typically involves, among other things, patients taking medications incorrectly or not at all, forgetting or refusing to make essential behavioral changes for their care, and persisting in behaviors such as smoking and high-risk sexual activity that jeopardize their health. As a result of their failure to adhere to recommended treatments, patients might become more seriously ill, and treatment-resistant pathogens may develop. Failing to recognize patients' nonadherence may prompt physicians to adjust medication dosages, and to be misled in their diagnoses. Practitioners and patients become frustrated by nonadherence, and the time and money spent on medical visits is wasted.

A great deal of research on nonadherence shows that although its prevalence varies with the type of regimen prescribed, at least a quarter of patients on average fail to adhere. Rates of nonadherence are quite high for long-term medication use in chronic disease (40–50%) and for lifestyle changes such as exercising or ceasing tobacco use (more than 75%). Adherence to treatment is most problematic when patients are quite ill with serious medical conditions (such as cardiovascular disease and end-stage renal disease) and their lives depend upon following complex treatment recommendations. Many of the regimens for these conditions are multifaceted and can include numerous medications with intolerable side effects, difficult dosing schedules, and restrictions on diet and activities. When patients are severely ill, frustration, pessimism, depression, cognitive deficits, and limited availability of social support may combine to threaten patients' continued adherence to treatments designed to manage their diseases.

It is important that both primary and specialty care providers recognize the potential for nonadherence among all patients, and avoid being judgmental toward them. Following medical treatments correctly can interfere with patients' quality of life and serve as constant and disturbing reminders of the illness. Patients need emotional and practical support, information, and guidance in order to be adherent; patients typically do only what they understand, believe in, and are able to do. The most important ingredients in achieving patient adherence are effective communication and patients' informed collaboration with their physicians.

AWARENESS OF NONADHERENCE

Nonadherence is often difficult to recognize (Table 17-1), but should always be considered whenever a patient is not responsive to treatment or when the clinical picture is confusing and does not appear to make sense. Rarely do patients readily admit to having difficulties following their treatment regimens, and few patients tell their providers that they have no intention of following recommendations. Patients may weigh their physician's recommendations against their own beliefs and what they have learned from other sources, and may reject recommendations if the benefits of adhering do not appear to outweigh the interference in their quality of life.

Patients who are passive, uninvolved, and unquestioningly obedient are often the least adherent. Passive patients are more likely to disregard medical directives than are patients who ask questions, offer opinions, and even attempt to negotiate more acceptable regimens. Any hints of patient depression should be considered "red flags" regarding adherence. The physician plays an integral role in fostering adherence because he or she can talk with the patient in a participatory fashion to determine adherence challenges and the patient's health beliefs. The establishment of rapport can facilitate greater adherence and the patient's feeling that he or she has a choice in care.

CASE ILLUSTRATION

Matt is a 54-year-old unmarried stockbroker in an urban brokerage firm. He has recently experienced a myocardial infarction due to uncontrolled hypertension and atherosclerosis. Prior to Matt's heart attack, many stressful factors in his life affected his health behaviors. He rarely exercised because he worked more than 80 hours per week with little quality sleep. His eating habits involved a pattern of fast food, both high in fat and salt content, and he continued the smoking habit he formed in his twenties. Matt often recognized that his profession was a source of high strain and stress, but he felt compelled to succeed.

Following his heart attack, Matt underwent coronary artery bypass surgery. While Matt was in the hospital recovering, his physician outlined the following goals: (1) beginning a dialogue with Matt about the stressful factors in his life that affect his health behavior, (2) educating Matt about the dangers of excessive weight and hypertension, and (3) developing a treatment regimen that he can believe in and integrate into his life. These tasks must be accomplished while maintaining Matt's trust and commitment to improving his health. Once a therapeutic alliance is established, Matt's emotional experience must be understood and support provided so that he can begin to accept that nonadherence could lead to another heart attack. The physician can then work with Matt to negotiate an acceptable treatment regimen, including a number of prescription medications and a strict exercise regimen. Matt is not overweight, but he has rarely found time for exercise, and a sedentary lifestyle has contributed to his poor cardiovascular health. Matt's physician also addresses the stress of Matt's current profession, and suggests various options including doing some work from home. It is hoped that Matt can develop healthier eating choices and more opportunities for quality sleep and better stress management. The physician also encourages Matt to join a smoking cessation program. Effective physician–patient communication will help to ensure his adherence to these major lifestyle changes.

UNDERSTANDING ADHERENCE PROBLEMS

The most important step in dealing with adherence problems is to talk openly with a patient about illness and its treatment while maintaining respect for the patient's beliefs. The fact that Matt's physician addressed some of the psychosocial factors connected with his heart problems

Table 17-1. Typical clues to nonadherence.

- Patient passivity and lack of involvement
- Appearance of unquestioning obedience
- Patient depression
- Lack of response or inconsistent response to treatment
- Confusing or indistinct clinical picture

demonstrates recognition of these issues in Matt's life. A further step would be to educate Matt about the connection between his lifestyle and poor health. By working together to understand the psychosocial challenges that Matt faces, they can identify possible obstacles to adherence. Matt may have misconceptions about heart disease, and he may not understand the connection between sedentary lifestyle, lack of sleep, and poor heart health.

Psychological Mechanisms

Problems with adherence are not caused by patient personality type, gender, ethnicity, social class, or educational attainment. Very affluent and highly educated patients can be as nonadherent as those who are poor and uneducated. The primary causes of nonadherence (Figure 17-1) are poor provider–patient communication, lack of understanding of the treatment and its importance, lack of trust and mutual caring in the therapeutic relationship, and provider behavior that is controlling and paternalistic. Nonadherence occurs when patients do not understand the costs, benefits, and efficacy of the recommended

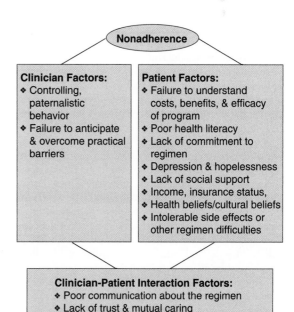

Figure 17-1. Causes of nonadherence.

regimen; when patients do not believe the regimen is valuable and worthy of commitment; and when physicians fail to anticipate and help patients overcome barriers to adherence (such as feelings of hopelessness and depression, the inability to afford costly medication, lack of social support, a hectic or irregular daily schedule, and lack of health insurance or good access to health care).

Nonadherence can sometimes be the patient's strategy for restoring a lost sense of control felt in the face of illness and a challenging medical treatment regimen.

Assessing Adherence in Practice

Studies show that physicians are consistently poor at recognizing problems with adherence. Some physicians assume higher levels of adherence among their patients than actually occur, and many cannot identify which of their patients have difficulties with adherence. A patient's apparent passive acceptance of the regimen, while likely to be interpreted by the physician as a sign of commitment, is instead a warning of nonadherence. Although agreeing verbally, the patient's body language—crossed arms, stiff posture, lack of eye contact, depressed affect—may indicate the opposite. Problems with adherence can be particularly challenging to detect if they are viewed by the physician as aberrant behavior rather than as rational choices. It should be assumed that every patient is potentially nonadherent, often for good reasons. Providers might think back to their own personal instances of nonadherence to gain perspective on how reasonable such a choice might sometimes seem to be. Patients often hide difficulties with adherence because of the social and normative pressures to be "good patients," particularly if they anticipate any criticism from their providers or negation of their right to make choices. Conversely, providers might be reluctant to inquire about nonadherence for fear that such revelation would be awkward or require additional time. The goal in questioning patients about their adherence is not to assert physician authority or reprimand patients for adherence failures, but rather to improve patients' health and quality of life.

Physicians should recognize and accept that patients are autonomous and make personal choices to maximize their quality of life *as they see it*. Patients are experts about their own values, preferences, and capabilities, just as physicians are experts in medical diagnosis and treatment. The provider's task is to be a sensitive, supportive advocate, not an authoritarian adversary. The patient is a complex individual, psychologically and socially, with unique values, lifestyle, and beliefs about quality of life, all of which must be incorporated into treatment decisions.

Patient responsibility for adherence requires effective practitioner–patient communication and collaboration toward the goal of self-management. Collaboration involves inevitable but manageable conflicts with which providers and patients can create reciprocal relationships.

Patients who are informed about and involved in their care provide better histories, report important symptoms and medication responses to their physicians, and assume responsibility for their adherence.

MANAGING NONADHERENCE

Effective, Accurate Communication of Information

First, the provider must build the two essential elements of provider–patient communication: accurate transmittal of information between physician and patient, and emotional support of the patient as a unique person (see Chapter 1). Unfortunately, such communication is not the norm in medical practice; close to 50% of patients leave their doctors' offices not knowing what they have been told and what they are supposed to do to manage their health. Physicians regularly use medical jargon that patients do not understand, and patients may be unwilling or lack sufficient skill to articulate their questions. Although the vast majority of patients greatly value obtaining as much information about their conditions as possible, including various treatment alternatives, such information is rarely provided to them. Physicians may underestimate how much their patients want to know, and they often unwittingly discourage patients from voicing concerns and requests for information by exhibiting rushed behaviors such as interrupting patients. Despite confusion about technical terms and medical jargon used by their physicians, patients often fail to ask for clarification. Providing written information for patients, and explaining that written information to them, can encourage the accurate transmittal of information essential for adherence. Educating patients and answering their questions may initially take a few extra minutes, but that time is very well spent in the long run.

Emotional Aspects of Care

The second element of provider–patient communication involves empathy and interpersonal trust in the physician–patient relationship (see Chapter 2). Building rapport with patients has traditionally been perceived as taking too much time and something for which physicians have not felt adequately trained. Attending only to diseases and ignoring their patients' suffering, however, insures that physicians will fail to support their patients' adjustment and healing.

Physicians' behavior and communication style during office visits directly affect patients' trust in and satisfaction with their providers, their recall of medical information, and their subsequent adherence to prescribed treatment regimens. Emotional support of patients appears to enhance positive expectations for healing and patients' fulfillment of those expectations.

Providers who are more sensitive to and emotionally expressive with nonverbal communication have patients who are more satisfied and who are more likely to adhere to the recommended treatments. Recent research indicates that enthusiastic, warm, and competent physician voice tone is positively correlated with patients' self-reported medication adherence. Physicians can contribute a great deal to their patients simply by giving them their full attention and genuinely listening to their concerns. Providers who make patients feel rushed or ignored, devalue patients' views, fail to respect and listen to them, and fail to understand their perspectives, risk patient dissatisfaction, nonadherence, and, if the outcome of care is less than satisfactory, even malpractice litigation. It is important to note that there is empirical evidence that technical skill and health care outcomes are not sacrificed in developing the capacity to respond to patients' feelings. Studies show that there is a positive relationship between physicians' technical and psychosocial skills. In addition, the provision of quality psychosocial care for patients results in significantly greater patient satisfaction, as well as better patient adherence and treatment outcomes. Therefore, any additional time that psychosocial care may take is more than justified by improved health care outcomes for patients, and ultimately greater time savings.

Patients' Beliefs & an Acceptable Course of Action

The physician should assess and, if necessary, modify the patient's beliefs about the regimen. Patient commitment to the regimen depends on the patient's clear belief that it is worth following; that it is likely to be effective; and that the benefits outweigh the costs in time, money, discomfort, possible embarrassment, and lifestyle adjustment. Such a commitment by the patient requires detailed discussion about the recommendation, including its value compared with other courses of action and any potential risks or problems that might be encountered. Discussion of possible disadvantages should take place before the choice is made so that adverse effects do not result in abandonment of a regimen. It is well documented that a patient's cultural beliefs and ideas about illness can play primary roles in their adherence behaviors (see Chapter 12). Physicians may not always understand a patient's cultural illness representations. Language barriers combined with different perspectives can produce communication difficulties that hinder adherence. According to the Health Belief Model, patients' adherence to health behaviors is related to their perceptions of the severity of a potential illness or the consequences of not preventing or treating the illness. Furthermore, the seriousness of a patient's illness is related to adherence, as more severely ill patients may be less adherent to their regimens. This may seem surprising, but patients who are symptomatic with very severe illnesses may face both physical and psychological barriers to adherence, and may have lost their faith in the efficacy of the regimen. Physicians treating patients with severe illnesses should be mindful of how patients' health beliefs about their disease may affect their efforts to adhere to medical recommendations, and they should continue engaging and collaborating with patients even when they are very ill.

Improving Patients' Quality of Life

In choosing and reinforcing a treatment regimen, it is essential to focus on the patient's overall quality of life. The goal of treatment should not be to achieve the provider's agenda. Rather, it is essential to recognize that the patient is the one whose quality of life will be affected by the regimen; the patient will benefit if the regimen is a success and must live with the results if the treatment fails. Physician and patient should therefore explore together the chances of achieving their joint goals, choosing among various alternatives.

Negotiating the Treatment Regimen

The clinician must accept the inevitability—and the value—of disagreements with the patient. For example, patients tend to be more risk averse than their physicians, and they usually favor more conservative interventions. Choosing the best course of action to enhance a patient's quality of life and solve a medical problem will take some effort. The mutual exploration of alternatives can help clinician and patient learn to work together despite their likely differing perspectives on the clinical situation. Patient involvement in the decision process leads to more satisfactory outcomes; clinicians should engage in negotiation and collaborative decision making with patients, and recognize that the most effective decisions occur when each party fully understands the objectives and preferences of the other.

Physicians should explore their patients' assessments and feelings about proposed health behaviors and make it clear to patients that the therapeutic encounter is one in which differences can be resolved through negotiation. Physicians should state principles and goals on which doctor and patient agree, elicit patient's feelings and concerns about alternative methods, and respectfully acknowledge physician–patient differences while compromising whenever possible.

Helping Patients Overcome Barriers to Adherence

After a patient has truly come to understand and believe in the value of the regimen, and to make a commitment to following it, the clinician should work to incorporate the plan into the patient's life. Physician and patient must identify ways to overcome practical problems that serve as barriers to adherence (e.g., change from a medication taken four times a day to one that can be taken twice). A clinical regimen associated with regular activities or paired with a wristwatch alarm or a medication schedule posted on the refrigerator, should improve adherence. At this stage, enhanced adherence requires working with the patient to determine precisely how the regimen can be implemented for maximum clinical effectiveness. It helps to suggest practical reminder strategies such as pairing pill-taking with brushing teeth, putting pills on the bedside table for morning or bedtime doses, or posting a note on the refrigerator. Discussing and finding solutions for transportation problems that prevent the patient from keeping scheduled appointments can improve adherence. Patients can be helped to employ reward systems for appropriate diet and exercise behaviors, such as buying a new article of clothing or taking a fishing trip. Self-generated rewards can improve patient's psychological well-being and foster "ownership" of the adherence process.

It is important to work with the patient to develop methods for follow-up and continued health behavior maintenance, such as regular telephone calls and office visits to check on progress, solve inevitable problems, or modify the regimen when necessary. Reminder letters are also effective in helping patients keep their appointments. Some physicians write out brief contracts with their patients, specifying what the patient is to do (the details of the treatment regimen) and what the physician is to do in return (e.g., regular telephone contact for encouragement). With the patient's permission, the involvement of an encouraging and supportive family member of the patient's choice can also help to enhance adherence to treatment.

Patients who are involved in both choosing and planning the implementation of their treatment regimens are much more involved in their own care, ask more questions, and express greater satisfaction than those who are not. Involved patients also have greater alleviation of their symptoms and better control of their chronic conditions, less distress and concern about their illnesses, and better responses to surgery and invasive diagnostic procedures. They feel a greater sense of control over their health and their lives, and demonstrate better adherence to the treatment they have helped to choose. Adherence can improve outcomes such as quality of life, self-efficacy, and patient satisfaction. The process of adhering is good for patients, because it helps them to organize their health care activities and allows them to feel effective and proactive in managing their illnesses.

The health care team, which often includes nurses, pharmacists, medical assistants, or health educators, provides valuable care to patients. Additional referrals, such as to a nutritionist for dietary modification or an exercise counselor for fitness education and training can be very helpful. All of these avenues of care work best in coordination with one another and with the primary

Table 17-2. Essential elements of achieving patient adherence.

- Accurate transmission of information between patient and clinician
- Emotional support and understanding of patient
- Awareness and modification of patient's beliefs
- Help in choosing an acceptable course of action to which a commitment can be made
- Help in overcoming barriers to adherence (e.g., reminders)
- Acceptance of the value of clinician–patient negotiation
- Focus on the overall quality of life of the patient
- Development of a specific plan to implement the regimen
- Recognition and treatment of patient's depression and hopelessness

care physician in order to enhance the patient's adherence outcomes. These elements and others are outlined in Table 17-2.

Comorbidity Considerations

Recent research shows a substantial negative correlation between patient adherence and mild to moderate patient depression. Although severe depression might easily be recognized as a clear indication for referral, milder depression including feelings of sadness and hopelessness, withdrawal from social support, and/or impairment in constructive thinking can seriously limit adherence and should be examined. If necessary, the patient could be referred for cognitive-behavioral therapy, with or without antidepressant medication (see Chapter 22). In addition, although the clinician must avoid overinterpreting nonadherence as a behavioral or mental disorder, there are cases in which a patient's seemingly irrational nonadherence should be evaluated by a mental health professional, particularly if that nonadherence is life threatening. Finally, many patients with chronic diseases are likely to do well with a support group, in which ideas for coping as well as practical help may be provided by others with the same illness experience.

SUGGESTED READINGS

Atreja A, Bellam N, Levy SR. Strategies to enhance patient adherence: making it simple. *Med Gen Med* 2005;7(1):4.

DiMatteo MR. Social support and patient adherence to medical treatment: a meta-analysis. *Health Psychol* 2004;23(2):207–218.

DiMatteo MR. Variations in patients' adherence to medical recommendations: a quantitative review of 50 years of research. *Med Care* 2004;42(3):200–208.

Martin LR, Williams SL, Haskard KB, et al. The challenge of patient adherence. *Ther Clin Risk Manag* 2005;1(3):189–199.

Osterberg L, Blaschke T. Adherence to medication. *N Engl J Med* 2005;353(5):487–497.

Roter DL, Hall JA. *Doctors Talking with Patients/Patients Talking with Doctors.* New York, NY: Auburn House, 1992.

Smoking

18

Nancy A. Rigotti, MD

INTRODUCTION

Cigarette smoking is the leading preventable cause of death in the United States, responsible for an estimated 438,000 deaths per year, or one in every five deaths. Physicians often take care of the health consequences of their patients' tobacco use. It is equally important for them to prevent smoking-related disease by treating their patients' smoking habits.

The prevalence of cigarette smoking in the United States rose rapidly in the first half of the twentieth century and peaked in 1965, when 40% of adult Americans smoked cigarettes. Since then, smoking rates have declined, reflecting growing public awareness of the health risks of tobacco use and public health efforts to discourage tobacco use. By 2006, adult smoking prevalence had fallen to 20.9%. Smoking starts during childhood and adolescence; nearly 90% of smokers begin to smoke before the age of 20. The rates of tobacco use in men and women, once very different, are converging. In 2006, 18.1% of adult women and 23.9% of men smoked cigarettes. In the United States, smoking is more closely linked to education than it is to age, race, occupation, or any other sociodemographic factors. Educational attainment is a marker for socioeconomic status, and these data indicate that smoking is a problem that is concentrated in lower socioeconomic groups.

HEALTH CONSEQUENCES OF TOBACCO USE

Cigarette smoking increases overall mortality and morbidity rates and is a cause of cardiovascular disease (including myocardial infarction and sudden death), cerebrovascular disease, peripheral vascular disease, chronic obstructive pulmonary disease, and cancers at many sites, including the lung, larynx, oral cavity, esophagus, bladder, kidney, pancreas, and uterine cervix. Lung cancer, once a rare disease, has increased dramatically. It has been the leading cause of cancer death in men since 1955 and in women since 1986.

Smoking is associated with many pregnancy complications, especially low birth weight (<2500 g). This is primarily attributable to intrauterine growth retardation (IUGR), although smoking in pregnancy also increases the risk of preterm delivery. Other adverse pregnancy outcomes linked to smoking are miscarriage (spontaneous abortion) and stillbirth. Smoking during pregnancy affects children even after birth. Sudden infant death syndrome is two to four times more common in infants born to mothers who smoked during pregnancy. Cognitive deficits and developmental problems in childhood are also linked to maternal smoking during pregnancy.

Cigarette smoking also increases a woman's risk of postmenopausal osteoporosis and fracture. Smokers have higher rates of upper and lower respiratory infections, peptic ulcer disease, cataracts, macular degeneration, and sensorineural hearing loss than nonsmokers. Smokers have more prominent skin wrinkling than nonsmokers, independent of sun exposure. The majority of residential fire deaths are caused by smoking.

There is no safe level of tobacco use. Smoking as few as one to four cigarettes per day increases the risk of myocardial infarction and cardiovascular mortality. Smoking cigarettes with reduced tar and nicotine content does not protect against the health hazards of smoking.

The health hazards of smoking are not limited to those who smoke. Nonsmokers are harmed by chronic exposure to environmental tobacco smoke (ETS). The children of parents who smoke have more serious respiratory infections during infancy and childhood, more respiratory symptoms, and a higher rate of chronic otitis media and asthma than the children of nonsmokers. Secondhand smoke exposure increases a nonsmoker's risk of lung cancer and coronary heart disease. A 2005 California Environmental Protection Agency study identified ETS as a source of carcinogens responsible for approximately 3400 lung cancer deaths per year in U.S. nonsmokers and up to 69,000 deaths from heart disease.

HEALTH BENEFITS OF SMOKING CESSATION

Smoking cessation has health benefits for men and women of all ages, even those who stop smoking after the age of 65 or who quit after the development of a smoking-related disease. Smoking cessation decreases the risk of lung and other cancers, heart attack, stroke, chronic lung disease, and peptic ulcer disease. After 10–15 years of abstinence, overall mortality rates for smokers approach rates of those who never smoked. The risk reduction for cardiovascular disease occurs more rapidly than the risk reduction for lung cancer or overall mortality. Half of the excess risk of cardiovascular mortality is eliminated in the first year of quitting, whereas for lung cancer, 30–50% of the excess risk is still evident 10 years after quitting and some excess risk remains after 15 years.

The benefits of stopping smoking translate into a longer life expectancy for former smokers compared with continuing smokers. Smokers who benefit the most are those who quit when they are younger, have fewer pack-years of tobacco exposure, and are free of smoking-related disease. The health benefits of smoking cessation far exceed any risks from the small weight gain that occurs with cessation.

SMOKING BEHAVIOR

Cigarettes and other tobacco products are addicting. Nicotine is capable of creating tolerance, physical dependence, and a withdrawal syndrome in habitual users. Nicotine withdrawal symptoms include: (1) cravings for a cigarette, (2) irritability, (3) restlessness, (4) anger and impatience, (5) difficulty concentrating, (6) anxiety, (7) depressed mood, (8) excessive hunger, and (9) sleep disturbance. These symptoms begin within a few hours of the last cigarette, are strongest during the first 2–3 days after quitting, and gradually diminish over a month or more. Other than craving for a cigarette, the symptoms are nonspecific, and many smokers fail to recognize them as nicotine withdrawal. The severity of nicotine withdrawal is variable and related to the level of prior nicotine intake. Smokers who smoke more than 25 cigarettes daily, have their first cigarette within 30 minutes of awakening, or are uncomfortable when forced to refrain from smoking for more than a few hours are likely to suffer nicotine withdrawal symptoms when they try to quit.

The discomfort of nicotine withdrawal is one reason smokers fail in their efforts to stop. However, the attractiveness of smoking is attributable to more than nicotine dependence. Smoking is also a habit, a behavior that has become an integral part of a daily routine. Smokers come to associate cigarettes with enjoyable activities, such as finishing a meal or having a cup of coffee. These actions trigger the desire for a cigarette in smokers who are trying to quit. Smokers also use cigarettes to cope with stress and negative emotions such as anger, anxiety, loneliness, or frustration. Quitting smoking represents the loss of a valuable coping tool for many smokers.

SMOKING CESSATION

Approximately half of living Americans who ever smoked have quit smoking. According to surveys, a majority of the remaining smokers would like to stop smoking and have made at least one serious attempt to do so. Forty-one percent of smokers attempt to quit each year, but few of them use the effective treatments available, and few achieve long-term cessation.

Surveys of former smokers reveal how and why they stop smoking. Fear of illness is the reason most often cited. However, awareness of health risks alone is not sufficient to motivate smoking cessation. Over 90% of current smokers know that smoking is harmful to their health, yet they continue to smoke. Many smokers rationalize that they are immune to the health risks of smoking until these risks become personally salient. Current symptoms (e.g., cough, breathlessness, chest pain), even if they represent minor illness rather than the onset of a smoking-related disease, stimulate change in smoking behavior more powerfully than does fear of future disease. Illness in a family member may also motivate smoking cessation. Another frequently cited reason for quitting is social unacceptability of smoking.

The majority of former smokers do not stop on their first try. About 30% of smokers who receive state-of-the-art treatment are not smoking 1 year later; most resume smoking within 3 months. In contrast, only 5% of smokers who try to quit without assistance succeed for 1 year. Behavioral scientists relate smoking cessation to a learning process rather than to a discrete episode of will power. Smokers learn from mistakes made during a prior attempt at quitting, thereby increasing the likelihood that the next attempt will succeed. Psychologists have identified a series of cognitive stages through which smokers pass as they move toward nonsmoking: (1) initial disinterest in quitting; (2) thinking about health risks and contemplating quitting; (3) preparing to quit in the near future; (4) currently taking action to stop smoking; and (5) maintained nonsmoking (see Chapter 16).

SMOKING CESSATION METHODS

Evidence-based clinical guidelines for smoking cessation were released by the U.S. Public Health Service in 2006 (www.surgeongeneral.gov/tobacco). The guidelines identified two methods as having strong evidence of efficacy: psychosocial counseling and pharmacotherapy. Their impact is synergistic. There is little evidence to support the efficacy of hypnosis for smoking cessation, and acupuncture is not effective.

Psychosocial

Cognitive-behavioral treatment methods address the barriers to quitting smoking that are rooted in habit. These methods are effective in aiding smoking cessation.

Counseling can occur in individual or group settings or can be provided by telephone. In a typical program, smokers monitor their cigarette intake to identify the things that trigger the smoking, change their habits to break the link between the trigger and smoking, and learn to anticipate and handle the urges to smoke when they occur. The counselor also provides social support to bolster the smoker's confidence in the ability to stop smoking. Cognitive-behavioral treatment techniques can also be packaged into booklets or videotapes for use at home.

Pharmacologic

Seven products have been approved by the U.S. Food and Drug Administration (FDA) as smoking cessation aids. Six of them are considered first-line drugs by the U.S. Public Health Service tobacco treatment guidelines (Table 18-1), five of these are nicotine replacement products. The sixth is bupropion, initially approved as an antidepressant. The seventh, varenicline, became available in 2006 and has not been formally reviewed by the clinical guidelines panel. Two other drugs, nortriptyline and clonidine, have shown efficacy for smoking cessation in clinical trials but are not approved by the FDA for this indication and are considered second-line drugs.

Nicotine Replacement Therapy

The rationale of nicotine replacement is to supply nicotine in a form other than a cigarette in order to block the symptoms of nicotine withdrawal. Nicotine replacement permits the smoker to break the smoking habit first and begin to taper off nicotine. Five forms of nicotine replacement are currently approved for use in the United States. Nicotine in the form of a gum, a transdermal skin patch, and an oral lozenge are sold without prescription. A nicotine nasal spray and an oral vapor inhaler are prescription-only products. Of all these products, the nicotine patch produces the most constant blood level of nicotine, a substantially different pattern from the fluctuating nicotine levels produced by cigarette smoking. The gum, lozenge, inhaler, and nasal spray produce nicotine levels that vary more than the patch but less than smoking a cigarette. They provide more control over nicotine level. The nicotine supplied by the gum, patch, or nasal spray is sufficient to reduce nicotine withdrawal symptoms but not to reproduce the rapid rise in nicotine blood levels caused by smoking a cigarette that contribute to nicotine dependence.

Randomized placebo-controlled trials demonstrate that nicotine gum, patch, lozenge, inhaler, and nasal spray all reduce symptoms of nicotine withdrawal at approximately double the rates of smoking cessation compared with placebo. Combining the patch with the other nicotine replacements is safe and, in most studies, produces higher rates of cessation than single agents. The effectiveness of all products depends on the instruction and counseling that accompany it. This is particularly true for the gum, nasal spray, and inhaler, which require careful instruction for proper use. Compliance is less of a problem with the nicotine patch. The most effective use of any product, however, requires that the physician provide the smoker with concurrent behavioral counseling of some type that teaches how to break the cigarette habit.

Nicotine replacement is safe to use in smokers with stable coronary artery disease. There are no data on its

Table 18-1. Pharmacotherapy for smoking cessation.[*]

Name	Dosage per Day	Recommended Duration of Use
Nicotine Replacement Products		
Transdermal nicotine patch		
24 hour	21 mg/24 h	8 weeks
	14 mg/24 h	
	7 mg/24 h	
16 hour	15 mg/16 h	8 weeks
Nicotine gum		
2 mg	9–12 pieces/day[†] (maximum 30)	2–3 months (maximum 6)
4 mg	9–12 pieces/day[†] (maximum 20)	2–3 months (maximum 6)
Nicotine nasal spray	1–2 doses/h (maximum 8/day)	3 months
Nicotine inhaler	6 cartridges/day	3–6 months
Nonnicotine Agents		
Bupropion SR	150–300 mg/day[‡]	3 months

[*]Products approved by the U.S. FDA as smoking cessation aid.
[†]Chew as needed or one piece every 1–2 h while awake.
[‡]Start 1 week before quit day. Use 150 mg/day for 3–5 days then 150 mg twice a day.

safety for use in smokers with unstable cardiovascular disease (myocardial infarction in the past 2 weeks, unstable angina, or life-threatening ventricular arrhythmias), although it is clearly safer than continuing to smoke; tobacco smoke contains carbon monoxide and other oxidant gases that are clearly detrimental to anyone with coronary heart disease.

TRANSDERMAL NICOTINE PATCH

The nicotine patch contains a reservoir of nicotine that is released at a fixed dose and is absorbed through the skin. The most common side effect is local skin irritation, which rarely requires discontinuation of treatment and can often be managed with topical steroids. Vivid dreams, insomnia, and nervousness have also been reported; they can be managed by removing the patch at bedtime or using a lower-dose patch.

The smoker applies the first patch on the morning of the quit day and applies a new patch to rotating skin sites each morning afterward. Data suggest that patch use should continue for 2 months. Lower starting doses are recommended for patients weighing under 100 lb or smoking fewer than 10 cigarettes per day. Long-term dependence on the nicotine patch is rare.

NICOTINE GUM

Nicotine gum is available without prescription in 2-mg and 4-mg strengths. To avoid side effects, the gum should not be chewed like regular gum. Careful instruction in proper chewing technique is essential for the nicotine to be absorbed through the oral mucosa rather than being swallowed. Initially, the gum should be chewed only long enough to release the nicotine, producing a peppery taste, then placed between the gums and buccal mucosa to allow for nicotine absorption. When the taste disappears, the gum is chewed again until the taste reappears, then "parked" again. After 30 minutes, it is discarded. No liquid should be drunk while the gum is in the mouth, and acidic beverages (e.g., coffee) should be avoided for 1–2 hours before gum use. Side effects are common but minor; they include those related to nicotine (nausea, dyspepsia, hiccups, dizziness) and to chewing (sore jaw, mouth ulcers). The product is approved for use as needed to handle urges to smoke; however, its onset of action is slower than smoking. Most patients chew fewer than the recommended 9–12 pieces daily. Consequently, many experts use fixed-dose schedules (e.g., chewing one piece for the first 30 minutes of every hour) to achieve blood nicotine levels adequate to prevent withdrawal. Long-term dependence on the gum is uncommon.

NICOTINE LOZENGE

A nicotine lozenge with similarities to the gum is also available for nonprescription sale in 2 mg and 4 mg doses. In randomized-controlled trials, it doubles cessation rates compared to a placebo lozenge. Like the gum, it is placed in the mouth. Nicotine in the lozenge is gradually absorbed through the oral mucosa over 30–40 minutes. The user cannot eat or drink when the tablet is in the mouth. The lozenge differs from the gum in that no chewing is required, making it easier to use properly. The lozenge can be used by people with dentures or poor dentition who generally cannot use the gum. The manufacturer recommends using 7–9 pieces per day as needed to control craving to smoke and to use it for 3 months.

NICOTINE INHALER

The nicotine inhaler, sold by prescription only, is a hand-held device containing nicotine in a plug that is vaporized when the smoker inhales. The nicotine is absorbed by the oral mucosa rather than in the lungs. Therefore, the bioavailability of the inhaler resembles that of nicotine gum, with peak nicotine levels reached 20 minutes after start of use. The inhaler mimics the hand-to-mouth behavior of cigarette smoking, a feature that may appeal to some smokers. The inhaler doubles the cessation rate compared to placebo in randomized trials. Side effects are minimal; throat irritation and cough are the most common.

NICOTINE NASAL SPRAY

Nicotine nasal spray is sold only by prescription. Nicotine is more rapidly absorbed from the nasal mucosa than it is through the oral mucosa, but less rapidly absorbed than through the lungs when a cigarette is smoked. The nicotine nasal spray doubles the cessation rate compared with a placebo spray in randomized-controlled trials, but has a high incidence of side effects (nose and throat irritation, watery eyes, sneezing, and cough). Careful instruction is required for its proper use. The dose is one spray in each nostril as needed; this delivers a dose of 1 mg of nicotine.

Bupropion

Bupropion is an antidepressant with dopaminergic and noradrenergic activity. In its sustained-release form (Zyban, Wellbutrin SR), bupropion doubles smoking cessation rates compared to placebo, and it is FDA approved for smoking cessation. The most serious side effect is a reduction in the threshold for seizure. The risk of seizure is 1 in 1000 patients or less, but the drug is contraindicated in patients with a seizure disorder or predisposition. Common side effects are insomnia, agitation, headache, and dry mouth. Doses of 150–300 mg/day for 7–12 weeks are effective for smoking cessation. The drug is started 1 week before the smoker's quit date to allow for blood levels to stabilize before quitting occurs.

Varenicline

Varenicline is a selective partial agonist at the α4β2 nicotinic receptor, the subtype of nicotine receptor in the brain that appears to mediate nicotine dependence. It is thought to have a dual mechanism of action. As a partial agonist, it relieves nicotine withdrawal symptoms. However, if a smoker using varenicline smokes a cigarette, the drug blocks the nicotine in cigarette smoke from binding to the nicotine receptor, thereby blocking the usual rewarding effect of smoking a cigarette. In two randomized-controlled trials comparing the drug with placebo and with bupropion, varenicline produced a higher long-term cessation rate than both. It nearly tripled the cessation rate compared to placebo. Nausea is the most common side effect, occurring in nearly 30% of subjects in clinical trials. Varenicline was approved by the FDA for prescription-only use in 2006. It is used for 12 weeks at a dose of 1 mg bid. The initial week's dose increases gradually to minimize nausea symptoms. The drug is started 1 week before the smoker's quit date to allow for blood levels to stabilize before quitting occurs.

Clonidine and Nortriptyline

A centrally acting α-adrenergic agonist, clonidine is used to treat craving for psychoactive drugs other than nicotine. In randomized, placebo-controlled trials, both oral and transdermal clonidine reduced withdrawal symptoms and increased rates of cessation. Clonidine is not FDA approved for smoking cessation and side effects (sedation, dizziness, and dry mouth) generally limit its use.

Nortriptyline, a tricyclic antidepressant, has demonstrated efficacy for smoking cessation in two randomized trials. It is not FDA approved as a smoking cessation aid. Hypotension and dry mouth are the most common side effects.

There is no evidence to support the use of any other antidepressants or any antianxiety agents for smoking cessation.

BARRIERS TO SMOKING CESSATION

Weight & Smoking Cessation

Smokers weigh 5–10 lb less than nonsmokers of comparable age and height. When smokers quit, 80% of them gain weight. The average weight gain of 10–15 lb (4.6–6.8 kg) poses a minimal health risk, especially when compared with the benefits of smoking cessation. Women and heavier smokers (>25 cigarettes per day) gain more than men and lighter smokers. The mechanism is incompletely understood, but a nicotine-related decrease in metabolic rate and possibly increases in food intake appear to be largely responsible. Although weight gain has been considered a trigger to relapse, some studies show that successful abstainers gain more weight than relapsers. The best approach to the problem may be to help smokers accept a small weight gain

and reassure them that the expected amount is less than they may fear. A vigorous exercise program reduces postcessation weight gain and promotes cessation. Smokers who use nicotine gum or bupropion gain less weight than those who quit with a placebo, although weight gain is delayed until after drug treatment stops. However, this may help weight-concerned smokers to quit.

Social Support

Smokers with nonsmoking spouses are more likely to quit than smokers whose partners smoke. Smokers whose efforts to stop are supported by partners, family, and friends are more likely to succeed than smokers without this support. Those who live with smokers can ask them to restrict smoking to outdoor areas in order to provide a smoke-free home. Formal cessation programs provide an additional source of social support.

Depression

Stopping smoking represents a loss for many smokers. Cigarettes have been reliable "companions" as well as coping tools. Transient sadness is common and requires no special treatment. Acknowledgment that this is normal can be helpful. There is, however, a strong association between smoking and mood disorders. Smokers have more depressive symptoms than nonsmokers and are more likely to have a history of major depression. Depressed smokers are less likely to stop smoking than nondepressed smokers. Clinicians should be alert to the possibility of depression in smokers. If present, it should be treated before cessation is attempted. Smokers with a history of depression should be watched for the reemergence of symptoms during smoking cessation.

Substance Use

There is a high rate of smoking among users of alcohol, cocaine, and heroin. As with depression, substance abuse should be considered as a potential comorbid disorder in smokers who repeatedly try and fail to quit. Even among smokers who do not abuse alcohol, drinking is frequently an ingredient in relapse situations. Smokers attempting to quit are commonly advised to avoid alcohol temporarily after quitting.

THE PHYSICIAN'S ROLE

Because smoking begins early in life, preventing young people from starting is a task for physicians who care for children and adolescents. The challenge for physicians taking care of adults is smoking cessation. Physicians have the opportunity to intervene with smokers, because each year they see an estimated 70% of the smokers in the United States. They also see smokers at times when their symptoms have caused them to be concerned about their health and therefore more likely to be willing to change their smoking behavior. For example, one-third of smokers stop smoking after a myocardial infarction; this can be increased with brief counseling by a physician or nurse. For women, pregnancy encourages smoking cessation. Approximately 25% of female smokers stop smoking while pregnant, although many resume smoking after delivery. Other smoking-related conditions may also provide "teachable moments" when smokers are more receptive to advice to stop smoking.

Providing brief advice to stop smoking to all patients seen in the office increases patients' rates of smoking cessation. Although advice alone is effective, randomized-controlled trials in general medicine and family practices have demonstrated that supplementing advice with brief counseling is more effective. Counseling smokers in an office practice is as or more cost-effective than other accepted medical practices.

SMOKING CESSATION COUNSELING STRATEGY FOR OFFICE PRACTICE

Evidence-based clinical guidelines for smoking cessation treatment by primary care providers recommend that the primary care of adults should include a routine assessment of smoking status in all patients, strong advice to all smokers to quit, assessment of a smoker's readiness to quit, assistance for those smokers who are ready to stop, and follow-up for all smokers. The guidelines have been organized into a five-step protocol for use in office practice (Table 18-2).

1. **ASK:** Physicians should routinely ask all patients at every visit whether they smoke cigarettes.
2. **ADVISE:** Regardless of a smoker's degree of interest in quitting, it is the physician's responsibility to deliver clear advice to each smoker about the importance of stopping. The message should be strong and unequivocal; for example, "Quitting smoking now is the most important health advice I can give you." If appropriate, advice should be tailored to the clinical situation, either current symptoms or family history. For example, smokers can be informed that they will have fewer colds or less asthma if they stop smoking. Advice is more effective when phrased in a positive way; for instance, emphasizing the benefits to be gained from quitting rather than the harms of continuing.
3. **ASSESS:** Assess a smoker's interest in stopping. Categorizing smokers in this way is a clinically useful approach that helps the physician to determine which counseling strategy is appropriate and to set achievable goals. Although the clinician's overall goal is to assist the smoker to stop permanently, a realistic goal for a single office visit is to move the smoker to the next stage of readiness to stop.
4. **ASSIST:** Help the smoker quit. The physician's approach should vary according to the smoker's readiness.
   - *If the smokers are interested in quitting,* the physician should ask whether they are ready to set a "quit date," a date within the next 4 weeks when they will stop smoking. If so, the date should be recorded in the chart and on material given to them to take home. The physician should discuss with the patient what approach is most likely to be successful considering the smoker's level of nicotine dependence and past experience trying to quit. Both behavioral treatment and pharmacotherapy should be offered. Behavioral treatment can be provided by a take-home booklet containing standard behavioral treatment strategies or by referring the smoker for group, individual, or telephone counseling for smoking cessation. Smokers can access free telephone counseling for smoking cessation nationwide by calling a central number (800-QUIT-NOW). The physician should be prepared to discuss the management of barriers to cessation if the smokers ask. More intensive treatment is indicated for smokers who have been unsuccessful in previous attempts. The options include referral to a formal smoking cessation program and pharmacotherapy. Smoking cessation programs provide intensive training in behavioral smoking cessation skills combined with social support from the counselor and other group members. Combinations of pharmacotherapy and behavioral counseling are more effective than either one alone.
   - *For smokers not interested in quitting or not ready to set a quit date,* the physician should elicit what the patient feels to be the benefits and harms of smoking. With this perspective, the physician can provide missing information about health risks and correct misconceptions about the process of smoking cessation. The discussion should focus on short-term benefits rather than distant risks, and the physician should be prepared to discuss common barriers to smoking cessation. The clinician should advise the smoker not to expose family members to passive smoke and suggest that help is available when they are ready to quit.
5. **ARRANGE:** Randomized trials have demonstrated that arranging follow-up visits to discuss smoking increases the success of physician counseling. Smokers should be asked to return shortly after the quit date to monitor progress; this is especially important for smokers using pharmacotherapy, so that side effects and nicotine withdrawal symptoms can be monitored.

Table 18-2. Smoking cessation counseling protocol for physicians.

1. **ASK**—about smoking at every visit: "Do you smoke?"
2. **ADVISE**—every smoker to stop.
   a. Make advice clear: "Stopping smoking now is the most important action you can take to stay healthy."
   b. Tailor advice to the patient's clinical situation (symptoms or family history).
3. **ASSESS**—readiness to quit: "Are you interested in quitting?"
4. **ASSIST**—the smoker in stopping smoking.
   a. For smokers ready to quit
      (1) Ask smoker to set a "quit date."
      (2) Provide self-help material to take home.
      (3) Offer pharmacotherapy.
      (4) Consider referral to a formal cessation program for smokers with other substance use, depression, poor social support for nonsmoking, or low self-confidence in the ability to quit.
   b. For smokers not ready to quit
      (1) Discuss advantages and barriers to cessation, from smoker's viewpoint.
      (2) Provide motivational booklet to take home.
      (3) Advise smoker to avoid exposing family members to passive smoke.
      (4) Indicate willingness to help when the smoker is ready.
      (5) Ask again about smoking at the next visit.
5. **ARRANGE**—follow-up visits.
   a. Make follow-up appointment 1 week after quit date.
   b. At follow-up, ask about smoking status.
   c. For smokers who have quit:
      (1) Congratulate!
      (2) Ask smoker to identify future high-risk situations.
      (3) Rehearse coping strategies for future high-risk situations.
   d. For smokers who have not quit:
      (1) Ask: "What were you doing when you had that first cigarette?"
      (2) Ask: "What did you learn from the experience?"
      (3) Ask smoker to set a new "quit date."

Source: Adapted from the U.S. Public Health Service Guideline Treating Tobacco Use and Dependence (www.surgeongeneral.gov/tobacco).

- *If smokers are not smoking at the follow-up visit,* they should be congratulated but warned that continued vigilance is necessary to maintain abstinence. The level of nicotine withdrawal symptoms should be assessed, and if indicated, treated by starting or increasing pharmacologic treatment. To help prevent relapse, patients should be asked to identify future situations in which they anticipate difficulty remaining abstinent. The physician can help to plan and rehearse coping strategies for these times. Further follow-up visits or telephone calls should be offered.
- *If the smoker has not been able to remain abstinent,* the physician's role is to redefine a failure into a partial success. The patient can be told that even 1 day without cigarettes is the first step toward quitting and be reminded that it takes time to learn to quit, just as it took time to learn to smoke. To help the patient learn from the experience, the physician should ask about the circumstances that preceded the first cigarette smoked after the quit date, what was learned from the experience that could be used for the next attempt to quit, and whether a new quit date should be set.

Health Care Organization

Smoking cessation counseling should not be limited to the physician. A systems approach is at least as effective and it reduces the burden on the individual practitioner. The patients' smoking status can be assessed by a staff member in the clinic or hospital before the physician sees the patient and a notation in the medical record can remind the physician to discuss smoking. The physician's prime role is to give advice, assess readiness to quit, direct the smoker to effective resources, offer to prescribe medication, and refer to community resources such as telephone quitlines and formal cessation programs. Other personnel may assist the physicians' efforts in referral and provide counseling and medication instruction.

SUGGESTED READINGS

Cigarette smoking among adults—United States, 2004. *MMWR Morb Mortal Wkly Rep* 2005;54:1121–1124.

Critchley JA, Capewell S. Mortality risk reduction associated with smoking cessation in patients with coronary heart disease: a systematic review. *JAMA* 2003;290:86–97.

Curry SJ, Grothaus LC, McAfee T, et al. Use and cost-effectiveness of smoking cessation services under four insurance plans in a health maintenance organization. *N Engl J Med* 1998;339: 673–679.

Gonzales D, Rennard SI, Nides M, et al. Varenicline, an $\alpha 4\beta 2$ nicotinic acetylcholine receptor partial agonist, vs sustained-release bupropion and placebo for smoking cessation: a randomized controlled trial. *JAMA* 2006;296;47–55.

Hajek P, West R, Foulds J, et al. Randomized comparative trial of nicotine polacrilex, a transdermal patch, nasal spray, and an inhaler. *Arch Intern Med* 1999;159:2033–2038.

Jarvis M. Why people smoke. *Brit Med J* 2004;328:277–279.

Jorenby DE, Hays JT, Rigotti NA, et al. Efficacy of varenicline, an $\alpha 4\beta 2$ nicotininc acetylcholine receptor partial agonist, vs placebo or sustained-release bupropion for smoking cessation: a randomized controlled trial. *JAMA* 2006;296;56–63.

Jorenby DE, Leischow SJ, Nides MA, et al. A controlled trial of sustained-release bupropion, a nicotine patch, or both for smoking cessation. *N Engl J Med* 1999;340:685–691.

Rigotti NA. Clinical practice: treatment of tobacco use and dependence. *N Engl J Med* 2002;346:506–512.

Schroeder SA. What do to with a patient who smokes. *JAMA* 2005; 294:482–487.

Tobacco Use and Dependence Clinical Practice Guideline Panel: A clinical practice guideline for treating tobacco use and dependence. JAMA 2000;283:3244–3254. (Full text of guidelines available at www.surgeongeneral.gov/tobacco.)

Tonstad S, Tonnesen P, Hajek P, et al. Effect of maintenance therapy with varenicline on smoking cessation: a randomized controlled trial. *JAMA* 2006;296:64–71.

Zhu A, Anderson CM, Tedescko GJ, et al. Evidence of real-world effectiveness of a telephone quitline for smokers. *N Engl J Med* 2002;347:1087–1093.

WEB SITES

Centers for Disease Control Web site. http://www.cdc.gov/tobacco (comprehensive web site of information about tobacco use, prevention, and cessation). Accessed September, 2007.

Society for Research in Nicotine and Tobacco Web site. http://www.treattobacco.net/home/home.efm (evidence based information on treatment). Accessed September, 2007.

U.S. National Cancer Institute Web site. http://www.smokefree.gov (tips for preparation, quitting and staying quit). Accessed September, 2007.

U.S. Public Health Service Tobacco Cessation Guideline Web site. http://www.surgeongeneral.gov/tobacco/ (U.S. clinical guidelines). Accessed September, 2007.

Obesity

19

Robert B. Baron, MD, MS

INTRODUCTION

Obesity is one of the most common problems in clinical practice. Defined as a body mass index (BMI) >30 kg/m^2, over 30% of adult Americans are obese. An additional 35% are overweight, with BMIs between 25 and 30 kg/m^2. Because obesity is at the center of chronic disease risk and psychosocial disability for millions of Americans, its prevention and treatment offer unique patient care and public health opportunities. If all Americans were to achieve a normal body weight, it has been estimated that the prevalence of diabetes would decrease by 57%, hypertension by 17%, coronary artery disease by 17%, and various cancers by 11%.

Obesity is often one of the most difficult and frustrating problems in primary care for both patients and physicians. Considerable effort is expended by primary care providers and patients with little benefit. Weight-loss diets, for example, even in the best treatment centers, result in an average 8% reduction in body weight. This lack of clinical success has created a never-ending demand for new weight-loss treatments. Approximately, 45% of women and 25% of men are "dieting" at any one time, spending billions of dollars each year on diet books, diet meals, weight-loss classes, diet drugs, exercise programs, "fat farms," and other weight-loss aids. The challenge for health care providers is to identify those patients with obesity who are most likely to benefit medically from treatment and most likely to maintain weight loss, and to provide them with sound advice, skills for long-term lifestyle change, and support. For patients not motivated to attempt a weight-loss program, health providers must continue to be respectful and empathic and focus on other health concerns. Whenever possible, providers should emphasize prevention of obesity and further weight gain and the importance of physical fitness independent of body size.

DEFINITIONS

Obesity is defined as an excess of body fat. Body fat can be measured by several methods including total body water, total body potassium, bioelectrical impedance, and dual-energy x-ray absorptiometry. In clinical practice, however, obesity is best defined by the BMI—body weight divided by height squared (kilograms per square meter). The BMI correlates closely with measures of body fat and with obesity-related disease outcomes. According to the National Institutes of Health (NIH), an individual with a BMI <18.5 kg/m^2 is classified as underweight, 18.5–24.9 kg/m^2 as normal, 25.0–29.9 kg/m^2 as overweight, and ≥30.0 kg/m^2 as obese. Obesity can be further classified as class I (BMI 30–34.9 kg/m^2), class II (BMI 35–39.9 kg/m^2), and class III or extreme obesity (BMI ≥40 kg/m^2). The term "morbid obesity" is best avoided for those with class III obesity since obesity-related morbidity can occur at any obesity level.

HEALTH CONSEQUENCES OF OBESITY

The relationship between body weight and mortality is curvilinear, similar to other cardiovascular risk factors. Most studies have demonstrated a J-shaped relationship, suggesting that the thinnest portion of the population also has an excess mortality. This is primarily due to the higher rate of cigarette smoking in the thinnest group except in the elderly, in whom malnutrition and being underweight is predictive of excess mortality independent of cigarette use. Recent analysis of the National Health and Nutrition Examination Study (NHANES) has suggested that overweight individuals may not have as much excess mortality as previously described and that the impact of obesity on mortality overall may be decreasing over time. Racial and ethnic factors may also impact the relationship of weight and mortality. In African Americans, the weight associated with the point of lowest mortality is greater than in whites, while in Asian Americans it is lower.

The increase in total mortality related to obesity results predominantly from coronary heart disease (CHD). Although it is not fully established that obesity is an "independent" risk factor for CHD, obesity is clearly an important risk factor for the development of many other CHD risk factors. Obese individuals aged 20–44, for example, have a three- to fourfold greater risk for type II diabetes, a five- to six-fold greater risk for hypertension, and twice the risk for hypercholesterolemia. The obese also have an increased risk for some cancers, including those of the colon, ovary, and breast.

As a result of these conditions, mortality from all causes for persons with class I obesity (BMI 30–34.9 kg/m^2) is 20% greater than for those with a normal BMI. Individuals with class II obesity, BMI 35–39.9 kg/m^2, have an 80% increase in mortality from all causes. Mortality for extreme obesity, although less well studied, is estimated to be at least double that of normal weight individuals.

Obesity is also associated with a variety of other medical disorders, including degenerative joint disease of weightbearing joints, diseases of the digestive tract (gallbladder disease, gastroesophageal reflux disease), thromboembolic disorders, cerebrovascular disease, heart failure (both systolic and diastolic), respiratory impairment including sleep apnea, and skin disorders. Obese patients also have a greater incidence of surgical and obstetric complications, are more prone to accidents, and are at increased risk of social discrimination. Several studies have also shown a rate of depression higher in the obese than in normal weight subjects and a very high rate (approximately 30%) of binge eating disorder.

In addition to the total amount of excess body fat, the location of the excess body fat (regional fat distribution) is a major determinant of the degree of excess morbidity and mortality due to obesity. Increased upper body fat (abdomen and flank) is independently associated with increased cardiovascular and total mortality. Body fat distribution can be assessed by a number of techniques. Measurements of skin folds (subscapular and triceps) reflect subcutaneous fat. Measurement of circumferences (waist and hip) reflect both abdominal and visceral fat. Computed tomography (CT) and magnetic resonance imaging (MRI) scans measure subcutaneous and visceral fat. Clinically, measurement of the waist and hip circumference is most useful, especially in individuals with BMI 25–35 kg/m^2. A circumference in men >102 cm (>40 in.) and in women >88 cm (>35 in.) can be used to identify individuals at increased risk of developing obesity-related health problems.

ETIOLOGY OF OBESITY

Numerous lines of evidence, including both epidemiologic studies of adoptees and twins and animal studies, suggest strong genetic influences on the development of obesity. In a study of 800 Danish adoptees, for example, there was no relationship between the body weight of adoptees and their adopting parents but a close correlation with the body weights of their biological parents. In a study of approximately 4000 twins, a much closer correlation between body weights was found in monozygotic than in dizygotic twins. In this study, genetic factors accounted for approximately two-thirds of the variation in weights. Studies of twins reared apart and the response of twins to overfeeding showed similar results. Studies of regional fat distribution in twins have also shown a significant (but not complete) genetic influence.

Genetic studies have confirmed a clear relationship between genetics and obesity in both animals and humans. In humans, at least 24 genetic disorders, such as the Prader-Willi syndrome, are associated with obesity. Studies suggest that genetic influences may impact both energy intake (control of appetite and eating behavior) and energy expenditure.

Differences in the resting metabolic expenditure (RME), for example, could easily result in considerable differences in body weight as RME accounts for approximately 60–75% of total energy expenditure. The RME can vary by as much as 20% between individuals of the same age, sex, and body build; such differences could account for approximately 400 kcal of energy expenditure per day. Recent evidence suggests that the metabolic rate is similar in family members, and, as expected, individuals with lower metabolic rates are more likely to gain weight. Differences in the thermic effect of food, the amount of energy expended following a meal, may also contribute to obesity. Although some investigators have shown a decreased thermic effect of food in the obese, others have not.

Environmental factors are also clearly important in the development of obesity. Decreased physical activity and food choices that result in increased energy intake also clearly contribute to the development of obesity. Medical illness can also result in obesity, but such instances account for less than 1% of cases. Hypothyroidism and Cushing syndrome are the most common. Diseases of the hypothalamus can also result in obesity, but these are rare. Major depression which more typically results in weight loss, can also present with weight gain. Consideration of these causes is particularly important when evaluating unexplained, recent weight gain. Numerous medications can also result in weight gain including antipsychotics such as clozapine, olanzapine, and risperidone, antidepressants such as amitriptyline and cyproheptadine, anticonvulsants such as valproate, carbamazepine, and gabapentin, and diabetic medications such as insulin and thiazolidinediones. Of note, each of these categories of medications includes drugs that do not cause weight gain. Weight gain is also common following smoking cessation. On average, patients gain 4–5 kg within 6 months of quitting smoking but some patients may gain much more.

PATIENT SELECTION FOR WEIGHT LOSS

Weight loss is indicated to assist in the management of obesity-related conditions, particularly hypertension, diabetes mellitus (type II), and hyperlipidemia, in any patient who is obese (BMI >30 kg/m^2). Many patients with BMI 25–30 kg/m^2 who have one of these conditions (particularly hypertension, diabetes, lipid disorders, or significant psychosocial disability) also often dramatically benefit from weight reduction.

Weight loss to prevent complications of obesity in patients without current medical, metabolic, or behavioral consequences of obesity is more controversial. In young and middle-aged individuals, particularly those with a family history of obesity-related disorders, treatment should be based on the degree of obesity and body fat distribution. Such individuals with upper body obesity (increased waist circumference) should be considered for treatment; those individuals with lower body obesity and no significant consequences of obesity can be reassured and monitored. Many such patients, however, desire weight loss for psychological, social, and cosmetic reasons. A careful discussion of the risks and benefits of weight loss in such instances helps patients make informed decisions about various weight-loss strategies.

A medical or psychosocial indication for weight loss is necessary but not sufficient to begin treatment. Treatment must be designed in the context of the patient's readiness to change. The Transtheoretical Model of Change, also commonly known as the Stages of Change Model, is a useful framework for helping patients modify behavior. Developed and applied initially in smoking cessation, the model has also been used to modify eating and exercise behavior, The model defines behavior change as a process of identifiable stages including precontemplation, contemplation, preparation, action, maintenance, and relapse. By understanding the patient's readiness to change, the clinician can work specifically with each patient to move him or her to the next stage. (See Chapter 18 for further discussion of assessment of patients' readiness to change.)

Clinical assessment should also focus on how the current attempt compares with previous attempts; a realistic assessment of the patient's goals for the amount and rate of weight loss; the extent to which outside stresses, mood disorders, or substance abuse might impair the attempt; and the degree to which others can provide support. Patient readiness to change can be further assessed by requiring the patient to complete specific pretreatment assignments. For example, patients can be asked to complete a 3-day diet record and to submit an exercise plan that includes both the type of aerobic exercise the patient plans to begin and how the patient plans to fit it into his or her schedule. When obesity coexists with other significant psychiatric disorders, particularly depression, binge eating disorder, and substance abuse, treatment should initially be directed at the concurrent disorder.

DIET THERAPY

The goal of diet therapy for weight loss is to achieve a daily energy deficit whereby energy intake is less than energy expenditure. Daily energy expenditure can be estimated based on age, gender, and activity level. Two thousand calories per day is often used as a reference level, but individual's requirements may vary by hundreds of calories per day. The goal of most weight-loss diets is to achieve an energy deficit of approximately 500 cal/day. Since a pound of fat equals approximately 3500 cal, this will result in approximately 1 lb of weight loss per week.

Meta-analysis of randomized studies of dietary therapy to achieve weight loss have demonstrated an average weight loss of 8% of the starting weight in patients followed for 3 months to 1 year. Follow-up for up to 5 years suggests average long-term weight loss of 2–4% of initial weight. Of note, all studies have a substantial variation of response. Some patients, approximately 20%, are able to lose substantially more weight and keep it off for longer periods of time. Studies of commercial weight-loss programs also demonstrate modest amounts of weight loss but with wide variations. Weight Watchers, for example, reports 3.2% weight reduction at 2 years.

The optimal composition for weight-loss diets has been the subject of numerous recent clinical trials and, of course, thousands of popular weight-loss books. Most clinicians, as well as federal nutrition guidelines such as the Dietary Guidelines, recommend a low fat, high fiber, "balanced" diet. This approach suggests keeping macronutrients in the "acceptable" range: the percent of the diet from fat, carbohydrates, and protein should be 20–35% of total calories, 45–65% of total calories, and 10–35% of total calories, respectively. These ranges are substantially wider than earlier federal guidelines and allow for flexibility in diet design. The DASH (Dietary Approaches to Stop Hypertension) Eating Plan, originally developed for treatment of hypertension, is an example of a balanced diet that meets these macronutrient ranges and is supported by federal guidelines. A Mediterranean-style diet can also be used to achieve an energy deficit for weight loss and remain within these ranges.

Recent clinical trials have compared this balanced approach with more extreme low carbohydrate diets such as the Atkins Diet. These studies have consistently shown equivalent amount of weight loss independent of the macronutrient composition of the diet. Rather than nutrient composition, weight loss was predicted by adherence to the diet. Similar findings have been published with comparisons of the very low fat Ornish diet, and the Zone diet.

An important alternative in the dietary treatment of obesity is the use of safe and effective very-low-calorie diets (VLCDs). Previously known as protein-sparing modified fasts and protein-formula liquid diets, these diets restrict calorie intake to ≤800 kcal/day. Patients ingest only prepackaged, often liquid, food that provides adequate protein, vitamins, and minerals. Additional intake is limited to 2–3 quarts of calorie-free beverages per day. The major advantage of these diets is the "complete removal of patients from the food environment" to facilitate short-term adherence. In addition, the significant energy deficit results in rapid weight loss, usually 2 lb/week, encouraging the patient to continue. Ongoing concerns about these diets include their cost, side effects, and long-term results. Clinical trials suggest that the use of 800-kcal VLCDs can lower cost and prevent most of the significant side effects associated with the lower-calorie (400–600) VLCDs, including gallstones and fluid and electrolyte disorders, with equal long-term efficacy.

As with standard diet therapy of obesity, VLCDs require adherence during the diet, and long-term nutritional and behavioral changes to maintain weight loss. Well-planned programs that combine VLCDs with nutrition education, behavior therapy, exercise, and social support report improved long-term results. For example, an average weight loss of 55 lb with 75% and 52% of the loss maintained at 1- and 2 1/2-year follow-up, respectively, and maintenance of an average of 24 lb after 2- to 3-year follow-up have been reported. Meta-analysis of published VLCD trials suggest that while initial weight loss is greater with VLCDs than standard diets both approaches have equal long-term results. As with other approaches, however, there is a wide variation of response with VLCDs and some patients can achieve long-term weight loss. Because of the quicker and greater amounts of weight loss, VLCDs may be particularly useful in situations in which rapid weight loss is clinically indicated such as preoperative treatment (joint replacement, transplant surgery, bariatric surgery) or for initial management of severe medical conditions (severe sleep apnea, poorly controlled diabetes, heart failure, coronary artery disease).

Recent studies have helped elucidate predictors of long-term weight maintenance after diet therapy for weight loss. Most important has been information from the National Weight Control Registry. This cohort of individuals who have lost an average of 33 kg and maintained the loss for 5 years report consumption of low calorie, low fat diets averaging approximately 1400 cal/day; high levels of physical activity averaging 60 minutes/day; regular self-monitoring of body weight; eating breakfast daily; and maintaining consistent dietary patterns on weekdays and weekends.

HEALTH CONSEQUENCES OF DIETING & WEIGHT LOSS

Surprisingly, few studies have examined the effects of weight loss on morbidity and mortality. Studies examining the effect of weight loss on cardiovascular risk factors generally show beneficial changes with weight loss as predicted. Descriptive studies on mortality, however, show inconsistent results. Such descriptive studies are unable to clarify if changes in mortality are caused by the weight change, if disease or other factors that contribute to disease, such as cigarette smoking, cause weight loss, or if both are related to a third factor. No randomized trials of long-term effects of voluntary weight loss on mortality have been published.

Because so many Americans are dieting at any one time, and having so little long-term success, considerable interest has been focused on the potential adverse effects of weight cycling ("yo-yo" dieting). Numerous adverse effects of weight cycling have been hypothesized, primarily from animal studies. These include making further weight loss more difficult, increasing total body fat and central obesity, increasing subsequent calorie intake, increasing food efficiency, decreasing energy expenditure, increasing levels of adipose-tissue lipolytic enzymes and liver lipogenic enzymes, increasing insulin resistance, increasing blood pressure, and increasing blood cholesterol and triglyceride levels. Most experts currently feel that these phenomena occur inconsistently, if at all. Descriptive studies that have addressed this question by looking at the impact of weight fluctuations on CHD incidence, CHD mortality, and total mortality have shown mixed results.

There is also debate over whether weight-loss diets cause eating disorders or binge eating. Although a history of dieting often precedes the development of eating disorders, there is no evidence proving a causal link. In addition, approximately 50% of individuals with binge eating disorder report that binging preceded dieting. There is also some evidence to suggest that successful weight loss may reduce binge eating in the obese (see Chapter 20).

Thus, there is only indirect evidence suggesting that dieting has negative health effects. This remains an important question, however, and reinforces the idea that casual attempts at quick weight loss should be avoided. At present, however, committed attempts at long-term weight loss should not be discouraged because of adverse health effects or the potential of regaining weight.

Dieting also has a significant effect on energy balance both during and after weight loss. As every successful dieter has observed, the rate of weight loss slows during the course of dieting. Because this can be quite discouraging to the unwary patient (or uninformed health care provider), it is important to inform the patient prior to initiating a weight-loss diet that this is likely to occur. Weight loss is most rapid during the initial days of hypocaloric feeding due to changes in sodium and water balance caused by early loss of glycogen and protein (both contain water) and, depending on the degree of calorie deficit and type of diet, loss of sodium associated with ketonuria. Following this initial phase, weight loss depends on the extent of energy deficit. With time, however, the rate of weight loss slows again as the body's metabolic rate decreases and the energy deficit becomes smaller. This change in metabolic rate can be two to three times greater than that predicted from changes in body weight. The lower the energy content of the diet, the lower the metabolic rate. Although it was initially suggested that exercise occurring during a period of hypocaloric feeding could prevent this decrease in metabolic rate, recent studies have suggested that it has no direct effect during hypocaloric feeding (but exercise does increase the postdiet metabolic rate by preserving lean body mass).

Following the period of hypocaloric feeding (resumption of normal energy intakes), the resting metabolic rate increases, but to a level below that observed before beginning the diet. This reduction is in part a reflection of the loss of lean body mass and in part due to additional, poorly understood effects on energy metabolism. Overall energy expenditure is further reduced due to a decrease in the thermic effect of food (the individual eats less) and in differences in physical activity (it takes less energy to perform the same amount of activity for a smaller person). Thus, to maintain weight loss, individuals need to consume less energy than before dieting and increase energy expenditure by increasing the amount of physical activity.

EXERCISE

Exercise offers a number of significant advantages to patients attempting to achieve long-term weight loss. First and foremost, exercise increases energy expenditure, helping to create the energy deficit necessary for weight loss. Unfortunately, the amount of energy expended during most aerobic exercises (e.g., walking, jogging, swimming) for the typical periods performed (30 minutes four to five times per week) is modest, approximately 500–1000 kcal/week. Thus, exercise can be predicted to have little effect on short-term weight loss. Clinical trials reflect this modest effect: some studies demonstrate weight loss with exercise alone or extra weight loss when exercise plus diet is compared with diet alone, but other studies do not show such an effect. In a recent meta-analysis of 43 studies, exercise combined with diet lead to 1.1 kg greater weight loss than diet alone. Studies comparing high intensity exercise to low intensity exercise demonstrated a 1.5 kg greater weight loss.

The importance of exercise for successful maintenance of weight loss is more clearly established. As discussed above, an hour per day of exercise was one of the predictors of long-term weight maintenance in the National Weight Control Registry. In addition to the cumulative effect of increased energy expenditure, exercise affects the composition of the body substance lost during weight loss. When exercise is directly compared with diet, or when exercise plus diet is compared with diet alone, exercise results in greater preservation of lean body mass. That is, for each pound of weight lost, less fat and more muscle are lost during weight-loss programs without exercise. This is particularly important as the body's RME (a major portion of the total daily energy expenditure) is closely correlated with lean body mass.

The observation that much of the long-term effect of exercise is through preservation of lean body mass has resulted in an increased interest in the potential role of resistance training (e.g., weight lifting, circuit training). Preliminary results suggest that resistance training during dieting does result in maintenance of lean body mass compared with the result from dieting alone. Thus, highly motivated patients can be instructed to add resistance training to their aerobic exercise program.

Regular aerobic exercise results in a number of other benefits to the obese patient, including improved cardiovascular training effect (increased exercise tolerance), decreased appetite (per calorie expended), a general sense of well-being, decreased blood pressure (in hypertensives), improved glucose metabolism and insulin action (in diabetics), improved blood lipids (in lipid disorders), and, in the long term, decreased mortality from cardiovascular disease and all other causes.

Young patients with mild-to-moderate obesity can be started directly on a regular aerobic exercise program. Patients are commonly instructed to select two exercises and to perform either one of them six times per week for 30–60 minutes/day. Patients are taught to take their pulse and to generate a sustained tachycardia at 70–80% of their maximum predicted heart rate. Sedentary patients, older patients, and patients with severe obesity are instructed to begin walking programs without initial concern about meeting target heart rates. In these patients, the focus is on frequency and duration, rather than intensity. As weight loss proceeds, and patients become used to exercising regularly, they can be advanced to formal aerobic programs.

BEHAVIOR THERAPY & SOCIAL SUPPORT

Sustained weight loss requires long-term changes in eating and exercise behavior. Patients must learn specific skills to facilitate decreased calorie intake and increased energy expenditure. Behavior therapy, combined with diet and exercise, forms the core of the most standard "lifestyle modification" approaches to weight management. Behavior therapy can be implemented in groups or in individual therapy. Trained psychologists and dieticians commonly lead such efforts, but office-based clinicians can often learn to use many of the same techniques. Intensity of interaction appears to be one of the predictors of success. In the highly successful Diabetes Prevention Project, for example, lifestyle modification was taught in 16 individual sessions over 24 weeks.

Meta-analysis of 36 studies of behavior therapy for weight loss showed that behavior therapy alone resulted in significantly greater weight loss, a decrease of 2.5 kg, than placebo. When behavior therapy was combined with diet and exercise and compared to diet and exercise alone, the combined treatment also resulted in greater weight loss in five of six studies. Two studies compared cognitive-behavioral therapy (CBT) plus diet and exercise with diet and exercise alone. In these studies, the combined treatment lost 4.9 kg more.

Standard behavior therapy relies on specific techniques to teach the skills needed to change problematic behaviors. (1) Goal-setting. Patients are taught to set specific quantifiable, realistic goals at the outset of behavior therapy and during each week of therapy. Succeeding at meeting realistic goals creates a sense of self-efficacy and can reinforce further change. (2) Self-monitoring. Patients are taught to monitor both food and beverage intake and physical activity. Specific attention must be directed at teaching patients how to estimate portion sizes since patients may underestimate intake by 50%. The context, degree of hunger, and emotional state of each time of eating is also recorded. This may allow eating-related factors to be targets for modification. Patients are also instructed to record all programmed physical activity. Additional monitoring of physical activity can be done with pedometers. (3) Stimulus control. Patients are instructed to identify stimuli that increase the likelihood of both desired and undesired behaviors. Particular emphasis is placed on attempting to modify nonfood cues that are associated with eating. Similarly, simple techniques such as keeping certain problem food out of the house may be useful. (4) Cognitive skills. Patients are taught skills for problem solving and cognitive restructuring. Patients are asked to identify problems, consider potential solutions, list the advantages and disadvantages of each, select a feasible solution, and evaluate the results. Cognitive restructuring involves identification of dysfunctional thoughts that interfere with goals and replacing such thoughts with more rational ones. Formal CBT can also be used as part of weight management. CBT places more emphasis on cognitive change, rather than behavioral change, as the primary focus of treatment.

Social support is an additional essential component for any successful weight-loss program. Most successful programs use peer group support. Diet partnerships are effective for some patients. Involvement of family members is also important. A comprehensive review of published results of weight-loss programs strongly suggests that close provider–patient contact is a better predictor of success than the particular weight-loss intervention.

MEDICATIONS FOR TREATMENT OF OBESITY

Medications for the treatment of obesity are widely available over the counter, via the Internet, and by physician prescription. A recent Centers for Disease Control survey suggested that 7% of Americans used nonprescription weight-loss drugs. Among young obese women and among those on prescription weight-loss medications the use of nonprescription weight-loss medications was 28.4% and 33.8%, respectively.

A variety of weight-loss medications are currently available by prescription in the United States. These include various amphetamines (Drug Enforcement Administration schedule II), benzphetamine and phendimetrazine (schedule III), and phentermine, diethylpropion, mazindol, sibutramine, and orlistat. Most obesity experts agree that there is no current role for the schedule II or III drugs. Only sibutramine and orlistat are approved by the Food and Drug Administration (FDA) for long-term use. Orlistat, at half the prescription dose, has been approved for over-the-counter use in the United States.

Considerable controversy exists about the efficacy of and indications for these medications. Numerous clinical trials, some up to 2 years in duration, demonstrate statistically significant weight loss in subjects who take an obesity medication compared with placebo. Total weight loss is modest, approximately 4 kg greater than placebo. There is no convincing evidence that any one of these medications results in more weight loss than others. Although some studies also show improvement in obesity-related metabolic abnormalities (e.g., blood sugar, blood pressure, lipids), these reductions are also small and are substantially less than those achieved with hypoglycemic, antihypertensive, or lipid-lowering medications. In addition, no studies have yet demonstrated that weight loss achieved with medications results in reductions in obesity-related mortality or cardiovascular disease outcomes.

Rimonabant, a selective cannabinoid-1 receptor antagonist is under ongoing investigation for release in the United States as a weight-loss medication. Four studies have compared rimonabant 20 mg/day to placebo. A 4.9 kg greater reduction in weight was observed with rimonabant at 1 year. Most common side effects include gastrointestinal effects such as nausea and vomiting and psychiatric effects including depression and anxiety. Forty percent attrition was noted at 1 year.

NIH guidelines state that FDA-approved weight-loss drugs may be useful as an adjunct to diet and physical activity for patients with BMI ≥27 kg/m² and obesity-related risk factors or diseases, and for any patient with BMI ≥30 kg/m². Based on the modest efficacy noted above, however, these guidelines have not been widely implemented by clinicians. Prescriptions for weight-loss drugs should be limited to patients adhering to weight-loss diets and physical activity. In addition, weight loss in the first month of use correlates highly with weight loss at 12 months. Thus, for patients in whom no weight loss is achieved within the first month of use, weight-loss medications should be discontinued.

SURGERY FOR WEIGHT LOSS

Surgery for weight loss is typically considered the last resort for patients with severe obesity. NIH guidelines state that weight-loss surgery may be an option for carefully selected patients with BMI ≥40 or ≥35 kg/m² with comorbid conditions. Such patients must be at high risk for obesity-related morbidity and mortality, must have failed medical therapy, must have stable psychiatric status, and must be fully committed to lifetime lifestyle changes.

In recent years, the use of surgery to treat obesity has grown substantially. With implementation of new techniques and the use of less invasive approaches, obesity surgery is now one of the fastest growing operations in the United States. A majority of procedures are now done laparoscopically and some are being done as an outpatient procedure.

Available surgical procedures include malabsorptive procedures such as duodenal switch and biliopancreatic diversion, restrictive procedures such as vertical banded gastroplasty and adjustable gastric band, and combined procedures such as roux-en-Y gastric bypass. Most centers have avoided malabsorptive procedures, despite excellent weight loss, due to concerns of potential metabolic and nutritional sequelae analogous to those observed with jejuno-ileal bypass procedures in the past. Restrictive procedures, particularly the laparoscopic adjustable gastric band, are gaining in popularity. Advantages include reduced perioperative morbidity and mortality compared to other procedures. Weight loss is less than other procedures, however, and intermediate and long-term complications are greater. Complications include prolapse of the stomach through the band, infected reservoir sites, heartburn and regurgitation, and severe esophagitis. Approximately one-third of banding procedures require conversion to a roux-en-Y bypass. The roux-en-Y bypass is the most common bariatric procedure in the United States. Weight loss, approximately one-third of initial weight, is greater than with purely restrictive procedures. Serious perioperative complications are greater however, and

include bleeding and gastrojejunostomy leaks. Perioperative mortality occurs in 0.5% of cases, even in the best centers, and has been shown to be substantially higher in older and sicker patients. Nutritional complications include deficiencies of fat-soluble vitamins, especially vitamin D, iron, B_{12}, folate, and calcium. The only long-term study reports significant weight regain over time. Weight loss at 10 years decreased from 38% at year 1 to 25% at year 10.

MANAGEMENT OF OBESITY IN THE HOSPITAL

Due to the increasing prevalence of obesity, the high rate of obesity-related morbidity, and the increasing use of operative procedures to treat obesity, such patients are increasingly cared for in inpatient and critical care settings. In most respects care is similar to that of nonobese patients; however, severely obese patients require special attention in several aspects of care. Technical procedures may be more difficult in the obese patient including intubation, tracheostomy, and vascular access. Blood pressure monitoring requires use of cuffs with bladders large enough to cover 80% of the arm circumference. Undersized cuffs can overestimate blood pressure significantly. Medication dosing of some medications must be adjusted in obese patients due to the larger volume of distribution for lipophilic drugs. Some drugs, such as digoxin, beta-blockers, and penicillins, should be dosed according to the ideal body weight rather than the actual weight. Other drugs, including heparin and succinylcholine, are dosed based on the actual body weight. A third group including aminoglycosides and vancomycin are best dosed at a dosing weight intermediate between the actual and ideal weight. The dosing weight is equal to the ideal body weight + 0.4 (actual weight − ideal weight). Similar issues are encountered with nutrition support in the obese patient. Use of the actual body weight in common energy estimation equations such as the Harris-Benedict equation is likely to overestimate energy requirements. If indirect calorimetry is not available to measure energy expenditure, the use of the ideal body weight, or an intermediate dosing weight as calculated above, is less likely to result in complications of overfeeding.

SUMMARY

The rapidly increasing prevalence of obesity is creating a major public health crises. Currently available treatments with diets, exercise, and behavior therapy provide limited efficacy for most patients. Some patients, however, can achieve long-term weight loss. Currently approved medications also demonstrate limited efficacy. Surgical treatment of obesity is the most effective treatment but is associated with substantial risk and long-term complications. Given the lack of effective therapy, preventive measures are essential. Broad and ambitious public health approaches are required to impact the obesity epidemic. For most individual patients, dietary changes that emphasize calorie reduction by consuming smaller portions, more plant foods, fewer high calorie beverages, and less fast food are necessary even to maintain current weight. Similarly, striking increases in daily physical activity are needed to maintain body weight and achieve fitness.

SUGGESTED READINGS

Dansinger ML, Gleason JA, Griffith JL, et al. Comparison of the Atkins, Ornish, Weight Watchers, and Zone diets for weight loss and heart disease risk reduction: a randomized trial. *JAMA* 2005;293(1):43–53.

Fabricatore AN. Behavior therapy and cognitive-behavioral therapy of obesity: is there a difference? *J Am Diet Assoc* 2007;107(1): 92–99.

Flegal KM, Graubard BI, Williamson DF, et al. Excess deaths associated with underweight, overweight, and obesity. *JAMA* 2005; 293(15):1861–1867. PMID: 15840860.

Gilden Tsai A, Wadden TA. The evolution of very-low-calorie diets: an update and meta-analysis. *Obesity (Silver Spring)* 2006;14(8): 1283–1293. PMID: 16988070.

Howard BV, Manson JE, Stefanick ML, et al. Low-fat dietary pattern and weight change over 7 years: the Women's Health Initiative Dietary Modification Trial. *JAMA* 2006;295: 39–49.

Kendrick ML, Dakin GF. Surgical approaches to obesity. *Mayo Clin Proc* 2006;81(10 Suppl):S18–S24. PMID: 17036575.

Shaw K, O'Rourke P, Del Mar C, et al. Psychological interventions for overweight or obesity. *Cochrane Database Syst Rev* 2005;(2): CD003818.

Shaw K, Gennat H, O'Rourke P, et al. Exercise for overweight or obesity. *Cochrane Database Syst Rev* 2006;(4):CD003817. PMID: 17054187.

Tsai AG, Wadden TA. Systematic review: an evaluation of major commercial weight loss programs in the United States. *Ann Intern Med* 2005;142(1):56–66.

Wadden TA, Berkowitz RI, Womble LG, et al. Randomized trial of lifestyle modification and pharmacotherapy for obesity. *N Engl J Med* 2005;353(20):2111–2120.

Wing RR, Phelan S. Long-term weight loss maintenance. *Am J Clin Nutr* 2005;82(1 Suppl):222S–225S. Review. PMID: 16002825.

Eating Disorders

20

Steven J. Romano, MD

INTRODUCTION

The eating disorders, including anorexia nervosa and bulimia nervosa, are receiving more clinical and research attention than ever before, paralleling an increase in their prevalence over the past few decades. Such disturbances in eating behavior are, of course, not new. Historical documentation of anorexia nervosa dates back to the early Christian saints. Binging and purging, although distinct from our current concept of bulimia nervosa, took place in the lives of ancient Romans.

The eating disorders are best viewed as clinical syndromes rather than specific diseases, as they do not result from a single cause or follow a single course. As psychiatric syndromes, they are defined largely by a constellation of behaviors and attitudes that persist over time and have characteristic complications contributing to physical and psychosocial dysfunction. Because of the complexity and breadth of contributing factors, as well as the extent of comorbid psychopathology, knowledge of the behavioral characteristics of the eating disorders can lead to improved recognition and implementation of effective treatment strategies. In light of the complicated interplay of psychiatric, psychosocial, and medical consequences, treatment beyond initial medical stabilization generally requires referral to specialists.

MULTIDIMENSIONAL MODEL

A comprehensive multidimensional model best illustrates the role various factors play in the genesis of clinically significant eating disturbances. In this schema, also referred to as a stress-diathesis model, psychological, biological, and sociocultural stressors contribute to the development of the syndrome.

Psychological factors include personality features, such as the anorectic's obsessive-compulsive qualities, constrained affect, and sense of ineffectiveness, and the bulimic's impulsivity. They also include the influence of developmental stressors and family dynamics.

Biological factors are most often due to the adverse effects of starvation, malnutrition, and purging behaviors, including vomiting and the misuse of laxatives and diuretics. Restrictive dieting and subsequent malnourishment may contribute to the development of comorbid psychiatric conditions, such as anxiety and depression. In addition, a preexisting biological vulnerability is supported by neurophysiologic investigations showing dysfunction of serotonin, dopamine, and norepinephrine neuromodulators; a small number of patients with anorexia develop amenorrhea preceding significant weight loss.

Sociocultural factors figure prominently in the etiology of the eating disorders. The idealization of thinness contributes to dieting behavior, often beginning in early adolescence. Of note, dieting is almost always present as a precipitant to the development of an eating disorder. Other precipitants include periods of illness leading to weight loss; in vulnerable individuals this may be followed by willful dieting.

THEORETICAL CONSIDERATIONS

Conceptual models aid in understanding the etiology and possible sustaining factors involved in the genesis and persistence of eating-disordered behavior. Important models include those derived from learning theory and neurophysiologic abnormality or dysfunction.

Cognitive-behavioral theory, which is derived from learning theory, states that cognition influences behavior in a predictable manner. Cues, both internal and external, can provoke behavioral outcomes through activation of cognitive sets. A change in negative cognition therefore influences a change from dysfunctional to healthy behavior. Thoughts that overvalue weight, food, and diet, especially the idealization of thinness, lead to the perpetuation of compromising responses, such as heroic dietary measures and abuses of substances believed effective for weight reduction. The coupling of such cognitions and behaviors affects self-esteem and may severely impair an individual's psychological state. Cognitive-behavioral therapy has been effective in achieving symptom reduction and improvement in both medical and psychological status.

The search for specific biological markers that may help identify patients with eating disorders has focused increasingly on neurotransmitters and other neuromodulators. Research findings suggest that dysfunction in various neurotransmitter systems, including serotonin, dopamine, and norepinephrine, as well as opioids and cholecystokinin (CCK), might play a role in the development and maintenance of the eating disorders. Rationale for the examination of these hormones and other substances derives from our understanding of the pathways modulating appetitive behavior, including hypothalamic regulation and the known connection between the gastrointestinal tract and the central nervous system. The complexity of these disorders, including the stress of eating-disordered behavior on physiology, however, makes it unlikely that a neurophysiologic hypothesis alone can explain the etiology and maintenance of these complex syndromes.

ANOREXIA NERVOSA

CASE ILLUSTRATION 1

Amy, a 15-year-old high school sophomore, presented to her pediatrician at her mother's insistence with vague complaints of abdominal pain and bloating, particularly after meals. Though she answered all questions posed, she was rather reserved and hesitant to embellish her responses. A review of systems revealed infrequent constipation and a history of two nonconsecutive missed periods over the last 6 months, a departure from her generally regular periods since onset of menses at age 13. Vital signs were notable for a pulse of 54 and a sitting BP of 85/60. She was 5 ft. 4 in. and 102 lb, 9 lb less than was recorded at the time of her annual exam approximately 8 months ago. Physical examination was without significant findings. In particular, there were no findings suggested of focal abdominal pathology.

In private, Amy's mother told the pediatrician that Amy was less socially engaged over the last several months, preferring solitary activities such as studying or going out with friends or family. She also noted that Amy appeared to be using a treadmill in the basement for extended periods of time, and was concerned that she may have lost "a few pounds" recently. This wouldn't ordinarily concern her, but Amy was also skipping meals with the family and had become "so picky" with regards to food choices. She was concerned that Amy was establishing unhealthy eating and exercise habits.

When presented with her mother's concerns and the clinical information by her pediatrician, Amy insisted that there was nothing to worry about, and denied voluntary attempts to lose weight. She did admit, though, that she was concerned about the amount of food her mother was serving at dinner, and that she had begun to avoid "fattening" foods and desserts, insisting that it was for health reasons. She reluctantly added that she was concerned that her hips were "too large" for her frame, and was hoping that continued exercise might minimize this perceived defect. She was unconcerned about her irregular periods, even though the pediatrician explained that it was unhealthy and likely due to her recent changes in weight, exercise, and eating habits. Following discussion with Amy and her mother, the pediatrician gently insisted that Amy and her family speak to a psychiatrist with experience in diagnosing and treating eating disorders, as he was concerned that Amy was developing anorexia.

Description

Anorexia nervosa is a relatively rare disorder affecting less than 1% of young women and a much smaller percentage of young men. Its most striking behavioral manifestation is the willful restriction of caloric intake secondary to an irrational fear of becoming fat, frequently in concert with a grossly distorted view of one's self as overweight, even in the presence of severe emaciation. Patients often exhibit a phobic response to food, particularly to fatty and other calorically dense items. They develop an obsessive preoccupation with food, eating, dieting, weight, and body shape and frequently exhibit ritualistic behaviors involving choosing, preparing, and ingesting meals (e.g., cutting food into very small pieces or chewing each bite a specific number of times).

Early in the course of the illness, patients begin to restrict many food items, as is typical of most dieters. As the disorder progresses, though, the anorectic's menu becomes grossly constricted and she demonstrates greater rigidity. Minor variations in meal content can produce tremendous anxiety. Unlike the average dieter, the anorectic continues her pursuit of thinness to an extreme and becomes dependent on the daily registration of weight loss. This fuels even more restrictive dieting. Extreme dieting is often complicated by other weight-reducing behaviors. Exercise is frequently compulsive, and hyperactivity in underweight patients is a curious but often-encountered concomitant. Weakness, muscle aches, sleep disturbances, and gastrointestinal complaints, including constipation and postprandial bloating, are common physical findings. Amenorrhea, reflecting endocrine dysfunction secondary to malnourishment, is generally present.

Some anorectics engage in bulimic behaviors, including binging and purging. This binge–purge subtype of anorexia nervosa contrasts with the purely restricting subtype described earlier. Often, purging behavior, such as self-induced vomiting or the misuse of laxatives and diuretics, is seen in the absence of binging. The coupling of purging with self-starvation compounds the medical consequences of the disorder. Furthermore, anorectics, particularly adolescents, generally minimize their symptoms and the negative consequences of their disorder and are thus rarely motivated for treatment. The characteristics of the illness, both medical and psychological, are intensified with weight loss, further frustrating attempts at engaging the patient in a meaningful therapeutic process. Family and friends become increasingly anxious, angry, and at times alienated, as their loved one regresses. Superficial compliance, as is sometimes seen, belies a profound resistance. Anorectic patients can be challenging to treat as they cling tenaciously to their beliefs and behaviors.

Psychosocial dysfunction is common in patients with anorexia. Although educational performance may not be affected in adolescent patients, social relations become increasingly constricted, and sexual interest is generally diminished or absent.

Differential Diagnosis

The pathognomonic features of anorexia nervosa, namely the intense fear of becoming fat coupled with the relentless pursuit of thinness, are generally absent in other medical and psychiatric conditions. The term *anorexia*, which itself refers to absence of appetite, is a misnomer in the case of the syndrome of anorexia nervosa. True anorexia, such as encountered in many medical conditions or diseases, would be accompanied by other signs or symptoms of those illnesses (as in gastrointestinal disease or many cancers).

Lack of appetite or decreased intake, with or without subsequent weight loss, is encountered in a number of psychiatric disorders. These include depression, hysterical conversion and other psychosomatic disorders, schizophrenia, and certain delusional disorders, but each of these is associated with a cluster of other substantiating symptomatology. Some patients with obsessive-compulsive disorder (OCD) may exhibit what appears to be bizarre behavior around food, eating, or meal preparation, but, on further exploration, their behavior is in response to obsessional ideation, for example, the fear of contamination. Such patients, in contrast to those with anorexia nervosa, generally admit their discomfort with the need to perform such compelling and often excessive or senseless acts.

In summary, although comorbid psychopathology may be encountered in patients with anorexia nervosa, including symptoms of depression or OCD, the hallmark of anorexia nervosa (the morbid fear of becoming fat and the relentless pursuit of thinness) is absent in the other psychiatric syndromes. In none of these syndromes does the goal of weight loss drive the behavior.

Medical Complications & Treatment

Treatment of anorexia nervosa is initially directed at correcting the acute medical complications and is followed by supportive nutritional rehabilitation. Most medical consequences resolve with nutritional rehabilitation and the discontinuation of purging behaviors. Exceptions include persistent osteopenic changes in those who have experienced extended periods of malnourishment and suppression of growth in severe cases of adolescent anorexia.

In most cases of anorexia associated with significant weight loss (15–20% or more of ideal body weight) a structured inpatient facility is necessary to maintain an adequate level of medical surveillance and sustain a steady rate of weight gain. On admission to an inpatient treatment facility, laboratory screening should include tests for electrolytes, liver function, amylase (elevated in patients who purge), thyroid function, a complete blood count with differential, and a urinalysis. Common laboratory findings include leukopenia with a relative lymphocytosis, metabolic alkalosis with associated hypokalemia, hypochloremia and elevated serum bicarbonate levels, and, occasionally, metabolic acidosis in patients who abuse large amounts of stimulant-type laxatives. An electrocardiogram should also be obtained since emaciation and associated electrolyte disturbances can contribute to significant cardiac abnormalities, especially in those who purge. Hypokalemia can lead to arrhythmia and the risk of cardiac arrest.

Acute medical conditions generally requiring immediate attention include electrolyte disturbances and dehydration, both of which are readily reversible. In most cases, initiating oral intake of fluids and food reverses minor disturbances in electrolytes and establishes adequate hydration. More severe cases, for example, patients with significant hypokalemia, may require intravenous hydration and parenteral replacement of depleted electrolytes, with daily electrolyte checks until the patient's condition stabilizes. Care should be taken to avoid overhydration and the consequences of excess fluid retention in vulnerable individuals. Importantly, treatment must ensure prevention of purging behaviors in patients with this history, as persistence of purging will alter electrolyte and fluid balance.

In patients who are significantly underweight, use of a liquid supplement, initially as replacement for solid food, helps ensure necessary caloric intake. When given in divided feedings throughout the day, it may decrease the patient's sense of postprandial discomfort and early satiety, both frequent consequences of extended caloric restriction and semistarvation. Further, this approach to refeeding decreases the inevitable manipulations around food choices. Replacement of solid food with a liquid supplement may also lessen the patient's phobic avoidance of food and the subsequent anxiety around meal choices.

Psychotherapeutic Interventions

Given the lack of motivation and strong resistance to treatment exhibited by the majority of patients with anorexia, it is helpful to initiate behavioral strategies as soon as any acute medical condition is stabilized. Initial behavioral interventions, tied to daily weight gain in increments of no less than 0.25 lb or 0.1 kg, include obtaining visits from family or friends, lessening physical restrictions, and increasing involvement in activities on and off the unit. It is important that all contingencies be tied to daily weight gain, which is measured each morning at the same time and in like manner, as this is a quantifiable observation not open to argument or discussion. A milieu supportive of such interventions helps to motivate the patient and exerts pressure toward positive change.

As the patient reaches a target weight range and establishes some degree of commitment to treatment, solid food can replace the liquid supplement. The ability of the patient to maintain weight through normalization of intake marks a transition to less structured treatment, such as a partial hospitalization program or outpatient follow-up.

Other treatments applicable to both inpatient and outpatient settings include individual psychotherapy and family intervention. The initial focus in family therapy should be on psychoeducation and obtaining the support of family members. The dynamics that may be contributing to the patient's eating disorder should be identified and, when possible, resolved. Such treatment often requires extensive contact beyond any acute interventions.

Individual psychotherapy is of limited value in the early stages of treatment, as the anorectic individual is generally unmotivated and, due to cognitive disturbances secondary to self-starvation, not capable of meaningful therapeutic work. Supportive therapy during this acute stage is often helpful in allaying anxiety and encouraging compliance. The more focused cognitive-behavioral and interpersonal therapies are generally more effective when the patient has begun to gain weight and is beyond acute medical risk. Cognitive-behavioral therapy focuses on the particular disturbing or distorted thoughts that contribute to the patient's maladaptive behavior and helps the patient establish more effective behavioral alternatives. It may also be effective in dealing with the central psychological features of anorexia nervosa, such as disturbance in body image. Interpersonal therapy may also be helpful. It focuses on interpersonal conflicts rather than specific eating disturbances. Following stabilization and resolution of the acute crisis, including achievement of

weight restoration, patients often require longer-term psychotherapeutic interventions.

Pharmacotherapy

Pharmacologic therapy can play an adjunctive role in the management of both primary eating symptoms and their comorbid psychiatric features, including anxiety and depression. Such treatments should focus on particular target symptoms or behaviors. No single medication is consistently effective in managing the primary psychiatric disturbances of anorexia nervosa. Antidepressants, especially the selective serotonin reuptake inhibitors (SSRIs), can alleviate depressive symptoms and, due to their ability to regulate obsessive-compulsive symptomatology, may help reduce the preoccupations and ritualistic behaviors encountered in most anorectics. Low doses of antipsychotics may sometimes be employed in severely obsessional or agitated patients. Anxiolytics in general, especially benzodiazepines, should not be given to anorectics as they are prone to development of addiction.

BULIMIA NERVOSA

 CASE ILLUSTRATION 2

Cynthia, a 28-year-old single attorney with no significant medical or surgical history, presented to her primary care physician with complaints consistent with gastroesophageal reflux. Symptoms included substernal burning sensations and regurgitation occurring several times a week, particularly following a large meal. She also reported occasional sharp chest pains lasting only a few seconds, not associated with shortness of breath or other signs or symptoms suggestive of cardiac origin. Other complaints noted on review of symptoms were general myalgia and fatigue, both experienced "a few days a week." She was on oral contraceptives, and stated that she took the suggested dose of an over-the-counter (OTC) laxative for constipation one or two times a week. Vital signs were normal, and she was afebrile. The only positive finding on physical examination was bilateral, nonpainful enlargement of the parotid glands. An electrocardiogram showed normal rate and rhythm, with nonspecific T-wave changes. Routine blood work was drawn, and a prescription for a proton pump inhibitor was given for symptoms of gastroesophageal reflux.

A review of Cynthia's laboratory values the next day revealed an elevated amylase and a serum potassium of 2.7. The laboratory abnormalities, together with the enlarged parotids and her presenting complaints, suggested self-induced vomiting. During a telephone call to Cynthia that day, her physician expressed concern and probed for confirmation. Cynthia hesitantly admitted to having a 5-year history of binging and purging, the latter by both self-induced vomiting and the use of a diuretic, furosemide, which she had been receiving from her OBGYN for menstrual complaints. She reluctantly agreed to return to the office for repeat electrolytes, as well as for a referral to an eating disorders clinic nearby.

Description

Bulimia nervosa affects approximately 2–3% of young women and 0.2% of young men, although bulimic behaviors may be encountered in many more patients. Bulimia nervosa is generally precipitated by periods of restrictive dieting. Bulimic individuals engage in regular episodes of binge eating, followed by compensatory behaviors to counteract the weight gain from ingested calories. Binge eating is characterized by the rapid consumption of large amounts of food over a short time, usually 1–2 hours. It is associated with a sense of being out of control and is often followed by feelings of guilt or shame and other dysphoric affective states, such as depression or anxiety. Some patients report alleviation of dysphoria or even emotional numbing during or immediately following the episode, although this is short-lived. During a binge, a few thousand to as many as 15,000 kcal or more may be consumed. Sometimes trigger foods, often a fattening sweet such as chocolate, precipitate a binge, although the overall content of food consumed, by macroanalysis of nutritional content, varies. The bulimic individual generally binges in private; grossly overeating is humiliating. Embarrassment can lead to varying degrees of social avoidance or isolation.

Contributing further to avoidance behavior is the need to compensate for eating, frequently by purging. Most bulimic individuals induce vomiting during or after a binge, and some also use laxatives or diuretics. A minority of patients employ laxatives or diuretics alone. Nonpurging compensatory behaviors include compulsive exercising and restrictive dieting or fasting between binges.

Another characteristic of bulimia nervosa is patient dissatisfaction with body shape or weight. This may evolve into a significant degree of obsessional preoccupation, with self-evaluation overly influenced by these physical concerns. It can have a profound effect on self-esteem and is evidenced in part by comorbid depressive symptomatology in the majority of patients. Impulsive behavior is encountered in many individuals with bulimia nervosa and at times leads to substance abuse, sexual promiscuity, and theft.

Differential Diagnosis

Few medical or psychiatric disorders can be confused with bulimia nervosa. More frequently, signs of self-induced vomiting or use of diuretics or laxatives in a young woman who does not admit to binging or purging behaviors lead the primary care clinician to search for another primary medical diagnosis. Signs and symptoms associated with gastritis, esophagitis, dehydration, or electrolyte disturbances result in primary care or emergency room visits, postponing psychiatric consultation. If the patient is underweight, amenorrheic, and is binging and purging, she has anorexia nervosa of the binge–purge subtype rather than bulimia nervosa.

Medical Complications & Treatment

The majority of medical complications due to bulimia nervosa are consequences of purging behaviors. Self-induced vomiting can lead to gastritis, esophagitis, periodontal disease, and dental caries. Gastric dilatation and gastric or esophageal rupture are rare medical emergencies. Metabolic alkalosis with the development of clinically significant hypokalemia in patients who vomit is not unusual, and serum electrolytes show typical indices. When present, electrocardiographic changes are significant. Arrhythmias can lead to cardiac arrest if hypokalemia and related disturbances are not corrected. Use of diuretics cause similar disturbances. Metabolic acidosis can develop in patients who use a significant number of stimulant-type laxatives. Dehydration, sometimes requiring intravenous hydration, can accompany each of the aforementioned purging behaviors. More often associated with bulimic behaviors are general physical complaints such as fatigue and muscle aches. Long-term use of the emetic ipecac can lead to myopathies, including cardiomyopathy, the latter a rare cause of death in patients with bulimia.

Most patients with bulimia nervosa can be treated as outpatients or in more structured partial hospitalization programs. An individual with an acute medical condition, however, such as dehydration or symptomatic hypokalemia accompanied by electrocardiographic changes, requires hospitalization for medical stabilization. Patients who have failed outpatient treatment and continue to binge and purge frequently, and those with significant depression and associated suicidal ideation, may require inpatient treatment.

Psychotherapeutic Interventions

Helping patients recognize the negative consequences of their behavior and dispelling myths about the efficacy of many of their dietary maneuvers, especially the usefulness of laxatives, diuretics, and self-induced vomiting, may be enough to motivate them to decrease the frequency of bulimic behaviors. Similarly, self-monitoring intake with the use of food diaries and normalization of meal patterns can lead to short-term gains in control of bulimic symptoms. Time-limited psychotherapy, focused specifically on the disturbed eating patterns, can be conducted in an individual or group format and is often useful. More traditional exploratory psychotherapies, which are generally not time limited, do not predictably affect outcome but may play a role in the treatment of underlying or persistent difficulties following improvement or resolution of bulimia.

Cognitive-behavioral therapy is an established treatment for bulimia nervosa and can lead to both acute reduction in symptoms of binging and purging and longer-term maintenance of gains. It targets the behavioral manifestations and challenges the cognitive distortions typically encountered in these patients. In cognitive-behavioral therapy, identifying disordered behaviors is the first step toward productive intervention, because behavioral consequences follow specific cues. To intervene, one must recognize the various cues and respond to them deliberately rather than automatically. Cues affecting eating-disordered patients are either internal or external. Internal cues include physiologic ones, most significantly hunger, as well as emotions and thoughts. External cues encompass a broad array of experiences from sensual, such as sight or smell, to situational. Cues lead to consequences that are either positive or negative, both can be reinforcing.

Following the identification of cues, associated responses can be addressed more specifically and in greater detail. Responses consist of thoughts, feelings, and behaviors. Helping the patient understand that thoughts and feelings affect behavioral responses to a cue is of great significance because both thoughts and feelings can be altered through cognitive-behavioral techniques. For each cue identified, patients are taught to delineate the various response components and to evaluate the appropriateness of each. Although schematically simple, many eating-associated responses are automatic, and learning to identify the cues and various responses requires much practice.

During cognitive-behavioral therapy patients are taught to recognize that behaviors follow cues and responses to cues can be broken down into thoughts, feelings, and behaviors. What a patient thinks and feels about a cue dictates whether her response is adaptive or maladaptive. How she feels is influenced by how she thinks, therefore the restructuring of thoughts is of primary importance. Eating-disordered patients manifest certain patterns of distorted thinking; these patterns negatively influence feelings and fuel the maladaptive behaviors. These various styles of thinking are identified, and strategies to challenge and ultimately to alter the distortions are developed.

A simple example helps illustrate the applicability of cognitive-behavioral therapy. A common cue that frequently leads to a bulimic response is the normal sense of fullness. Rather than recognizing satiety as a normal physiologic response, the eating-disordered patient often misinterprets this cue, stating instead, "I feel fat." This distorted thought, unchallenged, is associated with negative feelings and often leads to dysfunctional behaviors. Rather than the appropriate response to fullness, understanding that it is temporary and will pass, the patient believes she must compensate for being "fat" and rids herself of the meal through purging or compensates for the caloric intake through exercise. Such a response causes the cycle to reassert itself.

Pharmacotherapy

Pharmacologic management may play a significant role in treatment and, unlike in anorexia, can more predictably affect outcome. Many antidepressants, including SSRIs, monoamine oxidase inhibitors (MAOIs), and tricyclic antidepressants (TCAs) are effective in treating bulimia. (Dietary proscriptions limit the usefulness of MAOIs and lethality in overdose limits treatment with TCAs.) They reduce symptoms of depression and anxiety as well as the frequency of binging and purging. Bupropion is the only antidepressant that is contraindicated, as the metabolic imbalances precipitated by purging can make the patient more prone to seizures.

SUMMARY

Eating disorders represent a broad spectrum of psychopathologic features. They are best understood in terms of multiple etiologic factors influencing the development of clinical syndromes. Understanding the complexity of these disorders, the behaviors associated with them, and their comorbid psychiatric features aids in their recognition and treatment. Focusing initially on control of these primary eating disorder behaviors helps reduce the likelihood of psychological morbidity. It also limits the medical complications that frequently develop in these conditions. Interventions to control behavior range from response prevention (for patients placed on special inpatient wards) to cognitive-behavioral therapies for more motivated patients. Behavioral control may be augmented through pharmacologic management as well as other psychotherapies (psychoeducational and interpersonal) that help reduce the role that sustaining factors play in the maintenance of these disorders.

SUGGESTED READINGS

Fairburn CG, Wilson GT, eds. *Binge Eating: Nature, Assessment, Treatment.* New York, NY: Guilford Press, 1996.

Goldstein DJ, ed. *The Management of Eating Disorders and Obesity,* 2nd ed. Totowa, NJ: Humana Press Inc., 2005.

Halmi KA, ed. *Psychobiology and Treatment of Anorexia Nervosa and Bulimia Nervosa.* Washington, DC: American Psychiatric Association Press, 1992.

Halmi KA. Eating disorders. In: Hales KE, Yudofsky SC, Talbott J, eds. *American Psychiatric Press Textbook of Psychiatry,* 2nd ed. Washington, DC: American Psychiatric Association Press, 1994, pp. 857–875.

Hsu LKG. *Eating Disorders.* New York, NY: Guilford Press, 1990.

Mitchell JE. *Bulimia Nervosa.* Minneapolis, MN: University of Minnesota Press, 1990.

Walsh BT, Devlin MJ. Psychopharmacology of anorexia nervosa, bulimia nervosa, and binge eating. In: Bloom FE, Kuffer DJ, eds. *Psychopharmacology: The Fourth Generation of Progress.* New York, NY: Raven Press, 1995, pp. 1581–1589.

WEB SITES

Academy for Eating Disorders Web site. http://www.aedweb.org/. Accessed October, 2007.

American Psychiatric Association, Psychiatric Practice Web site. http://www.psych.org/psych-pract. Accessed October, 2007.

Alcohol & Substance Use

21

William D. Clark, MD

INTRODUCTION

CASE ILLUSTRATION

Jim is a 50-year-old factory worker with high blood pressure. He has a follow-up visit with the doctor who has been his primary care physician for the past decade. He mentions that he recently received his second "driving under the influence" (DUI) citation and considers it unfair. His probation officer ordered Jim to undergo alcohol counseling at the local alcohol treatment center. Jim has no interest in counseling but he thinks he must attend to keep his driver's license, needed to get to his job.

Physicians are well aware of the harm that the use of drugs and alcohol brings to their patients and families. The prevalence of substance-use disorders exceeds 20% in ambulatory practices and is higher in hospitalized patients, and involves everyone from adolescents, teachers, and shipyard workers to doctors themselves. Physicians report that conversations with patients about drinking are stressful and conflict laden, and that patients are unmotivated to change their behavior. Physicians' negative feelings derive from family experiences or from encounters with intoxicated patients who are hostile, uncooperative, and often violent. Anyone entangled in the web of substance abuse is likely to act irresponsibly—driving while intoxicated, attempting suicide, engaging in high-risk sexual behavior, and sharing, dealing, and stealing illegal drugs—despite legal, moral, and family sanctions. These dynamics, combined with the sense that substance abuse may not really be a "medical" issue, tend to keep physicians from speaking up and prevent them from helping their patients.

Evidence from many sources provides reason for optimism, however, and shows that doctors who take a few moments to thoughtfully structure their interventions with patients succeed in reducing harm. In so doing, physicians not only lower medical care costs and morbidity for patients and their family members, but also strengthen family and social relationships, self-esteem, and emotional stability. Indeed the recovery rate from substance abuse, 30–40% of treated patients, exceeds that from most chronic illnesses. Recovering patients often credit their clinicians with being a primary factor in their recovery and with literally saving their lives. For physicians, participating in the reversal of substance abuse can be as gratifying as helping patients recover from leukemia or pneumonia. Of course, caring for patients with these problems is more like helping patients with depression, anxiety, elevated cholesterol, or arthritis than patients with acute problems that respond to surgery. In this chapter, we will discuss identification and management of substance-use problems, and how Jim's success in coping with his problems will be affected by his physician's interactions with him.

ETIOLOGY & PATHOPHYSIOLOGY

No person is immune to nervous tissue actions of alcohol and other drugs, and no one seeks to develop substance-use problems. People modulate use according to feedback from internal states such as shame or hangover, and external cues such as reprimands, criticism, and sanctions. They succeed or fail in limiting use because of the interplay of genetic, physiologic, psychological, and social/cultural factors.

CASE ILLUSTRATION (CONTD.)

Jim cannot remember his father, but knows he had serious drinking problems and left the family when Jim was 4.

When people do not limit their drug or alcohol use, the predictable and multitudinous brain effects of heavy use facilitate a vicious cycle of using more, developing problems, and discounting the role of drugs. The insidious development of tolerance to intoxication, cognitive deficits from high doses, and the dysphoric aspects of related states (hangover, for example) engender unhealthy social dynamics. These relationship problems are exaggerated because friends and family resent the (apparently) voluntary "having fun and being irresponsible" nature of overindulgence. People become adept at ignoring reality and suppressing negative feelings. Longer times spent in brain-altered states result in the dramatic neurophysiologic changes of addiction and withdrawal. Further, emotional isolation develops because people make excuses for their behavior, direct blame onto others, and show hostility whenever sensible limits are discussed. They select friends and partners who tolerate heavy use and tacitly agree to overlook the consequences.

 CASE ILLUSTRATION (CONTD.)

Jim began drinking as a teenager and got up to a 12-pack per day. He cut back once he got out of his twenties since "that was going nowhere" but still drinks four to six beers daily—at his club or playing pool or cards with his buddies, and up to two six-packs per day on the weekend. (Based on his self-report and national survey data, only 3% of American men drink more than Jim.)

WORKING EFFECTIVELY WITH PATIENTS

Chemical dependence (non-tobacco-related addictive disease) is a chronic, progressive illness affecting 10–15% of Americans at some time in their lives (lifetime prevalence) and 5–7% of Americans at any given point in time. The brain effects of addictive drugs vary in neurochemical mechanisms, timing, intensity, and potential toxicity. The illness of chemical dependency, a condition manifested by adverse medical and social consequences for users, their families and social networks, is similar across the various drug classes and specific drugs. Alcohol, heroin, cocaine, benzodiazepine, and other addictions are variants of the underlying disease of chemical dependence, not distinctive disorders. Healthcare communication differences are related to interaction dynamics that stem from the legal and social consequences of obtaining and using the particular drug, and its potential medical complications.

Consequently, screening, assessment, and management of drug addictions other than alcohol are similar to strategies in use for alcohol-use disorders. A caveat to these general principles relates to prescription drug abuse, which may involve physicians' interpersonal and intrapersonal vulnerabilities, beliefs, and prescribing preferences and habits.

Promoting Behavior Change

Several approaches for promoting behavior change in patients with substance-use problems have emerged from research, these include *brief intervention, motivational interviewing, shared decision making, relationship-centered care*, and *autonomy support* (see Chapter 16 for a full discussion of behavior change). The fundamental **principles** derived from this research are as follows:

- Generally speaking, the physician takes responsibility for calibrating and adjusting interventions so that patients can hear information and feedback that create or amplify differences between the way life is now and the goals and values patients espouse. Using an empathic and caring style, the physician shows that discrepancies between the actual and the potential might be minimized if patients change their drug-use patterns.
- Patients will not change until they are ready, and ambivalence about change and/or resistance to change is universal.
- Physicians can best promote change by maintaining an empathic and relationship-centered style. Taking a strongly persuasive stand usually fails to promote change.
- Only the patient can take responsibility for change and effect change. Physicians can promote change by providing information (both feedback about the patient's health and problems and information about resources), by showing attentiveness and listening carefully to the patient's ideas about both the pros and the cons of possible changes, and by helping boost the patient's self-confidence about change.

The fundamental **content messages** physicians should include in interviews are as follows:

- I am concerned that your drug use is hurting you and others you care about (or has the potential to hurt you).
- Most people use a lot less than you, or abstain.
- For better health, you should curb (or cease) your drug use.
- The key choices are up to you, you are the person who will decide what to do.
- I will give you my best advice, which is based on ideas from the experts and my experience with other patients with similar problems.
- Changing drug-use habits may turn out to be difficult and scary.

- I want to collaborate with you, even if progress is slow or intermittent.

The fundamental **process strategies** physicians should follow are as follows:

- Maintain dialog when giving information and recommendations; use a *tell, ask, tell* strategy.
- Make clear recommendations, but do not try to persuade patients.
- State explicitly that you will advise, but that the patient decides.
- Establish the patient's commitment to any plans on which you agree.
- Never argue with patients and do not try to overcome resistance, reluctance, rebellion, or rationalization. Use reflection to respond to these manifestations of ambivalence.
- Support the patient's self-confidence.

Two key steps can assist physicians in doing a better job with substance-abusing patients. The first is to intervene when any clue suggests that a drug-use problem might be present—do not wait for "better data." Physicians can better limit serious consequences of drug use by broadening their focus from the detection of dependence or addiction to include the detection of use and risk.

The second key step is to conduct those interventions using techniques specifically structured to promote behavior change. For patients who are compelled to hide symptoms, lie about shameful behaviors, or behave in hostile or attacking ways with their doctors, there are skills of proven value. These skills are more effective than supportive or persuasive strategies in use by most physicians. We will discuss first the process of deciding which patients require interventions, and then discuss the principles, content, and strategies of physician interventions.

DIAGNOSTIC CATEGORIES

Drug and alcohol problems exist on a continuum (Table 21-1); in an individual case, diagnosis may be elusive because of scant or imprecise information. Nevertheless, experts agree on an evidence-based classification system that is useful in guiding physician actions. Patients on the severely afflicted end of the continuum, with the prototype syndrome *alcohol* or *drug dependence* (often called *alcoholism*, or *drug addiction*, respectively), suffer medical and social consequences from uncontrolled use. A striking 5–10% of adults develop this syndrome. People with dependence are recognizable across genders, cultures, and nationalities because a distinctive, defensive interactive style develops in parallel with typical medical and social complications. People hide important facts, defend their "right" to use, and

Table 21-1. Descriptors for the continuum of drug and alcohol use.*

"Hazardous use" has approximately the same meaning as "at-risk" use.†

"Abuse" of alcohol or drugs is a maladaptive use pattern leading to impairment or distress.

"Dependence" on alcohol or other drugs is a maladaptive use pattern leading to impairment or distress, more pervasive and persistent than for abuse, and often (but not necessarily) including physical dependence and withdrawal symptoms.

*See Fiellin et al. (2000).
†See Table 21-4 for alcohol amounts; any use of illicit drugs is "at risk"; see text for prescription drug use.

respond with hostility and reticence to attempts to talk about drinking or drug use. **Physical dependence** and **withdrawal syndromes** imply *drug dependence* virtually 100% of the time.

People toward the center of the continuum, with problems of modest severity, have *drug abuse*, a maladaptive pattern which leads to impairment or distress. Note that what distinguishes the patient with drug abuse from the patient with drug dependence is not the **nature** of the problems, but the **frequency, persistence, and pervasiveness** of the problems. Thus, both *drug abuse* and *drug dependence* may include health problems (e.g., stroke from cocaine use, hypertension from alcohol use, oversedation from benzodiazepines), legal problems (e.g., arrests for DUI or violence), family dysfunction, and performance problems at school or work.

On the mild end of the continuum are "at-risk," or "hazardous," users. These people use too much, but have not developed important negative consequences. Physicians should intervene with them on the basis of the quantity of intake—in contrast, intervention with patients with "abuse" or "dependence" is made because of negative consequences and high quantity of use. Most, but not all people who experience serious life consequences use very excessive amounts, but the decision about how vigorous to be with interventions is made on the severity of problems, not on the amount consumed. The need to know about the amount to determine whether a patient is on the mild end and the need to know about consequences to determine whether a patient is on the severe end confuses physicians. Data about both amounts and consequences should be sought, but the full meaning of the data about amounts cannot be established until the physician obtains a clear picture of adverse consequences or lack thereof.

Regarding alcohol, expert consensus is that *moderate drinking* is defined by quantity of intake (not more than 14 drinks per week for men and 7 for women), a social setting for drinking, and intoxication (not more than four drinks per occasion for men and three for women). Drinking above these limits is called "at risk" or "hazardous," and is likely to cause harm, according to long-term studies.

"At-risk" prescription drug use includes patients on mood-altering drugs or prescription pain medications for more than 3 months. The majority of patients using long-term sedative drugs to manage insomnia, anxiety, depression, and other disorders, as well as those using narcotics to treat chronic pain, develop neither problems nor dependence. Similar to drinkers and users of illicit drugs, however, 10–20% do experience problems such as falls, oversedation, drug interactions, drug overdoses, or symptoms of dependence, such as taking more medication than prescribed.

IDENTIFYING SUBSTANCE-USE PROBLEMS

Studies show that "brief interventions" can be structured for "dependent" users as well as "at-risk" users and "abusers." Adjusting interventions to problem severity is helpful, and consequently we suggest simple strategies that not only separate healthy users from potentially problematic ones, but also help clinicians assess severity. Subsequent sections advise physicians what to do in each case.

History

Drinking or drug use is a behavior imbued with societal myths and stigmas. Talking about it is always a sensitive matter, even in the context of a medical interview. The physician's history-taking techniques strongly impact patients' subsequent willingness to participate in treatment activities. Closed rather than open-ended questions are helpful here, because if patients answer open-ended questions vaguely, forcing the clinician to ask clarifying questions, they may feel accused of lying and become defensive.

STEP ONE

Step one is to "**prescreen**" about alcohol or drug use. Prescreen every new patient with two questions: "Do you sometimes drink alcoholic beverages?" and "When was your last use of marijuana or other drugs?" If the answer is "No," "Never," or "Years ago," leave this topic. If patients belong to an abstinent subgroup with past problems, they often disclose this spontaneously.

STEP TWO

Step two seeks to identify patients who deserve more attention. Lives can be saved by screening, just as with hypertension or cervical cancer. The defensive style typical of people with dependence or serious abuse promotes minimization and cover-up rather than exposure. Consequently, physicians who do not use a structured screening strategy will miss opportunities, and at present physicians miss 60–80% of cases. We favor **a short screen for dependence** as the next step, while many experts suggest that Step two should be to assess quantity and frequency of use (see **Step three**). Experts agree, however, that *consistent use of any strategy* is the most powerful determinant of clinical effectiveness.

In screening for dependence, we like the simplicity of the **TICS** ("two-item screen") questions: "In the last year, have you ever drunk or used drugs more than you meant to?" and "Have you felt you wanted or needed to cut down on your drinking or drug use in the last year?" For clinicians, these are efficient and straightforward, but validation studies are limited.

The **CAGE** test (Table 21-2) is a thoroughly studied screen. It is less accurate for women and African Americans. Studies show that substituting "alcohol or drug" for "alcohol" in the screen is effective. Any positive response to **TICS** or **CAGE** means that the physician needs to conduct a more thorough assessment. Two positive responses to the CAGE indicate a high likelihood of dependence.

Clinicians should avoid asking the "natural" question "How much do you drink/use?" Not only is "How much?" a reminder to people of shameful overindulgence, but it invites vague answers and subsequent defensiveness (see "Working Effectively" section), and some research demonstrates that asking "How much?" limits patients' responses to subsequent questioning.

Screening questions for specific illicit drug dependence have not been widely tested in primary care settings. One potential strategy—"Have you used marijuana more than five times in your life?" (chosen from the National Institutes of Mental Health's diagnostic interview schedule)—might be repeated for narcotics, amphetamines, and other drugs of interest.

STEP THREE

If Step two is negative, ask the National Institute on Alcohol and Alcoholism (NIAAA) recommended **single question about quantity** (Table 21-3). If positive (more than 1 day with 5 or more drinks for men; 4 or more for women), quantify the drinking behavior. Determine a weekly average by asking: "On average, how many days a week do you have a drink?" and "On a typical day, how many drinks do you have?" Drinking

Table 21-2. CAGE screening test for dependence symptoms.

Have you ever felt that you should **Cut down** on your drinking?
Have people **Annoyed** you by criticizing your drinking?
Have you ever felt bad or **Guilty** about your drinking?
Have you ever had a drink first thing in the morning to steady your nerves or get rid of a hangover? (**Eye-opener**)

Table 21-3. NIAAA screening question on quantity and frequency of drinking.

How many times in the past year have you had five or more drinks in 1 day (men); 4 or more drinks in 1 day (women)?

above "safe limits" (Table 21-4) means the person is at least an "at-risk" user. Proceed to Step four.

If a person drinks below these limits, **and** Step two shows no positive response, **and** no other hints exist that the patient has alcohol problems, no urgent intervention is needed.

When withdrawal symptoms are apparent, or liver disease is accompanied by odor of alcohol, or the patient has signs of injection drug use, or the spouse confides about problems, "screening" is not needed, but many clinicians choose to use screening strategies to organize their data-gathering.

Step Four

If any dependency screen (e.g., the **CAGE**) is positive, or if intake exceeds safe limits, or if another clue from examination or the family suggests a drinking or drug problem, the clinician needs more detail to clarify the extent of the problems. A search for characteristic negative consequences is warranted and not time consuming if thoughtfully structured. The physician decides when to conduct this inquiry based on priorities for the present encounter; however, because alcohol and drug use produce many symptoms and affects many other illness conditions, at least a brief inventory when the issue initially surfaces is imperative. Asking the questions in Table 21-5 provides ample data for the primary assessment, and the NIAAA "Clinician's Guide" organizes this inquiry very well. This Guide includes the **AUDIT** Questionnaire, with suggestions for its use and scoring in clinical practice. Protocols for drug-use assessment are less well developed than those for alcohol. Patients can be assessed further by inquiring how much money they spend a week on drugs, the frequency of use, and how many days or weeks they have abstained in the past 12 months.

Interviews with others, including family, nurses, or social workers, enlarge the inquiry if the patient furnishes insufficient data. Records from other physicians or hospitals may contain unanticipated information

Table 21-4. "Hazardous" or "at-risk" alcohol intake limits.

Men: more than 14 drinks* per week, or more than 4 drinks per occasion.
Women: more than 7 drinks* per week, or more than 3 drinks per occasion.

*A drink is 12 oz beer, 5 oz wine, or 1.5 oz (bar shot) of hard liquor.

Table 21-5. Symptoms of alcohol abuse or dependence.

- Somatic: gastritis, trauma, hypertension, liver function disorder, or new-onset seizure
- Psychosocial: symptoms of anxiety, depression, insomnia, overdose, or a request for psychotropic medications
- Alcohol-specific: any spontaneous mention of drinking behavior, such as "partying" or hangover, family history, AA attendance, arrests for driving while intoxicated, withdrawal symptoms, tolerance, blackouts

that establishes a diagnosis. Obtaining a thorough evaluation allows the physician to discuss impressions in a compassionate manner. In fact, experimental data show that thoughtful diagnostic conversation itself produces beneficial therapeutic effects.

 CASE ILLUSTRATION (CONTD.)

You have asked Jim the CAGE questions in the past, and at that time he said that when he was a lot younger he needed to cut down, and he drank eye-openers in the morning, again in the distant past. He said he was not annoyed because of criticism of his drinking, and that he never felt guilty or remorseful after drinking. Now, as you ask questions, he seems irritated.

Responding Effectively to Challenge, Resistance, & Ambivalence

We introduce the skill of "reflection"—paraphrasing the patient's message or meaning—(Table 21-6) at this moment because quite frequently, as physicians ask screening and clarifying questions, patients show resistance and challenge. Physicians can improve the quality of the data as well as minimize tension by responding to irritation or resistance with reflections.

Table 21-6. Reflection.

Description: Tell the patient the message you heard (or perceived nonverbally). Always statements, not questions, agreement or disagreement, judgment, and so on. Always brief: reflector may have to choose among several messages to be brief.
Examples: "I see, you think that none of your problems is related to drug use." "Alcohol really helps you to sleep." "You are saying that it confuses you when I say that your abnormal liver tests are from alcohol, because you don't really drink large amounts." "You seem irritated with my continuing to discuss drug use."

Physicians who can gently reflect back the resistance, ambivalence, or challenge they receive from patients generate an atmosphere of alliance and partnership. Reflection shows a desire to fully understand the patient, demonstrating acceptance of the person and a willingness to listen more. Reflection is neither aggressive nor defensive, and helps to minimize arguing, hostility, and negativity. Simple reflection gives the patient full choice over what to say next (whereas questions seek answers, and giving advice stakes out a position, as does agreement or disagreement, and statements of values). In fact, studies demonstrate that reflecting negative, resistant, or reluctant statements helps engage patients in dialog (see Chapter 1).

Especially when the patient seems negative or hostile, reflection is not an intuitive response. Studies show that doctors usually respond by asking questions, giving advice, persuading or arguing the point, or shifting the interview focus. With practice and attentiveness, physicians can reflect back patients' expressions of ambivalence, resistance, or challenge.

> **Patient:** I drink a lot because of the neuropathy and pain in my feet, so that I can sleep.
>
> **Doctor:** So, alcohol helps you a lot.
>
> **Patient:** Well, it's probably not so good for my liver.
>
> **Doctor:** You feel some conflict about getting sleep at the expense of hurting your liver.
>
> **Patient:** The drink seems to produce nothing but problems.

Physicians can equally reflect a patient's statements about feeling, thinking, attribute, choice, action, or behavior. Reflection helps the physician by encouraging patients to share more of their perspectives, feelings, and thoughts, and reflection thus engenders more trust and a feeling of safety in both persons. As patients who initially show disinterest, hostility, a sullen demeanor, or confusion reveal more of themselves, physicians become less judgmental and critical, more inclined to join patients and to support them. Patients who feel joined become better able to listen to their doctors, and have more strength to take responsibility for attempting change that might at first seem unimaginable. Reflection is useful in all interview stages, whether the physician seeks more information about drug use and its consequences, additional psychosocial information, or wishes to develop sensible management strategies for a patient.

CASE ILLUSTRATION (CONTD.)

You decide to begin your assessment of Jim's current situation by asking him the CAGE questions again. You ask about cutting down:

Jim: Look, doc, my father may have been alcoholic, and many of my buddies drink a lot more than me, but I'm not an alcoholic, and I can take it or leave it.

Rather than confronting him with the considerable evidence already available that indicates his situation qualifies as at least alcohol abuse and possibly dependence, you decide to use an empathic style and reflect his apparent feeling state as well as the content of his declaration.

Doctor: Jim, I see this is a sensitive topic, as it is for most people, and I get it that you are convinced that drinking is not a problem for you.

Jim: I quit several times when my wife complained, no problem. But 2 years ago she took the kids and left, saying that they couldn't live with me unless I quit drinking. I don't understand women!

You have important new data about drinking and about Jim's life, and Jim feels understood rather than interrogated.

PHYSICAL EXAMINATION & LABORATORY STUDIES

Physical and laboratory examinations are useful adjuncts to structured interviewing. *Odor of alcohol* is alarming, and distinctly abnormal in medical encounters. If alcohol is easily smelled in the room, the blood alcohol level (BAL) is likely greater than 0.125 mg/dL, and a less dramatic odor indicates a BAL between 0.075 and 0.125 mg/dL. The nose is a good breath analyzer. Alcohol on the breath is a convincing sign, and always signals a serious alcohol disorder.

Intoxication (slurred speech, incoordination, and/or emotional lability) in any encounter is worrisome, and means a high likelihood of drug or alcohol disorder, even in the emergency department. To underscore this important point, assume that the alcohol- or drug-dependent 10% of the population are intoxicated once a week (it is often more than once), and assume that the 60% who are not abusers or dependent are intoxicated once yearly (it is often less than once). Thus, in a year, from a population of 100, 30 abstainers yield no episodes of intoxication, 60 users (not in trouble) yield 60, and 10 dependent people yield 520! Further, moderate users seldom become as intoxicated and are more likely to use in controlled environments (e.g., where someone else can drive). Intoxicated people in the emergency situation are not healthy users or drinkers who "have had one too many."

Further, with respect to alcohol, if the odor of alcohol is apparent, and if the patient manifests no evidence of intoxication, *tolerance* to alcohol effect is present. Tolerance indicates brain adaptation to intoxicating alcohol levels, which is caused by heavy drinking, is inevitably toxic, and usually means that the patient has *alcohol dependence*. Withdrawal symptoms (see "Management of Withdrawal," below) indicate additional brain dysfunction, and are easier to discern than tolerance. The same reasoning holds for drugs other than alcohol, but our ability to quantify their use or blood levels, as well as our ability to detect intoxication (except for sedatives or opiates), is limited, so tolerance must be inferred less directly from the patient's history.

Other physical and laboratory findings (see general medicine textbooks for the multitudinous possibilities) are poor screening tests, as they have either low sensitivity or specificity, or both. Once again, more data are available about alcohol than for other drugs. Alcohol has a broad range of toxic effects and an abnormality may prove useful in context. First, an unexplained finding may begin a fruitful investigative process. For example, despite a negative CAGE test, the concerned physician of a young woman with palmar erythema continued the assessment, allowing the patient to reveal her alcohol problem. Second, in the presence of a clue, physical or laboratory findings substantially raise the posttest probability, and physicians should order appropriate tests, such as mean corpuscular volume (MCV) and liver enzymes (include a γ-glutamyltransferase [GGT], the most sensitive to alcohol intake). For example, a 55-year-old man with chronic pulmonary disease was admitted for atrial fibrillation. His wife complained about his drinking, and an elevated MCV, aspartate aminotransferase (AST), and EKG confirmed not only alcoholism, but also "holiday heart" (alcohol-induced arrhythmia after binge drinking). In a sedated patient with few clues, a response to naloxone confirms opiate intoxication.

Illicit drugs are readily detectable in urine; however, the ability to identify them varies with the technique used. Drugs that may not be included in routine panels include oxycodone, methadone, anabolic steroids, and short-acting designer drugs. Marijuana can be detected for up to 30 days in the urine of daily smokers (for 1–3 days in intermittent smokers), but all other illicit drugs are cleared within 72 hours; for example, a positive test for cocaine indicates use within the past 2–3 days. Simply being near a marijuana smoker never produces a positive urine test (it can be detected by mass spectroscopy, but levels are well below the cut-off levels of routine urine testing).

CASE ILLUSTRATION (CONTD.)

On repeated checks over the past couple of years, Jim has had an elevated MCV, but the rest of his complete blood count, metabolic panel, and liver function panel are repeatedly normal. He tells you his blood alcohol concentration was 0.22 (220 mg/dL, .08% is now the "legal limit" in most states) when he was cited.

MANAGEMENT OF WITHDRAWAL

Treatment of alcohol or drug withdrawal is of special concern to the medical practitioner. Other urgent complications such as arrhythmia, alcohol or viral hepatitis, bleeding, gastritis, pancreatitis, skin abscess, sepsis, and overdose are covered in appropriate medical textbooks. Alcohol and opiate withdrawal are the most common withdrawal disorders, and physicians can manage many patients in outpatient settings if the withdrawal syndrome is mild in severity. Important parameters that patients should meet for adequate treatment in the outpatient setting include a commitment to abstaining from all mood-altering drugs during withdrawal (except as prescribed for withdrawal) and an expressed willingness to engage in continuing treatment. Homeless people or others not living with someone who can help monitor medication and symptoms in case of adverse events, those with significant polysubstance use, and those with important or unstable medical or psychiatric illness should not be treated as outpatients.

With regard to alcohol, when physical dependence develops, initial withdrawal symptoms of anxiety, sleep disorder, and tremor are mild, sometimes not attributed to alcohol, and easily relieved by drinking. As time passes, alcohol less reliably controls symptoms, and intoxication is fleeting, occurring only at high BAL (>250 mg/dL). Withdrawal is not an all-or-nothing state, and addicted patients experience symptoms whenever their BAL falls. The altered neurophysiology in the brain "perceives" a drop in BAL as disruptive to the new steady-state condition of addiction, and expresses the disruption through withdrawal symptoms. Soon, the person drinks steadily to alleviate withdrawal, but relief is brief. The range of BAL at which the individual feels "not sick" diminishes, and severe withdrawal, even delirium tremens, may develop despite a BAL of 300 mg/dL or more.

Outpatient treatment can be attempted in mild withdrawal. Physicians should hospitalize patients with clouded sensorium, fever, hyperventilation, a concomitant medical problem (e.g., hepatic failure, pancreatitis), or if the patient has three risk factors for severe withdrawal (Table 21-7). Degree of tremor, anxiety,

Table 21-7. Risk factors for severe alcohol withdrawal.

- Drinking around the clock
- Daily consumption of a fifth of liquor, a case of beer, or more than a half-gallon of wine
- Heavy drinking for more than 5 years (on most days)
- Poor nutrition
- Heavy sedative, cocaine, or opiate use
- History of severe withdrawal within the past 2 years

Table 21-8. Medication for outpatient alcohol withdrawal.

Day 1: Give 25–75 mg chlordiazepoxide initially, then 25–50 mg every 4–6 hours, if needed.
Day 2: Give 25 mg chlordiazepoxide every 4–6 hours.
Day 3: Give 25 mg chlordiazepoxide every 6–8 hours.
Anticipate 400 mg for worst case (16 doses of 25 mg): 200 mg day 1, 125 mg day 2, 75 mg day 3. Admit for inpatient withdrawal treatment if the patient drinks or uses other drugs.

---

tachycardia, and stomach symptoms are poor predictors of need for inpatient care. When outpatient management is feasible, pharmacologic support helps with symptom relief (Table 21-8) and must be integrated with patient education and referral options designed to help patients change entrenched behaviors.

With regard to opiate withdrawal, physicians can be helpful. Patients who use high doses of opiates, particularly those who inject heroin, experience intolerable craving during withdrawal and few patients succeed in outpatient settings. Except for specially licensed physicians who dispense buprenorphine, doctors should never give any opiate drugs for treatment of withdrawal. Provision of opiates by well-meaning clinicians is never successful, and federal law prohibits the prescription of opiates for treatment. People who are ready to stop abusing oral opiates (especially prescription pain medications) can sometimes avoid hospitalization if treated with clonidine, benzodiazepines, and antiemetics for a few days to a week or two (Table 21-9 for a suggested regimen). Patients should check with the physician face to face every 2–3 days until symptoms are minimal, and during the withdrawal process make initial contact with a professional treatment program. The patient will relapse unless support in coping with psychosocial aspects of dependence is available, because the dependence pattern becomes ingrained over months to years, and always involves a substantial network of other users and supply sources.

Table 21-9. Medication for outpatient opiate withdrawal.

Day 1: Give 0.1 mg clonidine every 1 or 2 hours until dizzy or maximum of 0.6 mg is given; give 5–10 mg diazepam up to four times daily, including at bedtime.
Day 2: Give 0.1 or 0.2 mg clonidine three times daily, and repeat the diazepam regimen.
Days 3–5: Repeat day 2.
Do not go higher as an outpatient. Suppository of prochlorperazine or equivalent may help if nausea/emesis is severe, and Lomotil or equivalent if diarrhea is prominent.

We underscore this crucial point: treatment of withdrawal is not treatment of drug dependence.

Patients with a high tolerance who are taking the equivalent of more than 60 mg of diazepam a day are not candidates for outpatient treatment. Equivalent doses for other benzodiazepines are 300 mg chlordiazepoxide, 12 mg lorazepam, and 5 mg alprazolam. Sedative or tranquilizer dependence is best managed by addiction professionals, as pharmacologic treatment must be individualized and closely monitored as an inpatient.

INTERVENTION STRATEGIES

Early intervention is more important than certainty about diagnosis or having "all the facts." Physicians should always share their concern when they perceive a potential problem with drugs or alcohol. Effectiveness is more dependent on intervening early with the style and skills we discuss, rather than waiting to get the diagnosis exactly correct. Habits and addictive cycles are complex and entrenched, so starting earlier with effective brief interventions is better than waiting.

Assess Patients' Commitment About Change

As we move from data gathering to sharing information and planning, we like to begin with an assessment of interest.

 CASE ILLUSTRATION (CONTD.)

Your physical examination shows Jim's blood pressure is controlled, and you find no evidence for new medical problems or active withdrawal from alcohol. You agree to continue the lisinopril:

Doctor: *We have talked about alcohol quite a bit today, Jim. On a scale of 0–10, how interested are you in quitting drinking at this time, where 0 means not at all and 10 means quitting is a top priority?*

Jim: *I'm quitting until I get my license back, no problem.*

Doctor: *You feel you are in full control of your alcohol intake.*

Jim: *I'm fine, doc, and thanks for checking.*

Doctor: *I am pleased that you are ready to quit now, and I know you have been successful in the past. Also, I'm concerned, because I think you may have an alcohol use disorder that will require your attention even after you get the license back . . . What are your thoughts about that?*

In other cases, assessment of commitment might sound like this:

Doctor: How interested are you in making a change in your marijuana use at this time, on a scale of 0–10.

Doctor: From a medical point of view, I must cut back on your oxycodone dosage. How interested are you in working with me to accomplish a reduction at this time, on a scale of 0–10.

Support Autonomy

Patients must make commitments and decisions in an atmosphere that genuinely tolerates and respects the full expression of ambivalence, resistance, and uncertainty, with respect to both facts and feelings. Physicians create such an atmosphere when they show they are listening to patients' perspectives without judgment by simply reflecting what they hear, and by reminding patients that they are in charge of all the important decisions, and free to take whatever action (or inaction) they choose. That is, physicians recognize patients' autonomy, while simultaneously offering their own expertise, clear recommendations and support. A more explicit autonomy supportive statement (to Jim, above) could have been:

Jim: I'm quitting until I get my license back, no problem.

Doctor: It is your choice whether you wish to make any change in your drinking. I will always give you my best advice, and you make the final decisions.

CREATE DIALOG

True dialog is difficult in conversations that involve substantial differentials in perspectives, expertise, and/or power. Patients tend either to defend a point of view or to be passive and silent. Clinicians can encourage dialog by consciously employing a format of "tell, ask, tell, ask," which supports taking turns and results in a dialog. Briefly provide (i.e., "tell") advice or information, and then "ask" patients what they think about it, or how it feels to hear it, or what they intend to do about it. Keeping the "telling" brief helps clarity, and "asking" allows the patient to choose a "change-enhancing" or "change-obstructing" response. The manner in which patients respond to the "ask" also suggests which next steps will likely be helpful. Generally, "change-enhancing" responses include statements of agreement, commitment, or optimism, and these suggest that exploring the facts might be helpful. Generally, "change-obstructing" responses, such as statements of disagreement, reservation, pessimism, defensiveness, noncommittal statements, and all questions that do not

ask for clarification of meaning, suggest that the clinician should reflect back the response as the next step in the conversation. Reflection invites patients to look inside themselves, and encourages motivation and discrepancy. Both "asking" and making reflections foster exploration and choice.

Dialog About Information

Tell information about what is known about drug problems in an impersonal "objective" or "scientific" way. Here are some examples:

- "Research shows that treatment helps," or
- "Steady drug use changes brain function," or
- "Having a high tolerance for alcohol means that a person is deprived of the early warning system that tells him to stop drinking before the alcohol level gets so high as to be dangerous," or
- "95% of men drink less than 35 drinks per week," or
- "Many people are terrified to imagine stopping drug use," or
- "Being sick in the morning until after a drink means a person's brain has become hooked on alcohol," or
- "Men with any close relative with drinking problems have an almost 50% chance of developing serious problems themselves," or
- "Guidelines from extensive research show that drinking more than 14 drinks a week is risky."

Next, *ask* what patients think of this information, and how it might apply to their situation.

Tell information about the patient's situation as a fact, a number, or score, rather than a conclusion:

- "Three of your liver tests are abnormal," rather than "alcohol has damaged your liver," or
- "Your alcohol level when you arrived in the emergency room was 0.160," rather than "You were drinking heavily before you came into the emergency room," or
- "You have a serious infection in your arm," rather than "You got this infection because you were injecting," or
- "You mentioned three important things—that your relationship with your wife is going poorly, that you are having a lot of stomach trouble, and that you lost your license to drive," rather than "Alcohol is wrecking your marriage, your career, and your body," or
- "You are very shaky and sick to your stomach until you can get another pill," rather than "You are addicted to tranquilizers," or
- "You have quit drinking several times," rather than "Your relapses show you are addicted."

Next, *ask* what the patient thinks of this information. Think about whether the patient's response to the "*ask*" is "change-obstructing" or "change-enhancing."

Dialog About Recommendations; *Tell* Advice Clearly, but not Harshly

Then, after discussing relevant information, *tell* advice tentatively, as part of a search for a suitable and attainable action option before the next visit. "Wagging one's finger," actually or figuratively, tends to push patients into a corner, it highlights any feelings of shame or stigma, and it inhibits discussion. Physicians who display a posture of "I know what is right for you," without regard to cautions that apply to science (today's truth is tomorrow's fiction, and every case is unique), make patients defensive, and encourage arguments.

Useful *tell* advice has two other characteristics. First, give an objective rationale derived from a broader database than this case; and second, make your advice consistent with your assessment of your patient's willingness to consider it. The following specific examples illustrate these ideas.

- "The option that I recommend, based on data in the medical literature, and my experience with experts who have advised me about similar patients, is that you stop drinking all alcohol. Of course, no one can be certain that this is the right thing for you to do, or that it will work for you," or
- "Most people find that talking with people in Alcoholics Anonymous is helpful. AA might or might not be right for you. I recommend you go there," or
- "No one asks to get hooked on tranquilizers, it always sneaks up on people. Usually, people in this situation find that talking with an expert is helpful. I recommend that you talk with the person with whom I frequently consult about these problems, Dr. Mack."

Ask what the patient thinks of the advice. Commanding or ordering instead of checking the result of giving advice ensures poor adherence, as patients will not do things that they do not choose to do. If clinicians push ahead and try persuading patients in spite of reluctance, they foster continued ambivalence, raise resistance to change, and begin an enervating downward spiral in which both participants become further demoralized and discouraged.

> **Doctor:** Jim, one option that I recommend, based on my experience with experts who have advised me about similar patients, is that you take this opportunity to stop drinking all alcohol, and actively participate in the counseling. Of course, no one can be certain that this is the right thing for you to do, or that it will work for you.
>
> **Jim:** Thanks for your concern, Doc, but I know I'm OK; I'll quit for now, zoom through the stupid counseling thing, and get my license right back.

> **Doctor:** We have different perspectives, Jim. Your focus is on the license, while mine is on the big picture of alcohol effects over the years.
>
> **Jim:** Doc, you know me pretty well, so maybe there is some truth in what you say.
>
> **Doctor:** Since alcohol can have important effects on blood pressure, let's check your pressure while you are off alcohol and then continue our conversation about your license and drinking as well.

Here is another example of how this discussion might proceed.

> **Jim:** Thanks for your concern, Doc, but I know I'm OK; I'll quit for now, zoom through the stupid counseling thing, and get my license right back.
>
> **Doctor:** Jim, I appreciate that you are thinking about this matter, but are not interested in making a longer commitment right now. Before your next check with me, which I will schedule for about 6 weeks, I wonder if you would be willing to take careful note of both the good things about drinking and the not-so-good things about drinking? Think a bit about the good things and the not-so-good things about NOT drinking, too. Then, I'd value the chance to seek a deeper understanding of the total picture, and help you make the best decision you can for yourself, as time goes by.

(Jim's response might surprise you)

> **Jim:** You know, a fellow at work has been pushing me to go to AA, and I almost went with him after I got my OUI (operating under the influence; suggesting that Jim is or was more worried than he declares now).

(You might act on this hypothesis)

> **Doctor:** It seems that we agree that it might be good to do something differently right now. Many people learn a lot about themselves when they go to a few AA meetings with an open mind. Would you be willing to go to one meeting a week until I see you again in a month or so?

Confirm Results of Dialog

Finally, physicians need to be explicit that agreement has been reached on a specific plan. Check with patients that they are indeed committed to the plan, and confident that they can carry it out.

> **Doctor:** "So, you are going to abstain until you get your license, and we'll meet to check your pressure and talk in about a month, right?"

Doctor: "You plan to go to six A A meetings in the coming month, and we will talk about what you learn at your next appointment."

Doctor: "You decided to seek buprenorphine treatment from the city clinic. I'll send them a note about your diabetes and anemia, and I look forward to seeing you again after you get started there."

MAINTENANCE CARE

Many patients come to physicians having already made changes in drinking and drug use. These patients will benefit from thoughtful physician follow-up of those changes. Begin by acknowledging that change is difficult, and support any positive change, or efforts to change. Listen to patients' perspectives on their situation, and encourage reflection about both goals and strategies. Reaffirm your willingness to assist and talk, address any coexisting psychiatric disorders, and renegotiate the goals and plans when appropriate.

PHARMACOLOGIC CONSIDERATIONS

Disulfiram and naltrexone can be useful adjuncts to treatment of alcohol abuse and dependence. Although randomized treatment studies are mostly negative, they usually involve selected populations. Many addiction specialists agree that each drug can be helpful for patients who commit to abstinence, and cannot remain sober. Because patients may imagine that these medications will provide a miraculous cure, the physician should promote this additional step toward abstinence, and also steer the patient toward an improved recovery regimen. The primary care physician should refuse to prescribe unless the patient undertakes additional action steps, for example, toward more involvement with addiction professionals or self-help groups.

Disulfiram provokes acetaldehyde accumulation after alcohol ingestion, producing a toxic state manifest by nausea, headache, flushing, and respiratory distress. Severity depends on dose of alcohol and blood level of disulfiram. Achievement of adequate blood levels requires several doses of disulfiram, and one must wait 4–7 days after discontinuation to avoid the alcohol reaction. We recommend two 250 mg tablets daily for 4 days, then one daily. Naltrexone diminishes craving, and treated patients who do drink usually have shorter drinking episodes. Because of possible nausea and other side effects, start naltrexone at half-dose, 25 mg daily for 4 days, then increase to 50 mg. Monitoring of liver function tests is suggested. Patients should commit to use in 3-month blocks so as to help them avoid undermining their commitment to abstinence by frequently asking themselves, "Have I used this long enough; can I stop now?"

WHICH PATIENTS SHOULD BE REFERRED

Treatment programs provide patients with specialized care, and physicians should refer any patients who do not make good progress on changing substance-use patterns. Whether patients are making progress is more important to the need for referral than the apparent level of problem or the specific diagnosis of at-risk use, abusive use, or dependent use. Substance-dependent patients may benefit from access to detoxification services and multidisciplinary counseling opportunities. Treatment programs can help patients initiate contact with community-based self-help organizations, halfway houses, and intensive counseling, sometimes in an inpatient setting. Programs with dual-diagnosis treatment capabilities are able to serve patients with additional psychiatric problems (40–60% of all referrals in most programs) more comprehensively than any physician's office. Physicians in treatment programs are better prepared to prescribe and monitor medications of specific utility, such as buprenorphine, disulfiram, naltrexone, and clonidine.

Patients will often resist following through on a referral for specialized treatment. A helpful strategy is to confirm the patient's intention and commitment to follow through, as discussed in the sections above on making choices, supporting autonomy, and giving advice. An additional strategy is to emphasize your need for a second opinion from a specialist, just as might be the case with referral to a cardiologist. Set up the appointment before the patient leaves the office. Tell the patient you will send a referral letter summarizing your views and asking for advice from the specialist. Let the patient know that you will speak with the specialist after the assessment, and that you would like to participate in the treatment plan and provide follow-up with visits to your office, if everyone agrees to this.

Many communities have programs for patients with special needs, such as adolescents, women, abusers of particular drugs (methadone treatment for opiate abuse is the best-known example), and patients with severe psychiatric problems. Self-help alternatives to AA exist in many communities; Rational Recovery is one example and Women for Sobriety is another.

SUGGESTED READINGS

Clark W, Parish S. Alcohol: interviewing and advising. In: Clark W, Daetwyler C, Novack, D, et al., eds. *Doc. Com. An Interactive Learning Resource for Healthcare Communication.* (www.web-campus.drexelmed.edu/doccom; Accessed September, 2007.)

Fiellin D, Reid C, O'Connor P. Outpatient management of patients with alcohol problems. *Ann Intern Med* 2000;133: 815–827.

Friedmann P, Rose J, Hayaki J, et al. Training primary care clinicians in maintenance care for moderated alcohol use. *J Gen Intern Med* 2006;21:1269–1275.

NIAAA. *Helping Patients who Drink Too Much: A Clinician's Guide.* Washington, DC: Government Printing Office, January 2005. (NIH;(301):443–3860; www.niaaa.nih.gov).

Reiff-Hekking S, Ockene JK, Hurley MS, et al. Brief physician and nurse practitioner-delivered counseling for high-risk drinking. Results at 12-month follow-up. *J Gen Intern Med* 2005;20(1): 7–13.

Saitz R. Unhealthy alcohol use. *N Engl J Med* 2005;352:596–607.

UKATT Research Team. Cost effectiveness of treatment for alcohol problems: findings of the randomized UK alcohol treatment trial (UKATT). *Brit Med J.* 2005;331(7516):544–548.

U.S. Preventive Services Task Force. Screening and behavioral counseling interventions in primary care to reduce alcohol misuse: recommendation statement. *Ann Intern Med* 2004; 140: 554–556 (and more detail in pages 557–568).

Williams E, Kivlahan D, Saitz R, et al. Readiness to change in primary care patients who screened positive for alcohol misuse *Ann Fam Med* 2006;4:213–220.

WEB SITES

American Academy on Communication in Healthcare Web site. www.aachonline.org. Accessed September, 2007.

American Society of Addiction Medicine Web site. www.asam.org. Accessed September, 2007.

National Institute on Alcohol Abuse and Alcoholism Web site. www.niaaa.nih.gov. Accessed September, 2007.

National Institute on Drug Abuse Web site. www.drugabuse.gov. Accessed September, 2007.

SECTION IV
Mental & Behavioral Disorders

Depression

22

Steven A. Cole, MD, John F. Christensen, PhD, Mary Raju Cole, RN, MS, APRN, BC,
Henry Cohen, MS, Pharm D, FCCM, & Mitchell D. Feldman, MD, MPhil

INTRODUCTION

Depression is common, disabling, and often unrecognized in general medical practice. Even when recognized, physicians frequently do not provide systematic, longitudinal evidence-based management. And from the perspective of the patient, stigma and other psychosocial barriers often diminish adherence to treatment recommendations. Therefore, despite robust documentation that depression is quite treatable and the widespread availability of evidence-based guidelines, overall outcomes remain poor.

This chapter focuses on the core knowledge and skills needed by general medical practitioners to effectively assess and manage major depressive disorder (MDD). We briefly address several other related mood disorders: dysthymic disorder, adjustment disorder with depressed mood, depression secondary to general medical conditions, bipolar disorder/bipolar depression, and melancholia. Of core importance, we emphasize the routine use of a brief patient self-assessment tool, the nine-item Patient Health Questionnaire (PHQ-9), for diagnostic and ongoing management purposes. Widespread adoption of this one practice innovation may provide the pivotal leverage needed to improve outcomes for depression.

MOOD DISORDERS: MAJOR DEPRESSION & RELATED CONDITIONS

Major depressive disorder is associated with considerable disability, morbidity, and mortality. Epidemiologic studies demonstrate that depression causes as much, and often

more, physical disability and social and role impairment than most other chronic illnesses, such as diabetes, arthritis, hypertension, and coronary artery disease. The World Health Organization has identified major depression as the fourth leading cause of disability worldwide and projects it will become the second leading cause of worldwide disability by 2020. Major depression is also a well-documented and common comorbidity in most other chronic conditions: for example, heart disease, stroke, diabetes mellitus, cancer, Parkinson disease, arthritis, pulmonary disease, and others. Furthermore, when present as a comorbidity, depression accounts for significant increases in disability, morbidity, and mortality.

The etiologic and sustaining relationships between depression and these other conditions appear bidirectional. For example, preexisting depression has been established as a predictor of future atherosclerotic coronary artery disease, cerebrovascular disease, diabetes, and osteoporosis, and conversely, significant physical illness predicts higher prevalence of major depression compared to individuals without the physical illness. Depressed patients with heart disease (coronary artery disease, congestive heart failure) have worse medical outcomes including increased risk of reinfarction (after myocardial infarction [MI]) and up to a threefold increase in all-cause mortality (especially after MI), even after controlling for all other identifiable and measurable cardiac risks (such as overeating, sedentary lifestyle, smoking, and other predictors of poor outcome). Patients with diabetes and depression have worse glycemic control, more microvascular and macrovascular complications and greater all-cause mortality.

Major depression is associated with adverse health habits, such as smoking, poor diet, overeating, and sedentary lifestyle, all themselves contributing to the onset of general medical illness and/or poor outcomes in illness. Conversely, functional impairment stemming from these chronic illnesses predispose to development of new depression. From an etiologic perspective, variables such as genetic vulnerability, childhood adversity (neglect and abuse), and stressful life events all contribute to the development of depression itself as well as to lifestyle risks such as obesity, sedentary behavior, and smoking that themselves predispose to chronic general medical illnesses.

Chronic care of general medical illness requires self-management behaviors to optimize treatment, for example, special diets, exercise regimens, medication changes, daily glucose monitoring, blood pressure checks, and limiting potentially harmful behaviors, such as smoking and risky drinking. Studies show that depression adversely impacts self-management, at least partly due to the fact that depressed patients are three times more likely to be nonadherent than nondepressed patients. Depressed diabetic patients have decreased adherence to diet and suffer more lapses in refills of oral hypoglycemic medications. Depressed patients with heart disease or stroke show decreased adherence to treatment recommendations such as taking daily aspirin and participating in exercise rehabilitation programs. This nonadherence in post-MI patients predicts increased rehospitalizations and mortality. Depressed patients with HIV have decreased adherence to anti-retroviral therapy.

MDD, with or without general medical comorbidity tends to present a chronic, recurring pattern of illness, with varying cycles of exacerbation and remission. Furthermore, these exacerbations or new episodes of depression tend to occur more frequently and with greater severity as the patient ages.

Dysthymic disorder is a less severe but more chronic form of depressive illness that is also associated with significant disability, and is even more likely to go undiagnosed than major depression. This disorder is diagnosed when depressed mood and at least two other symptoms of depression have been present "more than half the days" during the previous 2 years. Dysthymic disorder has been shown to respond to treatment with antidepressant medication. Patients with dysthymic disorder have an increased risk of experiencing a major depressive episode, at which point the condition is often labeled, "double depression." A useful screening question for dysthymia developed by one of the authors (SAC) but not yet validated is: In the past 2 years, have you felt depressed or sad most days, even if you felt okay sometimes? Yes/No. This question can be added to the end of the PHQ-9 to include a screen for dysthymia.

Adjustment disorder with depressed mood involves a reaction to an identifiable stressor, such as divorce or job loss. It presents with a sad or depressed mood, a level of impairment greater than expected for most individuals facing that specific stressor and is diagnosed within the first 6 months after the stressor has occurred. A "normal" reaction to a distressing life event should not be diagnosed as an adjustment disorder. When a stressor precipitates a depressive condition that meets the severity and symptom criteria for major depression, the diagnosis of major depression is made, regardless of the condition's etiologic relationship to an identifiable stressor.

Mood disorders due to a general medical condition (or substance) refers to psychiatric syndromes judged to result from the direct physiologic consequence of a general medical condition (e.g., hypothyroidism), substance use (e.g., amphetamine withdrawal), or medication (e.g., interferon). Treatment focuses on resolution of the underlying general medical problem or withdrawal of the offending medication, although specific psychiatric treatment may also be useful.

Bipolar disorder is a common and severe mental illness, occurring in about 3–4% of the general population, causing significant disability, and carrying 80–85% genetic heritability. Bipolar I disorder refers to patients with a history of at least one episode meeting full criteria for major depression and at least one other distinct episode meeting criteria for mania. Other bipolar spectrum disorders such as bipolar II disorder (a condition marked by episodes of major depression and at least one documented episode of hypomania, not mania) and cyclothymic disorder (no episodes meeting full criteria for either major depression or mania/hypomania) are probably much more common, thought to occur in approximately 4–6% of the population.

Bipolar depression refers to an episode of illness meeting criteria for major depression in a patient with a history of either mania or hypomania. It can be very difficult for physicians to differentiate an episode of major depression from an episode of bipolar depression because the two conditions are phenotypically identical, that is they present the same signs and symptoms. It is extremely important, however, to distinguish between major depression and bipolar depression because the two conditions, though they present with the same symptoms, should be treated very differently. Studies in primary care indicate approximately 25% of patients presenting with symptoms suggesting the diagnosis of major depression actually suffer from bipolar depression.

Evidence for the best treatment of bipolar depression, however, is still somewhat limited and controversial. Only two medications, quetiapine and a combination product (olanzapine and fluoxetine) have received Food and Drug Administration (FDA) approval for the treatment of bipolar depression. Lamotrigine has FDA approval for maintenance treatment of bipolar depression, but is not yet approved for acute bipolar depression. Many experts recommend treating bipolar depression with a combination of a mood stabilizer (e.g., lithium, valproate, or carbamazepine) plus an antidepressant. However, a recent large and methodologically rigorous randomized-controlled trial (Sachs et al., 2007) determined that combination therapy (mood stabilizer plus antidepressant) was no better than mood stabilizer plus placebo for the treatment of bipolar depression (about 25% in both groups experienced a durable recovery).

Experts agree, however, that bipolar depression should *not* be treated with an antidepressant alone. Such "unopposed" treatment (i.e., antidepressant without mood stabilizer) increases the likelihood of precipitating an affective switch from depression to mania. Failure to elicit a history of mania or hypomania by the physician can lead, therefore, to potentially serious consequences by (mis)treating the condition with an antidepressant alone, thereby increasing the chances of a "switch" into mania or hypomania, with attendant risks of erratic or irrational behavior, poor judgment in social, occupational, economic, or interpersonal situations, psychosis, and even suicide. The section below on differential diagnosis provides physicians with some guidelines to help them make the diagnosis of bipolar depression in patients presenting with the symptom profile of major depression.

Melancholia is a severe form of major depression, often but not necessarily, associated with psychosis ("psychotic depression"). The symptom profile of melancholia includes lack of mood reactivity to usually pleasurable stimuli, loss of pleasure in all (or almost all) activities, distinct quality of depressed mood, diurnal variation in mood (worse in the morning), early morning awakening, marked psychomotor retardation or agitation, significant weight loss, and excessive or inappropriate guilt. This subtype of major depression is most closely associated with the so-called "biological markers" of depression, that is, nonsuppression of endogenous cortisol after administration of exogenous dexamethasone (DST), blunted thyroid-stimulating hormone (TSH) response to exogenous IV administration of thyrotropin-releasing hormone (TRH), and characteristically abnormal sleep physiology (including prolonged sleep latency, early onset rapid eye movement [REM], increased total REM, and increased REM density). It appears that presence of melancholic features may predict preferentially better response to tricyclic medications (vs. the selective serotonin reuptake inhibitors [SSRIs]). The presence of melancholic features predicts a positive response to electroconvulsive therapy (ECT).

EPIDEMIOLOGY

Epidemiologic studies demonstrate a lifetime prevalence of major depression in 7–12% of men and 20–25% of women. The point prevalence of major depression in a community sample is 2.3–3.2% for men and 4.5–9.3% for women. Reasons for these gender differences have not been fully elucidated, but both biological and sociocultural factors are involved. Numerous studies report a 10–15% prevalence of major depression in ambulatory medical settings with a substantially higher rate (20–40%) in patients with coexisting medical problems, particularly in those with diseases associated with strong biological or psychological predispositions to depression (e.g., stroke, Parkinson disease, traumatic brain injury, diabetes, coronary atherosclerotic disease, pancreatic cancer, and other terminal illnesses).

Prevalence of depression varies among age groups. Recent data point to a cohort effect through which current "baby boomers" experience the highest rates of depression of any previous generation. Although the most current epidemiologic findings show a surprisingly low 1-year prevalence rate of major depression in the elderly (1–2%), the rate of major or minor depression in elderly patients who seek treatment in primary care practices is 5%, with rates ranging from 15 to 25% in nursing home residents. Major depression is often misdiagnosed in elderly primary care patients as signs of aging, and cognitive impairment may also complicate accurate diagnosis. Some medications commonly prescribed in the elderly population may actually precipitate the onset of depression or cause symptoms like fatigue and poor concentration, which may mimic depressive symptoms.

Because the usual age of onset of depression is under 40, an apparent first episode of depression in an older patient should prompt a thorough evaluation to exclude other underlying disease and/or medication effects.

ETIOLOGY

Major depressive disorder represents a heterogeneous group of disorders. It is likely that future research will eventually provide diagnostic specificity to these disorders, leading to more targeted and effective treatments. For present purposes, however, the clinical manifestation of a major depressive episode should be considered a final common psychobiological pathway among multiple candidate etiologic determinants. Dramatic advances, however, in genetic, anatomic, physiologic, and immunologic studies already point the way toward a more precise biological understanding of this common and disabling condition.

THE EMERGING BIOLOGY OF DEPRESSION: ADVANCES IN GENETICS, ANATOMY, PHYSIOLOGY, & IMMUNOLOGY

Recurrent major depression has been shown to have a heritability of 35–40% and genetic linkage studies have begun to identify specific regions of the genome thought to be candidates for carrying depression susceptibility. One particularly interesting candidate gene is the serotonin transporter gene (5-HTT), which makes functional sense since many antidepressants seem to work through binding to the 5-HTT protein. Recent gene by environment studies have shown that individuals homozygous or heterozygous for the short allele of this gene are more likely to develop depression in response to negative life events than individuals with two long alleles.

Twin studies on depression in women indicate that genetic factors play the strongest etiologic role in depression, followed by recent (as opposed to early environmental) negative life events. Animal studies, on the other hand, demonstrate that early environmental stress predisposes to biological abnormalities associated with depression that may not emerge until adult life.

Postmortem pathologic studies, along with functional and structural imaging studies, converge in locating anatomic loci of depressive illness in the hippocampus, the dorsolateral prefrontal and the anterior cingulate cortex. Animal and human studies confirm volumetric decreases in the hippocampus in depressive illness and, even more remarkably, the ability of antidepressant medications to induce neurogenesis (increases in volume) in the hippocampus, possibly through increases in BDNF (brain-derived neurotrophic factor).

From the physiologic point of view, a considerable body of emerging evidence now conceptually and experimentally points to dysregulation of neuronal signaling and second messenger abnormalities as the underlying neurobiological abnormalities in recurrent mood disorders. This contrasts with earlier, somewhat oversimplified theories postulating that straightforward monoamine neurotransmitter deficits (e.g., decreases in norepinephrine, serotonin, and/or dopamine) serve as the biological substrate of depression. Lastly, immunologic studies have consistently found abnormalities of cytokines associated with depressive illness. Advances in all these biological correlates of depression hold great promise for the development of more specific and more effective treatments of depressive disorders in the not too distant future.

SOCIAL & PSYCHOLOGICAL FACTORS

High Stress & Low Support

From a societal perspective, significant life stress and/or lack of social support predisposes to development of MDD. Life stress that involves loss, for example, death of a parent or spouse, the end of a relationship, and events involving loss of self-esteem, such as termination from a job, create particular vulnerability for depression. Low social support, both independently and in the face of significant stress also predisposes to depressive disorder. Low *perceived* social support, that is, the extent to which an individual *believes* himself or herself

to lack a supportive social network creates a higher risk than any absolute or objective measure. (It is worth noting that these same risk factors of high stress and low support tend to increase risk for all illnesses, whether psychiatric or general medical illnesses.)

The stress caused by natural disasters also increases the vulnerability of survivors to depression. While the psychiatric impact of such disasters includes increased prevalence rates of posttraumatic stress disorder (PTSD), substance abuse, and other conditions, the increased rate of depression itself is significant and measurable. For example, children and adults in the tsunami-affected areas of southwestern Thailand showed significantly increased and persistent rates of depression: ranging from 6 to 30% depending upon level of exposure and level of life disruption. Similarly, war has always been a stressor with major mental health consequences. For example, the U.S. ground troops in Iraq have shown an increase in prevalence of depression from 11.4% prior to deployment to 15.2% after deployment.

With increased life expectancy and the aging of the population in the United States, spousal caregiving of persons with disability, including dementia, is increasing. Caregivers (most often the female partner) of spouses with chronic neurodegenerative illnesses (e.g., Alzheimer disease) experience extreme physical and emotional burden. The role of caregiver presents a situation of both high stress and increasingly low support (as the caregiver progressively loses any emotionally meaningful relationship with the patient). Up to 40% of caregivers of patients with progressive dementia suffer from significant depressive symptoms or major depression.

Postpartum "blues" typically occurs in 50–80% of women within 1–5 days of childbirth and lasts up to 1 week. This "normal" reaction should be distinguished from postpartum psychosis, which occurs in 0.5–2.0/1000 deliveries and typically begins 2–3 days after delivery. It is also distinct from nonpsychotic depression, which occurs in 10–15% of women in the first 3–6 months after childbirth.

DIAGNOSIS

The *Diagnostic and Statistical Manual of Mental Disorders, 4th edition, Text Revision (DSM-IV-TR)* criteria for major depression require that five of nine symptoms be present for a 2-week period (Table 22-1). One of these nine symptoms must be either a persistent depressed mood (present most of the day, nearly every day) **or** pervasive anhedonia (loss of interest or pleasure in living).

Clinicians should realize that a depressed mood is not synonymous with major depression and is neither necessary nor sufficient for a diagnosis of major depression. Sadness (or tearfulness) does not constitute major depression (four other symptoms described in the following paragraph are necessary), and, conversely, major

Table 22-1. Diagnosis of major depression.

1. Depressed mood
2. Anhedonia (lack of interest or pleasure in almost all activities)
3. Sleep disorder (insomnia or hypersomnia)
4. Appetite loss, weight loss; appetite gain or weight gain
5. Fatigue or loss of energy
6. Psychomotor retardation or agitation
7. Trouble concentrating or trouble making decisions
8. Low self-esteem or guilt
9. Recurrent thoughts of death or suicidal ideation

Five symptoms from the above are required to make the diagnosis of depression and must include depressed mood and/or anhedonia. The symptoms must have been present most of the day, nearly every day for 2 weeks.

depression can be diagnosed without the presence of depressed mood (if pervasive anhedonia is present).

Clinical evaluation can be facilitated by organizing these nine symptoms into clusters of four hallmarks: (1) depressed mood; (2) anhedonia; (3) physical symptoms (sleep disorder, appetite problem, fatigue, psychomotor changes); and (4) psychological symptoms (difficulty concentrating or indecisiveness, guilt or low self-esteem, and thoughts of death). Physical symptoms predict a favorable response to biological intervention. For example, when middle insomnia is present (awaking at 3 or 4 A.M. with an inability to return to sleep) and when a diurnal variation in mood is present (feeling more depressed in the morning), patients are more likely to respond to biological interventions.

The Fallacy of "Good Reasons"

Depression is often mistakenly believed to be an "expected" result of stressful life events. Studies of individuals under stress (e.g., terminal cancer or natural disaster) do show rates of major depression above the general population rate, but these rates do not exceed 50%. Although sad or depressed affect is an expected accompaniment of a stressful event, the full syndrome of major depression certainly does not appear in everyone. Thus, life stressors may seem to provide "good reasons" for sadness, but a stressful event, in itself, should not be considered a sufficient explanation for a subsequent major depression. If such a syndrome emerges following a stressful life situation, the medical provider should consider the diagnosis of major depression and treat it appropriately.

The term *reactive depression* has historically suggested a mild syndrome without a biological substrate, resulting from a psychosocial precipitant, and treatable with psychotherapy alone. None of these assumptions is true. Stressful events can precipitate very severe depressions; a

biologically predisposed individual may suffer major depression in response to a minor life event; a major depression following a life stressor may develop a biological substrate; and a major depression from a life stress may respond to biological therapy as well as or better than it responds to psychotherapy. *Thus, the presence or absence of identifiable precipitants is irrelevant to the diagnosis of major depression,* which can be treated pharmacologically whether or not the condition resulted in part from psychological stressors. One author (SAC) developed the concept of the "fallacy of good reasons" to describe this tendency of patients and clinicians to "explain away" a depression that has been precipitated by a clear environmental trigger. Depression is a frequent, but *not* an inevitable consequence of a stressful life event. When major depression is present, it should be treated aggressively.

The Confound of Overlapping Etiology

A comorbid general medical condition (such as cancer or Parkinson disease) may seemingly "cause" many of the physical symptoms of major depression, such as fatigue, anorexia, or psychomotor retardation. These symptoms may lead clinicians to discount their relevance and thus disregard the possibility of a treatable depression. However, a physical symptom may be "caused" by a physical illness (e.g., cancer) or by a major depressive illness or both. The *DSM-IV-TR* emphasizes the importance of *including* these symptoms in the initial diagnostic approach to depression in the medically ill, and excluding them *only if they are clearly and fully accounted for by the physical illness.* Although this "inclusive" approach might seem to result in the overdiagnosis of major depression; studies in stroke, Parkinson disease, hospitalized elderly, and traumatic brain injury indicate that the problem of overdiagnosis is, if anything, quite low (around 2%).

THE MEDICAL INTERVIEW
Build Trust by Responding to Distress

The medical interview holds the key to the assessment of major depression. Efficient assessment involves attention to data-gathering as well as rapport-building functions of the interview. Physicians should always be alert for nonverbal cues of depression: for example, a sad mood may be communicated by downcast eyes, slow speech, wrinkled brow, or tearful affect. When a depressed mood is detected or emotional distress is suspected, physicians should first respond empathically to this distress, by demonstrating a caring attitude, and using attentive silence or direct reflective and empathic statements, such as "I can see you're having some trouble," or "It sounds like you've been under a lot of stress lately," or "You seem pretty down right now." Responding directly to the patient's distress in this way builds trust and encourages the patient to more openly share his or her feelings that may underlie a depressive illness.

Use Direct, but Open-ended Questioning

Use open-ended questions and facilitation techniques to provide patients with the opportunity to discuss the issues that may be troubling (see Chapter 1). In gathering data for assessment, physicians should focus on *anhedonia* (e.g., "What do you enjoy doing these days?") and *depressed mood* (e.g., "How has your mood been the last few weeks?" or "Have you been feeling sad, blue, or down in the dumps?"). These simple questions can effectively uncover an underlying depression in most patients, despite the fact that most depressed patients in the general medical setting initially present with chief complaints more related to physical and bodily symptoms (e.g., headache, fatigue, insomnia, and so on).

Involve the Family

Optimal assessment and management of the depressed patient is enhanced by involvement of one or more significant other(s). A spouse, a partner, a parent, or others can help the physician gather useful information regarding the patient's mood, activities, behaviors, and history. In fact, because of stigma, denial, and other psychosocial barriers, other persons often provide much more accurate information regarding depressive illness than the self-report of the patient himself or herself.

The Patient Health Questionnaire: Screening, Assessment, Engagement, & Monitoring

The U.S. Preventive Services Task Force (USPSTF) supports screening for depression "in clinical practices that have systems in place to assure accurate diagnosis, effective treatment, and careful follow-up." Although many tools to screen for depression are available, USPSTF recommends the use of a straightforward two-item ("yes/no") screener for major depression that is as effective as longer screening instruments. When administered verbally, clinicians can ask:

1. "Over the past 2 weeks, have you ever felt down, depressed, or hopeless?" and
2. "Over the past 2 weeks, have you felt little interest or pleasure in doing things?"

A positive answer to either of these two questions requires a full diagnostic assessment for major depression. This screener has over 90% sensitivity but relatively low specificity (many false positives). From an operational point of view, therefore, this relatively high "signal-to-noise ratio" can present time consuming and potentially inefficient implementation.

To increase specificity of the screening process, some systems have turned to the use of the PHQ-2 for screening. The PHQ-2 refers to the first two questions of the PHQ-9 (Appendix 22-A) for screening. Scores of 3 or greater on the PHQ-2 (possible scores range from 0 to 6) are associated with 70–90% sensitivity/specificity for the diagnosis of major depression. Positive scores on the PHQ-2 can be followed by administration of the full PHQ-9 itself.

Alternatively, many experts now advocate administration of the full PHQ-9 itself to "red flag" patients, that is, patients likely to be at high risk of major depression. "Red flag" patients generally include those with chronic medical illness (e.g., diabetes), and patients with persistent unexplained medical complaints. This one-step approach, combining screening and assessment, can simplify operational strategies.

The PHQ-9 is an assessment and severity tool that has been validated for use in general medical as well as specialty psychiatric settings. A score of 10 or more has been demonstrated to have 88% sensitivity and 88% specificity for the diagnosis of major depression. Furthermore, the tool can also be used effectively as a severity tool to track patients' symptom severity and improvement over time. (The instrument and scoring key are in Appendices 22-A and 22-B. Pfizer holds the copyright for this tool, but it can be used in the public domain for clinical purposes or research. Readers are also referred to the web site of the MacArthur Foundation Initiative on Depression in Primary Care for materials related to the use of this instrument, www.depression-primarycare.org.) Use of the PHQ-9 is now endorsed by the Robert Wood Johnson Foundation, the MacArthur Foundation, the Institute for Healthcare Improvement, and the Bureau of Primary Healthcare.

BARRIERS TO DIAGNOSIS

Patient Barriers: Somatic Presentations & Stigma

Patients in general medical practice with major depression typically present with physical complaints such as pain (headache, backache), fatigue, insomnia, dizziness, or gastrointestinal (GI) problems. Many of these patients are willing to acknowledge feelings of depressed mood and to consider the possibility that biologically mediated depression may also cause or exacerbate their physical problems. There are many somatically preoccupied patients, however, who actually do not experience any depressed affect at all, and, without this self-appraisal of sadness, they are reluctant to consider the possibility that depression may contribute to their physical problems. In these patients, evaluating both general medical and psychiatric problems simultaneously saves time, expense, and frustration for both physician and patient. In addition, many patients and families (particularly in some cultures) are reluctant to accept the diagnosis of depression because of associated social stigma. Physicians can help overcome this barrier by understanding and explaining to patients and families that depression is a common and treatable illness, like other medical illnesses. They may explain that depression represents a chemical imbalance that can, like diabetes and other medical conditions, be corrected or managed with adequate treatment.

Clinician Barriers

Depression is often undetected or is not adequately treated in the medical setting. Some physicians avoid depression diagnoses because they harbor the same stigmatizing attitudes toward depression that many of their patients feel. In addition, inadequate knowledge and skill, lack of time, reluctance to "open up" new domains of emotional distress, and misaligned financial incentives all operate as barriers to physician recognition and treatment. However, early recognition of behavioral and psychiatric disorders is time efficient in the long run while minimizing the cost and risk of extended, unnecessary workups for nonspecific physical complaints.

SUICIDE

Suicide risk must be evaluated in all patients with symptoms of depression. It is one of the top 10 causes of death in all age groups, and one of the top 3 causes in young adults and teenagers. Risk factors for completed suicide include gender (elderly white males are at highest risk), alcoholism, psychosis, chronic physical illness, lack of social support, and use of generally lethal methods (e.g., gun rather than overdose of pills). Increased risk of suicide has also been noted among depressed adolescents and among gay and lesbian patients. Explicit suicidal intent, hopelessness, and a well-formulated plan indicate relatively higher risk. Many patients who eventually commit suicide visit a primary care physician in the weeks before they take their lives.

Physicians are sometimes reluctant to explore suicidal ideation in the mistaken belief that asking about suicide may actually increase a patient's risk. To the contrary, assessment of suicidal tendencies usually reassures patients, reduces anxiety for both patient and provider, and facilitates partnership in suicide prevention.

The assessment of suicidal ideation is best approached gradually, with general questions like, "Do you sometimes feel that life is not worth living?" and then asking more specifically about a history of suicide attempts, any specific current plans, hopelessness, and any specific current intentions. A straightforward 5-question algorithm (Table 22-2) presents an evidence and consensus-based tool developed by the first author (SAC) that can be found on the MacArthur Foundation web site as part of the toolkit for depression in primary care (www.depression-primarycare.org). Once a patient reveals suicidal ideation, the physician must consider psychiatric consultation and hospitalization. If outpatient management is considered, some experts suggest that physicians consider use of a "no suicide contract." The no suicide contract involves asking the patient to promise that he or she will contact the physician (or other appropriate caregiver) if there is a danger of losing control of a suicidal impulse. In using such a "contract," however, physicians need to realize that there is no convincing empirical evidence to support its validity. In fact, other experts specifically advise against its use, arguing that a mechanistic pursuit of obtaining a "contract" can functionally undermine an open relationship and provide physicians with a false sense of security.

In all cases, when treating depression, physicians must evaluate suicidality at the initiation of treatment and throughout the treatment program.

Routine use of the PHQ-9 can aid in assessing suicide risk at the initiation of treatment and, of equal importance, can also aid in the recognition of any subsequent or treatment-emergent suicide risk. Because the risk of suicide sometimes increases within the first few weeks of treatment and can emerge at any point in the subsequent treatment, regular and routine use of the PHQ-9 can function as an efficient and effective suicide reassessment tool.

PHYSICAL EXAMINATION

There are no specific diagnostic signs of depression. A careful medical history and physical examination are required for the evaluation of depression at all ages, but especially in the elderly. Some medical "mimics" of depression (e.g., hypothyroidism and Cushing syndrome) present with classic physical signs.

LABORATORY STUDIES

No current laboratory studies can be used to diagnose major depression reliably or specifically. A general laboratory screen (complete blood count, chemistry profile, urinalysis, TSH, and vitamin levels), however, may be useful in selected patients to rule out other conditions that may mimic or exacerbate depression. In treatment-resistant cases, or when indicated, brain imaging, an electroencephalogram (EEG) or lumbar puncture (LP) can be considered, but these studies are not part of the standard workup. Patients over age 40 usually require an electrocardiogram (ECG) to rule out conduction disturbances or bradycardia if treatment with a tricyclic antidepressant (TCA) is anticipated.

Table 22-2. Suicide risk assessment (PHQ-9 follow-up); 5 questions.

Use the following 5 follow-up questions for the patient who gives *any* positive response to item #9 on the PHQ-9 "In the past 2 weeks, have you had thoughts you would be better off dead (passive ideation) or of actively hurting yourself in any way (active suicidal ideation)?

1. Determine active vs. passive suicidal ideation

"Have you had thoughts of actually hurting yourself?" (Circle one)

         YES   NO

*Please describe these thoughts*_____

2. Determine presence of a plan

"Have you thought about how you might actually hurt yourself?" (Circle one)

         YES   NO

Please describe this plan_____

3. Past history

"Have you ever attempted to harm yourself?" (Circle one)

         YES   NO

*"When was this? What happened?"*_____

4. Thoughts vs. behavior

"There's a big difference between having a thought and acting on a thought. Do you think you might actually make an attempt to hurt yourself in the near future?" (Circle one)

         YES   NO

Please explain_____

5. Plan ("contract") for safety*

"If you feel out of control, will you contact me (... or the ER, etc)?" (Circle one)

         YES   NO

Please explain_____

Risk Assessment

<u>"Yes" to question 4: acute suicide risk</u>
"Yes" on question 4 should be considered an acute suicide risk. Further evaluation or action should be undertaken immediately.
<u>"Yes" to questions 1, 2, or 3: moderate suicide risk</u>
"Yes" on questions 1, 2, or 3 represents a moderate suicide risk.
"No" on questions 1–4, represents a low suicide risk.

*Caution must be exercised when using a "no suicide contract." Many experts consider it clinically useful, but there are no substantive data to support its validity.
Cole SA, unpublished document, October 2003.

DIFFERENTIAL DIAGNOSIS

Mental Disorders

Other mental disorders often present with symptoms similar to depression; in addition, depression often presents in combination with other mental disorders. Thus, knowledge of other mental disorders common in medical practice is essential for adequate assessment and management of depression. In the presence of psychiatric comorbidity, effective treatment of depression may lead to improvement in the other condition as well. Modifications of treatment, however, may be necessary depending on the particular comorbidity present.

Major Depressive Disorder Versus Bipolar Depression

One of the most important, yet difficult, differential diagnostic questions facing the physician is to distinguish MDD from bipolar depression (discussed earlier). The clinical signs and symptoms of the two disorders are exactly the same. The differential diagnosis hinges on one and basically only one crucial historical question: *Did the patient ever experience clinical mania or hypomania?* The symptoms of a manic episode are listed in Table 22-3, the most common of which include an elated or irritable mood, racing thoughts, poor judgment in interpersonal, sexual, or financial situations, and excess energy. Criteria for hypomania are the same, but are less intense and not disruptive of normal functioning. To uncover a possible history of mania/hypomania, the physician should ask about any personal or family history of treatment of mania/hypomania/bipolar disorder and whether the patient has ever experienced any distinct period when he or she experienced racing thoughts, markedly decreased need for sleep, especially high energy or unusually poor judgment, out of character to the patient's usual behavior. The MDQ (Mood Disorders Questionnaire) can be added to the physician's diagnostic armamentarium as a guide (Table 22-4), though its sensitivity and specificity are not high enough to rely on as a stand-alone tool.

Anxiety Disorders

Anxiety and depression commonly co-occur in medical patients. Most patients with depression suffer from anxiety symptoms or a formal anxiety disorder and most patients with an anxiety disorder have depressive symptoms or meet criteria for major depression. The most common anxiety disorders in medical outpatients are post traumatic stress disorder (PTSD), generalized anxiety disorder (GAD), panic disorder (PD), and obsessive-compulsive disorder (OCD). Central features of these disorders include pervasive and disabling anxiety (GAD), discrete panic attacks (PD), or the presence of unreasonable, uncontrollable, and repetitive behaviors (e.g., compulsions such as hand-washing or checking the stove) or the presence of intrusive, uncontrollable, and disturbing thoughts (e.g., sexual and violent obsessions in a patient who has no history or risk of such behaviors). Treatment of the major depression by itself, however, often helps to resolve or improve these other coexisting conditions (see Chapter 23), especially since many antidepressant medications have proven safe and effective for treating some common anxiety disorders.

Medically Unexplained Symptoms & Somatoform Disorders

Because depression often presents with unexplained bodily complaints, the differentiation between a depressive illness and disorders with medically unexplained symptoms, for example, a somatoform disorder can be difficult (see Chapter 25). Depressive disorders are highly treatable, but somatoform disorders can be more chronic and refractory to treatment. Somatoform disorders are usually best managed conservatively with a focus on improved functioning, whereas depression should be treated aggressively with the goal of complete recovery. Any of the somatoform disorders (conversion, somatization, hypochondriasis, body dysmorphic disorder, and somatoform pain disorder) can present comorbidly with major depression. Approximately 50% of patients with persistent unexplained physical complaints suffer from depression. Effective treatment of major depression usually improves the severity, intensity, and functional impairment of a comorbid somatoform disorder.

Substance Abuse

Patients with alcohol dependence or other substance use disorders commonly present with major depression. Likewise, all patients diagnosed with depression should be screened for comorbid substance use disorders, particularly alcohol. Physicians should be cautious about treating major depression in the context of continuing substance use. On the other hand, major depression even in the context of substance dependence deserves treatment in its own right, as long as the treatment plan attends to potential complications from continuing substance abuse. Furthermore, effective treatment of depression may help ameliorate the alcohol problem itself and does not generally lead to increased complications. Some

---

Table 22-3. Criteria for manic episode (from DSM-IV-TR).

A. A distinct period of abnormally and persistently elevated, expansive, or irritable mood, lasting at least 1 week (or any duration if hospitalization is necessary).
B. During the period of mood disturbance, three (or more) of the following symptoms have persisted (four if the mood is only irritable) and have been present to a significant degree:
  1. Inflated self-esteem or grandiosity
  2. Decreased need for sleep (e.g., feels rested after only 3 h of sleep)
  3. More talkative than usual or pressure to keep talking
  4. Flight of ideas or subjective experience that thoughts are racing
  5. Distractibility (i.e., attention too easily drawn to unimportant or irrelevant external stimuli)
  6. Increase in goal-directed activity (either socially, at work or school, or sexually) or psychomotor agitation
  7. Excessive involvement in pleasurable activities that have a high potential for painful consequences (e.g., engaging in unrestrained buying sprees, sexual indiscretions, or foolish business investments)

The mood disturbance is sufficiently severe to cause marked impairment in occupational functioning or in usual social activities or relationships with others, or to necessitate hospitalization to prevent harm to self or others, or there are psychotic features.

Table 22-4. The MDQ and scoring guide.

THE MOOD DISORDER QUESTIONNAIRE

Instructions: Please answer each question as best you can.

	YES	NO
1 **Has there ever been a period of time when you were not your usual self and …**		
…you felt so good or so hyper that other people thought you were not your normal self or you were so hyper that you got into trouble?	O	O
…you were so irritable that you shouted at people or started fights or arguments?	O	O
…you felt much more self-confident than usual?	O	O
…you got much less sleep than usual and found you didn't really miss it?	O	O
…you were much more talkative or spoke much faster than usual?	O	O
…thoughts raced through your head or you couldn't slow your mind down?	O	O
…you were so easily distracted by things around you that you had trouble concentrating or staying on track?	O	O
…you had much more energy than usual?	O	O
…you were much more active or did many more things than usual?	O	O
…you were much more social or outgoing than usual, for example, you telephoned friends in the middle of the night?	O	O
…you were much more interested in sex than usual?	O	O
…you did things that were unusual for you or that other people might have thought were excessive, foolish or risky?	O	O
…spending money got you or your family into trouble?	O	O
2 **If you checked YES to more than one of the above, have several of these ever happened during the same period of time?**	O	O
3 **How much of a problem did any of these cause you – like being unable to work; having family, money or legal troubles; getting into arguments or fights? Please circle one response only.**	O	O
No problem Minor problem Moderate problem Serious problem		
4 **Have any of your blood relatives (i.e. children, siblings, parents, grandparents, aunts, uncles) had manic-depressive illness or bipolar disorder?**	O	O
5 **Has a health professional ever told you that you have manic-depressive illness or bipolar disorder?**	O	O

Positive Screen (all three of the following criteria must be met) Questions 1: 7 of 13 positive (yes) responses + Question 2: positive (yes) response + Question 3: "moderate" or "serious" response

patients will benefit from referral to a specialty mental health or substance abuse facility for treatment of their substance dependence and some severely ill patients will need treatment in settings with the capacity to treat "dual diagnosis" patients.

Personality Disorders

Personality disorders represent enduring character patterns that are deeply ingrained and are not generally amenable to alteration (see Chapter 26). They often complicate the diagnosis and management of mood disorders. Because patients with personality disorders can be difficult and demanding, physicians often try to minimize contact with them. Unfortunately, this may lead to avoidance of emotional issues and failure to diagnose depression. Effective treatment of major depression often improves functioning when the depression coexists with a personality disorder, even if the underlying personality disorder is itself not fundamentally changed.

Dementia

In its early stages, dementia can be often difficult to distinguish from depression. Depression often leads to reversible cognitive impairment in the form of decreased concentration, memory difficulties, impaired decision-making ability, difficulty planning and organizing, and difficulty getting started on tasks. These are also impairments that can result from an insidious and irreversible neurodegenerative process. Likewise, the effect of dementia on a person's functioning can lead to a depressed mood. When diagnostic uncertainty exists, clinicians should treat the depressive component (with both medication and counseling) and observe for changes in the patient's cognitive symptom cluster.

The concept of "vascular depression" has emerged in recent years to characterize late-onset depression that seems to be associated with microvascular cerebrovascular ischemia (e.g., periventricular white matter disease on MRI) and a symptom profile including mild-to-moderate cognitive loss, particularly of effortful memory tasks (those tasks requiring attention and concentration) and impaired executive function (thinking and abstract reasoning). Late-onset vascular depression does not respond as well as early onset depression to first-line antidepressant medications and clinicians should consider cautious use of psychostimulants or novel treatments (e.g., pramipexole) in these patients.

The term "pseudodementia" is used to describe treatable depression in the context of some cognitive impairment. While it is useful for clinicians to understand that depression may be associated with cognitive impairment, clinicians should avoid use of this terminology. In actual practice, most patients for whom the concept of "pseudodementia" is considered actually suffer from both conditions. Furthermore, late-onset depression (even reversible late-onset depression) is itself predictive of future dementia.

Depression due to General Medical Conditions or Medications

Approximately 10–15% of all depression is caused by general medical illness, and is considered to be the direct physiologic result of a medical illness such as hypothyroidism or hyperthyroidism, pancreatic cancer, Parkinson disease, or stroke (Table 22-5). Because there are no clear criteria to help guide clinicians in their evaluation, this diagnosis is ultimately made by clinical inference, considering the timing of the depression in relation to the physical illness. Limited data seem to indicate that standard treatments for major depression are effective in these cases.

Similarly, depression can be caused by exogenous medications (Table 22-6). Approximately 50% of patients treated with interferon develop a full major

Table 22-5. General medical conditions with high prevalence of depression.

Disease/Condition
Lewy Body disease
End-stage renal failure
Parkinson disease
Stroke
Cancer or AIDS
Chronic fatigue
Diabetes mellitus
Chronic pain
Heart disease
Chronic lung disease
Following CABG surgery

Table 22-6. Medications that can cause depression.

- Interferon
- Antihypertensives
- Hormones
- Anticonvulsants
- Steroids
- Digitalis
- Antiparkinsonian agents
- Antineoplastic agents

depressive episode and the history of previous depression or the presence of even mild current depressive symptoms can reliably predict the development of subsequent depression during treatment with interferon. Evidence now supports the prophylactic use of antidepressants before initiating interferon treatment, especially in patients with histories of depression. No medication has been noted to "cause" depression in all patients, so it is therefore crucial to carefully evaluate the patient's clinical history and link the onset of depressive symptoms to the initiation of new medications or changes in the current regimen before this diagnosis is considered.

TREATMENT

Use Communication Skills, PHQ-9 Scores, & the Family for Engagement

Building on the patient's trust, the working alliance, and the doctor–patient relationship, the physician should integrate his or her understanding of the patient's symptoms and life situation into a clear presentation of the diagnosis to engage the patient for collaborative management.

In addition, the process of the clinician's communication with a depressed patient should be informed by an appreciation of the patient's slower rate of cognitive processing. Information should be given in small chunks, allowing adequate attentive silence for the patient to assimilate and respond. In addition, the physician should verify adequate assimilation of information by asking the patient to summarize what has just been communicated. The following statement would be appropriate:

"Doctors sometimes have a hard time communicating clearly with their patients. Just to be sure I have been able to make my thoughts clear to you, would you mind summarizing what we just went over."

By using the PHQ-9, practitioners can integrate these results into the engagement process. The first step is to check some of the symptoms with the patient to verify the validity of specific responses. After verifying that the actual score on the PHQ-9 appears to accurately capture the patient's symptoms, discuss the diagnosis and engage the patient for collaborative treatment planning. Because some patients may associate depression with stigma, it is often helpful to explain that major depression is a common biological disorder. Drawing a picture of a synapse and neurotransmitters may be helpful for some patients. It is may be helpful to name some famous historical persons (Abraham Lincoln and Winston Churchill) as well as many of the contemporary figures who have publicized their own depression and their successful treatment.

A crucial part of the engagement process involves instilling hope that this painful illness is treatable. The treatment involves mobilizing patient resources (see "Individual Office Counseling by the Physician" and "Support Patient Self-management: Use Ultrabrief Personal Action Planning," below) and/or external resources such as medication. Indicate that painful depressive symptoms can be relieved, and note that "others may notice improvements in you before you notice the change yourself." When adverse life circumstances play a role in the cause of major depression, the physician can acknowledge the role played by the stressors, but must also help the patient understand that treatment of the depression can help him or her cope better with life's adversities.

The physician who successfully involves the family (however defined) in treatment planning can be more efficient and effective in helping the depressed patient engage in collaborative management planning to attain full remission. For example, they can assist in involving the patient in treatment planning and can help ensure adherence to the collaborative plans. On the other hand, family and/or friends can as easily sabotage or undermine treatment and impede recovery. Approximately 40% of depressed patients suffer from some degree of discord in the relationship that contributes to illness onset and/or becomes a barrier to recovery. When discord is detected, it should be acknowledged and included in the overall treatment.

 CASE ILLUSTRATION

The following case illustrates many of the principles discussed earlier.

Mrs. Gladstone, a 45-year-old woman presents complaining of abdominal pain and fatigue. The abdominal pain is similar to episodes in the past of irritable bowel syndrome and after a very brief history, the physician is convinced that conservative management with added fiber in the diet and antispasmodic medication is appropriate.

Within the first 5 minutes of the interview, however, her physician also noted that her affect was flat and that she spoke with long latencies. She also complained of having trouble sleeping, frequently awakening after 4 hours with inability to get back

to sleep because of worries that she is not qualified for her new managerial position. Things are not going well at home either. Her husband is complaining that her work keeps her from her responsibilities to her adolescent children, to the household, and to him.

The physician then asked her to fill out the PHQ-9 (copies are in the examination room). After leaving the room for 2–3 minutes to return a phone call, the physician then returned and noted that the patient scored 16 on the PHQ-9, with significant symptoms including sleep problems, energy problems, low self-esteem, anhedonia, and sad mood. She did not endorse any suicidal ideation. Knowing that this score is associated with a high probability of moderate-to-severe major depression, the following dialogue represents one possible method for presenting the diagnosis and engaging the patient in treatment planning.

Physician: I see you answered positively to a lot of the questions on this form. I wonder what you think about the questions.

Mrs. Gladstone: I kind of surprised myself. I'm having trouble with almost everything on that form.

Physician: It seems like you're under a lot of stress.

Mrs. Gladstone: (Tearful) I am. When I go to bed, I dread the next day … I know I won't get enough rest and I get this sinking feeling I just can't do it—I'm not good at anything anymore—my work, my home, my marriage. And the stomach pain isn't going away.

Physician: I have some ideas for the stomach pain, but I wanted to check a few of your answers on this form before we come up with a plan for your stomach. It seems like you are feeling very sad almost all the time and there's no more fun in your life.

Mrs. Gladstone: (nods positively—with tears again). And I'm crying by myself a lot. I don't want the kids or my husband to see me.

Physician: It sounds like you're really struggling. The good news is that I think I know what is going on and I think I can help. Your score on this questionnaire is 16—which is a score that tells me you're probably suffering from depression—on top of everything else.

Mrs. Gladstone: Well, with the stress of the job, no sleep, the kids constant whining. and my husband's criticism, who wouldn't be depressed?

Physician: You're right. A lot of people would get depressed with this kind of stress. But now you've got a depression that reflects a chemical imbalance in your brain. And the good news is that there's a lot we can do to help you feel better. If that makes sense to you, you and I can start talking about different ways we might start to treat this problem and help you feel a lot better.

Treatment Goals: Defining Clinically Significant Improvement, Response, & Remission

A wide variety of biological and psychological therapies have been shown in randomized clinical trials to be effective for treatment of depression. The concept of "effectiveness," however, hinges on the demonstration of a "response" to treatment defined as "50% improvement in symptoms." A 50% improvement is certainly important clinically, but this criterion is broad enough to leave significant residual symptoms unresolved. The concept of "remission," therefore, has been introduced to underscore the importance of helping the depressed patient reach full return of function and achieve relative absence of all depressive symptoms. The goal of remission is a difficult one to reach. Many, perhaps most depressed patients don't reach full remission.

The following sections review broad treatment guidelines, psychotherapies, biological treatments, self-management support (SMS), and the need for objective monitoring of symptoms to help the patient attain full remission. Using the case example of Mrs. Gladstone, a 5-point decrease in her PHQ score from 16 to 11, would be considered a *clinically significant improvement* (the "minimally important clinical difference"). A decrease of 50%, from 16 to 8, would be considered a treatment "*response*," but the score of 8 reflects the persistence of residual symptoms of depression. Not until her PHQ score goes below 5, can Mrs. Gladstone be considered to be in *remission*.

General Treatment Guidelines: Close Monitoring, Persistence in Treatment Trials, & Chronic Reassessment

Recent studies indicate a disappointingly low overall 50% response rate and a 33% remission rate for the first antidepressant a physician selects for the treatment of depression. Using logical strategies to switch or combine antidepressants after the first failure, about 70% of all patients will eventually respond to treatment. And we also know now that depression is a chronic disease. At least 50% of patients with a major depressive episode will have a second episode, and patients who have had two or more episodes of major depression have a 75–90% likelihood of recurrence.

These results suggest the following 7-point treatment program to encourage close monitoring, persistence of treatment trials, and chronic care for patients suffering from major depression. These points are all aligned with current evidence-based guidelines.

1. Use the PHQ-9 to help confirm the diagnosis and establish baseline severity.
2. For those treated with medication, patients should have an "early follow-up" contact, visit or phone call (1–3 weeks) to check on adherence to treatment, side effects, or potential change in symptoms (e.g., emergent suicidality).
3. The first goal of treatment should be achieving a 5-point decrease in PHQ-9, which can be considered a clinically significant improvement. General target goal (which is very difficult to attain) should be achievement of a 5-point decrease in PHQ-9 score every month until a score <5 is attained.
4. Patients should be evaluated with a repeat PHQ-9 once per month until remission is achieved (PHQ-9 <5). In general, the treatment approach should be modified if the patient does not show continuing improvement in PHQ-9 scores. (Modifications could include, for example, adding medication to psychotherapy or the converse, increasing the dose of a medication, switching medication, augmenting medication, considering couple's therapy, re-evaluating the diagnosis, and so on.)
5. Once patients reach remission, treatment should be continued (current dose of medication(s), or decreased frequency of psychotherapy) for at least 6–12 months.
6. For patients achieving remission with medications, evidence is clear that maintenance therapy requires the same dose of medication used for recovery. For patients achieving remission with psychotherapy, evidence is less clear, but there is some indication that intermittent "refresher" maintenance psychotherapy sessions can help prevent recurrences.
7. Patients with a history of depression should receive PHQ-9 "check-ups" every 6–12 months for the rest of their lives.

Choosing Initial Treatments: Respect Patient Preferences

Evidence-based treatment for depression includes antidepressant medication, several forms of psychotherapy, a combination of medication and psychotherapy and, in refractory cases, ECT. ECT remains the single most efficacious treatment available for severe depression, and can be lifesaving.

Management of depressive illness, like any other chronic illness, should be collaborative. After providing basic education, physicians should offer patients realistic treatment options and respect patient preferences. Patients may need to be reminded that they deserve to feel better. They should also be told that without treatment, they will probably continue to suffer the same symptoms for a long time.

Support Patient Self-management: Use Ultrabrief Personal Action Planning

Evidence is increasingly clear that patients who learn to self-manage their own chronic illnesses achieve optimal outcomes. Physician SMS becomes one of the most important dimensions of treatment, in general. SMS generally includes active collaborative patient-centered goal-setting and joint problem solving. Physicians can utilize a rather straightforward form of SMS developed by the first author (SAC) called UB-PAP (ultrabrief personal action planning). This entails three basic steps:

1. Ask the patient what, very specifically, he or she would like to do for his or her health, or in this case, to help improve the depression. (This question can be asked after initial education about treatment options.) Use of a SMS tool (see Appendix 22-C) can help in goal-setting and problem solving.

   (Specific behaviors that patients might choose to help their depression could include things like taking medication regularly, attending regular counseling sessions, keeping a schedule, engaging in pleasant events, making plans with family, and so on.)

2. Ask the patient to assign a level of confidence to the plan just developed, on a scale from 1 (not confident) to 10 (very confident). For patients declaring levels of confidence below 7, efforts of collaborative problem solving can often lead to higher levels of confidence, or at least a level of 7, which is considered acceptable for behavioral outcomes.

3. Arrange follow-up to assess level of attainment of the personal action plan and to make new personal action plans for the next period between contacts.

CASE EXAMPLE: MRS. GLADSTONE CONTINUED

Let's consider the way the physician and Mrs. Gladstone might collaboratively agree on a management strategy and self-management plan.

Physician: OK, let's review the treatment options. The kind of depression you're struggling with responds well to antidepressant medication, counseling, or a combination of both medication and counseling. Often the combination works best, but if you are interested in either medication or counseling alone, that should work fine. Do you have any preferences?

Mrs. Gladstone: Well, I don't really like the idea of taking medication, but I have no time and no interest in psychobabble stuff. I'm OK with giving the medication a try, if you think it will help.

Physician: Great. That's fine. I'll get to the medication recommendation in another moment, but first I wonder if we could talk about some things you might want to do for yourself, to help manage your own illness.

Mrs. Gladstone: Sure, but I'm not sure what you mean.

Physician: Ok, let me explain. We have found that there are lots of things depressed patients can actually do themselves that can help them feel better ... and I wonder if you would be interested in doing something specifically that might help your depression.

Mrs. Gladstone: Sure, why not. I don't have anything to lose—but I don't have any time for anything anymore.

Physician: Ok, let me tell you a little about some things that have worked for other depressed folks and then you can let me know if any one of them sounds like something you might want to do.

Mrs. Gladstone: OK.

Physician: Well, taking your medication regularly helps, of course. Getting some exercise helps. Planning a schedule and including things you enjoy are helpful. Getting together with friends and family helps. These are some of the things that have worked for others. Would you like to make a plan to do one of these, or perhaps something else you think might help?

Mrs. Gladstone: Well, I already said I'm going to take the medication. The other things sound great but I don't think I'm ready to do anything like that—I just don't have the time or energy for any of them. Can we start with the medication first— maybe later I'll think of something else I can do.

Physician: Sure, that's fine. Let's see how the medication works for you. You will need to take it every day, once a day. Lots of people find it difficult to take their medication every day as prescribed. On a scale of 1 to 10, where 10 means you're sure you will take it every day, and 1 means you're not at all sure, how confident do you feel that you will actually take your medication every day.

Mrs. Gladstone: I want to get better. I am sure I'll take it—at least an 8 or 9.

Individual Office Counseling by the Physician

Despite the lack of randomized clinical trials, many experts agree that office counseling by the generalist physician can be helpful to patients with milder presentations of depression. At the very least, the physician can listen attentively to the patient's problems, express empathy, and make significant therapeutic progress by relying on UB-PAP (as described above) to support patient self-management activities targeted to depression.

Some physicians may want to engage in more specific counseling. The patient, however, should be notified that this interaction should not be considered formal psychotherapy, unless the practitioner has been adequately trained. Psychotherapeutic situations invariably arouse strong emotions in both patients and physicians. When complex interpersonal issues or strong feelings emerge during office counseling, the physician should seek supervision from a trained therapist or consultation from a colleague.

The acronym SPEAK was developed by one of the authors (JFC) to help physicians utilize office counseling for depressed patients (Table 22-7). The five components of **SPEAK** (**S**chedule, **P**leasurable activities, **E**xercise, **A**ssertiveness, and **K**ind thoughts about oneself) are grounded in core elements of evidence-based psychotherapies of depression including behavioral, interpersonal, and cognitive approaches. They provide a framework both for patient education and for ongoing supportive counseling by the physician. Following a *schedule* counteracts the motivational deficits and anergia that accompany depression. The physician can advise the patient to plan ahead and fill out a weekly schedule. The instructions are to follow what the schedule says, "whether or not you feel like it," thus making the patient's activities less mood dependent and more time contingent. The schedule should include *pleasurable activities* to counteract anhedonia and the tendency of depressed patients to withdraw from these types of activities. *Exercise*, depending on the medical condition and physical capabilities of the patient, has been shown to be a short-term mood enhancer and long-term prophylaxis against depression. The patient should be encouraged to exercise several times a week. *Assertiveness*, often difficult for depressed individuals because of low self-esteem and a tendency to doubt their own judgment and opinions, can be a key behavior in reversing depression. It is helpful to describe assertiveness as "being direct with others about your feelings, opinions, and intentions." The physician can encourage the patient to make small acts of self-assertion (with significant others, friends, strangers) and to reflect on both their mood and interpersonal outcomes. *Kind thoughts about oneself* is perhaps the most challenging element of the SPEAK approach for depressed patients. Patients can become more aware of the self-punishing nature of their thoughts and can be taught to trace the origin of a depressed mood to particular recurrent thoughts and to replace the self-punishing thoughts with more positive ones.

Office Couples Counseling

Practitioners who enjoy a trusting relationship with both partners (or who can develop one) can utilize some of the following interventions, all of which now have an emerging evidence-base. Again, make it clear to patient and partner that these interventions are not a substitute for therapy by a mental health specialist.

1. *Listen attentively* to the patient and partner, discuss their current life stresses and emotional difficulties. Allowing straightforward "ventilation" can be therapeutic in itself and you will learn the extent to which discord in the relationship may be a factor in the depression. In addition, by expressing empathy to each partner, the physician can model appropriate interpersonal behavior for the discordant couple and build mutual support and trust.

2. *Straightforward education about the biological nature of depression* is a necessary component of all treatment, but in the context of discord in a couple it can help both partners view the depression in a more "forgiving" manner. In a common, but painful and maladaptive "dance," the discordant partner typically expresses a blaming attitude toward the depressed partner, which the patient accepts wholeheartedly because it resonates with his or her own highly negative cognitive self-appraisal. By reframing the illness as an involuntary biological condition, the practitioner helps build the relationship and aids medication adherence (if antidepressants are part of the treatment plan).

3. *Encourage or facilitate joint problem solving.* Helping the depressed patient and partner identify two or three troubling life problems they face and helping them develop a shared, concrete behavioral solution can help build their alliance and contribute to recovery. On the other hand, continuing or persistent discord may undermine treatment or recovery and should be referred for formal couples counseling.

When involving the partner in assessment or management of depression, it is essential to obtain informed consent first. In cases where domestic violence or a power imbalance within the couple is suspected, couples counseling is generally discouraged (see Chapter 35).[1]

Role of Formal Psychotherapy

Cognitive-behavioral therapy (CBT) and interpersonal psychotherapies (ITP) have the broadest evidence-base for effectiveness in treatment of depression. There is also evidence that several variants of CBT, such as mindfulness-based cognitive therapy (MBCT) and cognitive-behavioral analysis system of psychotherapy (CBASP), as well as problem-solving therapy, behavioral therapy, and psychodynamic therapy may be effective

[1] We acknowledge the work of Shiri Cohen and Dan O'Leary in formulating this discussion.

Table 22-7. SPEAK approach to physician counseling for depression.

S	Schedule
P	Pleasurable activities
E	Exercise
A	Assertiveness
K	Kind thoughts about oneself

S Schedule:

Make a weekly schedule for yourself, with columns for each day of the week and rows for the hours of the day. Using a pencil (so you can make changes) make a plan for activities you will do each hour. Some of the times will already be structured for you, e.g., at work. Focus especially on the times that are currently unstructured. Start with things you know you usually do, e.g., eating meals, preparing meals. Include on the schedule time to do household chores and errands, but also include times for fun activities and exercise. Because temporarily you may not feel the motivation or desire to do any of these things, follow what the schedule says **whether or not you feel like doing it**. Sometimes you might feel like you are just going through the motions. When the time comes to switch to another activity, do so **whether or not you have completed the previous task**. You are making progress by putting in time on all these activities, not by getting through your "to do" list. Proceeding in this way will help you move out of depression by getting yourself moving through the day.

P Pleasurable activities:

Some of the items on your schedule should be activities that previously were fun for you before you became depressed. For the time being, you may feel you are just going through the motions in these activities. When we are depressed the part of the brain that allows us to feel pleasure is not functioning smoothly, so it is important to have a "jump start." You should plan something each day that would normally be fun and make yourself do it.

E Exercise:

Aerobic exercise increases oxygen and circulation to the brain and counteracts the hormonal changes caused by depression. It helps activate the natural pharmacy in your brain that will work with other parts of your treatment to help you come out of depression. Times for daily exercise should be included on your schedule. Running, swimming, bicycling, aerobic dancing, and walking are all forms of exercise that will help.

A Assertiveness:

This involves being **direct** with other people in your communication. Practice letting others know your feelings, needs, wants, opinions, and choices. This is more difficult when we are depressed, because we tend to doubt our own judgment. Or we might hold back because we are afraid others will think poorly of us. These thoughts are a product of depression, so it is necessary to act as if you were confident, even though inside you don't feel it. It takes more energy to hold in feelings than to express them. You might find that by stating clearly what you need or by saying "No" to what you don't want will help increase your energy and confidence. Read *Your Perfect Right* by Alberti and Emmons.

K Kind thoughts about yourself:

Since depression leads us to think self-punishing thoughts, it is very important to increase your awareness of when this is happening and to replace the negative thoughts with positive ones. Most of the time these negative thoughts are strongly held opinions that are not based on evidence. It is like carrying a negative, opinionated relative with you wherever you go. Once you become aware of this pattern of thoughts, begin to analyze them. You might write the most persistent negative thought on a 3×5 card. Then turn the card over and write three positive thoughts that you could replace it with. Carry this card with you and refer to it frequently. It takes about three positive statements to counteract the effect of one negative statement.

John F. Christensen, PhD.

---

in the treatment of depression. CBT attempts to identify and challenge long-held and deeply rooted pessimistic or self-critical thoughts ("schemata") that cause and/or sustain depression. Once these learned cognitive patterns are identified, behavioral strategies are deployed to help patients learn how to directly "combat" the negative thoughts and build more adaptive and realistic cognitive structures. ITP, on the other hand,

focuses on one or more of several interpersonal situations that may relate to initiating or sustaining depression: interpersonal conflict, role transition, grief, or social skills deficits. MBCT teaches patients to recognize and let go of ruminative thinking by enhancing "metacognitive awareness," which is a nonjudgmental observation of the passage of thoughts and feelings and how they are constructed. Patients undergoing this approach learn to experience negative thoughts and feelings as mental events, rather than as the self (see Chapter 7). Problem-solving therapy teaches patients to break down larger life problems into smaller elements and to identify specific steps to address these elements. Dynamic psychotherapy involves using the therapeutic alliance to gain an understanding of the ways maladaptive defense mechanisms have developed and contribute to depression and then working through these mechanisms in the effort to build more adaptive and less punishing defense mechanisms.

The evidence from many randomized clinical trials is that these psychotherapies are as effective as antidepressant medication (in mild-to-moderate MDD) in achieving a significant reduction of symptoms (over 50% response rate) after 10–16 weeks of treatment. Although the response to antidepressants is generally greater in the first 4 weeks, response to psychotherapy catches up and by 12 weeks the efficacy of medication and psychotherapy are roughly similar. There is some reason to believe that antidepressant medication and psychotherapy of depression achieve their benefits through different neurobiological mechanisms, so it is not surprising that combination treatments (medication and psychotherapy) have generally been found to be more effective than either one alone.

CBT is generally considered the treatment of choice for depression in children and adolescents, though one medication (fluoxetine) is FDA-approved for the treatment of child and adolescent depression. The clinical benefits of psychotherapy are usually seen in 8–12 weeks, and the duration of treatment is typically 6–16 sessions.

Given the strong association of depression with coronary heart disease, and the risk that depression plays in predicting future morbidity and mortality, it is possible that psychotherapeutic treatment of depression will show an influence on physiologic outcomes (including morbidity and mortality) relevant to heart disease. However, the ENRICHD (Enhancing Recovery in Coronary Heart Disease) study of psychotherapy after a heart attack (the largest controlled study of psychotherapy ever completed), did show the efficacy of CBT and support- enhancing therapy for depression after heart attack, but treatment did not affect physiologic outcomes and did not affect mortality.

Considerations for choosing psychotherapy in the acute phase of treatment are shown in Table 22-8. Besides being an adjunct to medication for the treatment of depression, psychotherapy may also have a role in prophylactic maintenance therapy for the prevention or delay of future depressive episodes in patients susceptible to recurrences. Psychotherapy can also be useful for women with major depression who want to become pregnant and bear a child in a drug-free condition or for other patients with major depression who must be

Table 22-8. Considerations for acute-phase treatment with psychotherapy alone.

- Less severe depression
- Prior response to psychotherapy
- Incomplete response to treatment with medication alone
- Chronic psychosocial problems
- Availability of trained, competent therapist
- Patient preference

medication free for limited periods. In mild to moderate depressions, psychotherapy alone may be as effective as psychotherapy combined with antidepressants.

Formal Marital Therapy

As mentioned above, marital or couple therapy may be an appropriate choice of psychotherapy, especially when marital problems are entwined with depression. Marital therapy for depressed women who are also in troubled relationships can be effective in alleviating the depression as well as in decreasing the marital discord.

A systematic review has found that marital therapy is no more or less effective than individual therapy, even when depression is associated with marital distress. While individual therapy for depression can be effective in decreasing the depressive symptoms even in the presence of marital discord, if the discord is not addressed relapse into depression is more likely. Moreover, it is useful for the physician to get some idea of what the patient believes caused the depression. If the patient believes that the marital discord caused the depression, then addressing the discord is even more important for the prevention of relapse.

Exercise & Physical Activity

Evidence from randomized clinical trials supports the benefit of moderate exercise in the treatment of depression. In the SMILE study, 16 weeks of aerobic exercise training was comparable to that of standard pharmacotherapy with sertraline and combined exercise and medication. In a 10-month continuation study, remitted subjects in the exercise group had significantly lower relapse rates than subjects in the medication group.

Self-help Books

For motivated, literate patients self-help books that increase understanding of depression and provide guidance on self-management strategies can be an effective adjunct to treatment. For patients without access to psychotherapy, the use of self-help materials can be a helpful substitute. A meta-analysis of studies examining the use of self-help books in the United Kingdom found that one book, *Feeling Good*, had a large treatment effect compared to delayed treatment.

Light Therapy

Light therapy has been used successfully in the treatment of seasonal affective disorder (SAD), a condition in which recurrent depressive episodes occur during autumn and winter alternating with nondepressive episodes during spring and summer. Phototherapy is based on the principle that the presentation of artificial light at a similar strength to natural sunlight will prevent the biological changes that mediate SAD during the winter.

ANTIDEPRESSANT PHARMACOTHERAPY

Evidence demonstrates that antidepressant medications are effective for the treatment of major depression and dysthymia. There are no compelling data, however, to support the use of antidepressant medication for patients with adjustment disorders or other minor depressive disorders. The initial treatment of choice for most patients with an adjustment disorder or other minor depressive episode depression is "watchful waiting," which consists of physician support, office counseling, and close observation, with repeat assessment to document improvement, remission, lack of improvement, or possible transformation into major depression. Physicians can also support patient self-management goal-setting and problem solving with UB-PAP (discussed earlier). Patients with minor depression who do not improve after 3–6 months of watchful waiting can be treated empirically with a trial of antidepressant medication or referred for psychotherapy.

Communicating With Patients About Medication

Patients initiating antidepressant medication for the first time sometimes are concerned about the stigma associated with their use. Some fear getting "hooked" on the medicine or that it will change their personality in some way. It is important to explain that antidepressants are nonaddictive medicine that can restore the natural balance of neurotransmitters in the brain. It can be helpful to inform the patient about the possibility of experiencing some of the known side effects of the particular antidepressant and to refer to those side effects as an indicator of the drug's potency to achieve the desired results. Finally, it is important to build a realistic expectation about the tempo of therapeutic effectiveness by letting the patient know that even though

the symptoms of depression may persist for a week or two after starting the antidepressant, the healing process has already begun.

Adherence to treatment has been shown to be enhanced when the physician-patient alliance is optimized, when the patient's attitudes toward and experience with treatment are thoroughly explored, and when the patient's opinion in treatment decisions is explicitly valued.

Pharmacotherapy Options

The Cyclic Antidepressants include the TCAs, SSRIs, serotonin norepinephrine reuptake inhibitors (SNRIs), and a noradrenaline and specific serotonin antagonist (NaSSa). The cyclic antidepressants are generally equally effective; however, due to the adverse effect profile of the TCAs, they have been supplanted by the SSRIs, SNRIs, and NaSSa agents. Nevertheless, TCAs are still commonly employed as second-line antidepressants in patients who do not respond to first-line agents and for augmentation therapy.

Antidepressants illicit immediate first-dose pharmacologic effects on the catecholamine reuptake system, however, these agents only begin to provide some symptom improvement after 1–2 weeks of treatment. An adequate trial of an antidepressant requires a minimum of 4–6 weeks at appropriate doses. Cyclic antidepressant response rates approximate 50–70%, hence, physicians should expect that up to half of the patients they treat with the first antidepressant may not respond. Patients with no response or minimal response should be switched to another agent. Patients with partial response can be managed with augmenting agents. If the first SSRI trial fails, patients may be switched to another SSRI (e.g., bupropion, venlafaxine, mirtazapine, or a TCA). Of note, 25–50% of patients who fail to respond to the first trial of an SSRI will respond to a different SSRI on a second trial. A list of antidepressant side effects, mechanisms of action, and dosages is listed in Table 22-9.

Tricyclic Antidepressants

The TCAs have fallen out of favor predominantly because of their adverse effects and toxicity profile in the overdose setting. Common antimuscarinic effects include dry mouth, blurred vision, constipation, urinary retention, and sinus tachycardia; histamine receptor blockade effects include sedation, drowsiness, and weight gain; and alpha-1 receptor blockade effects include orthostatic hypotension and sedation. The TCAs also possess quinidine-like effects such as QRS and QTc prolongation, which can predispose to ventricular dysrhythmias and torsades de pointes—especially in the overdose setting, or in patients with preexisting cardiac disease. A TCA overdose is a medical emergency, with

Table 22-9. Antidepressants: side effects, mechanisms of action, dosages.*

Antidepressants	Sedation	ACh Blockade	Orthostasis	SRI	NRI	Other Activity	Dosage (mg)
Tricyclics Tertiary Amines							
Amitriptyline (Elavil)	+++	+++	+++	++	+	0	75–300
Doxepin (Sinequan)	+++	+++	+++	++	+	0	75–300
Imipramine (Tofranil)	++	+++	++	+	++	0	75–300
Tricyclics Secondary Amines							
Desipramine (Norpramin)	+	+	+	0	+++	0	75–250
Nortriptyline (Pamelor)	++	++	++	+	++	0	50–150
SSRIs							
Citalopram (Celexa)	0	0	0	+++	0	0	20–60
Escitalopram	0	0	0	+++	0	0	10–20
Fluoxetine (Prozac)	0	0	0	+++	0	0	20–80
Paroxetine (Paxil)	+	+	0	+++	0	0	20–50
Sertraline (Zoloft)	0	0	0	+++	0	0	50–200
Other New Agents							
Bupropion (Wellbutrin)	0	0	0	0	+	DA/NE	150–450
Duloxetine (Cymbalta)	0	0	0	+++	++	0	40–60
Mirtazapine (Remeron)	+++	0	0	0	0	—†	15–45
Venlafaxine XR (Effexor XR)	0	0	0	+++	++	0	75–225

Abbreviations: ACh, acetylcholine; SRI, serotonin reuptake inhibition; NRI, norepinephrine reuptake inhibition; DA/NE, dopaminergic/noradrenergic activity.
*0, none; +, slight; ++, moderate; +++, marked.
†Blockade of α_2-NE, 5-HT$_{2A}$, 5-HT$_{2C}$, and 5-HT$_3$ receptors.

significant risk of lethality. TCAs lower the seizure threshold, with the potential for refractory seizures in overdose. To minimize the risk of lethal overdose in patients with suicidal ideation, principles of prudent care suggest that only limited amounts of TCAs should be prescribed at any one time (e.g., 7–10 days supply, especially in higher doses). Secondary amines such as desipramine and nortriptyline are favored over tertiary amines such as amitriptyline and imipramine because of a lower propensity to induce antimuscarinic adverse effects, less orthostatic hypotension, and less sedation. The adverse effects of the TCAs are dose related, and can be minimized by starting patients on low doses, and titrating upward slowly. Though the newer antidepressants seem to be generally as effective as the TCAs for the broad category of major depression, these older agents may be more effective for the more severe depressive disorders and, especially depression with melancholic features.

Selective Serotonin Reuptake Inhibitors

There are five SSRIs approved for major depression in the United States—fluoxetine, paroxetine, sertraline, citalopram, and escitalopram. The SSRIs have replaced the TCAs as first-line agents for major depression because they are generally better tolerated, and are not life threatening in overdose. SSRIs are virtually free of antimuscarinic, antihistaminic, and antiadrenergic side effects. All SSRIs are equally effective, therefore choice of any particular SSRI is generally based on side-effect profiles, pharmacokinetics, drug interactions, dosage forms, cost, formulary availability, and so on. Table 22-10 demonstrates comparative SSRI adverse effects. As a class, many SSRIs have also been shown to be effective for PD, GAD, OCD, social anxiety disorder, PTSD, premenstrual dysphoric disorder, and bulimia nervosa. Fluoxetine is the only SSRI with an FDA indication for the treatment of childhood or adolescent depression and fluoxetine peroxefine, and sertraline have FDA indications for the treatment of childhood and adolescent OCD. With the exception of fluoxetine and paroxetine, SSRIs show very little inhibition of liver isoenzyme systems. Because of a common SSRI discontinuation syndrome, marked by GI and autonomic signs and symptoms, physicians taking patients off these medications should taper them slowly. Withdrawal from paroxetine

Table 22-10. Comparative adverse effects of SSRIs.*

Drug	Nausea/ GI Upset	Insomnia	Somnolence	Weight Gain	Sexual Dysfunction	Anticholinergic Effects
Fluoxetine	+++	++++	+	+	+++	0
Sertraline	+++	++	+	+	+++	0
Paroxetine	+++	++	++	+++	++++	+
Citalopram	+++	++	+	Unknown	+++	0
Escitalopram	+++	++	+	Unknown	+++	0

*0, none; +, minimal; ++, mild; +++, moderate; ++++, severe.

seems to be more problematic than other SSRIs. Brief use of the long-acting SSRI fluoxetine (for several days) can be used to help "cover" SSRI withdrawal effects when discontinuing other SSRIs. In the overdose setting, SSRIs can cause dose-related toxicity, manifesting with nausea and vomiting, tremor, myoclonus, dysrhythmias, and seizures—plausibly all manifestations of the serotonin syndrome.

Gastrointestinal Adverse Effects

The SSRIs inhibit serotonin reuptake, thereby activating $5-HT_3$ receptors, which can cause nausea and vomiting in 10–15% of patients. Due to desensitization of the $5-HT_3$ receptors, tolerance to nausea and vomiting usually occurs within 1–2 weeks. Short-term use of cyproheptadine ($5-HT_3$ receptor antagonist) may decrease uncomfortable nausea and vomiting. To minimize GI irritation, nausea, and vomiting it is useful to administer the SSRIs with food. Dose-related diarrhea is also a common adverse effect of the SSRIs, with the possible exception of paroxetine which possesses mild-to-moderate anticholinergic effects and can cause constipation.

Weight Gain & Weight Loss

Both weight gain and weight loss have been reported with the SSRIs. The incidence of SSRI-induced weight gain greater than 5–10% of body weight can approach 25%, especially in females and, especially in patients using paroxetine (plausibly due to its anticholinergic effects). Addition of bupropion may decrease SSRI-induced weight gain. Anorexia and weight loss have also been reported during early treatment, especially in overweight individuals with carbohydrate cravings, underweight depressed patients, bulimics, or patients using fluoxetine.

Syndrome of Inappropriate Antidiuretic Hormone Secretion

A clinically relevant and underappreciated adverse effect of the cyclic antidepressants is the syndrome of inappropriate antidiuretic hormone secretion (SIADH). SIADH presents with serum hyponatremia and hypoosmolality, and urinary hypernatremia and hyperosmolality. This syndrome is caused by an excessive release of antidiuretic hormone, presenting with signs and symptoms such as nausea, vomiting, weakness, fatigue, confusion, and seizures. SIADH has been reported with all antidepressants, and is reversible upon dose reduction or discontinuation. Management also includes fluid restriction and demeclocycline. SIADH is more common in the context of tobacco use.

Bleeding Diatheses

Many physicians, including psychiatrists are still unaware of recent reports (mostly retrospective case-controlled studies) associating SSRIs with a plethora of bleeding diatheses including GI bleeding, epistaxis, petechiae, purpura, and ecchymosis. Approximately 95% of serotonin is stored in the platelets, and serotonin is one of many chemotactic factors responsible for platelet aggregation. SSRIs possess an aspirin-like effect and inhibit platelet aggregation, but the potency and duration of this effect is not yet well elucidated. When SSRIs are administered with nonsteroidal anti-inflammatory drugs (NSAID), the risk of NSAID-induced gastropathy can increase significantly. Physicians should be cautious when prescribing an SSRI in patients with a history of GI bleeding and in patients who are already taking other antiplatelet medications. In the context of concurrent NSAID, aspirin, or other antiplatelet therapy, physicians should consider adding a proton pump inhibitor for prophylaxis of gastropathy.

Sexual Dysfunction

Decreased libido, orgasmic difficulties or anorgasmia, penile anesthesia, and erectile dysfunction [impotence] are very common adverse effects associated with the SSRIs in men and women. Sexual side effects occur in 25–75% of all patients, a higher prevalence than reported in package inserts because of underreporting.

The only available cyclic antidepressants that are less likely to cause sexual dysfunction are bupropion and mirtazapine. Sexual dysfunction in males, especially erectile dysfunction has been successfully managed with phosphodiesterase type-5 antagonists such as sildenafil, tadalafil, and vardenafil. Other medications such as bupropion, yohimbine, amantadine, buspirone, bethanechol, neostigmine, and gingko biloba have all been utilized with mixed results, with no clear evidence of efficacy from randomized, placebo-controlled clinical trials. Some clinicians will attempt a *drug holiday*, and skip the dose of the SSRI 24 hours prior to sexual activity [not effective with fluoxetine because of its long half-life]. Because sexual dysfunction has such a significant impact on quality of life, this problem may be the most common limiting factor in use of SSRIs.

Serotonin Syndrome

Poison control centers report over 27,000 toxic exposures to SSRIs annually, with 15% of these reporting a serotonin syndrome. The serotonin syndrome can occur in overdose or when two or more serotonergic agents are combined. Table 22-10 lists common serotonergic agents. The serotonin syndrome presents as a clinical triad of autonomic dysfunction (e.g., hyperthermia, labile blood pressure), neuromuscular dysfunction (e.g., clonus, hyperreflexia), and mental status changes (e.g., agitation, delirium). This spectrum of clinical findings can be mild and transient and include akathisia, tremor, and altered mental status; however, it can progress to life-threatening symptoms such as sustained clonus, muscular hypertonicity, and hyperthermia approaching 40°C. Severe serotonin syndrome is a medical emergency. While it is important for physicians to be aware of the signs, symptoms, and risk factors for the serotonin syndrome, it is also important for physicians treating depression to understand that pharmacologic combination and augmentation treatment strategies often include the cautious prescription of two or medications with proserotonin effects. Bupropion does not have serotonin effects.

Venlafaxine

Venlafaxine is a bicyclic antidepressant, approved in 1994 as the first *dual-acting* antidepressant agent to inhibit the reuptake of both norepinephrine and serotonin. These agents are often referred to as SNRIs. At lower doses, venlafaxine exhibits relatively more serotoninergic activity, however, at doses above 150 mg daily the adrenergic and serotonergic effects become more balanced. Venlafaxine is also FDA approved for the management of generalized and social anxiety disorder and PD. The extended release form of the product (XR) has become preferred because it can be used once daily and has much lower propensity to cause nausea, vomiting, and increases in blood pressure (3% of patients on doses of 375 mg experience sustained elevation in blood pressure). Venlafaxine shows very low inhibition of liver isoenzyme systems and has much lower protein binding (about 30%) than most other antidepressants which are very highly protein bound. Discontinuation of venlafaxine is associated with an SSRI-like discontinuation syndrome, requiring gradual taper (or "covering" for withdrawal effects with fluoxetine).

Duloxetine

Approved by the FDA in 2004, duloxetine is a bicyclic SNRI antidepressant indicated for MDD, GAD, and diabetic peripheral neuropathic pain. Duloxetine, like venlafaxine can produce modest increases in blood pressure, nausea, sweating, insomnia, dizziness, and sexual dysfunction. Duloxetine is metabolized by CYP-1A2 and -2D6, and is a -2D6 inhibitor. Of clinical importance, physicians should be aware that when duloxetine is administered with 1A2 inhibitors such as fluvoxamine or ciprofloxacin or 2D6 inhibitors such as paroxetine, duloxetine serum concentrations can increase considerably. Duloxetine should not be used in patients with a creatinine clearance less than 30 mL/min due to significant accumulation of the parent (twofold) and numerous metabolites (ninefold). Duloxetine has been associated with hepatotoxicity; in controlled trials 1% of patients experienced elevations in liver enzyme tests three times the upper limit of normal. Duloxetine is best avoided in patients with a history of alcohol abuse or hepatic disease, and in patients receiving concomitant hepatotoxic agents.

Mirtazapine

Mirtazapine, a tetracyclic noradrenaline and specific serotonin antidepressant (a NaSSa agent), is a potent serotonin-2 (5-HT$_2$), serotonin-3 (5-HT$_3$), and central alpha-2-adrenergic receptor antagonist. Advantages of mirtazapine include the following: it is less likely to cause sexual dysfunction, may reduce sleep latency and prolong sleep duration, may have anxiolytic effects, is relatively devoid of alpha-1 blocking effects such as orthostatic hypotension, and may cause less GI adverse effects than the SSRIs. Mirtazapine is a potent appetite stimulant, causing substantial weight gain in many patients. This can be advantageous in patients who are cachectic and nutritionally deficient such as debilitated elderly, cancer and HIV patients. However, in obese, diabetic, and patients with cardiovascular diseases mirtazapine-induced weight gain is undesirable, and has been associated with deleterious effects on the lipoprotein profile (increased cholesterol and triglycerides). Patients should be warned about this side effect and often refuse to take it for this reason. Mirtazapine possesses significant antihistaminergic and minimal antimuscarinic effects, with the potential for considerable drowsiness, dry mouth, and constipation. Mirtazapine has a very low incidence of transient rise in liver enzymes (2%) and severe neutropenia or reversible agranulocytosis (0.1% incidence). It may be prudent for physicians to check white counts at initiation of the medication, semiannually, and with occurrence of infectious illnesses. Mirtazapine is unlikely to have clinically significant effects on the metabolism of other medications through liver enzyme systems.

Bupropion

The monocyclic antidepressant bupropion inhibits the reuptake of norepinephrine and dopamine into presynaptic neurons and is referred to as a norepinephrine dopamine reuptake inhibitor (NDRI). Bupropion does not inhibit serotonin reuptake and does not cause the serotonin syndrome. Bupropion is also indicated for smoking cessation under the trade name Zyban. Bupropion may enhance energy and motivation due to norepinephrine- and dopamine-induced activating effects. However, bupropion's activating effect can also cause agitation, irritability, aggression, vivid dreams, nightmares, and insomnia. Despite this pronorepinephrine and prodopamine effect, only 2% of patients on this medication demonstrate elevations in blood pressure. Bupropion may be used for sexual dysfunction, it may promote weight loss, and it has a lower propensity to induce mania in patients with a bipolar diathesis.

Bupropion is contraindicated in patients with seizure disorders, bulimia, anorexia, and alcohol withdrawal. Bupropion-induced seizure disorders are dose related, and total daily doses above 450 mg, or single doses above 150 mg of immediate-release or 200 mg of the sustained-release dosage forms increase the risk of seizures and should be avoided. Up to 450 mg of the XL form of the medication can be prescribed once a day, which is a major advantage for improving adherence. Bupropion has been shown to inhibit selective liver isoenzyme systems.

Black Box Warning on Antidepressant-induced Suicide Ideation in Children & Adolescents

In 2004, the FDA issued a "black box" warning that the use of antidepressant medication in children and adolescents may be associated with an increase in suicide ideation and suicide attempts. In 2007, the "black box" warning was expanded to include young adults to age 24 years. In brief, the warning results from a pooled analysis of 4400 subjects in 24 placebo-controlled drug trials with 9 different antidepressant medications in children and adolescents for treating depression or OCD. The study found prevalence rates of treatment-emergent suicidal thoughts or suicide attempts in 4%

of all patients in the active medication group, compared to 2% of patients taking placebo (a statistically significant difference). *There were no completed suicides in any of the studies.* Similar pooled analyses in adults found no difference between active drug and placebo in studies totaling more than 50,000 patients. The black box recommends that when prescribing antidepressant medication in children, adolescents, and young adults, physicians should warn patients and families to report immediately any increase in agitation or thoughts of suicide and physicians should monitor patients through regular and frequent follow-up visits.

Physicians should also be aware of some important general epidemiologic findings. In the decade before this warning was issued, suicide attempts and completed suicides decreased significantly in children and adolescents, somewhat paralleling the increased use of antidepressant medications in the population. Since 2004, however, use of these medications in children and adolescents have decreased 25%, and of interest and concern, rates of suicide attempts and completions in children and adolescents have increased for the first time in over a decade. Furthermore, large observational studies have documented that the risk of a suicide attempt actually decreases after patients begin taking medication and that communities with higher rates of antidepressant use have, on average, lower rates of suicide.

Drug Interactions

Whenever prescribing a new medication, practitioners must consider the possibility of drug–drug interactions. In addition, the use of the new drug in combination with another drug the patient is already taking may create a new condition of potential risk (e.g., additive sedative risks, or potential serotonin syndrome). Because antidepressants are in such common use, questions of potential antidepressant drug interactions become issues of daily importance to most physicians, especially in the medically ill or the elderly.

Physicians should routinely use an electronic database to check potential drug interactions whenever they prescribe a new medication. They should understand the basic principles of enzyme substrates and enzyme inhibitors to be able to better interpret the results they receive from such an electronic database check on drug interactions.

All antidepressant medications are metabolized by cytochrome P450 liver enzyme subsystems. That is, they are *substrates* for one or more major P450 isoenzyme systems 1A2, 2C9, 2C19, 2D6, and 3A4. While all antidepressants are metabolized in the liver, only some of the SSRIs are moderate inhibitors of either 2C19 (fluoxetine and sertraline) or 2D6 (fluoxetine and paroxetine). Fluoxetine and paroxetine, for example, are moderate 2D6 inhibitors. As such, these drugs inhibit the metabolism of drugs metabolized by the 2D6 subsystem, for example, several beta-blockers, some antipsychotic medications, most TCAs, some benzodiazepines, and the over-the-counter cough suppressant dextromethorphan. When dextromethorphan is combined with fluoxetine or paroxetine its plasma levels can increase significantly, which could theoretically increase the likelihood of a serotonin syndrome. Also, some SSRIs may inhibit the hepatic 2D6-mediated conversion of several prodrug-like opioids into their active analgesic metabolites such as codeine to morphine, oxycodone to oxymorphone, and hydrocodone to hydromorphone. Clinically, this inhibition could theoretically decrease the analgesic effect of the opiates listed above. Among the SSRIS, sertraline, citalopram, and escitalopram present the least inhibition of 2D6, while mirtazapine and venlafaxine also have little effect on 2D6.

Clinicians should evaluate the probability, outcome, and risk of drug–drug interactions prior to prescribing antidepressants. In most settings an alternative agent that does not interact can be prescribed. When patients are receiving drugs that can interact with each other, patients should be counseled on the signs and symptoms of toxicity, and clinicians should heighten monitoring techniques. Patients should be advised that using only one pharmacy allows the pharmacist to maintain a complete, comprehensive, and accurate medication profile and improves the likelihood that the pharmacist will also detect potential problematic drug–drug interactions.

Pharmacogenomics

Pharmacogenomics refers to the interaction of multiple genes in determining drug response. For example, genetic polymorphisms in the serotonin transporter gene have been associated with differential SSRI response rates. Some individuals have been shown to have differential activity levels of 2C19 and 2D6 isoenzymes—some patients are "extensive" metabolizers (high activity) and some are "poor" metabolizers (low enzyme activity). Of interest to researchers is that the prevalence rates of "poor metabolizers" varies by ethnicity: 30% of Asians, 10% of African Americans, and 5% of whites are poor metabolizers. From a clinical perspective, given the same dose of drug, poor metabolizers are likely to have much higher blood levels of the medication than extensive metabolizers. Why some individuals are more sensitive to lower doses of medication and/or respond better to lower doses, may be secondary to this genetically determined rate of metabolism, though how to apply this information clinically has not been clearly established.

The FDA has licensed and accredited several laboratories to provide DNA testing as well as blood tests for determination of CYP-2C9, -2C19, -2D6, and -1A2 genotypes. While these tests are currently available, they have not yet gained widespread acceptance. The next decade will probably witness great progress in pharmacogenomics, such that testing and genomic-based medication algorithms will become part of the routine practice of medicine.

Antidepressant Withdrawal

Abrupt withdrawal of SSRIs, usually within 24–48 hours may cause a *discontinuation syndrome* consisting of a constellation of somatic, neurologic, and psychological symptoms. These symptoms include GI complaints, headache, fever, malaise, vivid dreams, myalgias, paresthesias, "electric shock-like" sensations, worsened mood, irritability, anxiety, confusion, and forgetfulness. These symptoms can be extremely uncomfortable, even leading to emergency room visits, but they are not life threatening. The incidence of the SSRI *discontinuation syndrome* may be as high as 40%, but the most common and most severe withdrawal syndrome is the most commonly associated with paroxetine, probably due to its short half-life (21 hours) and the absence of any active metabolites. All of the SSRIs except for fluoxetine can cause this syndrome. Fluoxetine is unlikely to cause the discontinuation syndrome because of its long half-life (4–14 days, plus its active metabolite norfluoxetine), and hence has a self-tapering discontinuation mechanism. Venlafaxine, duloxetine, trazodone, and mirtazapine have also been associated with the discontinuation syndrome. Treatment of the discontinuation syndrome consists of reinstituting the SSRI and taper more slowly, or substitute the SSRI with one or two doses of fluoxetine (10–20 mg). In summary, all known antidepressants, with the possible exception of fluoxetine and bupropion should be withdrawn very gradually to avoid the discontinuation syndrome.

Antidepressant "Tolerance"

Despite the absence of clear evidence, clinicians commonly observe a tolerance phenomenon or *poop-out syndrome* that may occur in 10–20% of patients who have successfully responded to antidepressant therapy and remain compliant. Possible mechanisms for this observed tachyphylaxis include adaptation of central nervous system receptors via upregulation and decreased receptor density, disease severity or exacerbation, loss of a placebo effect, unrecognized rapid cycling, accumulation of a less potent or competitively antagonistic metabolite, or drug interactions. Enzyme inducing medications such as St. John's wort, phenytoin, barbiturates, carbamazepine, oxcarbazepine, rifampin, and rifabutin may increase the hepatic metabolism of non-CYP-2D6 substrate antidepressants, thus decreasing plasma levels. For example, phenobarbital has been associated with a 25% decrease in the area under the paroxetine serum concentration-time curve; St. John's wort has been associated with a 22% decrease in the area under the serum concentration-time curve of amitriptyline and a 41% decrease in its metabolite nortriptyline; and phenobarbital can decrease the plasma levels of mirtazapine by 60%. Additionally, clinicians should be suspicious of a lack of compliance in all patients with the poop-out syndrome. Management of the poop-out syndrome includes increasing antidepressant doses, switching to an alternative agent, or adding augmentation therapy.

Augmentation Therapy

After an antidepressant at maximal doses has produced only a partial response, with persistent residual symptoms, experts usually recommend consideration of augmentation therapy, which consists of adding another agent to the antidepressant currently in use. Quantitative assessment with the PHQ-9 can help clinicians make decisions about when to initiate augmentation therapy.

Clinicians can use the following guideline.

When a depressed patient experiences a significant clinical improvement (as manifested by a drop in PHQ-9 score by 5 points or more), but *fails* to reach remission (PHQ <5) within a minimum of 1 month after the dose of the initial antidepressant is raised to its maximum, then consider augmentation therapy.

The only two augmentation agents with a substantial evidence-base include lithium carbonate (300–1200 mg) and triiodothyronine (T3, 25–50 µg). More commonly used agents, however, include use of a second antidepressant from a different class (e.g., bupropion, venlafaxine, mirtazapine), buspirone (a $5-HT_{1A}$ receptor agonist, approved for GAD), pindolol (beta-blocker), atypical antipsychotics, and psychostimulants (e.g., methylphenidate, dextroamphetamine, modafinil).

ANTIDEPRESSANTS IN THE ELDERLY & MEDICALLY ILL: SAFETY, EFFICACY, IMPACT ON MORBIDITY, MORTALITY, & COST

Are antidepressant medications effective in the medically ill and the elderly? There have been surprisingly few randomized-controlled trials supporting the safety and efficacy of antidepressant medication in the medically ill and elderly. However, a recent systematic review of studies in specific medical populations such as post-MI, poststroke, cancer, diabetes, cancer, Alzheimer disease, as well as other recent studies in general medical populations and elderly medical populations all suggest the safety and efficacy of antidepressant medications in these populations. Physicians should be aware, however, that most studies suggest that concurrent

general medical illness is associated with somewhat lower overall depression response and remission rates compared to patients without concurrent medical illness.

Of particular importance, the SADHART study (Sertraline Antidepressant Heart Attack Trial) documented the safety of SSRI use (sertraline) immediately after heart attack, even in patients with severe cardiac disease and in patients using multiple other medications. Other recent studies now also document the safety and effectiveness of citalopram and of mirtazepine for depression after heart attack.

For many of the reasons enumerated earlier, the SSRIs and other new agents have become the agents of choice in the elderly and in the medically ill. When tricyclic agents are used, however, the safer ones are nortriptyline and desipramine, which are preferred because of their relatively lower anticholinergic and antiadrenergic side effects. Because of their quinidine-like effects, however, all TCAs are relatively contraindicated in patients with unstable cardiac disease or with recent MI. In depressed patients with diabetes, use of TCAs, compared to SSRIs has been associated with impaired glycemic control. Because of this finding, as well as their other autonomic side effects (constipation, postural hypotension, and so on), use of tricyclic medications such as amitriptyline should be used only with caution in diabetics, including for the treatment of neuropathic pain. For treatment of painful diabetic neuropathy, physicians could consider the preferential use of nortriptyline (a metabolite of amitriptyline) or one of the SNRIs (duloxetine or venlafaxine).

Dosing strategies in the elderly and medically ill should adhere to the general well-known guideline "start low and go slow." Pharmacokinetically, these agents are metabolized more slowly, resulting in accumulation and toxicity. Increased pharmacodynamic effects in the elderly may result from lower albumin levels, leading to higher levels of unbound drug.

Because depression is associated with increased morbidity, mortality, and cost in patients with concurrent general medical illness, it is reasonable to ask whether improvement in depression in medical patients leads to improvements in these other domains. There are limited and somewhat conflicting data on these questions, but some recent and notable studies point to potential decreases in morbidity, mortality, and overall health care costs with adequate treatment of depression. The SADHART study showed a trend (but not statistically significant) toward decreased rate of incident severe cardiac events and death in the sertraline group compared to placebo. A naturalistic outcome report of patients in the ENRICHD psychotherapy study noted that depressed patients treated with SSRIs (at physician/patient discretion, outside of protocol) had a statistically significant decrease in cardiac morbidity and mortality compared to the depressed patients who did not receive this treatment. A 2-year study of the collaborative care of patients with both depression and diabetes has shown an overall decrease in total health costs (general medical and psychiatric) in patients successfully treated for depression.

Electroconvulsive Therapy

Electroconvulsive therapy is still the most effective means available for the treatment of refractory depression. It is the treatment of choice for patients with psychotic depression, depression refractory to pharmacotherapy, and for some patients who are acutely suicidal. Despite prejudices and fears about ECT, new methods of administration have proven it to be a safe and effective treatment. In fact, ECT can be safer than antidepressant medication in the elderly. Some short-term memory loss is common, but research indicates that this reverts to normal in most patients. In some cases, ECT can be lifesaving and should not be denied to patients because of poor understanding or unrealistic fear. ECT does not lead to permanent remission of depression in patients susceptible to recurrence. Thus, patients with recurrent depression who receive ECT should receive either prophylactic medication after a course of therapy (as an outpatient) or maintenance ECT.

COLLABORATIVE CARE MODELS OF DEPRESSION

A generation of randomized, controlled health services trials indicate that systematic implementation of a "collaborative care model," or "chronic illness care" (or "chronic disease management") model of health care for depressed medical outpatients improves key processes and outcomes of care such as detection of depression; adequacy of depression treatment; patient adherence with treatment; improved clinical outcomes as assessed by measures such as PHQ-9 scores; and improved patient satisfaction. Key components of most of these new models generally include use of structured tools for assessment and management, utilization of care managers to help educate patients, support self-management, coordinate care and ensure follow-up, use of formal evidence-based guidelines and decision support tools and, finally, integration of behavioral health specialists into the medical team for consultation and ongoing support.

WHEN TO REFER

The criteria for referral to a mental health specialist depend a great deal on the experience and expertise of the primary treating physician. Patients should be informed that consultation with a mental health spe-

cialist may be necessary if the depression does not fully remit. This can make referral at a later stage much more acceptable. Because partial remission is a common occurrence, physicians should make every effort to establish clear indications of predepression functioning, and if full return to baseline functioning does not occur, referral to a specialist should be made. A baseline pretreatment PHQ-9 should be obtained and repeated at regular intervals to insure that the patient is responding appropriately to treatment. Patients with persistently elevated PHQ-9 scores (20 or above) or if scores are not reduced to at least 50% of pretreatment levels, should be evaluated by a mental health specialist. Other indications for referral include patients with active suicidality, bipolar disorder or psychosis; for evaluation of any patient in whom the diagnosis is in doubt; and for advice about pharmacologic management of patients with treatment-resistant depression. The primary practitioner should communicate with the mental health specialist and provide the following information: the nature of the depressive symptoms; baseline premorbid functioning, baseline and follow-up PHQ-9 scores; other treatments, including medication, that have been tried previously or are concurrent; and patient understanding and expectations about psychotherapy. Communication should be maintained with the mental health therapist about whether therapy is completed, since failure to follow through on a referral and/or premature discontinuation of psychotherapy is even more common than failure to comply with pharmacotherapy.

CONCLUSION

Of all the psychiatric conditions relevant to the general physician, major depression is arguably the most common and most important. Major depression is common, serious, often disabling, and associated with increased morbidity and mortality in general medical conditions. It is often missed and often inadequately treated. Recognition and adequate treatment is associated with response and remission and can often be provided adequately in the general medical sector. Increased understanding of the biopsychosocial etiology of major depression, the biopsychosocial manifestations of major depression, and the biopsychosocial treatment of major depression holds great promise for improving outcomes in this debilitating condition.

SUGGESTED READINGS

Bihme Z, Akiskal H. Do antidepressants threaten depressives? Toward a clinically judicious formulation of the antidepressant-sucid FDA advisory in light of declining national sucide statistics from many countries. *J Affect Discord.* 2006 Aug;94(1–3): 5–13.

Ebmeir KP, Donaghey C, Steele JD. Recent developments and current controversies in depression. *Lancet* 2006;367:153–167.

Hollon SD, Javrett RB, Nierenberg AA, Thase ME, Trivedi M, Rush AJ. Psychotherapy and medication in the treatment of adult and geriatric depression; which monotherapy or combined treatment? *J Clin Psychiatry* 2005 April; 66(4):455–468.

Mann JJ. The medical management of depression. *N Engl J Med* 2005;353(17):1819–1834.

Rush AJ. STAR*D: What have we learned? *Am J Psychiatry* 2007;164: 201–204.

PATIENT BIBLIOGRAPHY

Alberti RE, Emmons ML. *Your Perfect Right: Assertiveness and Equality in Your Life and Relationships*, 8th ed. Atascadero, CA: Impact Publishers, 2001.

Burns DD. *Feeling Good—The New Mood Therapy.* New York, NY: Avon Books, 1999.

Lewinsohn PM, Mufioz RF, Youngren MA, et al. *Control Your Depression.* Englewood Cliffs, NJ: Prentice-Hall, 1978.

Seligman MEP. *Learned Optimism.* New York, NY: Knopf, 1991.

WEB SITES

National Institute of Mental Health Depression Information Web site. http://www.nimh.nih.gov/publicat/depressionmenu.cfm. Accessed October, 2007.

The MacArthur Initiative on Depression and Primary Care Web site. http://www.depression-primarycare.org/. Accessed October, 2007.

Appendix 22-A. Patient Health Questionnaire—PHQ-9.

Name _____ Physician _____ Date _____

Over the last 2 *weeks*, how often have you been bothered by any of the following problems?

	Not At All (0)	Several Days (1)	More Than Half the Days (2)	Nearly Every Day (3)
1. Feeling down, depressed, or hopeless?	☐	☐	☐	☐
2. Little interest or pleasure in doing things?	☐	☐	☐	☐
3. Trouble falling or staying asleep, or sleeping too much?	☐	☐	☐	☐
4. Feeling tired or having little energy?	☐	☐	☐	☐
5. Poor appetite or overeating?	☐	☐	☐	☐
6. Feeling bad about yourself—or that you are a failure or have let yourself or your family down?	☐	☐	☐	☐
7. Trouble concentrating on things, such as reading the newspaper or watching television?	☐	☐	☐	☐
8. Moving or speaking so slowly that other people could have noticed? Or the opposite—being so fidgety or restless that you have been moving around a lot more than usual?	☐	☐	☐	☐
9. Thoughts that you would be better off dead or of hurting yourself in some way?*	☐	☐	☐	☐

10. If you are experiencing any of the problems on this form, how *difficult* have these problems made it for you to do your work, take care of things at home, or get along with other people?

☐ Not difficult at all ☐ Somewhat difficult ☐ Very difficult ☐ Extremely difficult

Office Use Only
Number of Symptoms: _____ _____ Severity Score: _____

If you have had thoughts that you would be better off dead or of hurting yourself in some way, please discuss this with your doctor, go to a hospital emergency room, or call 911.

Appendix 22-B. Scoring the PHQ-9.

How to Score the Patient Health Questionnaire (PHQ-9)

The PHQ-9 can assist in diagnosing depression, as well as planning and monitoring depression treatment. There are three steps to scoring the PHQ-9: Number of Depressive Symptoms, Severity Score, and Functional Assessment. The Number of Depressive Symptoms is used to aid in making the diagnosis of Depression. The PHQ-9 Severity Score and Functional Assessment are measured at initial assessment and regularly after treatment begins to determine the severity of depression and to evaluate patient progress.

Number of Depressive Symptoms (Diagnosis)

1. For questions 1–8, count the number of symptoms the patient checked as "More than half the days" or "Nearly every day." For question 9, count the question positive if the patient checks "Several days," "More than half the days," or "Nearly every day."
2. Use the following interpretation grid to diagnose depression subtypes:

0–2 PHQ symptoms	Not clinically depressed
3–4 PHQ symptoms*	Other depressive syndrome
5 or more PHQ symptoms*	Major depression

Severity Score

1. Assign a score to each response by the number value under the answer headings (Not at all = 0; Several days = 1; More than half the days = 2; and Nearly every day = 3).
2. Total the values for each response to obtain the severity score.
3. Use the following interpretation grid:

0–4	Not clinically depressed
5–9	Mild depression
10–14	Moderate depression
15 or greater	Severe depression

Functional Assessment

The final question on the PHQ-9 asks the patient how emotional difficulties or problems impact work, things at home, or relationships with other people. Patient responses can be one of four: "Not difficult at all"; "Somewhat difficult"; "Very difficult"; or "Extremely difficult."

- If the patient selects one of the last two responses, "Very difficult" or "Extremely difficult," his or her functionality at work, at home, or in relationships with other people is significantly impaired.
- If the patient has had difficulty with these problems for 2 years or more, consider the diagnosis of dysthymia (chronic depression).

*PHQ-9 items #1 or #2 must be one of the symptoms checked.
Steven A. Cole, MD, Stony Brook University Medical Center.

Appendix 22-C. Depression self-care action plan.*

Stay Physically Active.

Make sure you make time to address your basic physical needs, for example, walking for a certain amount of each time each day.
Every day during the next week, I will spend at least _____ minutes (make it easy, reasonable) doing _____
_____.

Make Time for Pleasurable Activities.

Even though you may not feel as motivated, or get the same amount of pleasure as you used to, commit to scheduling some fun
  activity each day, for example, doing a hobby, listening to music, or watching a video.
Every day during the next week, I will spend at least
_____ minutes (make it easy, reasonable) doing _____.

Spend Time With People who can Support You.

It's easy to avoid contact with people when you're depressed, but you need the support of friends and loved ones. Explain to
  them how you feel, if you can. If you can't talk about it, that's OK—just ask them to be with you, maybe accompanying you on
  one of your activities.
During the next week, I will make contact for at least _____
minutes (make it easy, reasonable) with
_____(name) doing/talking about _____
_____(name) doing/talking about _____
_____(name) doing/talking about _____

Practice Relaxing.

For many people, the change that comes with depression—no longer keeping up with our usual activities and responsibilities,
  feeling increasingly sad and hopeless—leads to anxiety. Since physical relaxation can lead to mental relaxation, practicing
  relaxing is another way to help yourself. Try deep breathing, or a warm bath, or just a quiet, comfortable, peaceful place and saying comforting things to yourself (like "It's OK").
Every day during the next week, I will practice physical relaxation at least _____ times, for at least _____ minutes each time.
  (make it easy, reasonable)

Simple Goals and Small Steps.

It's easy to feel overwhelmed when you're depressed. Some problems and decisions can be delayed, but others cannot. It can be
  hard to deal with them when you're feeling sad, have little energy, and not thinking clearly. Try breaking things down in to small
  steps. Give yourself credit for each step you accomplish.
The problem is _____

My goal is _____

Step 1: _____
Step 2: _____
Step 3: _____

How Likely are You to Follow Through With These Activities Prior to Your Next Visit?
Not Likely 1 2 3 4 5 6 7 8 9 10 Very Likely

---

*Kershnir Land Amann T: Unpublished documents. CoreSouth Carolina and CareOregon.

Anxiety

23

Jason M. Satterfield, PhD & Bruce L. Rollman, MD, MPH

INTRODUCTION

Anxiety is a common, normal emotion; most people experience occasional trepidation, fear, nervousness, "jitters," or even panic. Mild anxiety may aid mental sharpness as uncertainty or pressure mounts. For some individuals, however, anxiety occurs as part of an anxiety disorder that is a prominent, persistent, and disruptive aspect of their daily lives. Among the general population in the United States, about 25% will experience an anxiety disorder at some time in their life, making anxiety more common than depressive disorders. At over $50 billion per year, the direct and indirect annual costs associated with anxiety disorders in the United States are similar to, and may even surpass, the economic burdens attributed to mood disorders.

The major anxiety disorders are shown in Table 23-1. They are often comorbid with depression and with one another (e.g., panic disorder [PD] and agoraphobia). Similar to depression, patients with an unrecognized anxiety disorder tend to present to general medical or specialist settings, rather than to the specialty mental health sector, as they generally complain of the prominent physical symptoms of the anxiety disorder rather than its emotional symptoms.

It is important to distinguish among the various anxiety disorders and identify possible comorbidities because of differences in treatment, complications, and prognoses. Although cross-cultural epidemiologic research has shown that anxiety disorders are present in all cultures, ethnicities, and age groups, providers also must be alert to a variety of common medical conditions and medication side effects that can have symptoms resembling an anxiety disorder (Table 23-2).

DIAGNOSIS

Office-based screening instruments can improve the detection of anxiety and other mental disorders, and can be used to evaluate treatment response. Several instruments have been developed to aid in recognition of an anxiety disorder. A two-question screener, the GAD-2

subscale of the GAD-7, has been found to perform well as a rapid screening tool for the most common anxiety disorders. The GAD-2 questions are as follows: *Over the last 2 weeks how often have you been bothered by the following problems: (1) Feeling nervous, anxious, or on edge and (2) Not being able to stop or control worrying.* The Primary Care Evaluation of Mental Disorders (PRIME-MD) is a two-stage rapid screening and interview procedure that can also screen for such common anxiety comorbidities as depression, eating disorders, and alcohol abuse. Patients can complete the first-stage self-administered Patient Questionnaire (PQ) before seeing the provider. A single "yes" response to any of the three anxiety screening questions has a sensitivity of 94% and a specificity of 53% when compared to more formal assessment by a mental health professional. Positive screens are then followed-up with the PRIME-MD's second-stage Anxiety Module to determine whether the patient is experiencing a current episode of PD or generalized anxiety disorder (GAD). Overall, the two-part PRIME-MD has a sensitivity of 57% and a specificity of 97–99% for both PD and GAD, respectively. The Primary Care Posttraumatic Stress Disorder Screen (PC-PTSD) is a 4-item, self-administered questionnaire that maximizes sensitivity and specificity when three positive are used as a cutoff for further screening. Other clinically useful screening questions are listed in Table 23-3.

Early recognition of anxiety disorders can help identify patients suffering from treatable problems and provide the patient and the clinician with a formal diagnosis to better explain the patient's symptoms. It may also reduce patients' medical expenses and risk of iatrogenic complications by decreasing or eliminating unnecessary medical testing and referrals to specialists to evaluate unexplained physical and somatic symptoms, and various "treatment" trials of pharmacologic agents.

Symptoms & Signs

Understanding the signs, symptoms, and epidemiologic features of the various anxiety disorders can help the

Table 23-1. DSM-IV (*Diagnostic and Statistical Manual of Mental Disorders*, 4th edition) anxiety disorders.

Anxiety Disorder	Prevalence in Primary Care
ASD	3–5%
Agoraphobia	1–3%
GAD	4–9%
OCD	1–2%
PD	1–6%
PTSD	2–12%
Social phobia	3–7%
Specific phobia	8–13%
Adjustment disorder with anxiety	4.5–9.2%
Anxiety disorder due to a general medical condition	14–66%
Substance-induced anxiety disorder	Unknown prevalence
Anxiety disorder not otherwise specified (NOS)	Unknown

Adapted from American Psychiatric Association. *Diagnostic and Statistical Manual of Mental Disorders*, 4th ed. Washington, DC: American Psychiatric Association, 1994.

physician make an accurate diagnosis and initiate timely, appropriate treatment while avoiding invasive or unnecessary testing.

Anxiety disorders typically manifest with *emotional symptoms* (e.g., fear, nervousness), *cognitive symptoms* (e.g., worry, a sense of doom, or derealization), and *physical symptoms* (e.g., muscular tension, tachycardia, dizziness, and insomnia). General medical practitioners

Table 23-2. Selected medical conditions that can simulate an anxiety disorder.

- Cardiac
  Ischemic heart disease, mitral valve prolapse, arrhythmias
- Endocrine/metabolic
  Hyperthyroidism, hypoglycemia, pheochromocytoma, carcinoid
- Gynecologic
  Menopause, premenstrual syndrome
- Neurologic
  Transient ischemic attacks, seizure disorders
- Pharmacologic
  Caffeine, alcohol, sympathomimetic agents, amphetamines, corticosteroids, theophylline, illicit drugs
- Respiratory
  Asthma, chronic obstructive pulmonary disease

must therefore decide how much diagnostic investigation is both feasible and necessary to rule out other important nonpsychiatric diseases. For example, when should a patient with palpitations undergo cardiac monitoring, thyroid function studies, evaluation for pheochromocytoma, or referral for cardiac catheterization? When does a patient with episodic nausea and abdominal pain require upper and lower endoscopy?

 CASE ILLUSTRATION 1

Gwen is a 28-year-old woman who was admitted for a "rule out" and evaluation of syncope after presenting to the emergency department (ED) with shortness of breath, tachycardia, and a sensation that she is going to faint. The episodes started approximately 4 months ago, shortly after her husband was temporarily laid-off from his job, and are not associated with activity. They have been increasing in frequency to where she is now experiencing as many as four episodes per week lasting approximately 5–10 minutes each. Gwen is fearful that she may faint while driving or when out with her child. She is also worried about her heart, as her mother had heart disease in her early fifties.

Gwen was monitored overnight and had several tests, including thyroid function studies and a Holter monitor. She was told those test results were all "normal" and to follow up with her primary care provider who after reviewing the history and test results recognizes that the symptoms are consistent with PD. Further historical details eliminate other medical or substance-related illness, or new use of caffeine or over-the-counter herbal or other remedies. The physician then reassures Gwen that her symptoms are not unusual and that 2–4% of all people suffer from PD. Sensing Gwen might be embarrassed by a psychological diagnosis, the doctor explains the nature of PD emphasizing its biological basis and asks her if she thinks the new onset of her symptoms are possibly related to her concerns regarding her family's financial security. To help Gwen learn more about PD, the doctor gives her a booklet and a web site address to read about self-managing her anxiety symptoms (see "Suggested Readings," below) and schedules a follow-up visit in 2 weeks to review this information and see how she is doing.

At their follow-up encounter, Gwen asks about medication for her panic symptoms as she has become worried about experiencing new attacks Her physician recommends a selective serotonin reuptake inhibitor (SSRI), and advises that she use one-half a tablet for the first week and then increase

Table 23-3. Suggested screening questions for anxiety.

Disorder	Question
GAD	Would you describe yourself generally as a nervous person? Are you a worrier? Do you feel nervous or tense?
PD	Have you ever had a sudden attack of rapid heartbeat or rush of intense fear, anxiety, or nervousness? Did anything seem to trigger it?
Agoraphobia	Have you ever avoided important activities because you were afraid you would have a sudden attack like the one I just asked you about?
Social anxiety disorder	Some people have strong fears of being watched or evaluated by others. For example, some people don't want to eat, speak, or write in front of people for fear of embarrassing themselves. Is anything like this a problem for you?
Specific phobia	Some people have strong fears or phobias about things like heights, flying, bugs, or snakes? Do you have any strong fears or phobias?
Obsession	Some people are bothered by intrusive, silly, unpleasant, or horrible thoughts that keep repeating over and over. For example, some people have repeated thoughts of hurting someone they love even though they don't want to; that a loved one has been seriously hurt; that they will yell obscenities in public; or that they are contaminated by germs. Has anything like this troubled you?
Compulsion	Some people are bothered by doing something over and over that they can't resist, even when they try. They might wash their hands every few minutes, or repeatedly check to see that the stove is off or the door is locked, or count things excessively. Has anything like this been a problem for you?
Acute stress and PTSD	Have you ever seen or experienced a traumatic event when you thought your life was in danger? Have you ever seen someone else in grave danger? What happened?

to a full tablet in 7–10 days. The doctor also advises Gwen that it may take 4–6 weeks before she notices any improvement from the medication, and recommends another follow-up visit in 2 weeks to see how she is feeling, review the self-help recommendations, and answer any new questions she may have. After a month on the medication Gwen's symptoms resolve and she returns to full function.

Differential Diagnosis

Symptoms resembling an anxiety disorder can be triggered by use of or intoxication from over-the-counter cold preparations, caffeine, cocaine, theophylline preparations, amphetamines, and marijuana or withdrawal from alcohol, benzodiazepines, barbiturates, sedative-hypnotic agents, and other central nervous system (CNS) depressants. These conditions are commonly referred to as "substance-induced anxiety disorder" (Table 23-3). Therefore, the astute clinician must review the patient's list of medications and inquire about the use of over-the-counter medications including "herbal supplements" and performance-enhancing preparations (anabolic steroids), legal (alcohol, tobacco, caffeine) and illegal substances (cocaine).

Many medical conditions also have symptoms resembling those of anxiety (Table 23-2). Some are relatively common and obvious to practitioners (arrhythmias and asthma) and others are less so (insulinoma, pheochromocytoma, and carcinoid). Anxiety symptoms may also develop as a consequence of a medical condition. Examples include patients who experience anxiety symptoms following a myocardial infarction or following a pulmonary embolism. Clues to help sort medical from psychiatric patient presentations to guide diagnostic testing, if any, include patient age and gender, past medical and psychiatric history, family history, and social history. Indeed, people who have been in excellent physical health and develop new-onset anxiety symptoms after age 50 are more likely to have medical etiologies explaining their anxiety symptoms than those under 25 years old who have presented previously to several physicians and undergone extensive medical testing for evaluation of multiple unexplained somatic symptoms.

Etiology

The development of anxiety disorders involves multiple factors, including biological abnormalities, past and present psychological stressors, maladaptive cognitions, and environmentally conditioned behaviors. Abnormalities in the CNS associated with anxiety disorders relate to the γ-aminobutyric acid (GABA) receptor as well as to the locus ceruleus. Animal studies have shown that stimulation of the locus ceruleus produces hyperarousal states similar to those seen in anxious humans. GABA is an inhibitory neurotransmitter found throughout most of the CNS. It may decrease anxiety by inhibiting locus ceruleus activity and modulating the reticular activating system, another area of the brainstem thought to affect alertness and fear. Benzodiazepines, a class of medications commonly used to treat anxiety, bind to specific sites on the GABA receptor. When the benzodiazepine molecule binds the GABA receptor, the effect of GABA on the GABA receptor is enhanced, reducing anxiety. Two other neurotransmitters, serotonin and norepinephrine, are also under investigation based on therapeutic responses to medications that affect these systems (e.g., SSRIs and serotonin norepinephrine reuptake inhibitors [SNRIs]). Poor regulation of the adrenergic system is also suspected as β-adrenergic agonists induce symptoms of panic and α-adrenergic agonists decrease symptoms of anxiety.

Genetic factors are also likely to play a role in anxiety disorders, as evidenced by twin studies showing a higher concordance for PD and obsessive-compulsive disorder (OCD) among monozygotic twins than among dizygotic twins.

Cognitive-behavioral therapy holds that behavior is driven by underlying beliefs or *cognitions.* Patients with anxiety typically overestimate danger or threats and underestimate their ability to effectively cope. These patients subsequently feel "stressed" or anxious and select avoidant or other maladaptive coping strategies.

Conditioned learning may also play a pivotal role in the development of anxiety disorders and the resulting avoidance that often seriously compounds patients' anxiety-related functional impairment. For example, patients may notice some unusual autonomic arousal or physical sensation while driving a car. They may misinterpret this initially random and benign sensation as a life-threatening event (e.g., "I'm having a heart attack!"), which further intensifies the autonomic response, fuels the misinterpretation, and snowballs into a full-blown panic attack. They may learn to associate the physical sensation and the subsequent attack with the act of driving and feel heightened anxiety—fueled by catastrophic thinking—when they drive or anticipate driving. Initially, the association between driving and panic is coincidental (driving is not the event provoking the initial sensation or the panic attack). Eventually, however, a patient may completely stop driving for fear that another panic attack will occur. This conditioned learning between driving and panic may gradually become so strong that driving becomes a precipitant of panic attacks. Thus, the driver mistakenly becomes conditioned to fear driving.

Traumatic, highly stressful, and catastrophic life events are also key factors leading to anxiety disorders, particularly PTSD. PTSD and adjustment disorder with anxiety are examples of disorders in which these events play a specific causal role. Other research suggests that childhood trauma, sexual assault, battle-exposure, and terrorism can predispose individuals to develop hyperactive physiologic responses to everyday stressors, placing them at greater risk for developing anxiety and other mood disorders.

SPECIFIC DISORDERS
Panic Attacks

A panic attack is characterized by a discrete period of intense fear accompanied by the abrupt onset of several cognitive and somatic symptoms. Cognitive symptoms may include but are not limited to racing thoughts, preoccupation with health concerns, catastrophic misinterpretation of somatic symptoms, or believing one is going insane. Somatic symptoms may include a choking sensation, racing heartbeat, sweating, "jelly" legs, nausea, shaking, chest pain, numbness, or feeling detached or unreal. Frightening physical symptoms are commonly prominent and scare many patients into seeking urgent medical care. Primary care providers can usually be reassuring, as panic attacks are often infrequent, self-limited, and not related to any serious mental or physical disorder. Panic attacks are categorized as follows:

- Unexpected (untriggered or uncued),
- Situationally bound (always environmentally or psychologically cued), or
- Situationally predisposed (sometimes, but not invariably, cued).

Panic attacks can be comorbid with a number of other anxiety disorders including social and specific phobias, OCD, and PTSD. The presence and type of a panic trigger help clinicians make a correct diagnosis. Uncued panic attacks are characteristic of PD, whereas cued attacks suggest other psychiatric conditions such as the following:

- Social phobia (attack triggered by fear of embarrassment in social situations),
- Specific phobia (fear of places or things),
- OCD (triggered by exposure to the object of an obsession, such as contamination), or
- PTSD (triggered by an event resembling the original trauma).

Panic attacks are quite common; most people experience a subclinical, or limited-symptom attack at some time. Only about 9% of the general population ever experiences a full-blown panic attack.

Panic Disorder

DIAGNOSIS

Panic disorder is diagnosed when panic attacks are uncued and recurrent and are followed by a month or more of persistent fear of another attack or avoidance of situations because of fear of having another attack. Lifetime prevalence in the community is 2–4%, and about 3–8% of patients who present to primary care physicians meet current criteria. Community-based studies also reveal that suicide attempts are more common among patients with PD than among patients with major depression.

PD is a potentially debilitating disease with major complications. It leads to agoraphobia, a fear of being in a place or a situation where escape or rescue might be difficult if another attack occurs, in 30–50% of cases, most often within 6 months of the first panic attack. This fear may cause many patients to avoid important activities of daily living such as shopping or using public transportation.

MANAGEMENT

Treatments for several of the anxiety disorders have been developed and proven effective in clinical trials at reducing anxiety symptoms and in improving health-related quality of life and employment patterns. Appropriate treatment may also reduce substance abuse among patients who self-medicate with alcohol, benzodiazepines, or other substances in an effort to ameliorate their symptoms.

Initial management of the anxiety disorders begins with providing the patient with a clear understanding of the problem. This tends to ease anxiety, increase the strength of the therapeutic alliance, and the subsequent likelihood that the patient will adhere with the treatment plan. It is helpful to emphasize the biological nature of PD, as most patients find it reassuring and destigmatizing to know that they have a recognized, treatable biological syndrome that typically has a good prognosis. Patients should also be referred to self-help books, support groups, and cognitive-behavioral resources, which are widely available (see "Suggested Readings," below).

In tailoring the treatment of PD to the patient, several factors should be weighed, including the degree of avoidance present, the severity of physical manifestations, and the comorbidity of other psychiatric disorders. The clinician must balance patient education and supportive counseling with patients' beliefs about the cause of their symptoms. For example, if the physical symptoms are attributed to a cardiac problem, correcting this misinterpretation and emphasizing the biological basis of PD may help the patient accept the diagnosis and thus improve adherence to treatment. The primary physician has a vital role to play in many of the treatments, such as patient education, and advice to avoid possible triggering substances such as caffeine and cold medicines, supportive counseling, and initial management of pharmacotherapy which can appropriately be incorporated into routine office visits.

Patients with PD often focus on the somatic symptoms of the disorder, thus presenting to medical settings with chest pain, dizziness, abdominal concerns, and other unexplained complaints. Iatrogenesis and unnecessary medical costs can and often do result from unnecessary procedures and treatments. The dilemma for clinicians, therefore, is to decide whether and how extensively to evaluate the patient's specific symptoms.

One clinical strategy is to evaluate conservatively those symptoms that are potentially catastrophic, involve objective findings, or present as a classic constellation of symptoms. While the investigation is proceeding, the patient can be treated for PD and the symptoms periodically reassessed. Effective pharmacologic treatment can reduce the cognitive and physical symptoms of panic and lessen the patient's belief that the problem is caused by an undiscovered medical condition.

Medications used to treat PD include antidepressants, most commonly SSRIs and SNRIs, but tricyclic antidepressants (TCAs) and monoamine oxidase inhibitors (MAOIs) can also be used. Benzodiazepines (alprazolam, clonazepam) relieve symptoms rapidly, usually within the first week of treatment, and they have a relatively wide therapeutic index. Their main disadvantages are their potential for misuse and dependence, a high incidence of rebound panic attacks when the medication is discontinued, and interference with exposure-based cognitive-behavioral therapy. In contrast, SSRIs, SNRIs, and TCAs are not associated with dependence and may have a synergistic effect with cognitive-behavioral therapy, but generally take 3–4 weeks or longer before reaching maximum effectiveness. In addition, some antidepressants may exacerbate symptoms of anxiety during the first 1–2 weeks of administration.

A benzodiazepine can also be used in combination with either a SSRI or a SNRI (to avoid a "serotonin syndrome," SSRIs and SNRIs should not be used in combination). Given the availability of several potential first-line agents believed to be of similar efficacy (Table 23-4), the clinician is advised to first inquire about past personal and family experience with pharmacotherapy, side effects, brand preference, and insurance formulary restrictions before suggesting a particular medication.

A common practice is to initiate treatment with a low daily dose of a generically available SSRI (e.g., paroxetine, 10 mg orally each day), titrating the dose slowly upward to 20 mg daily over 1–2 weeks as tolerated until symptom relief or the maximum dosage is attained, whichever arrives first. If the panic symptoms are particularly troublesome or if they worsen in the

Table 23-4. Preferred anxiolytic medications for use in medical outpatients.

Generic Name	Class	Starting Dosage	Step-Up Dose	Target Dose	Top Dose/ day	Comment
First-line Agent						
Citalopram	SSRI	10 mg qd	10–20 mg/qd	20–40 mg/day	60 mg	Possibly fewer cytochrome P450 drug interactions; FDA-approved for PD
Duloxetine	SNRI	20 mg qd	20 mg/day	30 mg bid or 60 mg qd	60 mg bid	FDA-approved for depression
Escitalopram	SSRI	5 mg qd	5–10 mg qd	10–20 mg/day	20 mg	Enantiomer of citalopram; possibly fewer cytochrome P450 drug interactions; FDA-approved for GAD
Fluoxetine	SSRI	10 mg qd	10 mg/day	20–40 mg/day	80 mg	Most activating of SSRI class; slower onset of action; FDA-approved for depression, PD, OCD, and bulimia
Paroxetine	SSRI	10 mg qd	10–20 mg/day	40 mg/day	40 mg	FDA-approved for depression, PD, GAD, PTSD, OCD, social anxiety; slightly sedating
Sertraline	SSRI	25 mg qd	25 mg/day	100 mg/day	200 mg	FDA-approved for depression, PD, OCD, PTSD, social anxiety
Venlafaxine XR	SNRI	37.5 mg qd	37.5 mg qd	75–150 mg qd	225 mg	FDA-approved for depression, PD, GAD. Social anxiety; may increase blood pressure at higher doses
Second-line Agent						
Fluvoxamine	SSRI	50 mg qd	50 mg bid	50 mg bid	300 mg	FDA-approved for OCD
Bupropion SR	NDRI	100 mg/day	50 mg bid	150 mg bid	450 mg	FDA-approved for depression; favored if comorbid depression; may induce seizures at higher doses in seizure-prone individuals
Nefazodone	SARI	100 mg bid	50 mg bid	150 mg bid	600 mg	Sedation prominent at start; FDA-approved for depression
Alprazolam	BZD	0.25 mg bid-tid	0.25 mg bid	0.25 mg prn	4 mg	Short onset and duration of action; FDA-approved for anxiety and PD
Lorazepam	BZD	0.5 mg tid-qid	0.5 mg qd	1.0 mg tid	10 mg	Short onset and duration of action; FDA-approved for anxiety
Clonazapine	BZD	0.5 mg bid	0.5 mg qd	1.0 mg bid	4 mg	Longer onset and duration of action; FDA-approved for PD and anxiety
Third-line Agent						
Buspirone	Other	5 mg tid	5 mg qd	20–30 mg bid	60 mg	Moderate efficacy compared to SSRIs; no antidepressant effect; FDA-approved for GAD only

Abbreviations: BZD, benzodiazepine; NDRI, norepinephrine and dopamine reuptake inhibitor; SARI, serotonin agonist and reuptake inhibitor.

initial week of therapy, a benzodiazepine such as alprazolam or clonazepam can be added for more rapid control of symptoms and then tapered-off and discontinued when the SSRI or SNRI commences effect. As with treatment of major depression, to avoid symptom relapse experts currently recommend that anxiolytic pharmacotherapy be continued for a minimum of 9–12 months, and longer if the symptoms are particularly disabling or recurrent, or per patient preference and ability to tolerate relapse.

Adjunctive cognitive-behavioral interventions (e.g., relaxation training, challenging catastrophic thinking, and gradual exposures) can treat both the physical manifestations and avoidance behaviors and substantially decrease the likelihood of symptom relapse following discontinuation of pharmacotherapy. Patients should be helped to gradually face the situations and activities they feared and fully experience the physical sensations they once believed indicated a serious medical problem. For example, the patient in Case Illustration 1 would be encouraged to drive, shop, and manage other tasks outside her home while experiencing and eventually managing her shortness of breath, racing heartbeat, and sensation of fainting. If patients are at first overwhelmed by the prospect of doing this, they can first initiate exposure mentally, using relaxation techniques and guided imagery. The patient should be instructed to imagine a frightening but tolerable aspect of the activity (in this case, driving) while doing a relaxation exercise and to repeatedly visualize successfully coping with the activity. In some cases, it may be necessary to enlist the assistance of a cognitive-behavioral therapist who can design and manage successive "exposure" exercises for overly frightened patients.

Phobias

DIAGNOSIS

Specific phobias and social anxiety disorder (formerly known as social phobia) are characterized by episodic anxiety in response to specific precipitants. Stimuli for specific phobias include places, things, or events, such as airplane flights, heights, insects, snakes, or rodents. Affected individuals are aware that their fears are exaggerated or unreasonable; nonetheless, when exposed to the precipitant, patients experience intense, excessive fear subsequently leading to avoidance behaviors. Specific phobias are perhaps the most common but least disabling of the various anxiety disorders. Although many individuals have at least one, most experience only minor related dysfunction, and therefore seldom seek medical care. Indeed, when care is sought, the diagnosis is usually evident from the history and requires no further testing.

Social anxiety disorder involves excessive fear of embarrassment, failure, or humiliation before others. This may be manifested as a fear of speaking, performing, eating, or writing in public. Less often, it presents as a generalized type of anxiety that disables the patient in a wide range of social situations. Its physical symptoms include blushing, profuse sweating, trembling, nausea, and difficulty talking. Marked anticipatory anxiety can also cause avoidance behaviors that significantly disrupt patients' functioning.

 CASE ILLUSTRATION 2

Charlie, a man in his mid-thirties, presents to his primary care provider complaining of severe palpitations, sweating, and tremulousness. The symptoms occur when he is waiting in customs lines. As he approaches the front of the line, fear of evaluation and fear of talking with the customs official intensifies until the symptoms occur. Sometimes he flees to the end of the long line before he feels ready to face the customs official. Charlie realizes this cycle is silly and laughs anxiously as he describes it. This symptom is a major problem for him because his occupation is writing travel books. He has begun avoiding travel and is increasingly worried about his ability to meet writing deadlines and to continue working. A conservative medical workup is unrevealing, and the primary care provider makes the diagnosis of specific social anxiety disorder, prescribing a trial of alprazolam to be used a short time before standing in the customs line. Charlie is also given a self-help book and a tape on relaxation techniques and the use of guided imagery as a way of visualizing success in the customs line. Charlie uses these treatment approaches successfully on his next trip and realizes that the problem is controllable. He incorporates them into his routine work schedule, and within 2 months has returned to full occupational functioning.

MANAGEMENT

Treatment of specific phobias and social anxiety disorder almost always involves some form of cognitive-behavioral therapy such as systematic desensitization in which the patient is gradually exposed to the feared object or situation. Generally accepted pharmacotherapy guidelines have not been established for specific phobias. As noted in Case Illustration 2, patients with phobia and specific social anxiety disorder are often prescribed short-acting benzodiazepines to be taken prior to an anticipated exposure to the phobic stimulus. Benzodiazepines are often given for exposures to infrequent events that have no complex performance requirements (e.g., traveling by commercial airplane). Patients should be informed of the risk of anterograde amnesia, or blackouts, associated with some of these drugs. Sertraline, paroxetine, venlafaxine have all been Food and Drug Administration (FDA)-approved for the treatment of social anxiety disorder. Although less data are presently available, the other SSRI and SNRI medications may be similarly effective at treating this disorder.

Obsessive-Compulsive Disorder

DIAGNOSIS

Patients with OCD experience regular, intrusive, anxiety-provoking thoughts—called obsessions—or are driven to repeatedly perform seemingly unnecessary or bizarre rituals—called compulsions. Aggression, sex, and religion are common obsessional themes. Compulsions may involve mental tasks, such as counting or praying, or they may involve physical rituals, such as repeated hand-washing or checking the state of an object. In patients with both obsessions and compulsions, the ritualized compulsions are usually performed to control the anxiety generated by the obsessive thoughts (e.g., obsessive fear about germs is eased by compulsive hand-washing). Although patients' level of insight is typically high—they generally experience obsessions and compulsions as intrusive, upsetting, and silly—such insight may diminish acutely when they are faced with the focus of an obsession. They may also become so preoccupied with their obsessions and compulsions that they become extremely anxious, slow, and disabled. In one instance, a patient wrung her hands so constantly she could not cook, work, or sleep. Another washed his hands every 10–15 minutes which interfered significantly with his normal business and social activities.

Until the introduction of effective pharmacotherapies for OCD, the disorder was markedly underrecognized in both primary care and psychiatric practice. About 1–3% of the general population develops OCD during their lives. The disorder has been found to have a distinct biological component, a finding supported by the efficacy of biological therapies that selectively inhibit the reuptake of serotonin at CNS neurosynapses, and twin studies that show a significantly higher percentage of monozygotic twins with diagnostic concordance than dizygotic twins. Additionally, there is a distinct and reciprocal association between OCD and Tourette syndrome, a neurologic disorder involving persistent motor and verbal tics.

MANAGEMENT

Psychotherapy for OCD usually involves a form of cognitive-behavioral therapy called "exposure with response prevention" in which the patient is exposed to the anxiety-provoking obsessions or situation but does not engage in the subsequent compulsions or other maladaptive strategies to manage the anxiety. Patients are taught alternate ways of coping with the anxiety including diaphragmatic breathing and progressive muscle relaxation. The cognitive-behavioral therapist may also guide the patient in identifying faulty beliefs and assist the patient in testing those beliefs. The belief, "something terrible will happen if I don't check my lock a hundred times a day," is first rationally examined, then a behavioral test of that belief is collaboratively designed and executed—much as a scientist would design and run a test for any hypothesis.

SSRIs which inhibit presynaptic reuptake of serotonin appear to be effective in treating OCD in addition to clomipramine, the only TCA with this quality. SSRIs also have the advantages of ease of dosing and low toxicity in overdose. FDA-approved SSRIs for treatment of OCD include fluoxetine (Prozac), fluvoxamine (Luvox), paroxetine (Paxil), citalopram (Celexa), escitalopram (Lexapro), and sertraline (Zoloft). The dual SNRIs (venlafaxine and duloxetine) may also have efficacy in OCD. However, neither has yet been FDA-approved specifically for treatment of OCD.

Posttraumatic Stress Disorder & Acute Stress Disorder

DIAGNOSIS

Posttraumatic stress disorder and acute stress disorder (ASD) are the common mental sequelae of catastrophic trauma. ASD involves symptoms that occur within the first month after trauma. PTSD is essentially the same syndrome, but beginning or persisting beyond a month. Severe trauma of either ASD or PTSD entails an observed or experienced serious injury or attack (actual or threatened). By definition, the trauma experience is accompanied by feelings of intense fear, helplessness, or horror. Patients subsequently develop a mix of flashbacks, nightmares, persistent avoidance of stimuli resembling (concretely or symbolically) the precipitating event, numbing of general responsiveness (restricted range of affect, feelings of interpersonal estrangement, anhedonia), and persistent signs and symptoms of physiologic arousal. Secondary depression, panic attacks, substance abuse, unexplained physical symptoms, and aggressive behavior may also be present.

Epidemiologic studies suggest that about one-third of the population suffers some trauma, placing them at risk for PTSD, and one-fourth of those at risk will develop PTSD, usually within 1 year following exposure to the event, although on occasion, it may develop years after the event. While men experience more lifetime trauma, women in the general population are more likely to develop PTSD. They have a 10% lifetime prevalence of PTSD, double that of men. The prevalence of PTSD is considerably higher among certain groups including 18% among professional firefighters, 34% in adolescent survivors of motor vehicle crashes, 48% in female rape victims, and 67% in former prisoners of war.

 CASE ILLUSTRATION 3

Jacques was a successful accountant with no psychiatric history until he had mitral valve surgery at the age of 42. Subsequently, he became totally dysfunctional, losing jobs and clients. He now also suffers flashbacks about the postoperative period of pain and confusion. Jacques gradually became depressed, and his obnoxious, angry behavior alienated both friends and providers.

Jacques' primary care physician noted a change in his demeanor during a conversation at a routine follow-up visit to monitor his chronic anticoagulation therapy for his replacement valve. The physician asked Jacques how work was going for him since his return following surgery. Then Jacque began to disclose his personal fears and perceived failures triggered by the traumatic brush with serious illness and fear of a stroke caused by his replacement valve. His doctor then helped Jacques recognize the role of the surgical trauma event in his life and explained the potential for improvement with psychotherapy and pharmacotherapy for his symptoms. Jacques subsequently accepted referral to an established multidisciplinary treatment program for PTSD.

MANAGEMENT

Treatment of PTSD typically begins with a detailed evaluation and development of a treatment plan to meet the unique needs of the survivor. This is best accomplished with a multidisciplinary team that includes the primary care physician, a mental health professional, an addiction specialist, a social worker, and possibly community-based referral resources such as theme counseling groups (e.g., veterans groups and abuse-survivor groups). PTSD-specific treatment is typically begun after the patient has been safely

removed from the crisis situation. If the patient is still being exposed to trauma (e.g., ongoing domestic violence), or is severely depressed, experiencing extreme panic, suicidal, or is in need of drug or alcohol detoxification, then it is important to address these issues as a part of initial treatment.

It is generally helpful to label the problem as PTSD and thus legitimize the manifestations, as patients often blame themselves or others. Thus, the physician might say to the patient, "The kinds of feelings, thoughts, and problems you're having are not unusual—in fact they're fairly common among people who have gone through a catastrophe." Support groups of persons who have suffered similar trauma help patients feel understood and normalize their symptoms as they share their experiences and solve problems together. Cognitive-behavioral therapy is the nonpharmacologic treatment of choice for PTSD where patients are taught behavioral skills to manage their autonomic hyperarousal, and then are guided through repeated and desensitizing retellings of their traumatic experience.

Pharmacotherapy can reduce the anxiety, depression, and insomnia often experienced by patients with PTSD. Although no particular drug has emerged as a definitive treatment for PTSD and its associated flashback and nightmares, currently, only sertraline and paroxetine have been FDA-approved for the treatment of PTSD. Benzodiazepines have also been used to treat the anxiety, hyperarousal, and insomnia of PTSD. However, early and prolonged use of benzodiazepines to treat ASD may actually be associated with a higher rate of subsequent PTSD. Thus, it is recommended that benzodiazepines be reserved for time-limited treatment of extreme arousal, insomnia, and anxiety.

Generalized Anxiety Disorder

DIAGNOSIS

Generalized anxiety disorder consists of almost constant, nonepisodic worry and anxiety that affect patients for more than 6 months and interfere with normal functioning. The worry and anxiety are difficult for the patient to control and are associated with edginess or restlessness, easy fatigability, difficulty concentrating, irritability, muscle tension, or sleep disturbance. Worries typically involve multiple domains and may include concern about routine life circumstances, with the magnitude of worry being out of proportion to the severity of the situation. Symptoms must not be due to the physiologic effects of a medical problem such as hyperthyroidism or abuse of a medication or drug. Patients with GAD usually complain of feeling "up-tight" or constantly nervous. Physical symptoms such as muscle aches, twitching, trembling, sweating, dry mouth, headaches, gastrointestinal symptoms, urinary frequency, and exaggerated startle often accompany the disorder and are often the patient's presenting complaint.

GAD has a 4–6% lifetime prevalence, and two-thirds of those affected are women. The disorder tends to have a chronic, fluctuating course that worsens under stress. Approximately half of all cases are comorbid with depression.

MANAGEMENT

Short-term supportive psychotherapy can be helpful. Many patients with GAD have focal life conflicts or stressors for which psychotherapy may be helpful. Basic primary care strategies include empathic listening; encouragement; and assisting patients to identify problems, discuss possible solutions, and solve the problem. Cognitive-behavioral techniques can be used to help patients examine the catastrophic beliefs that underlie their unrealistic worries. Biofeedback and relaxation techniques are useful for improving patient control over muscle tension and other physiologic signs of anxiety.

Several SSRIs and benzodiazepines, venlafaxine, and the nonbenzodiazepine anxiolytic buspirone have all been FDA-approved for treatment of GAD. Benzodiazepine therapy at doses lower than those required for PD is usually rapidly effective with few adverse effects. Sedation is the most common side effect but diminishes over time. Tolerance to therapeutic effects is minimal. Minimum effective doses should be used, but care must be taken not to undertreat patients out of fear of making them drug dependent. As with benzodiazepine treatment for other anxiety disorders, rebound symptoms of anxiety are the rule as medication is discontinued. Often a lengthy (a month or more) taper is required.

Buspirone is a nonsedating medication specifically indicated for patients with GAD. It alleviates the symptoms of this anxiety disorder but like the SSRIs and venlafaxine, has a similarly slow onset of action to reach efficacy. Unlike these other medications, buspirone also requires twice-daily dosing which may adversely affect patient adherence. Importantly, it only has moderate efficacy compared with the SSRIs, and it lacks an antidepressant effect placing it at a disadvantage for patients with comorbid depression.

Adjustment Disorder With Anxiety

DIAGNOSIS

Adjustment disorder with anxiety should be considered in patients who are responding with maladaptive anxiety to a recent situational stressor but who do not meet the criteria for another mental disorder. The stressor may be a medical event (e.g., surgery, hospitalization, onset of an illness), but most often is a personal crisis such as a divorce, financial problems, or a job change. Symptoms usually begin within 2 months of the onset of the stressor and significantly impair social or occupational functioning. If symptoms persist for more than 6 months, then another diagnosis, such as GAD, is usually more appropriate. Sleeplessness and the physiologic aspects of anxiety predominate, and the patient may seek care for somatic complaints. Eliciting the history of the stressful life event and ascertaining the relationship of symptoms to that event help to establish this diagnosis.

MANAGEMENT

The fundamental management of adjustment disorder with anxious mood is supportive counseling, in which the patient discusses the stressful event and the provider helps the patient actively identify and solve problems and/or find ways to more effectively manage the stress (e.g., more effectively access social supports or engage in pleasant activities). Patients with adjustment disorder are generally well cared for by a primary care physician who has learned the details of the precipitating event and can incorporate brief supportive strategies into the office visit. Structured relaxation exercises and stress management or other support groups may also be helpful. Sometimes a brief trial of benzodiazepine (less than 3 weeks) can help improve patient coping by reducing the debilitating stress-related symptoms (e.g., insomnia or overwhelming fear). Referral to mental health professionals may help if patients do not respond quickly, are severely incapacitated, show a repetitive pattern of maladaptive coping, or specifically request a therapist.

Many studies suggest that there is a substantial group of primary care patients who present with relatively minor complaints of anxiety and depression. Although they do not satisfy criteria for a mental disorder, they do experience associated poor functioning. Often psychosocial stressors or chronic medical problems exacerbate the emotional symptoms. Generally speaking, effective management should emphasize supportive psychosocial rather than pharmacologic interventions.

MANAGEMENT OF ANXIETY: GENERAL PRINCIPLES

Several general principles pertaining to the primary care treatment of anxiety disorders are worthy of note.

Psychosocial Therapies

Primary care providers should not underestimate the importance of basic supportive measures that can easily be performed in the general medical setting. The relationship between the doctor and patient usually plays a pivotal role for anxious patients in need of reassurance. Patient–provider trust is especially important for anxious patients, enhancing timely and accurate history taking, physical examination, diagnosis, and treatment adherence.

Symptoms of anxiety are extremely distressing to patients, who often fear that occult disease is causing their symptoms. Clinicians must try to view the symptoms through the eyes and perceptions of the affected patient—what seems trivial to a provider may be overwhelming for the patient. Listening to patients, expressing empathy for their feelings and concerns, and providing information about anxiety disorders are crucial ways to improve patient rapport (see Chapters 1 and 2) and should be routine in the course of care.

Equipping patients with basic information about anxiety disorders is essential ("bibliotherapy"). Patients with anxiety are common in medical settings so hospitals and clinics should be prepared and knowledgeable with patient education resources such as brochures, and relevant web sites to enable patients to find high-quality information. Most patients find such explanations and self-management strategies from appropriate lay publications reassuring. A number of well-validated and available psychosocial treatments can be recommended (Table 23-5).

Pharmacotherapy

Pharmacologic treatment (Table 23-4) is appropriate when the patient's symptoms are severe enough to significantly interfere with functioning and the benefits of medication outweigh the risks for a given patient. The treatment must be carefully individualized, based on the patient's prior experiences with pharmacotherapy— if any, family experiences, brand-name preference, insurance formulary restrictions, symptom severity, complicating medical or substance-abuse problems, vulnerability to various side effects, and willingness to collaborate in a psychopharmacologic approach to treatment.

When medications are prescribed, it is important to recognize, track, and document specific target symptoms. We generally recommend treatment with a generically available SSRI or SNRI for treatment-naïve patients unless there is a compelling reason to use a branded medication as no medication within these classes have been proven more effective than another. The medication should be initiated at half the typical starting dosage for unipolar major depression, and then titrated upward at 1–3 week intervals so as to minimize both the target symptoms and bothersome side effects. Lower starting dosages are recommended for those 60 years and older because these drugs have longer half-lives in this age group, accumulation can easily occur, and sensitivity to unwanted cognitive and other toxic effects is greater. In addition, for this age group we recommend against use of TCAs to avoid the potential for cardiac side effects, and benzodiazepines to avert cognitive and physical impairment (e.g., falls).

It is critically important to speak to the patient by telephone or in the office within 1–2 weeks and then again approximately every 2 weeks after the start of pharmacotherapy. The purpose of these follow-up contacts are to: (1) promote medication adherence; (2) monitor for potential side effects; (3) assess for emerging suicidality; (4) monitor treatment response; and (5) answer any new questions or concerns the patient may have. Following complete symptoms remission, they may be extended to approximately every 1–2 months over the first year of treatment.

Although monotherapy is almost always preferable to medication combinations, a common exception is prescribing both ongoing antidepressants and 2–4

Table 23-5. Nonpharmacologic management of anxiety disorders.

Type of Treatment	Description	Indication
Education	Provides basic information and reassurance	Appropriate in all disorders Lay publications useful
Cognitive-behavioral therapy (e.g., systematic desensitization)	Gradually increases exposure to feared stimulus using relaxation techniques Helps patient reorganize way of thinking about symptoms	Useful in all disorders Particularly effective for PD
Relaxation techniques	Uses muscle-relaxation therapy, including hypnosis, biofeedback, meditation	Particularly useful in PDs, GAD, adjustment disorder with anxious mood

weeks of minor tranquilizers for patients with PD. This strategy achieves rapid reduction of symptoms, avoids the intensification of anxiety sometimes seen in early antidepressant treatment of anxiety disorders, and allows discontinuation of benzodiazepines before dependence occurs. If patients are being referred to cognitive-behavioral therapy, a benzodiazepine taper, typically a reduction by 25% of the daily dose every week, and discontinuation are recommended. Benzodiazepines should seldom be used in patients with a history of substance abuse.

INDICATIONS FOR REFERRAL

Multiple randomized, controlled trials have shown that pharmacotherapy and/or cognitive-behavioral therapy are effective treatments for most anxiety disorders. Patients should be considered for referral to a mental health professional under the following circumstances:

1. The patient has suicidal or homicidal thoughts or plans or exhibits intended suicidal or homicidal behavior.

2. The treatment does not lead to improvement in the patient's symptoms within the expected timeframe.

3. Diagnostic uncertainty. It is particularly important to differentiate patients who have bipolar disorder, alcohol abuse/dependence, or personality disorders from those with an anxiety disorder. Mental health consultation is appropriate if the primary care doctor is uncertain and the distinction has therapeutic implications.

4. Complicating substance abuse is suspected.

5. The provider has questions about appropriate administration or tapering of benzodiazepines and questions regarding possible dependence.

6. The patient has an especially complicated set of ongoing psychosocial stressors whose resolution requires greater time and expertise than can be provided in primary care.

7. When a multidisciplinary or more specialized treatment approach is indicated. Such conditions include, but are not limited to ASD, PTSD, and desensitization therapy for specific phobia.

In some circumstances, the primary care physician may be uncertain about whether a patient has another medical illness and believes a specialist is necessary to consider that possibility. It is helpful to select a specialist who understands anxiety disorders and will work with the referring physician to explain the nature of the specific anxiety disorder to the patient. It is imperative that the specialist brings a conservative approach to diagnostic studies, an understanding of the many physical manifestations of anxiety, and a respectful approach to treatment of the anxiety-disordered patient.

The accurate and prompt diagnosis of anxiety disorders can prevent unnecessary diagnostic testing, specialty referral, and iatrogenic harm. The primary care physician who is knowledgeable and skilled in the diagnosis and management of anxiety disorders can make an important contribution to the quality of patient care and to the appropriate use of health resources, particularly in the managed care environment. Nevertheless, delivery for appropriate care can be difficult in typical practice settings. To overcome patient, physician, and system barriers to provision of guideline-based treatment and provide sustained patient follow-up, "collaborative care" models have been developed and subsequently proven effective at improving clinical outcomes for panic and GAD. They typically involve a nurse or other allied health professional who follows an evidence-based protocol under the direction of a primary care physician with specialty back-up when necessary, who has the time to educate the patient about his or her disorder, provide monitor use of pharmacotherapy, and impart self-management skills either in person or via telephone. Still, more clinical trials are necessary to examine the effectiveness of this strategy at improving clinical outcomes for other anxiety disorders.

SUGGESTED READINGS

Kroenke K, Spitzer RL, Williams JBW, et al. Anxiety disorders in primary care: prevalence, impairment, comorbidity, and detection. *Ann Intern Med* 2007;146:317–325.

Lange JT, Lange CL, Cabaltica RBG. Primary care of post-traumatic stress disorder. *Am Fam Physician* 2000;62:1035–1040.

National Institute for Health and Clinical Excellence (NICE). *Anxiety: Management of Anxiety in Adults in Primary, Secondary and Community Care.* London, England: National Institute for Clinical Excellence, December 2004. Available at: http://www.nice.org.uk/page.aspx?o=cg22#documents.

Rollman BL, Belnap BH, Reynolds CF, et al. A contemporary protocol to assist primary care physicians in the treatment of panic and generalized anxiety disorders. *Gen Hosp Psychiatry* 2003; 25:74–82.

Schneier FR. Social anxiety disorder. *N Engl J Med* 2006;355: 1029–1036.

REFERENCE BOOKS FOR PATIENTS

Bourne EJ. *The Anxiety and Phobia Workbook*, 4th ed. Oakland, CA: New Harbinger Press, 2005.

Craske MG, Barlow DH. *Mastery of Your Anxiety and Worry*, 2nd ed. Oxford University Press, 2006.

Davis M, McKay M, Eshelman ER. *The Relaxation and Stress Reduction Workbook*, 5th ed. Oakland, CA: New Harbinger Press, 2000.

Foa E, Wilson R. *Stop Obsessing! How to Overcome Your Obsessions and Compulsions*. New York, NY: Bantam, 2001.

Zuercher-White E. *An End to Panic: Breakthrough Techniques for Overcoming Panic Disorder*, 2nd ed. Oakland, CA: New Harbinger Press, 1998.

WEB SITES

Anxiety Disorders Association of America Web site. http://www.adaa.org. Accessed October, 2007.

Cognitive-Behavioral Therapy Web site. http://www.abct.org/. Accessed October, 2007.

Consumer Nonprofit Web site. http://www.freedomfromfear.org. Accessed October, 2007.

National Institute of Mental Health Web site. http://www.nimh.nih.gov/publicat/anxiety.cfm#anx5. Accessed October, 2007.

Attention Deficit Hyperactivity Disorder

H. Russell Searight, PhD, MPH

Attention deficit hyperactivity disorder (AD/HD) is a condition first evident in early childhood. Symptoms include deficits in attention, concentration, and short-term memory. Behaviorally, children with AD/HD are overly active (as if "driven by a motor") and unable to remain seated, highly distractible, and impulsive. Concerns about AD/HD often initially arise during kindergarten or first grade, since these deficits significantly impair academic performance and are disruptive in a typical classroom.

Recent data suggest a 6–8% prevalence rate, though some believe it to be higher. AD/HD disproportionately affects males with a sex ratio between 3:1 and 9:1, with more conservative figures in clinic, rather than community, samples.

There are two essential clusters of AD/HD symptoms: inattentiveness and hyperactivity/impulsivity. To meet DSM-IV (*Diagnostic and Statistical Manual of Mental Disorders*, fourth edition) criteria for an AD/HD diagnosis, there must be six symptoms of either **inattention** (failing to give attention to detail, problems maintaining attention, not appearing to listen when spoken to directly, failure to follow through on instructions and to complete schoolwork or other tasks, problems with organization, avoiding activities requiring sustained concentration, losing important items, being easily distracted, and forgetfulness), or **hyperactivity/impulsivity** (fidgeting, inability to remain seated, inappropriate running and climbing, difficulty playing quietly, acting as if "driven by a motor," excessive talking, blurting out answers before questions are finished, difficulty taking turns, intruding upon others' activities and/or conversations), or of both clusters.

CASE ILLUSTRATION 1: PRESCHOOL CHILD

Four-and-a-half year old Ronnie has been dismissed from three preschools during the past 9 months. Ronnie's mother brings a teacher's note chronicling Ronnie's recent behavior:

- *2/25 = "Ran out of classroom and was on his way out of the building before I stopped him."*
- *2/28 = "Threw all of the students' coats on the floor … won't listen when he's told to hang them up."*
- *3/2 = "Would not sit through story time. Threw milk cartons during lunch time."*

In your examination room, Ronnie is laying across your stool face down yelling, "I'm flying," while pushing off from the walls with his feet. His mother, appearing exhausted, makes a few half-hearted attempts to get Ronnie to settle down but quickly gives up saying, "You see doctor, this is what it's like."

The two clusters of symptoms, inattentive and hyperactive/impulsive, lead to three basic AD/HD subtypes: inattentive type, hyperactive/impulsive type, and mixed type (with features of both the former types).

While there are no precise longitudinal figures, AD/HD is increasingly accepted as a lifelong condition for many, if not most, patients. Development, however, does affect the symptom picture. The DSM-IV criteria best reflect AD/HD in children from 5 years until early adolescence. Research indicates that at around age 9, hyperactivity and impulsivity begin to become less pronounced, while inattention and other cognitive deficits persist.

The DSM-IV criteria and accompanying behavioral examples have been criticized as primarily depicting the condition among children rather than adolescents or adults. The clinician will need to be somewhat creative in generating more developmentally appropriate examples. For example, "excessive running or climbing in situations where it is inappropriate" might be replaced with "has difficulty sitting through a full length movie" or "cannot listen to a lecture, sermon, or other speaker for more than 10 minutes without becoming restless and distracted." Others have suggested that the requirement of six symptoms is too stringent for older patients. A cutoff of four symptoms was able to accurately detect college students with AD/HD.

CASE ILLUSTRATION 2: EARLY ELEMENTARY SCHOOL CHILD

Christopher is a 7-year-old boy and first grader, who is accompanied by both parents. They bring several notes that the teacher has sent to them since school began several months ago. They also bring samples of Christopher's schoolwork. The teacher's notes describe situations in which Chris got up from his seat to sharpen his pencil 20 times in the course of a day, was repeatedly told to stop playing with the girl's hair who sits in front of him, and continued to yell out answers to the teacher's questions before she finished speaking. Christopher's parents say that he is not learning to read or spell because he is easily distracted and cannot follow the lessons. At home, they describe mealtime as a "hit and run" experience where Chris eats while alternately sitting and standing at the table for no more than 10 minutes, during which he frequently knocks over his milk. Christopher's mother says she no longer takes him shopping because he runs off from her in the store and she is afraid he will get lost.

CASE ILLUSTRATION 3: MIDDLE ELEMENTARY SCHOOL CHILD

Miranda, a 9-year-old fourth grader, is seen because of poor grades. Her teacher describes Miranda as "spacey" with difficulty concentrating, paying attention, and remembering. However, she

and Miranda's mother both describe Miranda as a "sweet, sensitive, and helpful girl" without any disruptive behavior. A Vanderbilt Scale confirms this picture. The teacher's version includes a comment that Miranda may have to repeat the grade unless her academic performance improves.

With children referred in preschool or the early grades, there is typically a high level of parental distress and urgency. Hyperactivity may take the form of an inability to remain seated for more than 5 minutes at school or during family meals. Even when seated, the child may be swinging their legs, rocking, or picking up any nearby objects. By the time they reach first grade, children may also have a number of scars on their legs, arms, and head, and can provide a number of stories about jumping off the garage roof, rear-ending a car with their bicycle, and running into countless pieces of furniture. Occasionally, parents may report sporadic aggressive acts. Upon further inquiry, these are impulsive rather than premeditated, and the child with AD/HD is typically remorseful afterward. The DSM-IV phrase "as if driven by a motor" captures the quality of the activity level. While the child, with adult urging, may sit relatively still for 2–3 minutes, they will begin moving around as if they cannot stop themselves. The hyperactive/impulsive behavior is not experienced as under the patient's control—particularly among younger children.

Impaired attention and concentration, distractibility, and short-term memory deficits are often misattributed to "laziness," poor motivation, or "not caring" rather than a central nervous system disorder. Parents frequently complain about having to tell their child "a hundred times" to do something before the request "seems to register." Multistep directions are particularly challenging for those of all ages with AD/HD. A mother tells her teenaged son to go upstairs and get his new pants to be hemmed, the sewing kit, and a piece of chalk. Fifteen minutes later, when he has not appeared, his mother goes upstairs to find him. He is in his room, trying on a shirt with his new pants in his hand having forgotten what he was asked to do.

CASE ILLUSTRATION 4: ADOLESCENT

Josh, a 15-year-old, is brought in by his father for a drug test. Yesterday, Josh was suspended from school after a baggie of marijuana was found in his locker. He readily admitted smoking it several times a week for the past 6 months to "help calm me down." Josh was diagnosed with AD/HD-mixed type at age 7 and responded well to stimulant pharmacotherapy until about a year ago. At that time, Josh's grades declined—largely because of missing assignments—and he has had several detentions because of being late to class. His father describes his son as increasingly fidgety, disorganized, and forgetful. During the seventh grade, Josh said he felt embarrassed about going to the school nurse's office for his second methylphenidate dose. Josh was switched from short-acting methylphenidate to an extended-release formulation that he only took once, in the morning, before school. When asked about how he was tolerating the current medication, Josh responded: "I don't like taking that stuff; it doesn't do anything for me. My friends don't have to take it." Josh's father adds, "Now that I think about it, we have at least two extra bottles full of pills at home. I don't think Josh is taking it every day."

At school, inattention and poor concentration lowers academic performance. Much of school success is still based on memorization. In order to encode material into longer-term memory for a test, it is necessary to pay attention to relevant information, relate it to existing knowledge, and rehearse in short-term memory. When this process is disrupted, retaining information from textbooks and classroom presentations is extremely challenging. In elementary school, a typical didactic process is that the teacher will present a lesson (e.g., steps involved in long division, identifying adverbs) with several examples of the concept and then students will individually work on exercises applying that particular concept. In the later elementary years through college, there is much greater emphasis on reading and retaining what is read. College students with untreated AD/HD often report that despite rereading material multiple times, they cannot remember it.

CASE ILLUSTRATION 5: ADULT

Jim, a 35-year-old male, comes to see you after a particularly poor performance evaluation at work. Jim is an auto salesman who was recently promoted to manager of a small group of junior sales people. On his evaluation, Jim's supervisor describes Jim as "...scattered, unable to set priorities; starts projects but doesn't finish them; paperwork late or lost." His supervisors describe him as a "nice guy" but "it's hard to know what he wants; he contradicts himself a lot."

At home, Jim's wife took over the family's schedule after Jim forgot several important dates, including her birthday. Many mornings, he dashes around

the house looking for misplaced car keys. Jim's wife has also become the primary disciplinarian of their two children because Jim had difficulty being consistent and following through with consequences.

Jim describes having a hard time getting through high school: "I did really badly on tests; I just couldn't memorize." Even in elementary school, "I was sent to the principal's office for being the class clown." College was a greater challenge. Jim had to repeat several classes and required an extra three semesters to graduate.

Among adults with AD/HD, work and family are affected by inattention and poor short-term memory. Birthdays and anniversaries are forgotten, as are commitments to attend children's school activities. Multiple auto accidents are also common. At work, multiple projects may be initiated but remain uncompleted. Phone calls, coworkers, and e-mail all pose distractions that make it particularly difficult to get back "on track."

Up to 70% of adolescents diagnosed with AD/HD continue to exhibit symptoms with a comparable adult rate of approximately 50%. Even when they no longer meet formal AD/HD diagnostic criteria, deficits are often present along with comorbid conditions, such as Oppositional Defiant Disorder (ODD) or Conduct Disorder (CD) in adolescence and substance abuse, Mood Disorders and Antisocial Personality in adulthood.

ETIOLOGY

Heritability for AD/HD is approximately 0.76. Adoption studies further support the strong role of genetics in the condition. Recent molecular genetic studies have attempted to locate specific neurotransmitter receptor sites. Specifically, the dopamine D4 receptor has been implicated. Most DRD4 studies have involved the Exon III 7-repeat allele that is associated with a blunted response to dopamine. This neurogenetic finding is generally consistent with the action of stimulant drugs that block the dopamine transporter. Genes involved in serotonergic transmission have also been implicated in the etiology of AD/HD.

Certain environmental exposures, while not specific to AD/HD, have been associated with increased prevalence. Lead exposure appears to be associated with AD/HD; however, most AD/HD children do not have elevated lead and, conversely, most children with elevated lead do not develop AD/HD. Pregnancy and delivery complications, including toxemia, maternal age, fetal postmaturity, long duration of labor, fetal distress, hemorrhage, and prematurity are all AD/HD risk factors. Alcohol use and maternal smoking during pregnancy also elevate AD/HD risk.

Frontal lobe dysregulation has been implicated in AD/HD. Reduced dopaminergic activity in the frontal brain region has been conceptually linked to core deficits of disinhibition and poor self-monitoring.

THE CLINICAL HISTORY

In obtaining a clinical history, there are several essential features regardless of age. First, the symptoms must be persistent and evident in at least two settings. Typically, parents report that hyperactivity was first evident at age 3–4 years. Inattention may not be apparent until a child is in elementary school. In many instances when evaluating AD/HD-inattentive type, the child's difficulties may not be apparent in school for several years— until the child is age 9 or 10. A recent onset of hyperactivity and inattention in an older child, adolescent, or adult is generally inconsistent with AD/HD and other diagnostic possibilities should be considered.

Among children, AD/HD symptoms are almost always evident in school. If a parent reports that inattention and/or hyperactivity are only demonstrated at home, an AD/HD diagnosis is unlikely. The physician's office cannot be used as one of the two environmental settings. The diagnosis cannot be ruled out from a parental report that the child can focus on video games for hours at a time. The constantly changing visual and auditory feedback unique to video games often engages the child with AD/HD.

Eliciting specific behavioral examples is important— particularly in evaluating hyperactivity/impulsivity. Parents and, at times, teachers often conceptually group all externalizing behavior under AD/HD. Significant, repeated aggression and/or property destruction, talking back, theft, lying, or refusal to do schoolwork are not core AD/HD symptoms. These behaviors suggest other diagnoses (CD or ODD) instead of or possibly comorbid with AD/HD.

Similarly, children with poor academic performance may be seen because school personnel and/or parents attribute a child's poor grades to AD/HD. Because of budgetary issues and the large number of children with learning and/or behavioral problems, adequate special education services are often not readily available. School personnel, hoping that if there is a problem it can be managed without additional educational resources, may encourage parents to seek an AD/HD evaluation (Table 24-1). Reviewing academic testing, report cards, schoolwork samples, as well as the developmental history may suggest a learning disability. Again, learning disabilities are frequently comorbid, with reading disorders the most common.

MENTAL STATUS TESTING

While detailed neuropsychological assessments are beyond the scope of the typical primary care setting,

Table 24-1. Process of AD/HD evaluation.

1. What are the symptoms?
   - Are they core AD/HD symptoms?
   - In self-diagnosed patients, are there other problems that the patient is misattributing to AD/HD?
2. How long have symptoms been present?
   - Must be present *continuously* since early childhood.
3. Do the symptoms impair daily functioning?
   - If symptoms do not, is there a plausible explanation?
4. Use rating scales.
5. Screen mental status in office.
6. Do symptoms seem to be better explained by another condition? If yes, treat that condition and reassess at later date.
7. If information is generally consistent with AD/HD diagnosis, initiate treatment.
8. If information is ambiguous, there is a complicated differential diagnosis or significant comorbidities, refer to psychologist or psychiatrist for further assessment.

there are several cognitive tasks that, when used along with other information, may be helpful. Attention and immediate memory may be assessed by saying a sentence (in the case of preschool children) or string of random numbers and asking the patient to repeat them. A task assessing concentration requires the patient to say the numbers immediately afterward but in reverse order. Words can also be used as the auditory stimulus with the request to spell them forward and backward. Vigilance may be evaluated by asking the patient to tap their finger every time they hear the letter "A." The examiner then says a string of random letters and frequently, yet at unexpected intervals, says "A." The ability to recall four words after a 5- to 10-minute delay tests short-term memory.

MEDICAL TESTING

There is no agreed upon set of laboratory tests to aid in diagnosing AD/HD, and they are usually unnecessary. In geographic regions with high levels of lead exposure, lead levels should be obtained since elevations have been associated with hyperactivity. Since hyperthyroidism may present with inattention, decreased recent memory, and increased motor activity, thyroid function tests are occasionally obtained—particularly with adults.

Obstructive sleep apnea is associated with impaired attention and concentration. A sleep study should be considered when other indications are present (loud snoring, brief breathing cessation, and so on).

RATING SCALES & CHECKLISTS

Attention deficit hyperactivity disorder children do not reliably report their own symptoms. While recognizing that they often got in trouble with their parents ("My parents often yell at me, but I don't know why"), children with AD/HD did not recognize their hyperactivity, impulsivity, inattention, or distractibility.

Because symptoms are often noticed by parents, teachers, and spouses rather than the patients, themselves, standardized behavioral ratings should be obtained. While these scales vary somewhat according to the instrument's developer and, more importantly, the age group to which they are applied, most instruments share basic properties. All require judgment about symptom frequency. The cognitive or behavioral symptoms must be nearly always present (observable everyday) to be considered a positive DSM-IV criterion. The scales may simply list the 18 DSM-IV symptoms or they may be intermingled with ODD or CD symptoms, as well as academic problems. The more recent Vanderbilt Scale also includes pediatric mood disorder symptoms, as well as a section for teachers and parents to rate the level of impairment created by the symptoms.

Since the classroom places demands on attention, concentration, organizational skills, and impulse inhibition, teacher ratings should always be obtained, if possible. Maternal child behavior ratings have been found to be strongly affected by the mother's level of emotional distress. Depressed mothers rate their children as having more behavioral problems.

Adult rating scales demonstrate greater heterogeneity, reflecting the greater emphasis placed on cognitive DSM-IV symptoms and more subtle forms of hyperactivity among older AD/HD patients. Distinct conceptual adult AD/HD models are also reflected in these scales. For example, the frequently used Brown Adult AD/HD Rating Scale emphasizes activation deficits—the ability to initiate and self-direct activities as a core deficit. Wender's Utah Rating Scale asks the adult to retrospectively rate behaviors exhibited in childhood. The Adult Self-Report Scale-V1.1 is a brief screening tool that can help primary care providers identify adult patients at risk for having AD/HD.

TREATMENT

Pharmacotherapy

STIMULANTS

Stimulant medications are the mainstay of AD/HD therapy. Historically, the most commonly prescribed treatment has been immediate-release methylphenidate given two to three times per day in doses of 5–20 mg. Methylphenidate typically begins working in 30–60 minutes, with effects peaking at 1–2 hours and an overall duration of 2–5 hours. The somewhat longer-acting D,L-amphetamine salts (Adderall) are equally effective in treating core AD/HD symptoms and are an alternative for patients who do not respond to methylphenidate.

A significant recent innovation in stimulant therapy has been the development of various longer-acting preparations. Metadate-CD, Ritalin-LA, and Adderall-XR all contain mixtures of immediate- and extended-release beads to simulate twice per day dosing. Concerta is given once per day and is designed to deliver methylphenidate at a constant rate, with duration of action of up to 12 hours. Ritalin-SR, despite its name, is actually a delayed-release medication with little action for the first 2 hours followed by 4 hours of activity. This issue is less of a problem with Metadate-ER; however, the duration of effect is only 6 hours—not long enough to help a child through a typical full school day.

Stimulants' adverse effects include appetite suppression, insomnia, and weight loss. Less common side effects include headaches and nervousness. Ritalin "rebound" is frequently experienced when the stimulant wears off and is characterized by fatigue and irritability. In some patients, irritability is less pronounced with longer-acting stimulants. Side effects occurring within 2 hours of ingestion are probably best addressed by reducing the dose. The stimulants, particularly amphetamine and methylphenidate, may have some cardiovascular risk, prompting the Drug, Safety and Risk Management Advisory Committee of the Food and Drug Administration (FDA) to issue a black box warning for these medications.

NONSTIMULANT MEDICATIONS

Nonstimulants are second-line therapies to be considered under certain circumstances such as: difficulty with stimulant side effects, comorbid conditions such as Tourettte syndrome or seizure disorders, concerns about stimulant abuse, or parents philosophically opposed to stimulant use.

Atomoxetine (Straterra), a norepinephrine reuptake inhibitor, has demonstrated efficacy relative to a placebo in reducing AD/HD symptoms. As a nonstimulant, atomoxetine is not associated with growth suppression, tics, or insomnia. It is also not a Schedule II drug and less tightly regulated. Adverse effects may include nausea, vomiting, weight loss, and sleep problems. After reports of serious liver damage in two patients taking atomoxetine, the FDA required a written warning that it should be discontinued when jaundice is present or there is laboratory evidence of liver disease. Atomoxetine does not demonstrate any abuse potential and is unscheduled. Its peak efficacy develops over 2–6 weeks. It is initiated at a dose of 0.5 mg/kg/day and then increased to 1.2 mg/kg/day in 2 weeks. There do not appear to be drug interactions between the stimulants and atomoxetine—a factor suggesting that the combination may be particularly helpful in treating refractory cases. Because atomoxetine is an antidepressant, it also has the standard black box warning about risk of suicide accompanying antidepressant medication, including the possibility of increased suicidal ideation. To date, suicide risk has not been a significant clinical concern with atomoxetine.

The alpha-2 agonists, guanfacine and clonidine, demonstrate some efficacy for AD/HD with comorbid conduct disturbance, particularly when angry outbursts and aggression are present. The alpha-2 agonists may also reduce headaches and "jitteriness" that are common stimulant side effects. Typically, they are prescribed along with a stimulant. Patients should be closely monitored for hypotension and sedation.

Other antidepressants, such as bupropion and tricyclic agents, have demonstrated some efficacy with AD/HD in open-label studies. Presently, these agents are more commonly used with adult rather than childhood AD/HD. The TCAs have associated cardiovascular risk, and children as well as adult patients with preexisting cardiac disease should, generally, avoid these medications. Since bupropion lowers the seizure threshold, this medication should be avoided in patients with seizure histories, as well as in patients with eating disorders.

Once pharmacotherapy has been titrated to optimal effectiveness, patients' comorbid conditions and residual difficulties are often more apparent. Learning disabilities, social skills deficits, and, in adult patients, communication and organizational skills may become a treatment focus.

Nonpharmacologic Treatment

Psychoeducational approaches for parents of AD/HD children may be beneficial for increased medication adherence, as well as decreasing school and family stress. Key components include: (a) an explanation of AD/HD's etiology as a biologically based condition, (b) reassurance to parents that they are not at fault or responsible for AD/HD, (c) distinguishing between impulsive, uncontrollable behavior and volitional acts, (d) the role of pharmacotherapy—specifically, the type of symptoms addressed and not treated by medication, (e) description of common medication side effects, and (f) the likelihood that medication doses may be changed and that trying different agents may be necessary before achieving optimal symptom control.

Encouraging parents to communicate frequently with their child's teacher helps identify problems early before they have significant academic consequences. If possible, a daily note home system should be established between the school and parents.

At home, high levels of structure and predictability will make AD/HD more manageable. Bedtimes, meals, and homework should ideally occur at preplanned times that rarely vary from day to day. Encouraging children to lay out all material needed for the next day, including wardrobe, will make mornings run more

smoothly. Older children should keep their desk or homework completion area free of distracting clutter, while younger children should pick up all of their play items before moving to another activity.

For children with AD/HD alone, the addition of behavior therapy to stimulant medication does not appear to add further benefit. However, for the high proportion of AD/HD children with comorbid CD or ODD, behavioral intervention is strongly indicated. Key elements of parent training include: (a) specifying no more than two to three target behaviors to address at one time, (b) establishing positive reinforcement for appropriately prosocial behavior, (c) developing a reasonable timeframe and frequency of target behavior so that the child will realistically receive early positive reinforcement, (d) responding to inappropriate behavior through ignoring or time out, and (e) clear communication of requests and expectations.

Adults with AD/HD benefit from making frequent lists, using planners and calendars, as well as palm pilots, to help organize activities and remember important events and deadlines. For those employed in office settings, going into work early before most coworkers arrive, will allow task completion without interruption.

Adult AD/HD can wreak havoc on intimate relationships. In many instances, marriage counseling may be valuable for addressing effects of long-standing forgetfulness, and the inability to actively listen and be psychologically present to one's spouse or partner. For the spouse without AD/HD, it is important to recognize that this pattern of neglect does not indicate a lack of loving concern but is a by-product of the condition that can be improved upon.

CONCLUSION: THE COST OF AD/HD

In addition to health care expenditures, AD/HD has economic, legal, and social costs. Youth with AD/HD have more outpatient physician office visits—even exceeding those for children and adolescents with asthma. Rates of accidental poisoning, as well as non-head injuries, are also higher among children with AD/HD. In addition to greater health care utilization, the high comorbidity of AD/HD with learning disabilities leads to more costly special education services.

By adolescence, there is also a marked rise in comorbidity. CD, when together with AD/HD, is particularly pronounced and contributes to property damage, theft, and harm to others. High school is particularly challenging for youth with AD/HD. Approximately one-third of adolescents with AD/HD do not complete high school; a disproportionate number are expelled compared with non-AD/HD teens. The high drop out rate may, in part, reflect the fact that by high school nearly half of AD/HD adolescents have repeated at least one grade. A significant percentage of AD/HD teens are having sexual intercourse by age 15 and with multiple partners, reflecting the brevity of their relationships.

By the time adulthood is reached, AD/HD has adversely impacted most significant life arenas. In the workplace, AD/HD adults change jobs and are fired at a rate two to three times greater than those without the condition. Performance evaluations are often poor.

Adults with AD/HD have three times as many sexual partners and are significantly more likely to have unplanned pregnancies, as well as to contract a sexually transmitted disease. A disproportionate number of parents with AD/HD no longer have custody of their children. Auto accident rates are disturbingly high with approximately 20% of AD/HD adults having had 12 or more traffic citations. Nearly one-third have three or more crashes.

Limited research suggests that treatment may reduce the likelihood of these adverse outcomes, for example, use of stimulant medication greatly reduced the number of errors in a driving simulator. Early identification and treatment may also greatly reduce later adverse outcomes. Recent studies suggest that adolescent substance abuse was more likely in children with AD/HD who were not treated compared with those receiving therapy, including medication.

SUGGESTED READINGS

Barkley RA. *Attention Deficit Hyperactivity Disorder. A Handbook for Diagnosis and Treatment*, 3rd ed. New York, NY: Guilford Press, 2006.

DuPaul GJ, Stoner S. *ADHD in the Schools*. New York, NY: Guilford Press, 2003.

Kessler RC, Adler L, Ames M, et al. The World Health Organization adult ADHD self-report scale (ASRS): a short screening scale for use in the general population. *Psychol Med* 2005;35: 245–256.

McGough JJ, Barkley RA. Diagnostic controversies in adult attention-deficit/hyperactivity disorder. *Am J Psychiatry* 2004; 161:1948–1956.

Murphy KRE, Adler LA. Assessing attention-deficit/hyperactivity disorder in adults: focus on rating scales. *J Clin Psychiatry* 2004; 65(Suppl 3):12–17.

Searight HR, Burke JM, Rottnek F. Adult ADHD: evaluation and treatment in family medicine. *Am Fam Physician* 2000;62: 2077–2086.

Searight HR, Evans SL, Gafford J. Attention deficit hyperactivity disorder. In: Mengel MB, Schwiebert LP, eds. *Family Medicine: Ambulatory Care and Prevention*, 4th ed. New York, NY: Appleton and Lange, 2005.

Wender PH. *Attention-Deficit Hyperactivity Disorder in Adults*. New York, NY: Oxford University Press, 1995.

Somatization

J. Jewel Shim, MD & Stuart J. Eisendrath, MD

INTRODUCTION

CASE ILLUSTRATION 1

Ms. A, a 57-year-old woman, makes an appointment with a new clinician. She presents with a 10-year history of multiple unexplained symptoms. She has seen many physicians over the past decade, including several primary care physicians and numerous subspecialists. Her principal complaints today include abdominal pain, chest pain, headache, palpitations, fatigue, and intermittent dizziness. She brings a thick stack of records from some of her prior physicians. These records include multiple laboratory tests and diagnostic procedures, none of which has identified any cause for her symptoms.

Clinician: How can I help you today, Ms. A?

Patient (sighing): I don't know. A friend of mine saw you a few months ago and said you were very good. I hope you can help me. I've had these problems for years now, and no one seems to be able to figure them out. Maybe you can. I know there's something wrong. I've been so sick.

Clinician: Why don't you tell me about your symptoms?

Patient: Well, it all began about 10 years ago....

Clinicians are taught that patients will present with symptoms (subjective complaints) and signs (objective findings) that suggest the presence of a pathophysiologic process. They are trained to recognize these presentations and to diagnose the underlying disease so that they may institute the appropriate treatment. Satisfaction for the care provider arises from the ability to perform these tasks proficiently and to see the patient benefit. Patients typically come to the clinician's office seeking an explanation for and relief from their symptoms. Difficulties arise in the relationship when the patient presents with symptoms and the clinician can find no explanation for them. Symptoms that lack discernible physical pathology have been referred to variously as medically unexplained, functional, or somatization.

The term *somatization* (as used in this chapter) refers to the experience and reporting of physical symptoms that cause distress but lack a corresponding level of tissue damage or pathology and are linked to psychosocial stress. In contrast to this broad and inclusive view of the process, psychiatrists have developed strict diagnostic criteria that define several distinct disorders, which are collectively referred to as the *somatoform disorders*. As such, clinicians should be careful to distinguish between somatization, as defined above, and somatization disorder, which is one type of somatoform disorder. In general, these conditions are chronic and reflect an enduring way for the affected individuals to cope with psychosocial stressors. However, it is much more common in the primary care setting to encounter patients who have somatization symptoms but do not meet the full criteria for a psychiatric diagnosis. In many individuals, the somatization might be a transient phenomenon during a particularly stressful period such as divorce consisting of an exaggeration of common physical symptoms such as headache. In other patients, the process may be more persistent and the symptoms may be disabling. The latter group of patients can be particularly difficult for clinicians. Although their symptoms are suggestive of an underlying medical or neurologic condition, no such etiology is discovered upon appropriate diagnostic evaluation. Some patients do find reassurance in the provider's statements that no medical cause for their symptoms has been found. Other patients may become upset and accuse the clinician of not believing them or of being incompetent. Some patients demand continued diagnostic testing or referral to specialists. Further, the somatization symptoms do not respond to medical treatments that are prescribed for the disease suggested by the symptoms; this apparent therapeutic failure can lead to demands for more testing and requests for referral or different treatment regimens. The combination of increasing demands made by patients and their failure to respond to treatment can be very frustrating for the clinician.

HISTORICAL CONCEPTS

The existence of medically unexplained symptoms has been recognized throughout the history of medicine. Each historical period has described syndromes composed of such symptoms. The scientific knowledge and theories of the time have shaped the etiologies proposed for these disorders. The treatments advocated by medical practitioners were directed at attempting to correct the abnormality assumed to cause the illness. Each of these syndromes were recognised by medical authorities of the time to lack the demonstrable, pathologically defined tissue changes that characterize most medical conditions.

Prior to the Renaissance, medical theories were based on limited understanding of anatomy or physiology and, as a result, seem quite primitive to modern practitioners. Diseases lacking an apparent cause were believed to result from gross disturbances in the function and behavior of bodily organs. For example, hysteria was attributed to a "wandering uterus" as early as 1900 B.C. The treatments for hysteria flowed from this conceptual model and included the application of ointments to the labia or manipulation of the uterus to return it to its "natural" position. It was not until after the Renaissance that medical practitioners began to implicate disturbances of the nervous system in the genesis of medically unexplained symptoms. However, despite this change in the understanding of these disorders, the treatments utilized by clinicians did not become significantly more advanced. For instance, some practitioners in the latter half of the seventeenth century advocated hitting patients who had symptoms of hysteria with a stick.

By the end of the seventeenth century, and continuing into the eighteenth century, clinicians increasingly recognized the role psychological factors played in the origin and maintenance of somatization symptoms. More importantly, their treatments were beginning to reflect this appreciation. Medical authorities no longer focused exclusively on somatic therapies in the care of afflicted individuals. Instead, practitioners were encouraged to inquire about and demonstrate an active interest in their patients' mental state and welfare. Further, clinicians recognized the need to attempt to promote optimism about recovery in their patients.

In the nineteenth century, despite many advances in the understanding of pathology, there was an awareness that patients suffering from somatization syndromes lacked discernible anatomic abnormalities. As a result, the medically unexplained disorders were attributed to a subtle or "functional" pathologic disturbance. This explanatory model of illness was associated with a return to predominantly somatic interventions for treating the symptoms. However, some practitioners maintained that psychological treatments were important for managing these patients. These clinicians also recognized that unless the therapy was delivered in a way that was consistent with the patients' belief that their illness had a physical etiology, the intervention would be rejected.

At the turn of the twentieth century, an exclusively psychological model for these disorders was developed. The idea of a functional pathologic lesion of the nervous system was replaced with the concept of psychogenesis (i.e., the somatization symptoms arose from the mind). Somatization was viewed as the means by which unconscious mental conflicts could be manifested in the form of physical symptoms. As a result, mental health practitioners became responsible for the diagnosis and treatment of these disorders. However, the idea of physical complaints originating from the mind was also associated with implications that the symptoms were not "real." Further, many patients were not convinced of the value of this explanatory model.

Medically unexplained syndromes have persisted as clinical problems for practitioners. Patients often present with many symptoms that are not associated with abnormalities demonstrable by physical examination or laboratory or radiologic studies. The symptoms are often clustered together as syndromes with a variety of proposed etiologies including environmental exposures, infections (e.g., *Candida*, Epstein-Barr virus), or multiple chemical sensitivity. In addition, the broad range of advocacy and educational groups that try to promote various agendas with regard to the disorders can make the evaluation of these syndromes difficult.

CASE ILLUSTRATION 2

Mr. B is a 32-year-old man who presents to his primary care physician with complaints about being tired, weak, and nauseated. He also complains about intermittent abdominal and chest pain as well as a feeling of "dizziness." He noted that he lived in an old building and was worried he had been exposed to lead or some other toxin. His physical examination and laboratory values were all normal. However, he was not reassured by these results and his complaints persisted. He began to phone frequently with questions about chronic Candida infections, postviral syndromes, and multiple chemical sensitivity syndromes. His physician discussed each process with him and continued to perform appropriate medical evaluations of Mr. B's symptoms. The patient began to research his symptoms on the Internet. He was convinced that he suffered from sensitivity to multiple compounds in his home and became involved in a number of "online" support groups. He resisted other explanations for his symptoms and gradually became dissatisfied with his primary care physician and chose to seek care from "experts" on his disorder.

ETIOLOGY

Somatization can be understood from a number of different perspectives, each of which proposes a cause for the symptoms. However, because the precise cause of these symptoms is not known, none of the following models is fully explanatory. Rather, each model provides practitioners with insight into the genesis of these symptoms and suggests possible treatments as well. Unfortunately, each model is able to explain the symptoms of only a select group of patients. A more comprehensive understanding of patients comes from incorporating more than one perspective.

Neurobiological

According to the neurobiological perspective, the somatization symptoms result from dysfunction in the neuroendocrine systems responsible for processing peripheral sensory and central emotional information. As a result, the affected individual misinterprets normal bodily sensations or emotional signals as indicating a dangerous somatic process. The mechanism by which dysfunction in the nervous or endocrine systems results in the preoccupation with somatic symptoms is unknown. There is growing evidence of the role of such abnormalities in these disorders. For example, researchers have recently suggested that hypocortisolism plays a role in posttraumatic stress disorder, fibromyalgia, chronic fatigue syndrome, and some chronic pain disorders. Although hypocortisolism has been found in groups of individuals with the above diagnoses, the precise relationship between a deficiency of cortisol and the production of these symptoms is not understood. Additional research has examined the ability of individuals with somatization symptoms to habituate to novel stimuli. Individuals with somatization syndrome reported higher levels of tension in novel situations and were less likely to habituate to the situation over time. In addition, the affected individuals had a slower return to baseline heart rate upon leaving stressful situations. These studies suggest a relationship between physiologic mechanisms involved in adapting to novel or stressful stimuli and the apparently psychological symptoms of individuals with somatoform disorders.

Psychodynamic

According to psychodynamic theory, the somatoform symptoms arise solely from the mind. They are believed to represent the outward expression of internal psychological conflicts. In support of this theory, studies have demonstrated that individuals with somatization symptoms have higher rates of prior emotional and physical abuse, depression, and anxiety than nonaffected populations. It is hypothesized that abuse places individuals at risk for the types of internal conflicts that result in somatoform disorders. For example, women who have suffered sexual abuse in childhood have increased rates of chronic pelvic pain when compared with nonabused populations. Depression and anxiety may be both a product and a cause of these internal conflicts. Other findings suggest that childhood trauma in women is associated with higher levels of somatization, mediated by the development of insecure attachment. Attachment theory predicts how individuals' interaction within interpersonal relationships is influenced by early experiences with caregivers. A four-category model of attachment has been proposed which describes four different types of attachment: secure, preoccupied, dismissive, and fearful. Research has examined the role of attachment style and its link to somatization and subsequent health care utilization. In particular patients with preoccupied attachment, where the individual tends to idealize others, is less self-reliant and needs more reassurance. In contrast those with fearful attachment, where individuals may be less trusting of others as well as less self-reliant, are more likely to be high in somatic symptom reporting and are higher users of medical resources.

 CASE ILLUSTRATION 3

Mrs. G is a 51-year-old woman who had suffered from abdominal pain and progressive loss of function over the past 1 1/2 years. She had failed conservative management and was admitted to the hospital for an exploratory laparotomy. However, there were no organic findings to explain her symptoms. Psychiatric consultation was requested to evaluate for a psychological component to her pain. At evaluation, Mrs. G denied any psychological stressors, but her husband shared that around the time of the onset of her symptoms, Mrs. G's mother, with whom she is very close, had moved out of state to care for another daughter who had become ill. Mrs. G was referred for psychotherapy to explore this perceived loss and to explore alternatives for support. Over the course of this treatment, Mrs. G's abdominal pain resolved.

Cognitive-Behavioral

According to cognitive-behavioral theorists, somatoform symptoms arise from incorrect beliefs about bodily sensations, for example, believing that mild gastroesophageal reflux (or panic symptoms) represents myocardial ischemia. These misinterpretations, in turn, result in certain maladaptive behaviors, such as going from emergency room to emergency room seeking evaluation of the symptom and reassurance that the heart is functioning normally. These symptoms are reinforced by factors in the individual's environment such as the responses of other people to the perceived illness. For instance, the affected individual may be excused from work or social obligations. As an example of this process, some researchers proposed that learning about a disease may lead certain individuals to attribute previously overlooked symptoms to the illness. The affected person seeks out confirmatory evidence of additional symptoms that both reinforces the belief in the illness and amplifies the somatic symptoms. The person's self-validating review of symptoms may be augmented by contact with advocacy or educational groups that promote awareness of the disease. The processing of bodily information gradually becomes colored by the belief that the person has a disease and this can result in the affected individual embracing the sick role.

 CASE ILLUSTRATION 4

Mr. C is a 53-year-old man who worked as a manual laborer. He had always been in good health. One day, while lifting a particularly heavy item, he experienced pain on the right side of his chest. A colleague said that his father had a similar experience and died of a heart attack shortly thereafter. Mr. C became focused on the idea that he has heart disease and began to visit a number of emergency rooms, primary care physicians, and cardiologists. His evaluations were always completely negative. However, his concern persisted and he now presents to a new clinician.

Clinician: How may I help you Mr. C?

Patient: Doc, I know that I have a problem with my heart.

Clinician: What are your symptoms?

Patient: Well, I sometimes feel like I am more out of breath and if I lift heavy things I can feel some pain in the muscle over my chest. Other times, I start to breathe fast and my fingers get tingly. I've watched programs on TV and they say those are things that can mean I have angina. I've stopped working because I don't want to stress myself out and have a heart attack.

Sociocultural

According to the sociocultural perspective, individuals learn to express disease and distress in culturally sanctioned ways. In any culture, the expression of certain bodily symptoms and illness behaviors are encouraged while others are discouraged. Although somatization is a universal process, an individual's culture can affect the manner in which somatic representations of emotional distress are utilized. Further, this theory maintains that because the patient and the clinician are often from different backgrounds, the cultural interaction between the clinician and the patient is important. This interaction often determines how the patient's symptoms are experienced and interpreted. The clinician's task in these meetings is to correctly recognize which of the patient's somatic complaints represent cultural idioms of emotional distress. Mistakes in this assessment can lead to misdiagnosis, unnecessary medical treatment or evaluation, frustration on the part of the provider when the patient does not respond as expected, and dissatisfaction on the part of the patient.

A DIFFERENT PARADIGM

Although the theoretical models discussed above have evidence to support them and have been used as the basis for treatment in cases of somatization, there is another way to conceptualize somatization and the associated disorders. This view begins with the clinician abandoning the either-or categories of "physical" and "psychological." That dichotomous framework leads to interactions in which the patient can feel that the clinician is rejecting them and the reality of their symptoms by concluding, "The doctor's saying it's all in my head." Instead, the provider adopts a more comprehensive view of disease based on the biopsychosocial model of illness. In this paradigm, all illnesses are understood to have biological, psychological, and social dimensions.

The western medical model focuses on the biological aspects of disease, and often ignores the psychological and social facets of the patient's experience. In addition, this model, often very effective for understanding and treating acute disease processes, may fail to explain much of the complexity of chronic illness. For example, pain researchers have found that psychological factors are more important than physical factors in predicting future disability. Such research has led to the development of new treatment paradigms that recognize the interplay between the biological disease process and the psychosocial impact of symptoms. Treatment is focused on both relieving the biomedical symptoms and modifying the thoughts, feelings, and behavior associated with the pain and disability.

Using the more comprehensive biopsychosocial model, illness can be understood as occurring along a spectrum with disorders characterized by predominantly somatic problems at one end and disorders with predominantly psychological or social manifestations at the other end. Therefore, evaluation of patients should routinely include inquiries into both the physical and psychosocial dimensions of their illness. Using the biopsychosocial framework, the somatoform disorders can be viewed as arising when the patient neglects the psychosocial components of their illness and focuses on viewing the problem solely from a somatic perspective. For example, an individual with a history of chronic pelvic pain who has undergone multiple thorough evaluations with no anatomic etiology identified but who insists on repeating the workup rather than discussing psychosocial facets of the symptoms is likely to be experiencing somatization. Somatization itself is not a single entity. Like most illnesses it can be understood to have a continuum of expression. At one end is the transient, stress-related exaggeration of common physical symptoms; at the other end are the serious, persistent complaints that leave the patient disabled.

Patient: I don't know. Maybe I am crazy . . . that's what everyone else seems to think.

Clinician: Let me assure you that you're not crazy. I hear your concern. Why don't we talk about this a little bit?

Patient: Well, a friend of mine had a disease called Cushing's. Do you think I might have that?

Clinician: That's a good question. There are a great many diseases that can present with symptoms like yours. I want you to know that as I've listened to you and examined you, I've tried to think of rare diseases. I don't believe any of them are very likely, especially since you've had your symptoms for so long. I do want to be honest with you, though. There's no way to be absolutely certain. There are so many different diseases that it would be impossible to get tested for all of them. Let's get a few laboratory tests done, though. If they're normal, let's not do any more tests, but I'll keep an open mind as to these possibilities as we get to know each other during the course of the next few months. If you develop symptoms later that suggest one of these rare diseases to me, I'll certainly order more tests. How does that sound to you?

Patient: Okay, that sounds like it could work.

Clinician: Are there other things going on that add stress to your life?

Patient: Now that you mention it, there are some stressful things going on....

In this brief dialogue the practitioner acknowledges uncertainty while communicating a sense of honesty and trustworthiness. By reinforcing the continuity of the relationship and the willingness to entertain different possibilities in the future, the provider helps the patient feel cared for without the need for multiple, and most likely unnecessary, diagnostic tests. Moreover, the clinician has helped the patient to entertain the idea of a connection between psychosocial and somatic factors in illness.

PREVALENCE

Somatization is frequently encountered in primary care clinics. Epidemiologic studies have demonstrated that 25–35% of the patients in primary care settings will meet criteria for a recognized psychiatric disorder with the most common disorders being anxiety or depression. In addition, research has shown that 50–80% of patients who meet criteria for an anxiety or depressive disorder initially present to health care providers with physical symptoms. Other studies have found that somatoform disorders can be diagnosed in up to 22% of patients in primary care outpatient clinics. One study found that no organic cause was found in 80% of primary care visits scheduled for the evaluation of common symptoms such as dizziness, chest pain, and fatigue. Similarly, studies of medical inpatients have found that between 20% and 40% of these individuals meet the criteria for a coexisting mental disorder. A recent study found that somatoform disorders were the most common psychiatric diagnoses in a population of medical inpatients. These results indicate that the phenomenon of somatization, as well as more rigorously defined somatoform disorders, is very common among patients presenting for medical services.

IMPACT & OUTCOMES

Somatization is not only common; it is also an expensive problem. One study estimated that patients with somatization disorder generate medical costs nine times those of the average medical patient. Other work has calculated total annual health care costs attributable to somatization in the United States to be over $250 billion, even after adjusting for comorbid psychiatric disorders. In addition, these patients often demand a great deal of time and attention and yet they frequently do not respond to the prescribed treatment. This can eventually lead to frustration for the practitioner and even feelings of incompetence or inadequacy. The patients' seemingly unending complaints can lead to feelings of anger at the individual or dread when their name appears on the appointment list. Thus, patients with somatization symptoms not only tax the health care system by disproportionately utilizing limited resources, but also burden health care providers who can feel overwhelmed by the needs of these individuals.

Research has consistently demonstrated that individuals who present with somatization symptoms have worse outcomes in regard to health status, physical functioning, and psychological well-being than those patients who do not manifest these symptoms. Patients with somatization symptoms have ongoing difficulties not only with their somatic complaints and concerns about physical illness, but also with emotional and social impairment and reduced quality of life. It is important to accurately diagnose these individuals so that appropriate management can be instituted.

DIFFERENTIAL DIAGNOSIS

Patients with somatization symptoms should be evaluated for a biomedical etiology. The nature of the evaluation will depend on the patients' medical history, presenting symptoms, and age. In evaluating patients, it is important to remember that the onset of multiple physical symptoms late in life is almost always due to a general medical condition; somatoform disorders generally start decades earlier.

The American Psychiatric Association *Diagnostic and Statistical Manual of Mental Disorders*, fourth edition, *Text Revision* (*DSM-IV-TR*) classifies a number of syndromes together under the heading of "Somatoform Disorders." This classification is based on the common feature that the affected individuals report symptoms suggestive of a general medical condition but appropriate workup either fails to reveal such a condition or, if the condition is present, does not explain the severity of the patient's complaints. In addition, the somatic complaints in these disorders are produced unconsciously and are not under the voluntary control of the patient (Table 25-1).

A number of other psychiatric disorders have been associated with somatization. These disorders should be considered when evaluating a patient who appears to have somatization symptoms. For example, panic attacks often involve symptoms in multiple organ systems such as palpitations, nausea, shortness of breath, and tingling in the extremities. Unlike symptoms of somatoform disorders, however, the symptoms of this disorder have an abrupt onset and are limited to the panic attack episodes. A careful history can often elicit this time course and prove helpful in making the diagnosis. Patients with generalized anxiety disorder may also present with multiple somatic complaints. Excessive worrying about multiple domains in life is the key feature of this disorder and helps to separate it from the somatoform disorders. Depressed patients often present to medical practitioners with unexplained physical symptoms, especially headache, pain, and gastrointestinal problems. In contrast to the somatic symptoms of

Table 25-1. Somatoform disorders.

- *Somatization disorder*: Begins before age 30, endures for many years, and involves a combination of pain, gastrointestinal, sexual, and pseudoneurologic symptoms. The defining feature of somatization disorder is the persistence of multiple system symptoms without the development of the structural abnormalities, laboratory abnormalities, or physical findings that are characteristic of the general medical condition suggested by the symptoms.
- *Undifferentiated somatoform disorder*: Characterized by the presence of one or more physical complaints that persist for 6 months or longer and cannot be explained by any known substance or general medical condition or are grossly out of proportion to what would be expected by history, physical examination, or laboratory evaluation.
- *Conversion disorder*: Characterized by the presence of symptoms or deficits affecting voluntary motor or sensory function that suggest a neurologic or other general medical condition. However, no underlying condition can be identified to explain the symptoms. It is important to emphasize that because many general medical etiologies for apparent conversion syndromes take years to become evident, the diagnosis should be viewed as provisional. In the past, studies have shown that up to 50% of patients with a presumed conversion disorder are later found to have a general medical condition. However, more recent studies suggest that this percentage is now less than 25%, perhaps because of improved diagnostic techniques and understanding of this disorder.
- *Pain disorder with psychological factors*: Characterized by pain in one or more anatomic sites as the focus of clinical attention. Psychological factors are judged to have an important role in the onset, severity, exacerbation, and maintenance of the pain.
- *Hypochondriasis*: Characterized by the preoccupation with or fear of having a serious disease based on the individual's misinterpretation of bodily symptoms.
- *Body dysmorphic disorder*: Characterized by preoccupation with an imagined or exaggerated defect in the individual's physical appearance.
- *Somatoform disorder not otherwise specified*: Refers to any disorder with somatoform symptoms that does not meet the criteria for any of the other more specific somatoform disorders (e.g., pseudocyesis—the false belief that one is pregnant often accompanied by signs of pregnancy such as missed menstrual periods and abdominal distention).

the chronic somatoform disorders, the physical complaints in depression exist only in the presence of the mood symptoms. In such cases, the depression and the somatic complaints resolve contemporaneously. Studies have demonstrated a high level of comorbidity between depression and somatoform disorders, so clinically both disorders may be present. Patients with obsessive-compulsive disorder whose beliefs focus on bodily functions or organs can appear to be suffering from a somatoform disorder. The key to diagnosis is a careful history about the presence of the obsessions and compulsions. Patients with psychotic disorders, such as schizophrenia, may also present with multiple somatic complaints. In contrast to the concerns in the somatoform disorders, psychotic symptoms tend to be bizarre or completely irrational (e.g., "My insides are rotting" or "I have pain from the dinosaur eggs in my stomach").

In contrast to the psychiatric disorders described above, there are conditions in which the individual's symptoms are consciously produced. Factitious disorders are diagnosed when the clinician determines that the symptoms are consciously or voluntarily fabricated or exaggerated. However, in these individuals there is no discernible external incentive to produce the symptoms such as financial compensation. The patient's only apparent goal is to assume the sick role. Malingering, on the other hand, is diagnosed when the clinician determines that the individual has consciously produced the symptoms for an apparent external gain, such as obtaining a monetary award, acquiring drugs, or avoiding a noxious situation such as military duty or incarceration. Malingering is not considered a mental disorder (Table 25-2).

EVALUATION

A stepwise, evidence-based approach is invaluable to the evaluation of patients with suspected somatization symptoms. This framework can help the clinician avoid

Table 25-2. Abnormal illness-affirming states.

Symptom	Production	Motivation
Malingering	Conscious	Conscious
Factitious disorder	Conscious	Unconscious
Somatization	Unconscious	Unconscious
Hypochondriasis	Unconscious	Unconscious
Pain disorder	Unconscious	Unconscious
Conversion disorder	Unconscious	Unconscious
Body dysmorphic disorder	Unconscious	Unconscious

Source: Data from Eisendrath SJ, Lichtmacher J. Psychiatric disorders. In: McPhee S, Tierney LM, Papadakis MA, et al., eds. *Current Medical Diagnosis and Treatment 2007.* New York, NY: Lange/McGraw-Hill, 2006:1072–1074.

unnecessary and costly diagnostic procedures or referrals to specialists. In addition, it can spare the patient potential iatrogenic complications from any of the evaluation procedures. The first step in evaluating the patient with multiple somatic complaints is a detailed and thorough history of the presenting problem. The clinician should, of course, include review of pertinent medical records in the history-gathering phase of the evaluation. The practitioner should then perform appropriate physical and neurologic examinations. The provider may then consider what tests are indicated to confirm the diagnosis or rule out a predominantly biomedical disease based on the information obtained. The urge to order a wide variety of tests should be resisted and a rational determination of the patient's needs should be made. Obtaining an informal consultation from a colleague can be useful in appropriately evaluating these individuals.

Once the provider determines that the patient's physical symptoms are not explained by any underlying pathologic abnormalities, the focus can turn to more predominantly psychological disorders. The assessment of psychiatric disorders can be accomplished through the use of a careful clinical interview or a semistructured interview tool or by referral to a mental health clinician. The clinical interview can be helpful in establishing the presence of psychiatric illness as well as in communicating to the patient that the clinician is taking an active interest in the individual's life. Instruments such as the PRIME-MD (Primary Care Evaluation of Mental Disorders), which are designed for use in primary care settings, can help the provider diagnose somatoform disorders as well as depression, anxiety, eating disorders, and substance abuse. Such instruments have the advantages of rapid administration and established validity. The Patient Health Questionnaire (PHQ) is a self-administered scale that is a version of the PRIME-MD that has also been used in primary care settings to diagnose common mental disorders. The PHQ-15 is a subscale of the PHQ that assesses somatization symptoms, and can be used to monitor symptom severity as well as symptom improvement. Such instruments are useful as many patients refuse referral to a mental health specialist because they fear that their complaints are being dismissed. Above all, when evaluating a patient the clinician should recognize and articulate the interplay between the physical and psychosocial realms.

> **Clinician:** Today I would like to talk about how you are doing.

> **Patient:** Well, my chest has been hurting again and I have been really worn down.

> **Clinician:** (after several pertinent questions about the symptoms) It sounds like this is the same pain you've had before, although I do understand that

it's a little worse. I wonder if there is anything else that has changed in your life recently besides the intensity of the pain?

Patient: Nothing . . . really. Well my wife and I are arguing about the mortgage again.

Clinician: Oh, I remember that's been a problem before when you've been having pain.

Patient: Yeah. I just get tired of her nagging and the stress of barely making ends meet.

Clinician: I think its possible that the stress you've been under may be taking its toll on your body and your sense of well-being.

TREATMENT

The treatment strategies to be described are not specific to a certain somatoform diagnosis. It is less important in most cases to make a specific psychiatric diagnosis of a somatoform disorder than it is to recognize that the patient's symptoms represent somatization. However, if a psychiatric disorder such as anxiety, depression, or psychosis is identified, specific treatments for the identified disorder should be utilized.

Treatments Designed for Primary Care Providers

Nonsomatic therapies are the primary treatments for the somatoform disorders. Patients with somatization symptoms most often present to the primary care setting and are resistant to psychiatric referrals. Techniques are required that are effective, acceptable to primary care clinicians, and useful in busy primary care settings. Finally, the intervention must be congruent with patients' beliefs about the nature of their illness so that they are willing to engage in the treatment.

The most important aspect of managing patients with somatization symptoms is the development of an empathic, trusting relationship. Although it is not easy to form such a relationship with these individuals, establishing a therapeutic alliance is critical to both diagnosis and treatment. It can be helpful to remember that patients with somatization are reacting in the best and, without treatment, only way available to them. Before considering specific therapies for these individuals, it is useful to consider basic techniques for interacting with them.

The practitioner should never challenge the reality of the patient's physical symptoms. Somatization is an unconscious process and therefore the somatic complaints are very real to the patient. Further, because most of the symptoms are subjective in nature, there is no means to

verify or dispute them. It can be helpful to explicitly acknowledge the patient's suffering to bolster the therapeutic relationship.

Clinician: I can see how much you've suffered with all of these symptoms.

Patient: You're the only one who seems to understand that.

Medical providers should avoid trying to convince the patient that the symptoms are psychological in origin. They should also avoid the use of psychological labels (e.g., depression, anxiety). Instead, they should try to use easily understandable and mutually acceptable language to discuss symptoms. Each appointment should begin with a discussion of the somatic complaint. The provider can then use descriptive physiologic explanations, which are more acceptable to these individuals, to describe the symptoms (e.g., "abnormally tense muscles in your neck go into painful spasm"). It is important to note that while such descriptors imply a physiologic component to the symptoms, they do not provide an etiology. Over time (often months or years), the patient and clinician may begin to explore possible explanations for the symptoms that integrate somatic and psychosocial aspects of the problem.

Patient: I just don't get why my neck keeps getting spasms.

Clinician: I have noticed that sometimes you mention this happening after your supervisor criticizes you. Sometimes our muscles react to emotions like anger or stress by tightening up. When this becomes extreme, they can spasm.

Patient: You know that makes some sense. When he comes around I can feel myself grit my teeth and begin to feel stiff.

Another management suggestion is to have the provider conduct an evaluation in an appropriate manner to rule out a somatic cause of the symptoms. Once somatization is identified, the clinician continues to schedule the individual for brief, regularly spaced intervals. These visits are time contingent; patients need not have new symptoms to be able to meet regularly with their medical practitioner. These visits allow for an initial brief check-in regarding the somatic symptoms followed by discussions of events in the patient's life and the patient's emotional well-being and relationships. The clinician can adopt a conservative approach toward new treatments or diagnostic workups when the patient presents with new or worsening symptoms. The goal is to focus the patient on behaviors promoting well-being and to help them discuss the psychosocial aspects of their life and illness. They are discouraged from pursuing new therapies or evaluations for their symptoms. At the same time, they are shown that the provider is taking an active interest in them. Moreover, they learn that they will receive this care and attention even without new symptoms or exacerbations of existing symptoms. The clinician may also ask the patient when they want to return for the next visit. This provides the patient with a sense of control and over time many patients will suggest lengthening the interval between appointments.

Establishing appropriate goals is also important when working with these patients. These disorders, like any chronic disease, are often not curable. However, clinicians often hope that another medication will relieve the symptoms or that one more diagnostic procedure will elucidate the cause of the patient's problem. However, these beliefs can lead to disappointment for both the patient and the clinician. Rather than aiming for complete resolution of the symptoms, it is better to set more realistic goals. For the primary care practitioner, these might include reducing the number of phone calls and visits with new symptoms, the number of requests for medications or referrals to specialists, and the number of emergency room visits. For patients, these goals might include an increased sense of control in their lives, improved social functioning, and better coping with day-to-day symptoms.

> **Clinician:** Today I would like to talk about what we should expect from each other in this relationship. From your perspective, I suspect that the best thing I could do would be to figure out what's causing these symptoms and make them go away completely. Given all of your years of suffering and the many doctors you've seen and the limited success of treatments so far, it might be more realistic for us not to focus so much on pursuing a cure but to look at how to improve how you feel and maximize your functioning. What do you think?

> **Patient:** Well, of course I was hoping that you could find a cure. So—does this mean that you can't help me?

> **Clinician:** No, I didn't mean to imply that. I do think I can help. First, I'd like to work on helping you learn to cope more effectively with your symptoms. We could also work to improve how you function from day to day. Whether or not we are immediately successful, I'm committed to helping you in the best way I can.

A novel treatment for somatoform disorders involves the use of a "written self-disclosure protocol." This therapy involves having the patient with somatoform symptoms periodically write in a journal format. The clinician convinces the patient to spend 20 minutes one time per week at home writing about distressing experiences in their lives. They are specifically encouraged to think about experiences involving relationships with others. The patients are also instructed to write about how these experiences have affected them in the past and how they may continue to affect them in the future. The journal may be shared with others if the patient wishes, but it does not have to be shared to have a benefit. This technique has been found to be acceptable by both patients and providers. It has also been found to be helpful, time effective, and cost effective. The patients do the writing outside of the office and have demonstrated decreases in health care utilization.

Another recently developed technique for treating patients with somatization symptoms in the primary care setting is designed to help general practitioners teach these patients to reattribute and relate physical symptoms to psychosocial problems. The clinician is encouraged to take a history of the patient's illness including related physical, mood, and social factors. The clinician then broadens the view of the problem and the necessary treatment by reframing the complaint using the biopsychosocial information provided by the patient. The practitioner then links the patient's distress and the physical complaint using a coherent explanation of how psychosocial factors can give rise to physical symptoms. This intervention model has been found to be both cost effective and clinically effective.

Despite all of these interventions, it may be necessary to refer the patient to a mental health specialist. Many individuals with somatization will resist such a referral. Although this reluctance on the patient's part can be frustrating, the primary care provider should remember that many of these patients have experienced such referral as the first step in the termination of their relationship with a health care provider. The primary care clinician can address this concern by making a follow-up appointment with the patient prior to the referral. Once the continuity of the relationship is ensured, the referral can be discussed. Further, a consultation model in which the patient is asked to see the mental health provider for one or a few visits in order to "advise and help the primary care provider do a better job" is often more acceptable to patients than a referral for ongoing treatment. The consultation can be useful in confirming diagnosis or in providing advice on the use of psychotropic medications.

> **Clinician:** I'd like to see you in a month. In the meantime, I'd like you to consider seeing Dr. R, the psychiatrist we've talked about. I know that you don't think that your chest pain is caused by your depression. But we've both agreed to try to treat the depression. I still don't know if we've found the right antidepressant, and I'd really value Dr. R's opinion. What do you think?

Psychotherapy

Cognitive-Behavioral Therapy (CBT) has been studied as a means of addressing medically unexplained somatic symptoms. This technique is based on the theory that incorrect beliefs about bodily functioning and related dysfunctional behaviors underlie these symptoms. The first task in therapy is to identify these beliefs and behaviors. Next, the patient is encouraged to challenge the beliefs and is taught to adopt more accurate ideas about bodily functioning. This change is paired with adoption of more appropriate behaviors. In a recent, randomized, controlled trial, investigators compared the outcomes of 10 sessions of CBT with standard medical care augmented by psychiatric consultation in two groups of patients with somatization disorder. After 15 weeks, researchers found that the group that received CBT had significantly reduced somatization symptoms as well as greater improvements in self-reported functioning and greater decreases in medical costs compared to the standard medical treatment group. This research suggests that CBT can be effective in patients with somatoform and related disorders.

Psychodynamic psychotherapy is based on the assumption that the individual is experiencing internal emotional conflicts and that the associated emotions cannot be expressed. As a result, the conflict is manifested through somatic symptoms. The therapy focuses on attempting to uncover these conflicts and having the patient express them openly in the therapy sessions. As the patient does this work, the somatic symptoms become unnecessary and resolve. Unfortunately, most somatizing patients are not enthusiastic about exploring unconscious conflicts. In general, the psychodynamic perspective is a long-term, time-intensive approach that requires a referral to a specialist and a commitment by the patient.

In family-oriented approaches to therapy, therapists must integrate the biological and psychosocial aspects of the patient's illness. The care provider must collaborate with the patient and the patient's family in treating the illness. Further, the clinician must demonstrate true interest in and curiosity about the patient's symptoms, family, relationships, and life. These therapies attempt to help the patients and their families break down the distinction between physical and psychological and move their thinking from "either-or" (e.g., it is either a physical problem or a mental problem) to "both-and" (e.g., the problem has both physical and mental facets). Relational therapists argue that effective therapy involves validating the illness, involving the family, working closely with the health care team, and enhancing the patient's curiosity about symptoms. They also emphasize demonstrating interest in the patient's somatic symptoms, helping the patient to see the relationship between the somatic symptoms and psychosocial stressors, and

Table 25-3. Management of somatization.

Interventions
1. Take a detailed history, perform a physical examination, and order appropriate diagnostic studies.
2. Screen individuals with multiple somatic complaints for psychiatric disorders.
3. Integrate the patient's physical and psychosocial concerns by inquiring not only about somatic symptoms but also about other events in the person's life.
4. Develop an empathic relationship.
5. Never challenge the validity of the patient's somatic symptoms.
6. Do not utilize psychological labels for the patient's symptoms.
7. Schedule the patient for appointments at regular intervals.
8. Establish realistic expectations.
9. Care for yourself.

using physical interventions (e.g., biofeedback and relaxation techniques) to form an alliance with the patient to deal with the illness.

Medication

Data on the efficacy of using medications to treat somatoform disorders are limited to studies in certain disorders. In particular, studies have shown in patients with body dysmorphic disorder, agents which enhance serotonergic transmission such as fluoxetine, citalopram, escitalopram, and fluvoxamine, appear to reduce somatization symptoms in addition to improving comorbid depression and anxiety. There is also evidence that St. John's wort is effective in treating somatoform disorders. A randomized, double-blind placebo-controlled trial in 184 subjects with somatization disorder, undifferentiated somatoform disorder, and somatoform autonomic dysfunction were given either 300 mg of St. John's wort twice daily or placebo. After 6 weeks, the group given St. John's wort demonstrated significantly superior improvements in all outcome measures, including somatization symptoms and overall self-assessment of improvement.

A summary of recommendations for managing patients with somatization symptoms is found in Table 25-3.

CLINICIAN–PATIENT RELATIONSHIP

Caring for individuals with somatoform disorders is difficult. The patients present with symptoms suggestive of a medical or neurologic illness and require an appropriate evaluation. However, at the completion of the evaluation the clinician is faced with an individual who, by definition, does not have a physical condition or who has a condition that cannot account for the level of symptoms or disability that the patient experiences. However, the patients view the symptoms as somatic and strenuously resist the idea that the symptoms have a psychological component. As a result, neither party is satisfied with the interaction.

Why is dealing with patients who experience somatoform disorders so difficult? One theory is that clinicians use terminology that was developed to promote communication with other health care providers. It is not meant to provide the patient with an explanation of or validation of their illness experience. Health providers focus on understanding the pathophysiology of disease in a scientific manner. Laypersons have different explanatory models of disease, and therefore, when they present to the clinician's office they may already have a theory about the origin of their symptoms. In the case of patients with somatization, this theory involves a physical cause. In contrast, the practitioner may feel that a physical cause for the symptoms is less likely than a psychological etiology. As a result, the patient and clinician possess models of illness that are not only competing but also conflicting. To work effectively with the patient, the provider must reconcile these theories.

> **Patient:** So you think I have "depression"? How is that causing me to be tired all the time? I don't understand how you can say that. I don't cry and I don't feel sad.
>
> **Clinician:** Depression is not just feeling sad. It is a medical illness, just like diabetes or epilepsy. It is caused by an imbalance in the chemicals in the brain that help the brain cells communicate with each other. When those chemicals, or transmitters, are out of balance the brain does not function correctly and people develop symptoms such as fatigue, sadness, changes in sleep and appetite, and changes in their ability to concentrate.
>
> **Patient:** Well what can be done?
>
> **Clinician:** The good news is there are a number of treatments. Medications can be very helpful by directly affecting the balance of the transmitters. Other treatments involve working with someone to help you train your brain to function better without medications.

It seems, then, that working with these patients is difficult because they do not share the clinician's explanatory models and they resist giving up their own model of illness. When providers are able to explain the patient's symptoms in a way that provides a holistic and empowering perspective, they are viewed as a positive and helpful influence. As a result, the patient is satisfied, an alliance is formed to address the symptoms in a collaborative manner, and the practitioner may feel more positive about the patient.

Research has also focused on the reasons clinicians experience certain patients as difficult. Patients who are rated as difficult by health providers have twice the prevalence of psychiatric disorders. Further, the presence of more physical symptoms, both those judged to result from medical causes and those judged to be somatoform in origin, contributes to the sense that the patient is difficult. In addition, clinicians expect physical symptoms to be associated with medical diagnoses and the lack of such an association leads to frustration over the "vagueness" of the symptoms and their own inability to make a diagnosis. Patients may have reasons for "holding onto" the symptoms. The assumption of the sick role may confer some benefits, through changes in social and family systems that are difficult for the provider to discern or understand. The practitioner may feel that the patient is consciously faking symptoms. Clinicians should attempt to understand the role that the symptoms play in the patient's family and social systems to gain insight into why the symptoms persist despite the lack of a somatic etiology.

CARING FOR THE CLINICIAN

The care of patients with somatoform symptoms is a draining experience and the clinician must take care not to burn out. The patient's unending physical concerns, resistance to treatment, and complaints that the clinician is not doing enough can easily overwhelm the provider. The practitioner is well advised to remember that these are chronic disorders. As a consequence, it can be helpful to set reasonable goals for treatment such as "care and not cure." Clinicians must remember that they can provide support and effective treatment but that the patient will likely have some residual symptoms. The practitioner should feel comfortable setting limits with their somatizing patients. Once the clinician and patient have committed to regular follow-up appointments, it is appropriate to set limits on calls and drop-in visits. For example, the patient can be asked to reserve all but emergency complaints for the regular visits. If the patient calls between scheduled sessions, the discussion should be limited to ascertaining that there is no emergency. If there is none, then the patient can be gently urged to defer further discussion until the next visit.

Outside of work, practitioners should take time for exercise, family, friends, and other interests. They may also wish to discuss difficult cases with colleagues to manage the powerful feelings these patients can elicit. In this way, they can maintain a healthy lifestyle and balance in their life. Clinicians must remember that the illness belongs to the patient and not to them. They must not allow the patient's frustration or demands make them forget this. The combination of empathic listening, conservative (but appropriate) evaluation, and gentle limit setting can not only benefit these patients, but also improve the primary care provider's satisfaction with these relationships.

SUGGESTED READINGS

Allen LA, Woolfolk RL, Escobar JI, et al. Cognitive-behavioral therapy for somatization disorder: a randomized controlled trial. *Arch Intern Med* 2006;166:512–518. PMID: 16864762.

Barsky AJ, Ahern DK. Cognitive behavior therapy for hypochondriasis: a randomized controlled trial. *JAMA* 2004;291:1464–1470. PMID: 15039413.

Duddu V, Isaac MK, Chaturvedi SK. Somatization, somatosensory amplification, attribution styles and illness behavior: a review. *Int Rev Psychiatry* 2006;18:25–33. PMID: 16451877.

Heinrich TW. Medically unexplained symptoms and the concept of somatization. *WMJ* 2004;103:83–87. PMID: 15622826.

Kroenke K, Spitzer RL, Williams JB. The PHQ-15: validity of a new measure for evaluating the severity of somatic symptoms. *Psychosom Med* 2002;64:258–266. PMID: 11914441.

Mai F. Somatization disorder: a practical review. *Can J Psychiatry* 2004;49:652–662. PMID: 15560311.

Muller T, Mannel M, Murck H, et al. Treatment of somatoform disorders with St. John's wort: a randomized, double-blind and placebo-controlled trial. *Psychosom Med* 2004;66:538–547. PMID: 15272100.

Rief W, Barsky AJ. Psychobiological perspectives on somatoform disorders. *Psychoneuroendocrinology* 2005;30:996–1002. PMID: 15958280.

Rosendal M, Olesen F, Fink P. Management of medically unexplained symptoms. *BMJ* 2005;330:4–5. PMID: 15626783.

Waldinger RJ, Schulz MS, Barsky AJ, et al. Mapping the road from childhood trauma to adult somatization: the role of attachment. *Psychosom Med* 2006;68:129–135. PMID: 16449423.

Personality Disorders

26

John Q. Young, MD, MPP

INTRODUCTION

Establishing successful relationships with patients who are suffering from personality disorders can be quite challenging for health care providers, yet these patients are common in medical practice. Complications associated with patients with comorbid personality disorders are myriad, including suboptimal utilization of medical care (over- and under-use), difficulty adhering to treatment plans, and more problematic relationships with clinicians. In addition, these patients are more likely to be hospitalized. An understanding of personality disorders allows physicians to anticipate the challenging interpersonal and behavioral problems that can arise in working with these patients and can help physicians work through the negative emotions that working with such patients may arouse. This facilitates the development and implementation of appropriate treatment plans, improved alliance between patient and clinician, and better outcomes.

The current edition of the American Psychiatric Association *Diagnostic and Statistical Manual of Mental Disorders*, 4th edition, *Text Revision (DSM-IV-TR)* defines personality disorder as:

> *an enduring pattern of inner experience and behavior that deviates markedly from the expectations of the individual's culture, is pervasive and inflexible, has an onset in adolescence or early adulthood, is stable over time, and leads to distress or impairment.*

People suffering from personality disorders have dysfunctional beliefs about self and others, and impaired capacity to establish and maintain relationships with others, function at work, and experience pleasure in life. These patients have difficulty negotiating complex situations and coping with stress and anxiety. The sick role and the demands of medical care can be particularly problematic for them. The stress of illness is often extreme and sets into motion defensive and inflexible emotional processes, cognitions, and behaviors—with negative consequences for their medical treatment. In addition, these patients' difficulties in relating to others manifest themselves in the doctor–patient relationship. They may be quite demanding or disrespectful of the needs of others, or they may experience such anxiety when they need to trust or confide in others that they avoid building relationships.

Personality theorists have long debated how best to understand and classify personality disorders. The debate has centered on two models. The **categorical model**, adopted by *DSM-IV*, views personality disorders as entities that are distinct from one another—that is, classified in separate categories—and also distinct from normalcy. This model blends more easily with traditional medical diagnosis than does the **dimensional model**, which views personality disorders as entities that overlap each other and that are not distinct from normalcy, so that the maladaptive traits of patients with personality disorders represent normal traits that are exaggerated.

In fact, both models hold some truth. Some personality disorders, such as schizotypal and paranoid, may belong to a spectrum of illness that includes psychotic Axis I disorders and are thus better explained by a categorical model. Other personality disorders, such as histrionic and obsessive-compulsive personality, may depict exaggerated normal traits, reinforcing the concept of a dimensional model.

DIAGNOSTIC CLASSIFICATION OF PERSONALITY DISORDERS

DSM-IV classifies personality disorders on a separate axis, Axis II, and groups them into three clusters based on descriptive similarities. Cluster A includes paranoid, schizoid, and schizotypal personality disorders—individuals who often appear odd or eccentric; cluster B includes antisocial, borderline, histrionic, and narcissistic personality disorders—individuals who often appear dramatic, emotional, or erratic; and cluster C includes avoidant, dependent, and obsessive-compulsive personality disorders—individuals who often appear anxious or fearful. Given the unique nature of any individual personality, a patient can exhibit traits of two or more personality disorders, or meet the full diagnostic criteria for more than one disorder. Hence, co-occurrence is very common. National survey data suggest that approximately 15% of the general population have at least one personality disorder. Table 26-1 indicates the prevalence of each personality disorder within the general U.S. population. It is important to remember that the prevalence is higher in medical patients.

Diagnosing a personality disorder can be difficult. To make an accurate diagnosis, it is usually necessary for the physician to get to know the patient over time, to learn how the patient reacts and relates to people in other situations, and to obtain collateral information from family and friends. Clinicians should attend to three key issues.

First, it is important to differentiate a true personality disorder from personality traits that become exaggerated under stress. The stress of illness often causes a patient to behave in maladaptive ways; because of this, many patients, at one time or another, seem to have a personality disorder. Patients who do not suffer from a true personality disorder, however, are usually capable of more adaptive functioning. The maladaptive behavior itself is less "enduring" and "engrained" and more situational and modifiable. In these cases, the physician can successfully intervene by supporting and strengthening these patients' own natural coping skills.

Second, it is also important to differentiate personality disorders from such Axis I disorders as major depression or generalized anxiety disorder. For example, patients with panic disorder may—out of sheer terror—become extremely dependent on their physician. If their panic disorder is diagnosed and treated, they may reveal an underlying independent and self-sufficient personality. Similarly, a patient's grandiosity and arrogance may stem largely from a bipolar mania rather than a narcissistic personality disorder. When patients who do have a personality disorder are evaluated, looking for Axis I disorders is particularly important as the latter are more frequent and difficult to treat if patients actually have a personality disorder. Treating an episode of major depression in a patient with borderline personality disorder, however, can alleviate suffering and lead to better coping with illness.

Third, it is important to distinguish personality disorders from personality changes caused by general medical conditions, such as head trauma, stroke, epilepsy, or endocrine disorders. Patients with one of these problems may exhibit many of the characteristics of a personality disorder. These behaviors can be distinguished from a true personality disorder, however, in that they typically represent a change from baseline personality characteristics. Medical conditions such as these at times may also exacerbate preexisting personality traits (e.g., obsessive mannerisms). Treatment of the underlying medical problem may bring about reversal of the personality changes.

Finally, personality disorder diagnoses, like other mental disorder diagnoses, are often misunderstood and may serve to stigmatize the patient. These diagnoses should therefore be made carefully, deferred in cases of uncertainty, and noted in medical records and correspondence only when their notation is likely to be helpful in enhancing patient care.

Doctor–Patient Relationship Issues

The primary care provider may find many challenges in working with patients with personality disorders. Personality disorders often significantly impair the quality of interpersonal relationships. Because the doctor–patient relationship requires effective communication about important health issues of a personal nature, tensions and at times overt conflict may develop between patients with personality disorders and their providers. These tensions may also affect other members of the

Table 26-1. DSM-IV personality disorders and their prevalence.

Cluster	Personality Disorder	Discriminating Feature	Prevalence in General Population
A: odd or eccentric	Paranoid	Suspicious	4%
	Schizoid	Socially indifferent	3.1%
	Schizotypal	Eccentric	3%
	Antisocial	Disagreeable	3.6%
B: dramatic, emotional, or erratic	Borderline	Unstable	2%
	Histrionic	Attention seeking	1.8%
	Narcissistic	Self-centered	0.5%
C: anxious or fearful	Avoidant	Inhibited	2.4%
	Dependent	Submissive	0.49%
	Obsessive-compulsive	Perfectionistic	7.9%

health care team and may be especially pronounced in the context of acute illness or crisis situations. In fact, the first diagnostic clues suggesting personality dysfunction or disorder may appear as difficulties in the doctor–patient relationship.

For patients with personality disorders, physical illness can cause exaggerated degrees of emotional distress, not always expressed to the provider. Although some patients do tell their providers about their emotional distress, others may instead manifest distress as noncompliance with the agreed-upon plan of evaluation or treatment or as changed, unexpected, or undesirable behavior (as judged by the physician) toward the physician.

In response to patients' actions or statements, physicians may have a significant emotional reaction to the patients and may change their behavior toward them. Even when they experience no subjective distress from a medical condition or the doctor–patient relationship, patients with personality dysfunction may have such aberrant expectations of others that their statements or behaviors are troubling or burdensome to the physician. Physicians must be aware of their own emotional responses to such patients so as to avoid reacting inappropriately. Physicians who deny their negative feelings toward the patients may fail to recognize a personality disorder or other psychiatric diagnosis, or fail to address the diagnostic and treatment needs of the patient with the necessary vigor and thoroughness. When clinicians recognize and deal with their negative feelings, they are better able to make thoughtful and appropriate responses to these patients' symptoms and behavior, minimizing the emotional strain for both patient and doctor and optimizing the quality of the medical outcome.

A clear understanding by both patient and doctor of the role each expects the other to play can aid in identifying problematic behaviors and can help to maintain the necessary degree of cooperation and collaboration, even when the patient has significant personality dysfunction. In this regard, it is important to understand how patients with different personality disorders vary in their needs and expectations in this relationship. Table 26-2 outlines typical responses to illness by patients with each of the most common personality disorders, details troublesome reactions by physicians, and suggests strategies to avoid further problems with these challenging patients.

Management of Patients with Personality Disorders

In most cases, a stable therapeutic alliance with patients who have personality disorders can be maintained by implementing the behavioral strategies suggested in the following sections. Sometimes other factors must also be addressed. As mentioned earlier, comorbid Axis I diagnoses must be treated (e.g., treatment of depression or anxiety disorders). Pharmacotherapy and psychotherapy are often more complex for patients with comorbid Axis I and II disorders. This is particularly evident when patients with personality disorders have concurrent substance-abuse problems or psychotic symptoms (e.g., hallucinations, delusions, paranoid ideation). In such cases, mental health consultation can be particularly helpful.

When a provider feels unable to continue productive work with a patient with a personality disorder, it may be appropriate to transfer the patient to another clinician. Although such transfers of care may be both necessary and helpful, they require consideration of the impact of the transfer on the well-being of the patient. Patients with certain personality disorders may experience such transfers as rejection or abandonment, perceptions that may exacerbate their emotional distress and potentially disrupt their medical treatment. Prior consultation with a mental health provider can be useful in determining whether such a transfer might be helpful and can aid in carrying it out smoothly.

The remainder of this chapter discusses the 10 personality disorders as they manifest in the medical setting, and management recommendations.

PARANOID PERSONALITY DISORDER

Symptoms & Signs

Patients with paranoid personality disorder (Table 26-3) have a long-standing pattern of distrust and suspiciousness. They perceive the behavior and motives of others as malevolent in nature and expect others, in many situations, to disappoint or take advantage of them. They are reluctant to confide in others and can be preoccupied with unwarranted doubts about the loyalty or trustworthiness of friends and associates. They may perceive seemingly benign or innocuous statements or behavior by others as threatening, insulting, or hurtful. To defend against their perceived vulnerability, they usually adopt a rigid, distanced, or guarded position. In general, persons with this personality structure find intimate relationships undesirable and difficult, which often leaves them without any significant social supports.

Differential Diagnosis

Long-standing psychotic symptoms, such as delusions and hallucinations, suggest a diagnosis of paranoid delusional disorder or paranoid schizophrenia. Although persons with paranoid personality disorder usually do not have frank paranoid delusions, at times of extreme stress they may develop such symptoms. Brief paranoid ideation may be associated with medical causes or with alcohol or substance abuse or withdrawal.

Table 26-2. Common personality disorders and typical manifestations.

Personality disorder	Paranoid	Schizoid	Schizotypal	Antisocial	Borderline
Prominent features of disorder	Distrust and suspiciousness of others, such that their motives are interpreted as malevolent	Pattern of detachment from social relationships and a restricted range of emotional expression	Odd beliefs, inappropriate affect, perceptual distortions, and desire for social isolation	Disregard for and violation of the rights of others, beginning in adolescence	Pattern of instability in interpersonal relationships, self-image and affects, and marked impulsivity
Patient's experience of illness	Heightened sense of fear and vulnerability	Threat to personal integrity; increased anxiety because illness forces interaction with others	May have odd interpretations of illness, increased anxiety because of interactions with others, may become overtly psychotic	Sense of fear may be masked by increased hostility or entitled stance	Terrifying fantasies about illness; feels either completely well or deathly ill
Problematic behavior in the medical care setting	Fear that physician or others may harm them Misinterpretation of innocuous or even helpful behaviors Increased likelihood of argument or conflict with staff	May delay seeking care until symptoms become severe, out of fear of interacting with others May appear detached and unappreciative of help	May delay care because of odd and magical beliefs about symptoms, may not recognize symptoms as a sign of illness May appear odd and eccentric and paranoid toward others	Irresponsible, impulsive, or dangerous health behavior, without regard for consequences to self or others Angry, deceitful, or manipulative behavior	Mistrust of physicians and delay in seeking treatment Intense fear of rejection and abandonment Abrupt shifts from idealizing to devaluing caregivers; splitting Self-destructive threats and acts
Common problematic reactions to patient by caregiver	Defensive, argumentative, or angry response that "confirms" patient's suspicions Ignoring the patient's suspicious or angry stance	Overzealous attempts to connect with patient Frustration at feeling unappreciated	Frustration about patient's misinterpretation of illness Not wanting to connect with an odd and eccentric patient	Succumbing to patient's manipulation Angry, punitive reaction when manipulation is discovered	Succumbing to patient's idealization and splitting Getting too close to, patient causing overstimulation Despair at patient's self-destructive behaviors Temptation to punish patient angrily
Helpful management strategies by caregiver	Attend to and be empathic toward patient fears, even when irrational in appearance Carefully detail care plan	Appreciate need for privacy and maintain a low-key approach Focus on technical elements of treatment; these are	Try not to be turned off by patient's odd appearance Try to educate patient about the illness and its treatment	Carefully, respectfully investigate patient's concerns and motives Communicate directly; avoid punitive	Don't get too close to patient Schedule frequent periodic check-ups Provide clear, nontechnical

(Continued)

Personality Disorder	Histrionic	Narcissistic	Avoidant	Dependent	Obsessive Compulsive
(continued)	for patient with advance information about risks of procedures/treatments Maintain patient's independence when possible and optimize the patient's control Not overly friendly, but professional, objective stance	better tolerated Encourage patient to maintain daily routines Do not become personally overly involved or too zealous in trying to provide social supports	Do not become overly involved in trying to provide social support	reactions to patient Set clear limits in context of medically indicated interventions	answers to questions to counter scary fantasies Tolerate periodic angry outbursts, but set limits Be aware of patient's potential for self-destructive behavior Discuss feelings with coworkers and schedule multidisciplinary consultations
Prominent features of disorder	Pattern of excessive attention seeking and emotionality	Pervasive pattern of grandiosity, need for admiration, and lack of empathy for others	Pattern of social inhibition because of fears of being rejected or humiliated by others	Pervasive and excessive need to be taken care of that leads to submissive and clinging behavior, and fears of separation	Pattern of preoccupation with orderliness, perfectionism, control
Patient's experience of illness	Threatened sense of attractiveness and self-esteem	Illness may increase anxiety related to doubts about personal adequacy and disrupts image of self as resilient and superior	Illness may heighten sense of inadequacy and worsen low self-esteem	Fear that illness will lead to abandonment and helplessness	Fear of losing control over bodily functions and over emotions generated by illness; feelings of shame and vulnerability
Problematic behavior in the medical care setting	Overly dramatic, attention-seeking behavior, with tendency to draw caregiver into excessively familiar relationship Inadequate focus on symptoms and their management, with over emphasis on feeling states May provide answers they believe physician wants to hear Tendency to somatize	Demanding, entitled attitude Excessive praise toward caregiver may turn to devaluation, in effort to maintain sense of superiority Denial of illness or minimization of symptoms	May not be forthcoming about symptom severity, may easily agree with physician out of fear of not being liked	Dramatic and urgent demands for medical attention Angry outbursts at physician if not responded to Patient may contribute to prolong illness or encourage medical procedures in order to get attention May abuse substances and medications	Anger about disruption of routines Repetitive questions and excessive attention to detail Fear of relinquishing control to health care team

Table 26-2. Common personality disorders and typical manifestations. *(Continued)*

Personality Disorder	Histrionic	Narcissistic	Avoidant	Dependent	Obsessive Compulsive
Common problematic reactions to patient by caregiver	Performing excessive workup (when patient is dramatic) or inadequate workup (when patient is vague) Allowing too much emotional closeness, thereby losing objectivity Frustration with patient's dramatic or vague presentation	Outright rejection of patient's demands, resulting in patient distancing self from caregiver Excessive submission to patient's grandiose stance	Feeling overly concerned for the patient, taking on a paternalistic role that may increase patient's sense of inadequacy May feel angry and betrayed by patient if the patient's symptoms turn out to be more extensive than initially reported	Inability to set limits to availability, thus leading to burnout Hostile rejection of patient	Impatience and cutting answers short Attempts to control treatment planning
Helpful management strategies by caregiver	Show respectful and professional concern for feelings, with emphasis on objective issues Avoid excessive familiarity	Generous validation of patient's concerns, with attentive but factual response to questions Allow patients to maintain sense of competence by rechanneling their "skills" to deal with illness, obviating need for devaluation of caregivers Present treatment recommendations in the context of their right to the best care	Provide reassurance, validate patient's concerns Encourage reporting of symptoms and concerns	Provide reassurance and schedule frequent periodic check-ups Be consistently available but provide firm realistic limits to availability Enlist other members of the health care team in providing support for patient Help patient obtain outside support systems Avoid hostile rejection of patient	Thorough history taking and careful diagnostic workups are reassuring Give clear and thorough explanation of diagnosis and treatment options Do not overemphasize uncertainties about treatments Avoid vague and impressionistic explanations Treat patient as an equal partner; encourage self-monitoring and allow patient participation in treatment

Table 26-3. Diagnostic criteria for paranoid personality disorder.

A. A pervasive distrust and suspiciousness of others such that their motives are interpreted as malevolent, beginning by early adulthood and present in a variety of contexts, as indicated by four (or more) of the following:
   1. Suspects, without sufficient basis, that others are exploiting, harming, or deceiving him or her
   2. Is preoccupied with unjustified doubts about the loyalty or trustworthiness of friends or associates
   3. Is reluctant to confide in others because of unwarranted fear that the information will be used maliciously against him or her
   4. Reads hidden demeaning or threatening meanings into benign remarks or events
   5. Persistently bears grudges, that is, is unforgiving of insults, injuries, or slights
   6. Perceives attacks on his or her character or reputation that are not apparent to others and is quick to react angrily or to counterattack
   7. Has recurrent suspicions, without justification, regarding fidelity of spouse or sexual partner
B. Does not occur exclusively during the course of schizophrenia, a mood disorder with psychotic features, or another psychotic disorder and is not due to the direct physiologic effects of a general medical condition.

Source: Reprinted, with permission, from American Psychiatric Association: *Diagnostic and Statistical Manual of Mental Disorders*, 4th edition, *Text Revision* (*DSM-IV-TR*). Washington, DC: American Psychiatric Association, 2000.

Illness Experience & Illness Behavior

Illness is difficult for individuals with paranoid personality disorder because illness makes them more dependent, and, hence, more vulnerable. Communicating personal information to the physician may challenge the self-protective, rigid way they approach social interactions. Patients may experience a heightened sense of vulnerability and fear of harm by the physician. In their fearful state, they may perceive innocuous or even overtly helpful behavior as threatening. They may then question or challenge the physician about the content of an intervention or the motives behind it. This can lead to possible conflict and argument between patient and doctor or to the patient disengaging from care.

THE DOCTOR–PATIENT RELATIONSHIP

Physicians confronted with such a paranoid stance may react in ways that exacerbate the situation. If they feel that their intentions are inappropriately suspect they might argue with the patient or become defensive, perhaps using an angry tone. This kind of reaction may frighten the patient and may be perceived as confirmation of the patient's suspicion. Although such a response should be avoided, ignoring the patient's distrustful or angry behavior can also be problematic; the patient's concerns, however irrational, may increase if not addressed.

Specific Management Strategies

It is essential to address the patient's concerns and fears empathically, however irrational they seem. Although the physician may see the patient's concern as unrealistic, to the patient the fear is real. Dismissing these patients' concerns or calling them paranoid will not address their emotional needs and may instead create distance in the doctor–patient relationship. A professional, "matter-of-fact" or objective stance is most reassuring to these patients. Excessive friendliness or reassurance may be misinterpreted

and may intensify their paranoia. It is important to give these patients detailed information about their proposed treatment plan, allowing them to feel they are in control of the treatment and can make independent decisions. Provide factual information about risks associated with the treatment, whenever possible, before any major procedures or changes in treatment.

 CASE ILLUSTRATION 1

Simon, a 42-year-old, single, male parking lot attendant, presents to the urgent care clinic complaining of 3 months of tension headaches and fatigue in the context of what he calls "job stress." The only notable finding in the physical examination is a mild elevation of blood pressure. The physician also observes that Simon seems angry and anxious. When asked about his job stress, Simon reveals anxieties about not being able to trust two new coworkers, along with fears that his supervisors are conspiring to dismiss him from his job. He also mentions, hesitantly, that he had not sought evaluation of his headaches sooner because he worried that the physician would dismiss his fears as unfounded or "crazy." Additional social history reveals difficulty with close relationships and recurrent problems adjusting to changes in the workplace.

The physician listens in a nonjudgmental and empathic manner. He responds with scientific curiosity asking specific and thorough questions in order to define the nature of the complaint. An over-the-counter analgesic for the headaches and buspirone for anxiety and agitation are prescribed after a discussion of the likely diagnosis and the pros and cons of each treatment option. The physician plans follow-up measurements of the blood pressure and suggests that Simon see a psychiatrist for further evaluation of his very stressful job situation.

Simon feels that his concerns have been seriously. He finds the referral to a psychiatrist acceptable because it has been proposed in a way that offers support and does not dismiss his fears as pathologic. The physician's matter-of-fact responses to Simon's somatic complaints help increase the patient's trust in the physician.

SCHIZOID PERSONALITY DISORDER

Symptoms & Signs

Individuals with schizoid personality disorder (Table 26-4) remain detached from social relationships and exhibit a restricted range of emotional expression in their interactions with others, often appearing cold or indifferent. Because patients with this disorder find emotions, intimacy, and conflict threatening, they tend to isolate themselves and avoid close or sexual relationships. They prefer dealing with technical or abstract concepts to contact with people, and so they may devote their time to pursuits such as mathematical games. Work can be problematic if it involves interactions with others, but many individuals can perform quite well if they work with some degree of independence.

Differential Diagnosis

Patients with schizoid personality disorder do not exhibit prolonged psychotic symptoms. They may, however, suffer a brief psychotic decompensation during times of extreme stress. In addition, schizoid personality disorder may in some cases precede the development of psychotic Axis I conditions, such as schizophrenia or delusional disorder. It can also coexist with schizotypal, paranoid, or avoidant personality disorders.

Illness Experience & Illness Behavior

Illness can be especially stressful for these patients because it gives rise to strong emotions that they are not prepared to cope with. The necessity of interacting with caregivers when ill, often around quite personal issues, forces them to do the very thing they systematically avoid. They may therefore delay seeking care until their symptoms become more serious. When they finally present for medical attention, they may appear indifferent or detached as a way of protecting themselves from overwhelming emotion. They may show little facial expression and may not respond in kind to caregivers' empathic nods or comments—which may make establishing a therapeutic relationship difficult.

THE DOCTOR–PATIENT RELATIONSHIP

Because these patients often appear cold or indifferent, physicians may consider them as unappreciative of help. They may also be puzzled or frustrated by their patients' delay in seeking medical care and their apparent passivity in the face of illness. As a result, caregivers may make overzealous attempts to connect with patients by trying to be especially empathic, a tactic that may instead frighten them away. On the other hand, providers may themselves draw back and lose their enthusiasm for helping patients who seem so unappreciative or uninvolved in their own treatment.

Specific Management Strategies

Understanding that individuals with schizoid personality disorder have difficulty tolerating emotions and intimate interactions is important. Physicians should appreciate their patients' need for privacy and should maintain a low-key approach, avoiding attempts to reach out by becoming too close or by insisting on providing social support. It is helpful to focus on the more technical aspects of treatment, as these are better tolerated, and encourage patients to maintain daily routines. Caregivers should remain available and provide steady but nonthreatening help.

Table 26-4. Diagnostic criteria for schizoid personality disorder.

A. A pervasive pattern of detachment from social relationships and a restricted range of expression of emotions in interpersonal settings, beginning by early adulthood and present in a variety of contexts, as indicated by four (or more) of the following:
  1. Neither desires nor enjoys close relationships, including being part of a family
  2. Almost always chooses solitary activities
  3. Has little, if any, interest in having sexual experiences with another person
  4. Takes pleasure in few, if any, activities
  5. Lacks close friends or confidants other than first-degree relatives
  6. Appears indifferent to the praise or criticism of others
  7. Shows emotional coldness, detachment, or flattened affectivity
B. Does not occur exclusively during the course of schizophrenia, a mood disorder with psychotic features, another psychotic disorder, or a pervasive developmental disorder and is not due to the direct physiologic effects of a general medical condition.

Source: Reprinted, with permission, from American Psychiatric Association: *Diagnostic and Statistical Manual of Mental Disorders*, 4th edition, *Text Revision* (*DSM-IV-TR*). Washington, DC: American Psychiatric Association, 2000.

CASE ILLUSTRATION 2

Ben, a 44-year-old computer programmer, is admitted to the University hospital for evaluation of nausea, anorexia, and a 30-lb weight loss occurring over the previous several months. When asked by the admitting resident why he hadn't sought treatment before, Ben states that he has always been healthy and thought he would probably regain the lost weight.

Throughout the interview, Ben makes poor eye contact and gives brief answers to questions. He appears to dislike being interviewed by both a medical student and a resident. He becomes more uncomfortable when asked questions about his personal life and how he likes spending his time. Ben states that he usually keeps to himself, with the exception of visiting his sister about once a month. He spends much of his time programming and playing with his computer.

Ben appears visibly anxious when the resident recommends a consultation by the gastroenterology service. He asks whether this is truly necessary. The resident emphasizes the importance of this consultation, and Ben seems to calm down a bit when the conversation focuses more on the possible tests that might be done to evaluate his symptoms, thereby distracting his attention from his concerns about having to see yet another doctor. The resident later explains to the medical student that it is important to minimize the number of doctors Ben sees over time and to avoid an overfriendly style, which might frighten him.

SCHIZOTYPAL PERSONALITY DISORDER

Symptoms & Signs

Patients with schizotypal personality disorder (Table 26-5) behave in an odd and eccentric manner, are socially inept and isolated, and experience cognitive or perceptual distortions. Their distortions include magical thinking, odd beliefs, ideas of reference, bodily illusions, or telepathic and clairvoyant experiences. These beliefs and distortions are inconsistent with subcultural norms, occur frequently, and are an important and pervasive core component of the patient's experience. The patient's enduring psychotic-like symptoms may worsen under stress. Patients often dress in an odd and peculiar fashion and their affect is often inappropriate; for example, they may laugh inappropriately during the visit while talking about their problems.

These patients are socially isolated and usually have few or no close friends. Their social isolation stems from their odd behavior as well as from their persistent social anxiety due to suspiciousness or paranoia toward others.

Differential Diagnosis

Schizotypal personality disorder shares the symptom of suspiciousness and paranoia with paranoid personality disorder and that of social isolation with schizoid personality disorder. However, the latter two disorders do not present with odd and peculiar mannerisms and behaviors and also lack cognitive or perceptual distortions.

The differential diagnosis includes schizophrenia (Axis I disorder). Although patients with schizotypal personality disorder lack signs and symptoms of overt

Table 26-5. Diagnostic criteria for schizotypal personality disorder.

A. A pervasive pattern of social and interpersonal defects marked by acute discomfort with, and reduced capacity for, close relationships as well as by cognitive or perceptual distortions and eccentricities of behavior, beginning by early adulthood and present in a variety of contexts, as indicated by five (or more) of the following:
   1. Ideas of reference (excluding delusions of reference)
   2. Odd beliefs or magical thinking that influences behavior and is inconsistent with subcultural norms (e.g., superstitiousness, belief in clairvoyance, telepathy, or "sixth sense"; in children and adolescents, bizarre fantasies or preoccupations)
   3. Unusual perceptual experiences, including bodily illusions
   4. Odd thinking and speech (e.g., vague, circumstantial, metaphorical, overelaborate, or stereotyped)
   5. Suspiciousness or paranoid ideation
   6. Inappropriate or constricted affect
   7. Behavior or appearance that is odd, eccentric, or peculiar
   8. Lack of close friends or confidants other than first-degree relatives
   9. Excessive social anxiety that does not diminish with familiarity and tends to be associated with paranoid fears rather than negative judgments about self
B. Does not occur exclusively during the course of schizophrenia, a mood disorder with psychotic features, another psychotic disorder, or a pervasive developmental disorder.

Source: Reprinted, with permission, from American Psychiatric Association: *Diagnostic and Statistical Manual of Mental Disorders*, 4th edition, *Text Revision* (*DSM-IV-TR*). Washington, DC: American Psychiatric Association, 2000.

psychosis, the disorder is considered a schizophrenia-spectrum disorder. This means that it may be related to schizophrenia. Family studies show an increased risk of schizophrenia in relatives of patients with schizotypal personality disorder and an increased risk of schizotypal personality disorder in families of patients with schizophrenia.

Illness Experience & Illness Behavior

Patients with schizotypal personality disorder may present late in the course of their illness because they may have odd interpretations of their illness and may, therefore, not recognize the serious nature of their symptoms. Also, like patients with schizoid personality disorder, they do not like to interact with and seek the company of others. Illness forces them to interact with health care providers and their support staff, something they may not be prepared to do. This may lead to increased paranoid ideation or overt psychotic symptoms.

THE DOCTOR–PATIENT RELATIONSHIP

These patients' eccentric appearance may cause the clinician to be hesitant in approaching them. Odd and weird interpretations of illness may lead to misunderstandings between patient and clinician. It may be challenging for the physician to improve these patients' understanding of their problems.

Specific Management Strategies

Clinicians should try to overcome their apprehension about treating these patients, often caused by their eccentric appearance. It is helpful to find out what these patients think about their symptoms and to help them obtain a better understanding of their illness. At the same time, the physician should not get overly involved in trying to increase their patients' social support or exposure to others. Knowing that patients with schizotypal personality disorder desire social isolation is important. Occasionally, assessing decision-making capacity can be complicated by odd or magical beliefs associated with the illness. Consultation can be helpful.

CASE ILLUSTRATION 3

Donna, a 35-year-old single female, has developed a cough, high fever, and chills and her family noticed that she started to look ill. She was brought to the emergency room by her mother. She is oddly dressed in a long and colorful country style wraparound shirt with military type boots. Her hair is unkempt and pinned up with a number of different hairpins. During the interview, Donna laughs in a silly manner while discussing her problem with the physician and the nurse. She says that she does not like to see a doctor because she prefers to walk in the woods by herself and communicate with the birds and insects.

The physician focuses on the patient's presenting symptoms and explains to her that she may suffer from pneumonia. He explains to her in simple terms what pneumonia is and that she needs sputum cultures and a chest x-ray to confirm the diagnosis.

While Donna has her chest x-ray taken, the physician and the nurse discuss how the health care team should help the patient understand her symptoms as well as the rationale for her medical workup and treatment. The physician also recommends focusing on the patient's problems and respecting her need for distance from others.

ANTISOCIAL PERSONALITY DISORDER

Symptoms & Signs

Persons with antisocial personality disorder (Table 26-6) demonstrate a disregard for others and behavior that violates others' rights. The diagnosis can be made only in persons over age 18, and it requires a history of conduct disorder prior to that age. Characteristics include lack of conformity to social norms and laws, using lies or other deceitfulness for personal gain, and impulsiveness and irresponsibility in many settings. These individuals may be threatening, manipulative, or harmful to others, and they are generally not remorseful. Their tendencies toward aggressive behavior may not be immediately evident, but contact with collateral sources frequently reveals a criminal record. These character traits affect relations with both strangers and family alike, as persons with antisocial personality disorder may engage in inconsiderate, angry, or harmful behaviors. These individuals may present themselves in a superficially grandiose manner, and they can also initially appear somewhat charismatic, until others recognize their charm as manipulative.

Differential Diagnosis

Antisocial personality disorder can overlap significantly with other personality disorder traits, most commonly narcissistic, histrionic, or borderline personality disorder. Because substance abuse is a frequent comorbid diagnosis, it is important to distinguish between the problems when making the diagnosis.

Illness Experience & Illness Behavior

To mask the fear that illness may cause, patients with antisocial personality disorder may unconsciously adopt

Table 26-6. Diagnostic criteria for antisocial personality disorder.

A. There is a pervasive pattern of disregard for and violation of the rights of others occurring since age 15 years, as indicated by three (or more) of the following:
  1. Failure to conform to social norms with respect to lawful behaviors as indicated by repeatedly performing acts that are grounds for arrest
  2. Deceitfulness, as indicated by repeated lying, use of aliases, or conning others for personal profit or pleasure
  3. Impulsivity or failure to plan ahead
  4. Irritability and aggressiveness, as indicated by repeated physical fights or assaults
  5. Reckless disregard for safety of self or others
  6. Consistent irresponsibility, as indicated by repeated failure to sustain consistent work behavior or honor financial obligations
  7. Lack of remorse, as indicated by being indifferent to or rationalizing having hurt, mistreated, or stolen from another
B. The individual is at least age 18 years.
C. There is evidence of conduct disorder with onset before age 15 years.
D. The occurrence of antisocial behavior is not exclusively during the course of schizophrenia or a manic episode.

Source: Reprinted, with permission, from American Psychiatric Association: *Diagnostic and Statistical Manual of Mental Disorders*, 4th edition, *Text Revision* (*DSM-IV-TR*). Washington, DC: American Psychiatric Association, 2000.

an excessively self-assured, entitled, or hostile stance. Irresponsible, impulsive, or dangerous health behavior may help these patients deny their vulnerability to illness. This behavior can occur without regard for medical consequences, and many patients show blatant disregard for the health care personnel and resources from which they have benefited. Patients may assume a privileged, self-deserving stance and can become antagonistic if they fail to obtain the desired response. They may attempt to manipulate their physician, malingering to obtain things such as drugs or inappropriate disability benefits. This behavior can be an embellishment of a real illness, or it can occur when they are not ill.

THE DOCTOR–PATIENT RELATIONSHIP

Because these patients often behave in ways that are noncompliant, ungracious, or dishonest, they are frequently irritating to health care providers. Physicians may become angry with these individuals or reject them if they see that the treatments in which they have invested their knowledge and energy have not been followed, or if they discover they have been manipulated by these patients.

Specific Management Strategies

Managing manipulative patients can be particularly challenging. If the patient tricks the physician, the outcome is usually detrimental to the patient's overall health (broadly defined). On the other hand, although recognizing the manipulative behavior may avert a detrimental health outcome, the physician's confrontation can alienate the patient. The more authoritarian the physician's stance, the more likely it is that the patient will become oppositional, reducing the possibility for development of an effective therapeutic alliance.

The key here is to maintain an objective, thorough, nonauthoritarian, and respectful approach to investigating the patient's presenting complaints. If the patient's presentation or motives are suspicious, the provider should gather corroborating data from collateral sources (other providers or family members) when needed. It is important to avoid becoming angry, punitive, or rejecting toward the patient; these behaviors may recapitulate behavior the patient experienced earlier in life that contributed to the development of the antisocial personality disorder. Such behavior by the physician can cause the patient to become hostile, with additional deterioration in the doctor–patient relationship. If confrontation or disagreement is necessary, it is essential to avoid humiliating the patient while identifying the attempted manipulation. Communication should be direct and factual with these patients, based on what is medically indicated, and clear limits should be set on the diagnostic or treatment plan.

 CASE ILLUSTRATION 4

On returning from vacation, the doctor's first patient is Randy, an angry 42-year-old man, well known to her for his problems with long-standing recurrent low back pain. Although his back pain is generally well controlled with back exercises and as-needed nonsteroidal analgesics, Randy frequently takes long motorcycle trips with friends, during which he does not exercise or take his analgesics. While the physician was away, Randy went on a motorcycle tour and had a recurrence of acute back pain. He then telephoned the clinic and became angry and abusive toward the on-call nurse practitioner, who would not submit to his demands for narcotics.

The physician, who has seen similar behavior from Randy in the past, listens carefully to his story, acknowledges his anger, and reflects empathically on how painful his back must be. She inquires, non-judgmentally, about the reasons for his failure to exercise. She then explains the benefits of a more preventive approach—using exercise and avoiding pain-inducing behaviors—compared with the long-term risks of relying on narcotics and failing to exercise. Finally, she offers him referral to a physical therapist for a review of the exercise plan, along with a refill of his nonsteroidal analgesic, emphasizing her view that this would offer the best long-term outcome. With some bitterness, Randy acknowledges the benefits of the physician's recommendations and agrees to try to follow through with them.

In dealing with Randy, the physician uses her past experience with him as a guide. Randy's self-destructive behavior, hostility, and disregard for others are met with clear limit setting by the physician, who responds in a calm and nonpunitive manner, emphasizing her concern for the patient's long-term well-being.

BORDERLINE PERSONALITY DISORDER

Symptoms & Signs

Patients with borderline personality disorder (Table 26-7) exhibit instability in their self-image, their affect, and their relationships with others. They can be quite impulsive and may engage in self-destructive behaviors, such as substance abuse, self-mutilation, and suicide attempts. These behaviors reflect a deep sense of emptiness and an intense fear of abandonment by others. On the other hand, patients with borderline personality disorder are often also fearful of closeness. They experience many contradictory emotions and feelings that are not integrated into a stable sense of who they are and that may be associated with rapid shifts in mood. This instability can cause frequent changes in goals and values. These patients usually have difficulty differentiating reality from fantasy and tend toward all-or-nothing thinking in their view of themselves and others, alternating between overidealization and devaluation.

Differential Diagnosis

Some patients with borderline personality disorder may suffer brief psychotic episodes when under stress. They may, for example, become very anxious or experience auditory hallucinations. The brief duration and specific association with stressors distinguishes these episodes from Axis I psychotic disorders. In addition, patients with borderline personality disorder also often suffer from a concurrent Axis I mood disorder, such as major depression or bipolar disorder, which should, of course, be treated. Other personality disorders (e.g., histrionic or narcissistic) may co-occur or be confused with borderline personality disorder.

Illness Experience & Illness Behavior

Patients with borderline personality disorder have difficulty distinguishing reality from fantasy, and they may have terrifying fantasies about illness. The complex and contradictory feelings engendered in response to illness can feel intolerable to these patients, so they may try to cope by pretending that they are completely well and denying the presence of illness. Alternatively, they may

---

Table 26-7. Diagnostic criteria for borderline personality disorder.

A pervasive pattern of instability of interpersonal relationships, self-image, and affects, and marked impulsivity beginning by early adulthood and present in a variety of contexts, as indicated by five (or more) of the following:

1. Frantic efforts to avoid real or imagined abandonment; *Note:* Do not include suicidal or self-mutilating behavior covered in criterion 5
2. A pattern of unstable and intense interpersonal relationships characterized by alternating between extremes of idealization and devaluation
3. Identity disturbance: markedly and persistently unstable self-image or sense of self
4. Impulsivity in at least two areas that are potentially self-damaging (e.g., spending, sex, substance abuse, reckless driving, binge eating); *Note:* Do not include suicidal or self-mutilating behavior covered in criterion 5
5. Recurrent suicidal behavior, gestures, or threats, or self-mutilating behavior
6. Affective instability due to a marked reactivity of mood (e.g., intense episodic dysphoria, irritability, or anxiety usually lasting a few hours and only rarely more than a few days)
7. Chronic feelings of emptiness
8. Inappropriate, intense anger or difficulty controlling anger (e.g., frequent displays of temper, constant anger, recurrent physical fights)
9. Transient, stress-related paranoid ideation or severe dissociative symptoms

Source: Reprinted, with permission, from American Psychiatric Association: *Diagnostic and Statistical Manual of Mental Disorders,* 4th edition, *Text Revision* (*DSM-IV-TR*). Washington, DC: American Psychiatric Association, 2000.

become convinced that they are deathly ill, even when suffering from a mild illness. Having felt wounded in earlier relationships, individuals with borderline personality disorder mistrust and fear caregivers. In an attempt to cope with their simultaneous intense wish for, and fear of, closeness, they tend to conceptualize caregivers as all good or all bad—a mechanism called "splitting." To complicate things further, these conceptualizations are not stable. Even an overidealized caregiver can abruptly be devalued if a borderline patient becomes angry and disappointed or feels abandoned. In addition, patients with borderline personality disorder may respond to feeling overwhelmed by engaging in impulsive and self-destructive acts, such as self-mutilation, substance abuse, and suicide gestures or attempts. They may also be noncompliant with treatment in order to test the limits of the clinician's availability, devalue the clinician, or even to remain ill and thus maintain an ongoing relationship with the caregiver.

THE DOCTOR–PATIENT RELATIONSHIP

A common mistake clinicians make in treating patients with borderline personality disorder is getting too emotionally close. This occurs when clinicians feel intensely drawn to help patients through their suffering and spend a great deal of time with them. This usually causes overstimulation of the patient's emotions, leading to initial idealization of the clinician and then increased instability and acting out. It should be noted that the patient's emotional behavior can cloud the clinician's judgment, causing the clinician to succumb to the patient's idealization and splitting. The borderline patient's self-destructive or often provocative behaviors can cause despair and helplessness in caregivers. Caregivers may also feel tempted to punish the patient, for example, by becoming uncharacteristically inflexible or even verbally hostile or by withholding needed (e.g., pain) medication or care (e.g., more frequent visits).

Specific Management Strategies

While providing basic support and reassurance, clinicians should be careful not to become emotionally overinvolved with the borderline patient. It is appropriate to counter the patient's frightening fantasies about illness and "overwhelming neediness" by scheduling frequent periodic check-ups and providing clear, nontechnical answers to questions. Caregivers may have to tolerate periodic angry outbursts, but it is appropriate to set firm limits on both the patient's disruptive behavior and on the caregiver's response. When a multidisciplinary team of clinicians is involved, meetings of all providers should be arranged, to allow them to vent their feelings about the patient and to reach consensus on a treatment plan. It is helpful to select a small number of caregivers to interact with the patient directly and to present the same clear and consistent plan. This approach often prevents

splitting. Finally, it is essential to remain aware of these patients' potential for self-destructive behavior and not to retaliate for their disruptions by displaying anger at them when setting limits.

 CASE ILLUSTRATION 5

A primary care resident expresses concern about her patient Amanda to her clinic's attending physician. She is scheduled to leave the clinic in 3 months and believes that Amanda will find transferring to a new doctor difficult.

Amanda is a 35-year-old temporary clerical worker with a long-standing history of migraine headaches. She often delays taking medication until her migraine headaches become severe, and then calls the resident, complaining of unbearable pain, sometimes stating that the pain is so intolerable that she wishes to die. She sometimes comes to the clinic without a scheduled appointment, demanding to be seen right away. On the other hand, she often misses regularly scheduled appointments. During her visits, she expresses a fear of becoming homeless; she house-sits at other people's homes but doesn't have a stable place of her own.

The resident asks for a psychiatric consultation to help her work with Amanda. She is particularly concerned about Amanda's periodic statements that she wishes to die.

Following the psychiatrist's recommendations, the resident continues to schedule regular, brief follow-up appointments, and encourages Amanda to keep these appointments. She explains that this is not a walk-in clinic, and that Amanda will have to seek treatment for acute pain in the emergency room. She also reminds Amanda that taking medication early will likely keep the headache from becoming very intense.

Other helpful interventions include providing increased support to Amanda by referring her to a psychotherapist and asking the team social worker to assist her in finding a stable residence. It is also important to monitor Amanda for suicidal ideation. If she expresses a wish to die, the resident assesses her suicidal ideation and intent. One afternoon, Amanda drops in at the clinic expressing suicidal ideation, and a nurse practitioner calls for an urgent psychiatric consultation. After talking to the psychiatrist, Amanda gradually calms down and denies any suicidal intent; however, she refuses a referral for ongoing psychiatric treatment.

Over time, Amanda continues to miss some appointments, and occasionally becomes demanding or complains bitterly about the resident to the nurse practitioner. When both the resident and the nurse practitioner, however, firmly and supportively continue to reiterate their treatment plan—to meet with the doctor for regular appointments, to treat migraines early, and to go to the emergency room for acute pain—Amanda's unpredictable visits and noncompliance diminish. Periodic meetings between the resident and the nurse practitioner help them both present the same coherent plan to Amanda, thus minimizing splitting.

In planning ahead for her departure from the clinic, the resident and the attending physician discuss some helpful strategies to facilitate this transition, such as introducing the new resident to Amanda ahead of time and involving the nurse practitioner—who is staying at the clinic—in the process.

In this case, regular meetings of the resident, the attending physician, and the nurse practitioner allow them to present the same coherent plan to the patient, minimize the splitting, and reduce the patient's anxiety and unpredictable behavior. This approach successfully combines increased support and limit setting.

HISTRIONIC PERSONALITY DISORDER

Symptoms & Signs

Histrionic personality disorder (Table 26-8) is marked by excessive attention seeking and emotionalism. These patients may present with dramatic, theatrical shows of feeling, or they may dress or behave in a sexually provocative fashion in an unconscious effort to engage others and draw attention to themselves. The emotions they express may be shallow and inconsistent, but the patients may still believe that the sharing of those feelings creates a special closeness (which they often exaggerate) with the physician. These patients have a tendency to prefer subjective and intuitive impressions over objective, linear, logical thinking. They often have somatic complaints, with impressive—but inconsistent—presentations.

Differential Diagnosis

Histrionic personality disorder may be difficult to distinguish from narcissistic or borderline personality disorder, and patients in each of these categories may exhibit traits common to patients in the others. Patients with histrionic personality disorder are deeply affected by perceived frailties in relationship bonds, as are patients with borderline personality disorder. The latter, however, display less emotional stability and are more impulsive and self-destructive. Patients with histrionic personality disorder may crave attention—as patients with narcissistic personality disorder crave admiration—but the former tend to be less grandiose, arrogant, and self-absorbed.

Illness Experience & Illness Behavior

Medical illness represents a particular threat to the emotional well-being of patients with histrionic personality disorder, who derive much of their sense of self-worth and personal desirability from their sense of physical attractiveness. To reduce the fear of being deemed less desirable by others, these patients may attempt to bolster their physical appearance or embellish their abilities.

As a result, patients of either gender may engage in flirtatious or seductive behavior. When they feel weak and vulnerable, they may express their emotions with more intensity, in an attempt to strengthen their bond with the physician. In addition, because these patients focus on feelings, rather than on carefully observed physical symptoms, they may present with a collection of loosely connected somatic complaints. Their descriptions of the symptoms may reflect their desire to capture the physician's interest.

Table 26-8. Diagnostic criteria for histrionic personality disorder.

A pervasive pattern of excessive emotionality and attention seeking, beginning by early adulthood and present in a variety of contexts, as indicated by five (or more) of the following:
1. Is uncomfortable in situations in which he or she is not the center of attention
2. Interaction with others is often characterized by inappropriate sexually seductive or provocative behavior
3. Displays rapidly shifting and shallow expression of emotions
4. Consistently uses physical appearance to draw attention to self
5. Has a style of speech that is excessively impressionistic and lacking in detail
6. Shows self-dramatization, theatricality, and exaggerated expression of emotion
7. Is suggestible, that is, easily influenced by others or circumstances
8. Considers relationships to be more intimate than they actually are

Source: Reprinted, with permission, from American Psychiatric Association: *Diagnostic and Statistical Manual of Mental Disorders*, 4th edition, *Text Revision (DSM-IV-TR)*. Washington, DC: American Psychiatric Association, 2000.

THE DOCTOR–PATIENT RELATIONSHIP

In working with the histrionic patient, the physician may be drawn in by the patient's dramatic and somewhat dependent style, become overly involved, and perhaps embark on an excessive workup. As the physician becomes increasingly engaged by the patient's style, the patient may then become anxious, distant, or noncompliant, puzzling and frustrating the physician. Alternatively, the physician may instead pursue too cursory an evaluation, because of a lack of objective information, or out of frustration with the patient's emotional and vague style.

Specific Management Strategies

Because the patient with histrionic personality disorder has a vague and global emotional (rather than a precise, logical) style and may display contrasting behaviors— that range from excessive anxiety about potentially minor symptoms to inappropriate indifference about significant medical problems—it is essential that the physician maintain an objective stance. The physician must offer a supportive and logical approach to the patient's problems. This requires being both sensitive to the patient's emotional concerns and sufficiently distanced to avoid any degree of closeness that the patient might misperceive as intimate or sexual.

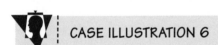 CASE ILLUSTRATION 6

Rita is 38-year-old, single, unemployed actress with lupus. She is excessively friendly and flirtatious with her 45-year-old male physician, calling him frequently with questions about her medical problems and dressing somewhat seductively for office visits. During these visits she asks for examinations of a variety of somatic complaints. Over time, the physician becomes increasingly uncomfortable. Finally, Rita complains that she would like more time to discuss her problems at each office visit, and asks the physician if he thinks her problems "deserve more time."

After reflecting on the chronicity of this pattern of behavior, the physician responds that Rita's medical problems are significant and deserving of attention. He states that he intends to evaluate each of them carefully, allocating time on the basis of his impression of their medical necessity. He also says that he understands that she would like more time to discuss her concerns, but that as a busy doctor he cannot make additional time available to her. He suggests, gently, that if he cannot provide adequate emotional support to her, he could refer her to a local clinic's health psychologist. Although she is rather disappointed, Rita is able to accept this limit setting and continues to work with this doctor.

This approach is successful because the physician shows positive regard for the patient and her problems— while clearly setting the limits of the doctor–patient relationship.

NARCISSISTIC PERSONALITY DISORDER

Symptoms & Signs

Narcissistic personality disorder (Table 26-9) is characterized by a long-standing pattern of grandiosity, with a need for praise and admiration that stands out in contrast to a lack of sensitivity to the feelings of others. These persons may have an exaggerated sense of self-importance and social status and require excessive admiration. They may be driven toward attaining an idealized position in terms of social, personal, romantic, or career accomplishment. In this regard, they may be envious and potentially devaluing of others whose accomplishments they perceive as exceeding their own. Beneath the grandiosity and devaluation exists an underlying view of self as inferior or inadequate. To avoid these beliefs and their associated painful effects, patients seek to convince self and others of their "specialness" or "unusual talent."

Differential Diagnosis

Narcissistic personality disorder may be difficult to distinguish from borderline, antisocial, histrionic, or obsessive-compulsive personality disorders, and in many cases it may overlap with these disorders. When the differentiation is unclear, identifying a high degree of grandiosity and a need for admiration can help clarify the diagnosis. In contrast to persons with borderline personality disorder, persons with narcissistic personality disorder have a more stable self-image and display less impulsiveness and sensitivity to relationship losses. In addition, persons with narcissistic personality disorder are generally less aggressive and deceitful than are persons with antisocial personality disorder, who also display evidence of childhood conduct disorder. Persons with histrionic personality disorder, in contrast, may be relatively more dramatic and emotional than those with narcissistic personality disorder. Although persons with narcissistic personality disorder, like those with obsessive-compulsive personality disorder, may be perfectionists, the former often have a higher self-assessment of their accomplishments.

Clinicians must be careful not to misdiagnose a person with transient hypomanic or manic grandiosity as having narcissistic personality disorder. Similarly, it is important to distinguish between narcissistic personality disorder and transient substance-related personality changes (e.g., from central nervous system stimulants) or personality changes caused by a general medical condition.

Table 26-9. Diagnostic criteria for narcissistic personality disorder.

A pervasive pattern of grandiosity (in fantasy or behavior), need for admiration, and lack of empathy, beginning by early adulthood and present in a variety of contexts, as indicated by five (or more) of the following:

1. Has a grandiose sense of self-importance (e.g., exaggerates achievements and talents, expects to be recognized as superior without commensurate achievements)
2. Is preoccupied with fantasies of unlimited success, power, brilliance, beauty, or ideal love
3. Believes that he or she is "special" and unique and can only be understood by, or should associate with, other special or high-status people (or institutions)
4. Requires excessive admiration
5. Has a sense of entitlement, that is, unreasonable expectations of especially favorable treatment or automatic compliance with his or her expectations
6. Is interpersonally exploitative, that is, takes advantage of others to achieve his or her own ends
7. Lacks empathy: is unwilling to recognize or identify with the feelings and needs of others
8. Is often envious of others or believes that others are envious of him or her
9. Shows arrogant, haughty behaviors or altitudes

Source: Reprinted, with permission, from American Psychiatric Association: *Diagnostic and Statistical Manual of Mental Disorders*, 4th edition, *Text Revision (DSM-IV-TR)*. Washington, DC: American Psychiatric Association, 2000.

Illness Experience & Illness Behavior

Health problems are a particular blow to patients with narcissistic personality disorder. Illness threatens these patients' unconscious attempts to maintain an intrapsychic and external image of untarnished well-being, resiliency, and superiority. Medical problems and physical limitations may disrupt this image, threaten their public personas, and leave them fearing disruption of their (unrealistically unchallengeable) sense of self. In an attempt to defend against this threat, patients may minimize the significance of symptoms or deny the presence of the illness. More commonly, as patients try to recapture their admired, idealized status, they may demand special treatment, second opinions, or transfer of care to more "senior" or "well-known" clinicians, or ridicule the physician caring for them. These patients may devalue, criticize, or question the behavior or credentials of the treating physician, or they may fail to comply with treatment recommendations.

THE DOCTOR–PATIENT RELATIONSHIP

Narcissistic patients' arrogant and grandiose behavior, combined with demands for special treatment, can be extremely irritating to physicians. Reactions to these patients can take many forms. Sometimes, in an attempt to avoid conflict, physicians submit to the demands. With particularly critical patients, providers may feel frustration, resentment, and even anger. Alternatively, they may feel devalued and question their own competence. Frustration may be especially great if the physician expends special energy on behalf of a charismatic or demanding patient, only to later become the butt of unfair criticism. Physicians may reject or avoid the patient, withhold treatment, or respond in an angry manner—responses that can harm both the patient and the doctor–patient relationship.

Specific Management Strategies

The most effective strategy for dealing with narcissistic patients is to be respectful and nonconfrontational about their sense of specialness and entitlement and to help them use their self-perceived talents in the service of their treatment. If narcissistic patients feel vulnerable and threatened by the illness, they are more likely to criticize and devalue the physician. Thus, physicians should not take this devaluation personally, and instead understand it as the patients' attempt to cope with their own intense insecurity. Providers can appeal to the patients' narcissism by explaining that they chose a particular course of action because they believe it represents the best possible care—a course of action they feel the patients deserve. Physicians can further support the patients by validating their concerns about the illness and pointing to their patients' ability to respond competently to its challenges. This approach helps the patients feel more secure and able, allowing them to ally confidently with—rather than defensively attack—their physicians.

 CASE ILLUSTRATION 7

Maggie, a 44-year-old married female lawyer who is quite prominent in the community, is an unusually demanding patient. She becomes very angry with her male physician, whom she accuses of not responding adequately to her complaints about menopausal symptoms. In fact, the physician has done all the necessary laboratory tests, has conferred extensively with the patient's gynecologist, and has answered numerous phone calls by the patient over a period of several months.

The physician, aware of Maggie's long-standing sense of entitlement and her extreme sensitivity to slights, responds by reviewing her concerns, discussing the treatment plan and rationale, and encouraging her to discuss some of her emotional reactions to this unexpectedly early menopause. He then emphasizes the special consideration he has put into her evaluation and treatment plan. He arranges more frequent office visits and tells Maggie that he predicts a relatively good response to treatment, given her active involvement in her own care.

This response is reassuring to the patient, because it validates her concerns and satisfies her narcissistic feelings of entitlement.

AVOIDANT PERSONALITY DISORDER

Symptoms & Signs

Patients with avoidant personality disorder (Table 26-10) have a long-standing pattern of excessive anxiety in social situations and in intimate relationships, and extreme hypersensitivity to what other people think about them. These patients desire relationships but avoid them because of fears of being rejected, humiliated, or embarrassed. If they do engage in social situations or relationships, they are constantly preoccupied with being rejected, criticized, and not being liked by others. As a result, these patients have low self-esteem, feel socially inept, have feelings of inferiority, and are shy and inhibited.

Differential Diagnosis

Patients with schizoid personality disorder also avoid social situations and relationships but they do desire social isolation. In contrast, patients with avoidant personality disorder strongly desire relationships but avoid them because of anxiety and fears of rejection and humiliation.

Avoidant personality disorder should be distinguished from social phobia (Axis I disorder). Whereas patients with avoidant personality disorder try to avoid social interactions in general, patients with social phobia usually have more specific concerns related to social performance, such as saying something inappropriate to unfamiliar people at a social gathering.

Illness Experience & Illness Behavior

Illness provokes anxiety and increases feelings of ineptness in patients with avoidant personality disorder. Patients may delay care out of fear of not being liked or being rejected by the caregiver. In their interactions with clinicians, they may be shy and not forthcoming about their problems out of fear of being rejected or humiliated by them. They may blame their physical discomfort on themselves and may actually not ask for appropriate pain relief. Because these patients feel that they may not deserve attention by their physician, they may be reluctant to undergo necessary medical procedures.

THE DOCTOR–PATIENT RELATIONSHIP

Physicians treating patients with avoidant personality disorder may initially not realize the full extent of their patients' symptoms. Because these patients are shy and easily agreeable to what their physicians propose, physicians may be prone to take a more paternalistic stance with them. If they discover later that the patient's symptoms are more severe than initially reported, clinicians may react with concern or feel betrayed by the patient for withholding information and for their passive attitude.

Specific Management Strategies

Patients with avoidant personality disorder need reassurance and permission to express their distress and concerns in a nonjudgmental environment. It is helpful for

Table 26-10. Diagnostic criteria for avoidant personality disorder.

A pervasive pattern of social inhibition, feelings of inadequacy, and hypersensitivity to negative evaluation, beginning by early adulthood and present in a variety of contexts, as indicated by four (or more) of the following:

1. Avoids occupational activities that involve significant interpersonal contact, because of fears of criticism, disapproval, or rejection
2. Is unwilling to get involved with people unless certain of being liked
3. Shows restraint within intimate relationships because of the fear of being shamed or ridiculed
4. Is preoccupied with being criticized or rejected in social situations
5. Is inhibited in new interpersonal situations because of feelings of inadequacy
6. Views self as socially inept, personally unappealing, or inferior to others
7. Is unusually reluctant to take personal risks or to engage in any new activities because they may prove embarrassing

Source: Reprinted, with permission, from American Psychiatric Association: *Diagnostic and Statistical Manual of Mental Disorders,* 4th edition, *Text Revision (DSM-IV-TR).* Washington, DC: American Psychiatric Association, 2000.

health care providers to explain that they are interested in knowing about the patient's problems.

 CASE ILLUSTRATION 8

Michael, a 45-year-old single office clerk, presents 45 minutes early for his annual check-up with his primary care physician. While signing in at the reception desk, he asks whether he has arrived on time for his appointment.

The physician finds a marked rash over the patient's elbows upon physical examination. The patient has a known history of psoriasis. Michael's face turns red out of embarrassment. He starts to explain that he applied the cream that his physician prescribed for him last year but that he ran out of the prescription some time ago. When asked why he did not call the physician's office for a refill, Michael states that he felt that he should not bother his physician for just a rash.

The physician expresses concern about the patient's rash. He writes a new prescription and asks Michael to call his office for a refill once he finishes the prescription. The doctor explains to the patient that he does not feel bothered by the patient's phone calls and that communication between patient and doctor is necessary to ensure appropriate medical care. He again requests that Michael call him for any refills or problems in the future.

This reassuring and supportive approach encourages the patient to communicate with his physician and not hold back out of fear of being rejected.

DEPENDENT PERSONALITY DISORDER

Symptoms & Signs

Patients with dependent personality disorder (Table 26-11) have a pervasive and excessive need to be taken care of. They experience intense fear of separation and abandonment and feel great discomfort when they are alone. This leads to submissive and clinging behavior in their interpersonal relationships. These patients have difficulty making independent decisions without a great deal of advice and reassurance, and they are afraid of disagreeing with others.

Differential Diagnosis

It is important to distinguish dependent personality disorder from the dependency that arises from panic disorder, mood disorders, or agoraphobia. Patients suffering from medical illnesses may also become very dependent on others, without having this disorder. Dependent personality disorder can sometimes be confused with other personality disorders, and dependent personality traits may be the result of chronic substance abuse.

Illness Experience & Illness Behavior

Patients with dependent personality disorder fear that illness will lead to both helplessness and abandonment by others. In their interactions with caregivers, they may become very needy and make dramatic demands for urgent medical attention. If the response is not what they wish, they may display angry outbursts at the physician. They may also blame their physical discomfort on others,

---

Table 26-11. Diagnostic criteria for dependent personality disorder.

A pervasive and excessive need to be taken care of that leads to submissive and clinging behavior and fears of separation, beginning by early adulthood and present in a variety of contexts, as indicated by five (or more) of the following:
1. Has difficulty making everyday decisions without an excessive amount of advice and reassurance from others
2. Needs others to assume responsibility for most major areas of his or her life
3. Has difficulty expressing disagreement with others because of fear of loss of support or approval. *Note:* Do not include realistic fears of retribution
4. Has difficulty initiating projects or doing things on his or her own (because of a lack of self-confidence in judgment or abilities rather than a lack of motivation or energy)
5. Goes to excessive lengths to obtain nurturance and support from others, to the point of volunteering to do things that are unpleasant
6. Feels uncomfortable or helpless when alone because of exaggerated fears of being unable to care for himself or herself
7. Urgently seeks another relationship as a source of care and support when a close relationship ends
8. Is unrealistically preoccupied with fears of being left to take care of himself or herself

Source: Reprinted, with permission, from American Psychiatric Association: *Diagnostic and Statistical Manual of Mental Disorders*, 4th edition, *Text Revision (DSM-IV-TR)*. Washington, DC: American Psychiatric Association, 2000.

including their physician. In addition, they may use addictive substances or overuse medications in a desperate attempt to obtain immediate relief from their suffering. Because receiving medical care may fulfill their wishes for attention from others, some dependent patients may unconsciously contribute to prolonging their illness, or—in some extreme cases—they may encourage unnecessary medical procedures.

THE DOCTOR–PATIENT RELATIONSHIP

Clinicians treating patients with dependent personality disorder may initially react with aversion to their patients' clingy and demanding behavior. Alternatively, clinicians may find it difficult to set limits on their availability and may try to provide reassurance by attempting to meet every demand, which ultimately leads to burnout or feelings of inadequacy. Eventually, caregivers may react in a hostile fashion and openly reject these patients.

Specific Management Strategies

Effective ways to provide reassurance to dependent patients and allay their fear of being abandoned include scheduling frequent periodic check-ups and being consistently available. It is nonetheless important to provide firm, realistic limits to this availability early in treatment or as soon as the patient's dependent traits become apparent. To prevent burnout, enlist other members of the health care team in providing support for the patient. In addition, physicians should help these patients find outside support systems to lessen fears of abandonment. They must also be alert to the patients' potential contribution to prolonging their illness or to their possible abuse of substances or medications.

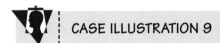

CASE ILLUSTRATION 9

Terry, a 50-year-old divorced secretary, repeatedly presents to her primary care physician complaining of various somatic symptoms, including dizziness, headaches, blurred vision, and leg pains. Repeated workups of her symptoms are negative, and her evaluation for major depression is negative. Further inquiry into Terry's life reveals that after her divorce 6 years ago, her daughter became the focus of her life. Even though her history of occasional somatic symptoms goes back to her teenage years, there had been no appreciable change until 2 years ago, when her daughter got married and left her home.

Terry makes frequent phone calls to her doctor. She usually sounds nervous, expresses concern about some new symptom, and asks for medication.

The doctor decides to schedule regular follow-up appointments to address Terry's concerns. Terry often complains during office visits that there is not enough time to evaluate all her symptoms and laments that her daughter no longer has much time for her. Her doctor listens in a supportive manner and acknowledges that the available appointment time is limited, explaining how he will ultimately address all the complaints. He also emphasizes the importance of continuing to meet for regular appointments. In addition, the doctor acknowledges Terry's increased sense of isolation after her daughter's marriage and evaluates her for possible major depression. He further suggests a referral to the clinic's social worker as a means of helping her pursue a volunteer activity and increase her social interactions.

This approach usually helps diminish the patient's anxiety and decreases the frequency of phone calls. If the patient's distress does not improve with such interventions, a referral for psychotherapy and evaluation for a possible underlying anxiety disorder are indicated.

OBSESSIVE-COMPULSIVE PERSONALITY DISORDER

Symptoms & Signs

Individuals with obsessive-compulsive personality disorder (Table 26-12) are preoccupied with orderliness, perfectionism, and control. They are excessively concerned with details and rules, tend to be overly moralistic, and are usually focused on work to the exclusion of leisure. They find it difficult to adapt themselves to others and instead insist that others follow their plans. Their general inflexibility and restricted emotional expression betray an underlying fear of losing control. Because they can be indecisive, they feel distressed when faced with the need to make decisions.

Differential Diagnosis

Obsessive-compulsive disorder (see Chapter 23) is distinguished from obsessive-compulsive personality disorder by the presence of actual obsessions (repetitive intrusive thoughts) and compulsions. Sometimes, however, both disorders coexist in one patient, and obsessive-compulsive personality disorder can also be confused with other personality disorders.

Illness Experience & Illness Behavior

Illness is threatening to persons with obsessive-compulsive personality disorder because it generates an

Table 26-12. Diagnostic criteria for obsessive-compulsive personality disorder.

A pervasive pattern of preoccupation with orderliness, perfectionism, and mental and interpersonal control, at the expense of flexibility, openness, and efficiency, beginning by early adulthood and present in a variety of contexts, as indicated by four (or more) of the following:

1. Is preoccupied with details, rules, lists, order, organization, or schedules to the extent that the major point of the activity is lost
2. Shows perfectionism that interferes with task completion (e.g., is unable to complete a project because his or her own overly strict standards are not met)
3. Is excessively devoted to work and productivity to the exclusion of leisure activities and friendships (not accounted for by obvious economic necessity)
4. Is overly conscientious, scrupulous, and inflexible about matters of morality, ethics, or values (not accounted for by cultural or religious identification)
5. Is unable to discard worn-out or worthless objects even when they have no sentimental value
6. Is reluctant to delegate tasks or to work with others unless they submit to exactly his or her way of doing things
7. Adopts a miserly spending style toward both self and others; money is viewed as something to be hoarded for future catastrophes
8. Shows rigidity and stubbornness

Source: Reprinted, with permission, from American Psychiatric Association: *Diagnostic and Statistical Manual of Mental Disorders*, 4th edition, *Text Revision* (*DSM-IV-TR*). Washington, DC: American Psychiatric Association, 2000.

intense fear of losing control over bodily functions and emotions. Patients may experience extremely unsettling feelings of shame and vulnerability. They may also feel anger at the disruption of their usual daily routines by medical appointments and treatments. They may fear having to relinquish control to health care providers. In the physician's office, their intense anxiety tends to drive them to ask repetitive questions and to pay excessive attention to detail.

THE DOCTOR–PATIENT RELATIONSHIP

Caregivers may react to patients with obsessive-compulsive personality disorder by becoming impatient at their repetitive questions, cutting their answers short. They may feel their competence challenged by their patients' insistence on knowing every single detail and reason for choosing a particular treatment. Clinicians may also inadvertently attempt to control treatment planning rather than making it a joint effort, without realizing how important it is for these patients to remain in control.

Specific Management Strategies

Helpful strategies in working with patients with obsessive-compulsive personality disorder include taking a thorough history, performing a careful diagnostic workup, giving patients a clear and thorough explanation of their diagnosis and treatment options, and providing and explaining laboratory test results. It is important not to overemphasize uncertainties about treatments or the patient's possible response to treatment. Patients find it reassuring when clinicians cite literature reports and avoid

vague and inexact impressionistic explanations. It is helpful to treat these patients as equal partners, encourage self-monitoring, allow their participation in treatment, and give them recognition for their clear reasoning and high standards.

 CASE ILLUSTRATION 10

Sam, a 42-year-old biochemist, requests an appointment with his primary care physician for evaluation of an uncomfortable lump in his left groin. The physician is familiar with Sam's mild nervousness during routine medical check-ups and his tendency to ask detailed questions about his health. After a physical examination, the doctor diagnoses an inguinal hernia and recommends a surgical consultation for further evaluation and possible surgery. Sam, in his usual formal and somewhat restricted manner—but this time appearing visibly more anxious—repeatedly asks several questions about surgical repair, whether the literature discusses any alternative treatments, and what guidelines physicians follow to recommend one treatment over another. He then asks questions about the risks of general anesthesia and whether this procedure can be performed under local anesthesia.

When the physician tries to reassure him that this is a routine procedure, Sam asks him whether he is sure of his diagnosis; he also asks him to list the criteria he used in diagnosing the inguinal hernia. Sam also talks at length about his responsibilities at work and expresses concern that surgery might disrupt ongoing projects at his laboratory, as several people depend on him for regular supervision. He also wants to know how long his doctor has known the recommended surgeon, and whether they have worked together in the past.

Reassurance is essential here. The doctor explains that the surgeon is both trustworthy and well known to him. He praises Sam for his thoroughness and initiative in finding out about treatment alternatives before making a decision. He answers basic questions in a precise manner and defers some questions to the surgeon, explaining that these will be better answered by a specialist. He reassures Sam that he will not wait for a written report but will personally contact the surgeon after the consultation to discuss treatment options. The physician also suggests a follow-up appointment to help Sam with his decision.

Although Sam continues to express concern that the surgery will disrupt his work, his anxiety decreases somewhat after the physician takes his concerns seriously. His questions are answered precisely, and the physician further suggests an article in the literature that he can read to learn more about the treatment of inguinal hernias.

TREATMENT OF PERSONALITY DISORDERS

Effective psychopharmacologic treatment do not exist for a given personality disorder. Nevertheless, pharmacotherapy plays an important role. Medication can be beneficial in targeting symptom clusters within the disorder and in treating comorbid Axis I disorders, such as major depression, bipolar affective disorder, substance abuse, posttraumatic stress disorder, panic disorder, social anxiety, and obsessive-compulsive disorder.

Symptoms such as paranoid ideation and suspiciousness in patients with cluster A disorders (paranoid, schizoid, and schizotypal personality disorder) may improve with low-dose antipsychotic treatment (e.g., haloperidol, risperidone, olanzapine, ziprasidone, quetiapine, aripiprazole). In case of overt psychotic symptoms, a psychiatric consultation and treatment with an antipsychotic medication should be considered.

Patients with cluster B disorders (antisocial, borderline, histrionic, and narcissistic personality disorder), who often appear dramatic and emotional, should be evaluated for prominent mood symptoms and the coexistence of an Axis I disorder, especially mood, anxiety, and substance-abuse disorders.

Patients with prominent depressive symptoms should be treated with selective serotonin reuptake inhibitors (SSRIs) antidepressants, such as fluoxetine, sertraline, paroxetine, citalopram, and escitalopram.

Patients with prominent mood swings, irritability, or impulsive behaviors may be candidates for treatment with a mood stabilizer (e.g., valproate or lithium) or a second-generation antipsychotic. However, a psychiatric consultation is recommended for this type of treatment. Medications have been most extensively used in patients with borderline personality disorder. Borderline patients with more affective dysregulation can be considered for treatment with an antidepressant, mood stabilizer, and/or low-dose antipsychotic medication. Antipsychotics can also be considered in borderline patients with dissociative or psychotic symptoms.

Anxiety and fear are the most dominant symptoms of patients with cluster C disorders (avoidant, dependent, and obsessive-compulsive personality disorder). Symptoms in these patients may improve by treatment with an SSRI. Time-limited symptomatic treatment with a benzodiazepine might be considered.

In addition to psychopharmacologic treatments, patients may be referred for various psychosocial and psychotherapeutic treatments, including dialectical behavioral therapy for borderline personality disorder, cognitive-behavioral therapy, and psychodynamic therapies..

SUGGESTED READINGS

Fogel BS. Personality disorders in the medical setting. In: Stoudemire A, Fogel BS, eds. *Psychiatric Care of the Medical Patient.* New York, NY: Oxford University Press, 2000.

Gabbard GO. Psychotherapy of personality disorders. *J Psychother Pract Res* 2000;9:1–6.

Geringer ES, Stern TA. Coping with medical illness: the impact of personality types. *Psychosomatics* 1986;27(4):251–261.

Giesen-Bloo J, van Dyck R, Spinhoven P, et al. Outpatient psychotherapy for borderline personality disorder: randomized trial of schema-focused therapy vs transference-focused psychotherapy. *Arch Gen Psychiatry* 2006;63(6):649–658. [Erratum in: *Arch Gen Psychiatry* 2006;63(9):1008.]

Grant BF, Hasin DS, Stinson FS, et al. Prevalence, correlates, and disability of personality disorders in the United States: results from the national epidemiologic survey on alcohol and related conditions. *J Clin Psychiatry* 2004;65(7):948–958.

Gross R, Olfson M, Gameroff M, et al. Borderline personality disorder in primary care. *Arch Intern Med* 2002;162:53–60.

Gunderson JD. *Borderline Personality Disorder. A Clinical Guide.* Washington, DC: American Psychiatric Publishing, 2001.

Linehan MM, Comtois KA, Murray AM, et al. Two-year randomized controlled trial and follow-up of dialectical behavior therapy vs therapy by experts for suicidal behaviors and borderline personality disorder. *Arch Gen Psychiatry* 2006;63(7):757–766.

Markovitz PJ. Related articles, links: recent trends in the pharmacotherapy of personality disorders. *J Personal Disord* 200418(1):90–101.

Marmar C. Personality disorders. In: Goldman H, ed. *Review of General Psychiatry.* New York, NY: McGraw-Hill, 2000.

Svraki DM, Cloninger RC. Personality disorders. In: Saddock B, Saddock V, eds. *Comprehensive Textbook of Psychiatry.* Philadelphia, PA: Lippincott Williams & Wilkins, 2005.

Dementia & Delirium

27

Bree Johnston, MD, MPH & Kristine Yaffe, MD

INTRODUCTION

Dementia is a common disorder with a prevalence that doubles every 5 years after the age of 60, thereby affecting up to 45% of those age 85 and older. Dementia is defined as an acquired, persistent, and usually progressive impairment in intellectual function, with compromise in multiple cognitive domains, at least one of which is memory. The deficits must represent a significant decline in function, and must be severe enough to interfere with work or social life for the diagnosis to be formally applied. As the disorder progresses, individuals with dementia often fail to recognize family members, are unable to express themselves clearly and meaningfully, and often undergo dramatic personality changes. Table 27-1 lists some of the more common causes of dementia.

Despite the high prevalence of dementia, the diagnosis is often missed by clinicians, particularly in the early stages. The primary care practitioner can play an important role in diagnosing and treating dementia. An early diagnosis can offer the opportunity to involve patients in meaningful advance care planning while they are still able to express their preferences clearly. In addition, potentially treatable causes, though rare, are more likely to be partially or fully reversed if diagnosed early. Later in the disease, the practitioner can work with other team members to manage difficult behaviors, ensure that the patient is as comfortable and safe as possible, recognize when referral for specialist care is needed, educate caregivers about the condition, and support caregivers in coping with their situations to the best of their abilities. Furthermore, with several pharmacologic treatments available for dementing illnesses, it has become more important for physicians to be proficient in diagnosing specific subtypes of dementia and knowing what therapies may (or may not) be helpful for that syndrome.

David M. Pope, PhD, and Alicia Boccellari, PhD, were authors of the first edition version of this chapter, and William Lyons, MD was author of the second edition version of this chapter.

TYPES OF DEMENTIA

Alzheimer Disease

Alzheimer disease (AD) is the most common form of dementia, accounting for about 60–70% of cases. The age of onset varies considerably, but most commonly symptoms arise after age 70. Incidence of the disease increases with age. Women may be at a slightly higher risk of developing the disorder than men. The rare patient with early onset of AD (before age 60) may have a genetic disorder with an autosomal dominant pattern of inheritance, and a good family history is important in these cases.

AD usually follows a slow, but progressive and insidious, course (Table 27-2). Life expectancy following the appearance of the disorder ranges from 3–15 years, but considerable variation may occur, and survival of up to 20 years has been reported. Memory deficits are prominent in all dementias, but especially so in AD. Typically, short-term episodic memory problems are the first and most obvious manifestation of the disorder. AD affects both the encoding and retrieval of new information to a profound degree, such that these patients do not appear to benefit from cueing and prompting of memory. For example, a patient asked to remember the words "piano," "carrot," and "green" may not be helped by hints such as "musical instrument," "vegetable," or "color." Although diagnostic certainty is less than 100% without pathologic examination, careful clinical and neuropsychological evaluation results in a reliable diagnosis of the disease in most instances. A computed tomography (CT) or magnetic resonance imaging (MRI) scan often shows cerebral atrophy and hippocampal volume loss; the electroencephalogram (EEG) may show diffuse slowing. These are nonspecific findings.

CASE ILLUSTRATION 1

Gertrude is 74 years old. She is brought by her family to a medical clinic for evaluation. Since the death of her husband 2 years ago, Gertrude has

Table 27-1. Common causes of dementia.

- Alzheimer disease (AD)
- Vascular disease (multiple infarcts and other cerebrovascular disease)
- Dementia with Lewy Bodies (DLB)
- Frontotemporal dementia
- Parkinson disease
- Metabolic and potentially reversible disease (e.g., chronic vitamin B_{12} deficiency, hypothyroidism)
- HIV/AIDS
- Neurodegenerative disorders (e.g., Huntington's chorea, progressive supranuclear palsy)

become increasingly absentminded, withdrawn, and sedentary. Her family assumed at first that she was grieving and would eventually readjust. Gertrude's condition, however, has continued to deteriorate. Now she is confused and disoriented and has difficulty recognizing family members. Her general physical examination is normal, but her mental status examination reveals multiple deficits. For example, given three words to remember, she

is unable to recall any of them after several minutes. She cannot give the correct month and year and thinks she is in the city where she had lived many years ago. Asked to repeat several sentences, she makes a number of verbal slips. When she is given a geometric design to copy, her drawing is distorted and unrecognizable. Her laboratory examinations are normal, a CT scan of the head shows mild cerebral atrophy, and no other potential explanations for her deficits are found. A diagnosis of AD is eventually made.

In retrospect, her family recalls that Gertrude had been having some mild difficulties in memory and functioning prior to her husband's death and had been dependent on him for helping her to manage things. Recognition of Gertrude's emerging dementia had been made more difficult by her grief and possible depression after her husband's death.

The physician spends some time with family members discussing the nature of Gertrude's condition and options for future care. She inquires about immediate concerns such as agitation and other behavioral disturbances, none of which is currently present. The physician then refers the family to a

Table 27-2. Stages of Alzheimer disease.

Stage	General Change	Specific Change
Early	Patients show relatively subtle changes in memory, along with declining clarity of thought and ability to perform everyday tasks. These changes may go largely unnoticed by the patient and significant others. Patients typically retain some ability to compensate for the cognitive changes.	• Mild memory problems such as missed appointments, failure to pay bills. • Occasional mild and transitory confusion and disorientation. • A "slowed-down" quality to thinking, personality, and lifestyle. • An increase in personal rigidity and intolerance of changes. • Social isolation, loss of interest in usual activities. • Possible increase in restlessness and impulsivity.
Middle	Cognitive deficits become more prominent during this stage and the loss of functioning becomes obvious to others.	• Severe memory impairment. • Frank and persistent confusion and disorientation. • Aphasia, apraxia, and visuospatial disturbances. • Serious difficulties in the ability to manage everyday activities. • Agitation, simple paranoia, other delusions.
Late	In the third, and terminal, stage of the disorder, the patient becomes very inactive, is extremely withdrawn, and loses nearly all ability to engage in purposeful activities.	• Profound loss of short- and long-term memory. • Severe confusion and disorientation. • Bladder and bowel incontinence. • Patient eventually is bedridden and nonresponsive. • Primitive reflexes such as grasping, rooting, and sucking. • Seizures. • Signs of gross neurologic impairment, such as hemiplegia, tremor, pronounced rigidity. • Bodily wasting in the face of adequate nourishment just prior to death.

Note: The signs and symptoms of dementia include the progressive loss of cognitive abilities, especially memory, and a decline in everyday functioning. Dementia is generally a deteriorating condition, and its progression is best described in terms of several stages. The stages outlined above are based on the most common form of dementia, AD.

social worker specializing in geriatric issues and indicates the availability of groups such as the Family Caregiver Alliance for education and support. She also advises Gertrude not to drive, and, in accordance with the law in her state, notifies the health department of the new diagnosis of dementia. Finally, the physician initiates a trial of donepezil, which is associated with no obvious benefits at 3 months, according to the family. The physician and family elect to continue treatment for another 3 months and re-evaluate the treatment at that time.

Dementia With Lewy Bodies

Dementia with Lewy Bodies (DLB) is reported to be the second most common cause of dementia in autopsy studies, accounting for 15–30% of cases. It is defined by the presence of cognitive impairment, parkinsonism, prominent (often bizarre) hallucinations or other psychotic symptoms, and fluctuations in alertness, although patients may not have all of these symptoms. Patients with DLB are often intolerant of traditional antipsychotic medications, and their use can induce severe parkinsonism or even death. At least one randomized-controlled trial suggests that cholinesterase inhibitors such as donepezil may be useful in treating the disorder.

Vascular Dementia

Previously known as multi-infarct dementia, vascular dementia is characterized by the development of cognitive impairment in association with single or multiple areas of infarction and/or subcortical ischemia. Not surprisingly, the risk factors for vascular dementia are identical to the risk factors for cerebrovascular disease, including smoking, hypertension, diabetes mellitus, coronary artery disease (CAD), and previous history of stroke. A patchy and inconsistent pattern of deficits may be seen initially, with relative preservation of some cognitive areas. Because vascular dementia can result from insults to a variety of cortical or subcortical areas, the neuropsychological profile of patients with vascular dementia can be quite varied.

Focal neurologic signs are more common in vascular dementia than in AD, and lateralized motor and sensory findings may be seen. CT and MRI scans frequently reveal multiple areas of infarction in the brain, often with diffuse subcortical white matter changes. Later in the course of the disorder atrophy from loss of brain tissue may be seen.

A number of diagnostic criteria for vascular dementia have been proposed, but none are sensitive or specific enough to rule the diagnosis in or out with certainty. Many elders show diffuse white matter changes

on brain imaging, and yet are cognitively intact. Other demented elders, who were thought by their clinicians to have vascular dementia because of cognitive decline following cerebral infarcts, are subsequently found to have Alzheimer's pathology at autopsy in addition to the known infarcts. Such individuals, with elements of both AD and vascular dementia, are considered to have mixed dementia. In short, current diagnostic instruments and criteria are often inadequate for clinicians confidently to employ or reject the "vascular dementia" label.

Other Causes

Frontotemporal dementias (FTD) are a group of disorders characterized by personality change (e.g., apathy, or socially inappropriate behavior), hyperorality, and cognitive decline especially involving language and executive function. FTD tends to affect individuals at a younger age than AD, with many persons receiving the diagnosis in their 50s or 60s. Imaging studies may show marked atrophy in frontal and temporal lobes.

Advanced Parkinson disease commonly results in dementia. These patients frequently display mental sluggishness and a general lack of spontaneity. Language functions (compared with those of AD patients) are relatively preserved.

Chronic alcohol abuse can result in serious cognitive deficits if drinking is severe and prolonged, although it is not clear whether the dementing process occurs in the absence of coexisting thiamine deficiency. Severe head trauma can also result in permanent cognitive impairment, which might be viewed as static dementia.

Human immunodeficiency virus (HIV)-1-associated dementia (HAD) is caused by the direct infection of the brain by the HIV-1 virus. It is associated with late-stage AIDS and is generally seen in individuals whose T cell count has fallen below 200. Features of this form of dementia are summarized in Table 27-3. HAD is discussed further in Chapter 33. Creutzfeldt-Jacob disease is a rare infectious cause that should be suspected when a nonelderly person develops a rapidly dementing illness associated with other neurologic deficits such as myoclonus.

Table 27-3. Signs and symptoms of advanced HAD.

- Impaired attention and difficulty learning new information
- Slow, soft, and impoverished speech
- Ataxia, decreased manual dexterity, and motor slowness
- Poor judgment
- Flat and unspontaneous facial expression with fixed gaze
- Personality changes that may include apathy or increased impulsivity

---

Reversible Conditions

A number of medical conditions can result in cognitive impairment. These may be treatable, but full or partial reversal of dementia is relatively rare, even with appropriate treatment. However, because dementia is such a devastating diagnosis, assessing the patient for these conditions is an important part of the dementia workup. Fully or partially reversible dementia syndromes are usually the result of depression, medication, or a toxic or metabolic disorder. The most common types of primary and secondary syndromes are listed in Table 27-4.

Differential Diagnosis

Persons suspected of having dementia are encountered in a number of medical settings. For example, a patient who presents to the emergency department with confusion, disorientation, and hallucination should be evaluated for delirium (e.g., from infection, metabolic derangement, or use of or withdrawal from medications or recreational substances) and psychotic disorders. An older adult with a history of recent bereavement, withdrawal, and increased forgetfulness may indeed be demented, or may be suffering from cognitive deficits related to major depression. Other problems that initially may be confused with dementia include sensory deficits (severe visual or hearing impairment), aphasia, developmental disability, and low levels of literacy or education.

Normal Aging

As people age, some degree of decline in cognitive functioning is common. The presence of mild memory impairment among older adults has been reported to occur among a very wide range (11–96%) of participants in various research studies. Normal aging often brings minor word-finding difficulties, slowed memory

Table 27-4. Treatable syndromes that impair cognition.

Hydrocephalus	Chronic subdural hematoma
Metabolic disorders: hypercalcemia, hyper- & hypoglycemia, hyper- & hyponatremia, hyperuricemia	CNS infection (meningitis, encephalitis, abscess)
Myxedema	Medication side effects or toxicity
Hepatic encephalopathy	Vitamin deficiencies: B$_{12}$, thiamine, niacin
Depression	Delirium
Status epilepticus	CNS malignancy

retrieval, and some changes in the speed and efficiency of thought. These changes, however, typically do not cause significant problems in everyday functioning or produce confusion or disorientation, which are signs of impaired cognition (see Chapter 11).

Some individuals demonstrate greater-than-expected cognitive decline for their age, yet they do not meet the criteria for a formal diagnosis of dementia. The label of mild cognitive impairment (MCI) has been applied to this group. These patients tend to have subjective complaints of forgetfulness and objective evidence of memory impairment or deficits in other cognitive domains. Nevertheless, they often have normal overall cognitive function and capabilities for performing activities of daily living. Importantly, such individuals are at substantially increased risk of subsequently becoming demented. The American Academy of Neurology recommends that these patients be identified and monitored by their providers. There is no documented treatment of MCI, although one study suggested that cholinesterase inhibitors may slightly delay the progression of MCI to dementia.

Dementia Versus Delirium

 CASE ILLUSTRATION 2

George is an 80-year-old man who is admitted through the emergency department with a fracture of the femoral neck. He undergoes an open reduction and internal fixation. On the second postoperative day, he develops agitation, pulls out his IV, and is restrained. Physical examination reveals an elderly man who is inattentive, moaning, and seeming to drift in and out of the conversation. The consultant notes that the patient was given 50 mg of diphenhydramine as a "sleeper" the night before, and he now appears to have a distended bladder. Placement of a Foley catheter, around the clock treatment with opioids, low-dose haloperidol, and having family members at his bedside, all seem to help calm him down. Over the next 3 days, he receives no further diphenhydramine, his pain improves, his catheter is removed, and his mental status clears somewhat, but not to his baseline level.

The family says that George had very mild dementia, but seemed to be functioning well at home prior to his hip fracture. Following hospital discharge, he goes to a nursing home for short-term rehabilitation, but he never seems to regain his former level of cognition or functioning. He lives in a nursing home for the remaining year of his life. He dies of apparent aspiration pneumonia after a period of progressive functional and cognitive decline.

Delirium is a state of cognitive impairment that is acute in onset and associated with fluctuations in mental status and behavior, inattention, disorganized thinking, and an altered level of consciousness. Because dementia is a significant risk factor for delirium, the two syndromes are closely linked (see Table 27-5). It is not uncommon for delirious patients to be incorrectly labeled as demented by an inpatient team with no prior knowledge of the patient. Optimized communication between inpatient and outpatient teams, good baseline mental status testing on elderly outpatients, and/or collateral information from family and friends, can often be critical in trying to determine how likely it is that the delirious patient will "clear" enough to be able to live independently following hospital discharge. Unfortunately, some patients, like George, never return to their prior level of functioning following an episode of delirium.

Delirium is usually caused by toxic and metabolic derangements or infections. In determining the cause, a clinician should consider reviewing the medication record (looking for recent changes); checking blood cell counts, electrolytes, renal function, glucose, calcium, and urinalysis; and reviewing a chest film and electrocardiogram. In general, workup does not need to include neuroimaging or lumbar puncture unless routine labs or medication review are unrevealing, or focal neurologic deficits or fever are present.

Most studies have suggested that prevention of delirium is more effective than treatment. Preventive strategies include avoiding anticholinergic medications (like diphenhydramine); treating pain adequately; promoting normal sleep patterns; keeping patients active, stimulated, socially connected, and oriented during the day; making certain vision and hearing aids are available; promoting adequate hydration; and avoiding unnecessary tubes and catheters. Established delirium, if disruptive to care, is probably best treated with low-dose haloperidol, 0.5 mg once or twice daily. If the delirium is related to alcohol or benzodiazepine withdrawal, benzodiazepines are the treatment of choice.

Dementia Versus Depression

Especially among older adults, symptoms of depression may masquerade as dementia (Table 27-6) making it difficult to distinguish between "true" dementia and the dementia syndrome of depression (DSD, formerly called "pseudodementia"). It has become increasingly apparent that depressed patients who present with cognitive impairment are much more likely to go on to develop true dementia within a few years. Formal neuropsychological testing and/or an empiric trial of antidepressant medication may provide the best means of distinguishing between dementia and DSD.

Dementia Versus Psychotic Disorders

The symptoms of psychotic disorders such as schizophrenia or bipolar disorder may resemble the disorganization, confusion, delusions, and agitation that sometimes accompany dementia. The typical presence of more consistent and systematized delusions and the increased likelihood of previous psychosis and a family psychiatric history among individuals with nondementia-related psychotic disorders are important in making this differentiation.

Table 27-5. Delirium vs. dementia: signs and symptoms.

Delirium	Dementia
• Rapid onset; short duration	• Insidious onset; progressive deterioration
• May show heightened autonomic arousal	• No impairment in autonomic arousal
• Clouded consciousness or gross confusion	• Alertness retained in early stages
• Prominent waxing and waning	• Consistently impaired mentation except in late stage dementia
• Often restless, agitated, hypervigilant, or lethargic	• Agitation less prominent; varies with stress
• Gross perceptual distortions and hallucinations common	• If psychotic, usually vague paranoid ideas

Table 27-6. Differentiating between dementia and DSD.

Dementia	DSD
History	
• Slow, insidious onset	• Rapid onset
• Precipitating event not necessarily present	• Recent stress, loss
	• Previous depression
• Family complains of problem	• Patient complains of problem
	• Multiple somatic complaints
Evaluation	
• Often indifferent or anxious	• Sad, withdrawn, hopeless
• Willing to put forth good effort on mental status examination	• Little motivation, poor effort on mental status examination
• Excuses or denies deficits	• Complains of deficits
• Psychotic symptoms usually not with depressive content	• If psychotic, has depressive quality

DIAGNOSTIC WORKUP

A dementia workup should include a careful history (Table 27-7) and physical, neurologic, and mental status examinations. In many cases, additional tests and procedures may be helpful; these are discussed later.

History

A complete history should be elicited from both patients and their families. In many cases, it is helpful to ask both about the same topics. Although many demented individuals are unreliable historians, they may be able to provide much useful information, including symptoms of which family members are not aware. In addition, patients' abilities to provide a coherent and organized account of their complaints and recent history can often tell you much about their conditions.

A complete social and family history that includes native language; family history of dementia; and educational, marital, and employment background can also be useful. An educational and occupational history, for example, may provide information about a patient's previous level of functioning. A quality of vagueness in patients' reports or inconsistency in the information supplied may suggest less blatant memory deficits. Particular attention should be paid to patients' accounts of more recent events. Individuals with mild or moderate dementia often show intact recall for older, overlearned information (e.g., family, education, work) but cannot provide accurate information about the immediate past.

Ask patients about their regular activities, appetite, and sleep habits, as well as any physical or cognitive complaints. Information about their mood can be gained not only by inquiring directly, but also by asking about things that they enjoy and look forward to, any worries or concerns they may have, and their plans for the future.

Family members may be able to supply a more complete and balanced impression of the patient's symptoms, behavioral changes, and level of functioning. Individuals with dementia typically lack insight into their cognitive problems and minimize or deny any difficulties. In fact, it is the family that most frequently raises concerns about the patient. Because family members may feel more comfortable discussing their observations away from the presence of the patient, they should be interviewed separately. It is especially important to inquire about both current and potential safety issues, such as driving (Table 27-8).

Physical & Neurologic Examinations

In addition to a routine physical examination, a complete neurologic examination should be done, although the results of the latter are generally unremarkable in cases of early AD. Parkinsonian signs may be apparent during the later course of many dementing illnesses. Individuals with a developing vascular dementia may show focal signs on the neurologic examination.

The Mental Status Examination

Because cognitive impairment is the hallmark of dementia, it is necessary to add additional screening items to the traditional mental status examination. Several brief dementia-screening instruments offer the advantages of both a structured format and a scoring system. These instruments must be used with caution, however, for the reasons discussed here.

The Mini-Mental State Examination (MMSE)© is the most commonly used dementia-screening instrument (see Table 27-9). It takes about 5 minutes to administer and samples a wide range of functions, including orientation, immediate and delayed memory, concentration, basic language and reading functions, and visual construction abilities. Patients are asked to count backward by 7, write a sentence, follow concrete directions, and copy geometric figures. A maximum score of 30 is possible; a score lower than 24 (some clinicians recommend 27) is suspicious for dementia. Because the MMSE is not sensitive for early dementia, a significant number of false-negative results occur among individuals with mild disease. Conversely, low scores may be obtained from individuals who are not demented but are uncooperative, psychiatrically impaired, not formally educated, or lacking in English proficiency. Consequently, results should be interpreted cautiously. Other brief dementia-screening instruments include the Mini-Cog, the Blessed Dementia Scale, and the Neurobehavioral Cognitive Status Examination.

Table 27-7. Dementia workup: history.

- Time course and nature of symptoms and functional decline
- Slow and insidious vs. more sudden/dramatic changes
- Current ability to function
- Accompanying mood or personality changes
- Presence or absence of confusion, agitation, and disorientation
- Psychotic symptoms
- Complicating factors, such as alcohol or substance abuse

Table 27-8. Dementia workup: potential safety issues.

- Ambulation and balance
- Dizziness
- Ability to live independently
  - Leaving stove or running water unattended
  - Wandering behavior
  - Confusion/agitation
  - Ability to manage finances
- Ability to drive
- Level of supervision available

Table 27-9. Dementia workup: MMSE.

Function	Question or Task	Maximum Score
Orientation	What is the year, season, date, day, month? (5 points)	10
	Where are we: state, county, town, hospital, floor? (5 points)	
Registration	Name three objects and ask the patient to repeat the names of the objects (correct response = 1 point). Repeat the names of the three objects until the patient learns them.	3
Attention and calculation	Ask the patient to recite serial 7s backward from 100. Stop the patient after five responses (correct response = 1 point).	5
Recall	Ask the patient to repeat the names of the three objects learned above (correct response = 1 point).	3
Language	Show the patient two common objects, e.g., a pencil and watch, and ask the patient to identify them (2 points). Ask the patient to repeat "no ifs, ands, or buts" (1 point). Instruct the patient to follow the three-stage command: "take a paper in your right hand, fold it in half, and put it on the floor" (3 points). Ask the patient to read and obey the following: "close your eyes" (1 point). Instruct the patient to write a sentence (1 point). Ask the patient to copy a design (1 point).	9

Source: Reprinted, with permission, from Folstein MF, Folstein SE, McHugh PR. "Mini-Mental State": a practical method for grading the cognitive state of patients for the clinician. *J Psychiatr Res* 1975;12:189–198.

Other Tests

The American Academy of Neurology recommends that structural neuroimaging (with noncontrast CT or MRI) be employed in the initial evaluation of most patients with dementia, as some 5% of such patients have been found to have important but clinically unexpected structural lesions. We believe that in cases of long-standing dementia that is consistent with AD, there may be instances when the burdens of neuroimaging outweigh the benefits, particularly in a patient who becomes agitated in unfamiliar settings. An EEG is helpful if the differential diagnosis includes status epilepticus or postictal confusion. On the other hand, the major dementing disorders, especially early in their course, do not generate characteristic EEG patterns, and a normal EEG cannot be taken as definitive evidence of the absence of brain pathology.

Lumbar punctures are indicated when there is a question of an infectious process or when a rapidly progressing condition is present. In rare instances brain biopsy may be employed to help with diagnosis. See Table 27-10 for other recommended laboratory tests.

Neuropsychological Testing

Neuropsychological testing involves the use of psychometric tests designed to detect and characterize a wide variety of cognitive problems. The testing requires the patient to be able to attend for a minimum of 20–30 minutes; some patients may be too agitated, withdrawn, or resistant to comply. Consider referring a patient for neuropsychological testing in the following circumstances:

- When the reported deficits are subtle or equivocal and the impairment is mild.
- When the differential diagnosis is difficult to resolve (e.g., distinguishing between dementia and depression).
- When a baseline is needed to measure the degree of cognitive deterioration over time.
- When a greater understanding of the patient's everyday level of functioning, limitations, potential safety issues, and the appropriate level of supervision is needed.
- When deficits or competency issues must be documented, such as in conservatorship proceedings.
- To monitor effects of treatment.

Table 27-10. Dementia workup: recommended laboratory tests.*

Complete blood count	Calcium
Thyroid studies	Albumin
Blood urea nitrogen	Vitamin B$_{12}$
Creatinine	Electrolytes

*Consider: liver function, rapid plasma reagin, HIV serology, glucose, medication serum levels, toxicology screens, folate, urinalysis, and lumbar puncture.

TREATMENT & MANAGEMENT ISSUES

Treatment of dementia consists of identifying and addressing a treatable basis for the underlying condition (if one exists), treating secondary disorders such as anxiety or depression, educating patients and their families as to the nature of the condition, and assisting caregivers with safety and management issues. In addition, clinical trials have demonstrated benefits of pharmacologic agents that may directly improve cognition and functional capacity of AD patients, or at least slow their decline. Table 27-11 summarizes overall principles of dementia management.

Behavioral Issues

Management of patients with dementia involves matters of self-care, safety, and communication. Individuals with dementia are characteristically disorganized, forgetful, and inefficient in many of their activities. They have difficulty following directions, in managing everyday activities, and in expressing themselves clearly. They may be impulsive, have limited insight into their abilities, and fail to learn from experience. Emotionally, they may be labile and unstable, irritable, or anxious; they may be fearful, easily frustrated, or apathetic and withdrawn. Because of circadian rhythm disturbances, patients with AD may tend to be awake and wandering during the night, leading to sleep deprivation in caregivers.

These traits create special problems in managing and caring for patients with dementia, and many interactions with family and caregivers therefore focus on day-to-day management issues and behavioral problems. The following sections provide some general guidelines for addressing these issues. It is useful in many situations to refer patients and their families to groups that can provide counseling, home evaluations, and case management. (In some instances, there may be no more important knowledge for the primary doctor than familiarity with the capabilities of local support agencies.)

Table 27-11. Overall principles of dementia management.

- Periodically assess safety and self-care function
- Assess caregiver each visit
- Address advance directives early
- Educate patient and caregivers about dementing condition
- Refer to Alzheimer's Association and supportive community organizations
- Treat secondary disorders (anxiety, depression)
- "Fine-tune" comorbid illnesses (e.g., congestive heart failure)
- Consider a trial of cholinesterase inhibitors for mild-to-moderate AD
- Consider a trial of memantine for moderate-to-severe AD

SELF-CARE

This area includes dressing, grooming, and hygiene. The best approach is to provide sufficient structure and guidance so that the patient can manage, while allowing some preservation of independence and choice. Individuals with MCI often get by with prompts and reminders. For individuals with more severe impairment, caregivers should offer a limited choice of clothing, food, or activities; use signs or pictures to identify important objects and locations; and emphasize routine and predictability. Breaking down complex and potentially overwhelming activities such as bathing into simple one step tasks may keep these activities manageable well into the course of the illness. The caregiver may need to modify clothing, for example, by incorporating sweatshirts to avoid buttons, and using shoes with Velcro closures rather than laces.

SAFETY ISSUES

Individuals with dementia are at increased risk for accidents because of their problems with attention, perception, and judgment. The following guidelines are designed to minimize the risk of household accidents:

- Carefully supervise use of medications.
- Keep things simple: reduce clutter; keep passageways clear.
- Install railings and other safety equipment, such as shower chairs and tub rails.
- Use a night-light where necessary.
- Remove stove and oven controls if necessary.
- Use safety gates or install keyless locks on exterior doors if wandering is a problem.
- Make sure patients wear medical and personal identification bracelets.

Another important safety issue concerns driving and dementia. Deficits in attention, reaction time, visual spatial abilities, and judgment typically impair the ability of individuals with marked cognitive deficits to operate a motor vehicle safely. Individuals with advanced dementia who continue to operate a car seriously endanger others as well as themselves. Unfortunately, patients with dementia may insist on driving because of their lack of insight into their problems, and caregivers may be reluctant to press the issue. Because driving is symbolic of independence, this often becomes an emotional issue for everyone involved.

Confidentiality must be weighed against issues of competency, safety of the public, and the duty to warn. Legal requirements vary considerably between states. For example, in California physicians are required by law to report patients who are unable to operate a motor vehicle because of "Alzheimer's or other related dementias." In the case of accident or injury, physicians who have failed to make such a report may be legally

Table 27-12. Tips for communicating with the cognitively impaired.

- Make sure you have patients' attention when you speak with them. Keep distractions, such as television, radio, or other conversations, to a minimum by meeting with patients in a quiet place.
- Keep communications brief, simple, and concrete. Break more complex information down into smaller pieces.
- Give patients several options to choose among, or phrase questions in multiple-choice format.
- Have patients paraphrase back the information to make sure they have understood what was said.

---

liable. Clinicians should inform themselves of the legal requirements in their own state regarding this issue.

COMMUNICATION

Individuals with brain impairment may have specific deficits in language comprehension and expression similar to the various forms of aphasia that occur in stroke patients. More common may be a generalized difficulty in communication secondary to a short attention span, memory problems, or confusion. Some guidelines for communicating with the cognitively impaired are presented in Table 27-12.

Drug Therapy

MEDICATION FOR COGNITIVE DEFICITS

No drug has been shown to prevent or reverse dementia, although intensive research efforts are currently underway. Aggressive treatment of vascular risk factors can help reduce the risk of stroke, and it is a reasonable strategy for patients with vascular risk factors who are at risk for vascular dementia.

Cholinesterase inhibitors have been the class of drugs most extensively studied for use with AD patients. Currently, there are four Food and Drug Administration (FDA)-approved medications, but only three are commonly in use: donepezil, rivastigmine, and galantamine.

Most studies have tested these agents in patients with mild-to-moderate dementia, which may roughly correspond to MMSE scores of 10 to 24. On the whole, statistically significant benefits have been demonstrated, but clinical effects tend to be modest, equating to about a 1-point difference in MMSE score after 2 years of treatment. Patients, families, and caregivers should not expect dramatic results. Table 27-13 gives dosing recommendations for the four medications. The drugs have not yet been studied in head-to-head comparisons, so drug choice may best be made based on half-life and side effects. If a patient is started on one of these drugs and shows no benefit (as gauged by clinicians' and caregivers' impression of behavior and function, and confirmed by some form of neuropsychological testing, such as the MMSE) after a few months, the drug should be discontinued. For this purpose, "benefit" might practically be defined as a slowing in the rate of decline, if not frank improvement. These medications have also shown some efficacy in vascular dementia, DLB, and possibly, for the behavioral disturbances of dementia. For more advanced AD, memantine, a *N*-methyl-D-aspartate (NMDA) antagonist, with or without concomitant use of a cholinesterase inhibitor may produce modest benefits. For vascular dementia, treatment of vascular risk factors may reduce the incidence of future stroke.

MEDICATION FOR SEVERE BEHAVIORAL AND PSYCHIATRIC PROBLEMS

When serious psychiatric symptoms occur, such as severe depression, agitation, or psychosis, psychotropic medications may be indicated. Some general guidelines should be followed:

- Because these medications have the potential to further disrupt cognitive processes and worsen the problem, use considerably lower doses than those used for younger or nondemented individuals. Older adults are particularly susceptible to side effects from these medications, especially when there are concurrent medical problems.
- Avoid benzodiazepines, especially for more than brief periods, as they have significant potential for causing sedation, confusion, and ataxia.

Table 27-13. Cholinesterase inhibitors for AD.

Drug	Initial Regimen	Dose Escalation
Donepezil	5 mg orally every day	10 mg orally every day after 4–6 weeks
Rivastigmine	1.5 mg orally twice a day	Adjust every 2 weeks to 3 mg orally twice a day, then 4.5 mg orally twice a day, maximum 6 mg orally twice a day
Galantamine	4 mg orally twice a day	Adjust every 4 weeks to 8 mg orally twice a day, maximum 12 mg orally twice a day
Memantine	5 mg daily	Increase to 5 mg bid after 1 week, increase by 5 mg weekly until maximum 10 mg bid

- A recent randomized controlled trial suggested that donepezil had no benefit when used to treat agitation in Alzheimer disease. However, if a medication such as a cholinesterase inhibitor or memantine is being considered for cognition, it is reasonable to see if it has an impact on behavior, as well. If at all possible, we recommend delaying the prescription of second agent (e.g. antipsychotic or other psychoactive medication) until the impact of the cognitive agent medication can be evaluated.

- If behavioral approaches fail, it may be necessary to try an antipsychotic medication. All antipsychotic medications appear to be modest in efficacy but carry some risk, so should be used with caution. Haloperidol (Haldol), an older "typical" antipsychotic agent, is often used at an initial dosage of 0.5 mg orally every night or twice daily, with gradual and slow increases if symptoms persist. Newer "atypical" antipsychotics such as risperidone (starting 0.5 mg orally every night) and olanzapine (starting 2.5 mg orally every night) may be less likely to produce extrapyramidal side effects than "typicals" when used at lower dosages. However, all atypicals carry a "black box" warning because their use in patients with dementia is associated with an excess risk of stroke and death. Although typical antipsychotics such as haloperidol do not have a black box warning (at least at the time of this review), they may also be associated with excess mortality. If antipsychotic medications are being considered, the potential risks and benefits should be discussed with the caregiver, and their efficacy and side effect profiles should be frequently re-evaluated.

- If the problem continues, consider another agent or obtain consultation with a psychiatrist, preferably one specializing in geriatric psychiatry.

- Nonpsychotic agitation deserves careful evaluation before a drug is prescribed. New agitation may represent delirium, undertreated pain, depression, a distended bladder, or fecal impaction. If these disorders are not contributing and if nonpharmacologic approaches are inadequate, an empiric trial of analgesics such as acetaminophen, an antidepressant medication, or a mood stabilizer may be worthwhile. However, any empiric trial should be time limited, and consultation with a geriatric psychiatrist is recommended in recalcitrant cases if at all possible.

Caregivers

Caring for cognitively impaired individuals is often exhausting and stressful. Primary care providers should ensure that caregivers also attend to their own needs and guard against fatigue and burnout. A number of support services, such as the Family Caregiver Alliance (web site http://www.caregiver.org), offer education, support groups, and information about resources. Specialized case management and home consultation services can also be very helpful in assessing patient and family needs and locating additional services. Respite-care and day-activity programs may be invaluable in allowing stressed families and caregivers time off and providing needed stimulation and increased structure for the patient. Many experienced clinicians often assess stressed caregivers at each clinic visit.

Nursing Home Placement

In the management of demented patients, the issue often arises as to whether the patient can continue to be managed at home. This is an area fraught with strong feelings on the part of patient and caregiver alike, and it is often difficult to make objective decisions. Major predictors of nursing home placement include the presence of behavioral problems, dementia severity, and extent of caregiver burden. Some important considerations related to nursing home admission are as follows:

- Can the necessary level of supervision and care required by the patient be realistically and dependably supplied at home? Such issues as wandering and the potential for neglect and abuse should be considered here.

- Is sufficient assistance available to caregivers for them to continue to care for the patient without becoming overstressed and burned out?

- What financial resources are available for the patient's care?

All things being equal, many patients and caregivers prefer to remain in their own home. In many cases, however, doing so creates other significant problems, and however desirable this goal, it must be carefully weighed against issues of safety and practical limitations. In the advanced stage of dementia, when the patient becomes mute, bedbound, and incontinent, very often the services of a skilled nursing facility are required to ensure that the patient receives proper care. Nursing facilities should be chosen carefully; obviously, cost must be considered, but the quality of care must also be investigated. Information about both complaints and compliance with state regulations can be found through government agencies, advocacy groups, published reviews, and organizations (e.g., geriatric care programs) that frequently place patients in such facilities. Although definitive data are lacking, some studies suggest that Alzheimer's special care units reduce behavioral disturbances and use of restraints. Some patients do better in structured environments such as Alzheimer's special care units or Alzheimer's day care programs than in less structured home settings.

Dementia is a terminal disease, and in late stages the patient may become bedbound, unable to recognize family, and have difficulty swallowing. In these instances, hospice care is often appropriate (see Chapter 37).

SUMMARY

Dementia is an increasingly common syndrome characterized by a progressive loss of cognition and functioning. Given the aging of the population, it is essential that clinicians become comfortable with diagnosis, counseling, community and specialist referral, and treatment. Early diagnosis may allow for identification of (unfortunately rare) reversible causes, improved symptom management, and planning for the future.

When patients present with cognitive complaints, the clinician must consider differential diagnoses including dementia, delirium, depression, and psychosis. Diagnostic workup includes a careful history from patient and family, physical examination, mental status examination, lab work, brain imaging, and on occasion, referral or neuropsychological testing or other specialized assessment.

Treatment and management consist of ruling out treatable conditions, treating secondary disorders such as anxiety or depression, providing information to patients and families, and assisting caregivers with safety and management issues. Use of medications may modestly slow the rate of cognitive decline or help with management of severe psychiatric symptoms, but interventions also consist of adjusting the environment to make the patient as comfortable and safe as possible and providing support for caregivers.

Taking care of demented patients and their caregivers can be extremely rewarding. Further, with abundant research efforts under way, there is reason to be optimistic that improved methods of preventing and treating dementing disorders are just over the horizon.

SUGGESTED READINGS

Borson S, Scanlan JM, Chen P, et al. The Mini-Cog as a screen for dementia: validation in a population-based sample. *J Am Geriatr Soc* 2003;51(10):1451–1454. PMID: 14511167.

Clarfield AM. The decreasing prevalence of reversible dementias: an updated meta-analysis. *Arch Intern Med* 2003;163(18): 2219–2229.

Courtney C, Farrell D, Gray R, et al. Long-term donepezil treatment in 565 patients with Alzheimer's disease: (AD2000): randomized double blind trial. *Lancet* 2004;363:2105–2115. PMID: 15220031.

Howard RJ, Juszczak E, Ballard CG, et al. Donepezil for the treatment of agitation in Alzheimer's disease. *N Engl J Med* 2007;357:1382–1392.

McKeith I, Del Ser T, Spano PF, et al. Efficacy of rivastigmine in dementia with Lewy bodies: a randomized, double blind, placebo controlled international study. *Lancet* 2000;356: 2031–2036. PMID: 1145488.

Modrego PJ, Ferrandez J. Depression in patients with mild cognitive impairment increases the risk of developing dementia of Alzheimer type: a prospective cohort study. *Arch Neurol* 2004; 61(8):1290–1293. PMID: 15313849.

Petersen RC, Thomas RG, Grundman M, et al. Vitamin E and donepezil for the treatment of mild cognitive impairment. *N Engl J Med* 2005;352(23):2379–2388. Epub 2005; Apr 13. PMID: 15829527.

Petersen RC, Stevens JC, Ganguli M, et al. Practice parameter: early detection of dementia: mild cognitive impairment (an evidence-based review). *Neurology* 2001;56:1133–1142.

Reisberg B, Doody R, Stoffler A, et al. Memantine in moderate-to-severe Alzheimer's disease. *N Engl J Med* 2003;348:1333–1341. PMID: 12672860.

Schneider LS, Dagerman KS, Insel P, et al. Risk of death with atypical antipsychotic drug treatment for dementia. *JAMA* 2005;294: 1934–1943.

Sink KM, Holden, KF, Yaffe K. Pharmacologic treatment of neuropsychiatric symptoms of dementia: a review of the evidence. *JAMA* 2005;293:596–608. PMID: 15687315.

Trinh NH, Hoblyn J, Mohanty S, et al. Efficacy of cholinesterase inhibitors in the treatment of neuropsychiatric symptoms and functional impairment in Alzheimer's disease: a meta-analysis. *JAMA* 2003;289:210–216. PMID: 12517232.

Wang PS, Schneeweiss S, Avorn J, et al. Risk of death in elderly users of conventional vs. atypical antipsychotic medications. *N Engl J Med* 2005;353:2335–2341.

Wilkinson D, Doody R, Helme R, et al. Donepezil in vascular dementia: a randomized placebo controlled trial. *Neurology* 2003; 61:479–486. PMID: 12939421.

WEB SITES

Alzheimer's Association Web site. http://www.alz.org. Accessed October, 2007.

Alzheimer's Disease Education and Referral Center Web site. http:// www.alzheimers.org. Accessed October, 2007.

American Geriatrics Society Web site. http://www.americangeriatrics. org. Accessed October, 2007.

Assessment instruments for dementia and related disorders available at Society for Hospital Medicine Web site. http://www.hospitalmedicine.org/geriresource/toolbox. Accessed October, 2007.

Blessed Dementia Scale Web site. http://www.strokecenter.org/trials/ scales/blessed_dementia.html. Accessed October, 2007.

Brain Injury Association of America Web site. http://www.biausa.org. Accessed October, 2007.

Eldercare Locator (nationwide toll-free service helps older adults and caregivers to fine local services for seniors) Web site. http://www. eldercare.gov. Accessed October, 2007.

Family Caregiver Alliance Web site. http://www.caregiver.org. Accessed October, 2007.

Gerontological Society of America Web site. http://www.geron.org. Accessed October, 2007.

Mini-mental state exam Web site http://www.minimental.com. Accessed October, 2007.

Sleep Disorders

28

Clifford M. Singer, MD & Garrick A. Applebee, MD

INTRODUCTION

Thirty-five percent of adults in the United States experience sleep-related symptoms over the course of a year, making insomnia and daytime sleepiness among the most common symptoms seen in medical practice. Ten to fifteen percent of these adults will suffer chronic insomnia and will be frequent visitors to health care providers. Sleep disorders also pose a major public health threat. Chronic insomnia is associated with doubling of mortality rate over time. Sleep deprivation increases risk for chronic disease, including hypertension, diabetes and depression. Daytime sleepiness impairs work performance and increases the risk of industrial and motor vehicle accidents. Sleep loss due to sleep-related breathing problems leads to profound sleepiness and life-threatening cardiovascular and pulmonary diseases. Sleep medications themselves carry morbidity such as falls, daytime anxiety, and worsened sleep apnea.

Normal Sleep Physiology

ADULTHOOD

The sleep–wake cycle is a complex electrophysiologic process consisting of alternating periods of wakefulness, rapid eye movement (REM) sleep, and non-REM sleep. Each of these periods has a characteristic electroencephalogram (EEG), peripheral muscle, and autonomic nervous system pattern that can be documented by polysomnographic (PSG) recording in hospital-based sleep laboratories, although newer technology allows in-home recordings. PSG allows clinicians to make specific diagnoses based on electrophysiologic monitoring of EEG, electrooculogram, electromyogram, nasal airflow, ear oximetry, and electrocardiogram.

Sleep has a structure, or architecture, that consists of four stages of non-REM and REM sleep cycles. The wake EEG contains low-voltage, high-frequency waveforms that become dominated by alpha waveforms (8–12 cps) as a person becomes drowsy. Stage 1 sleep is defined by the disappearance of the alpha pattern, the establishment of theta waveforms (2–7 cps) and slow, rolling eye movements. Stage 2 is defined by the appearance of low-frequency, high-amplitude discharges (K complexes) and brief high-frequency (12–14 cps), variable-amplitude discharges (sleep spindles) on a background of theta waveforms similar to stage 1. The emergence of slow waves (high-amplitude, low-frequency [0.5–2 cps] delta waveforms) heralds stage 3 sleep, when they make up at least 20% of sleep time, and stage 4 sleep when they comprise more than 50% of sleep time. These two stages are known as the "deep stages" of sleep, because they are associated with high-arousal thresholds. REM sleep is a distinct state of sleep characterized by wake-pattern EEG, skeletal muscle paralysis, and rapid, conjugate eye movements.

With the initiation of sleep, the healthy adult will descend through the non-REM stages within 45–60 minutes before beginning the first REM cycle, which tends to be brief. As the night progresses, less time is spent in slow-wave sleep and REM cycle duration increases, eventually comprising 20–25% of total sleep time. The non-REM/REM cycle typically lasts 90–110 minutes, with about four complete cycles per night.

The timing and duration of sleep are controlled by many factors. Although most adults have some control over when to go to sleep and when to wake up, they have less control over how much sleep they need and when they become sleepy. Although stimulants such as caffeine and habituation to a state of chronic fatigue can help people cope with inadequate sleep, they must ultimately pay the price of diminished energy and mental efficiency. Individual sleep requirements vary; while most people need 6–9 hours of sleep per night, the human range is thought to be from 3 to 12 hours. Children generally need more sleep than adults, but after adolescence, daily sleep requirement remains fairly stable until late life. In old age, sleep need may increase or decrease, but the most dramatic changes are in sleep quality and duration. There is a gradual reduction in the amount of time spent in deep sleep as we age, plus a tendency to have more awakenings at night and more naps during the day.

The body clock (hypothalamic suprachiasmatic nucleus), functions as the circadian pacemaker. It superimposes a rhythm of sleepiness and alertness to days and nights and determines whether a person is a night owl, morning lark, or somewhere in between. The light–dark cycle and nightly rhythm of melatonin secretion by the pineal gland act synergistically to keep the body clock synchronized with the day–night cycle, allowing alertness during the day and sleepiness at night.

CHILDHOOD

Newborns typically spend about 70% of each day asleep, with more time in REM than older children and adults. A circadian pattern of wake and sleep does not usually develop until 1–2 months of age, rhythmic melatonin secretion being identified at 12 weeks. Of great interest to parents, sleeping through the night is one of the first maturational milestones. Sleep continues to be polyphasic, with decreasing amounts of daytime napping until the child is 4 or 5 years. From ages 5 to 10 years, children are usually consummate sleepers with few arousals. Total sleep time gradually decreases throughout childhood, but for hormonal and psychosocial reasons the amount and quality of sleep drops sharply with puberty. This is exacerbated by a high incidence of delayed sleep-phase syndrome (DSPS), which puts adolescents at odds with their environment and in subsequent chronic sleep deprivation.

There is ongoing debate over household arrangements for children's sleep. Some anthropologists point out that isolating a newborn in a separate bedroom is unique to western cultures and that co-sleeping with infants is more natural and may be beneficial. Recent studies have linked bed sharing with Sudden Infant Death Syndrome (SIDS), however, and the current recommendation of the American Academy of Pediatrics (2005) is to place infants in a separate sleeping area in the same room with the parent. Sleeping alone in a separate room is a desirable mark of independence, but at what age this should occur varies considerably depending on the child and the family.

OLD AGE

As people age, sleep tends to be lighter, with more frequent awakenings and the near disappearance of deep or slow-wave sleep. Sleep onset and awakening come earlier. Sleep disorders also increase with age, including insomnia and disorders causing excessive daytime sleepiness, such as obstructive sleep apnea (OSA) and periodic leg movements.

CLASSIFICATION OF SLEEP DISORDERS

Sleep disorders are generally grouped into three categories: disorders of initiating and maintaining sleep (insomnias), disorders of excessive daytime sleepiness

Table 28-1. The sleepless patient: disorders of initiating and maintaining sleep.

Category	Disorder
Insomnia	Transient and chronic insomnia, chronobiological insomnia, comorbid insomnia (secondary to RLS, periodic leg movements, mood and anxiety disorders, alcohol and drugs, and medical disorders affecting sleep)
Hypersomnia	Sleep apnea syndrome, narcolepsy, idiopathic CNS hypersomnolence, delirium, advanced dementia, and traumatic brain injury
Parasomnia	Pavor nocturnus (sleep terrors), nightmares, somnambulism (sleepwalking), and RBD

(hypersomnias), and abnormal sleep behaviors (parasomnias) (Table 28-1).

Every review of systems should include screening patients for daytime sleepiness and nighttime sleep problems. Three basic questions give clinicians a head start in diagnosing sleep disorders and determining whether they are severe enough to warrant treatment:

- How are you sleeping?
- How much sleep do you get in a typical night?
- Do you feel alert during the day?

Follow-up questions should sharpen the differential diagnosis of specific disorders.

The Sleepless Patient: The Insomnias

TRANSIENT AND PERSISTENT INSOMNIA

Insomnia is one of the most common complaints in primary care practice. It is best to think of insomnia as a symptom rather than a diagnosis. Many factors combine to produce insomnia, which often occurs when a delicate balance is tipped; for example, a constitutionally light sleeper may be fine until he or she enters a period of stress or uses a medication that has alerting effects. It may be necessary to deal with several causative factors concurrently to restore a natural sleep cycle.

Insomnia is often described as initial insomnia (trouble falling asleep), and middle or terminal insomnia (trouble staying asleep during the night or early morning awakening). Insomnia may be transient (self-limited) or chronic (persistent or relapsing). Transient insomnia can evolve into chronic insomnia by a number of perpetuating factors.

Transient insomnia caused by stress, environment (cold, noise, new baby), acute illness, or pain is easy to identify and usually needs no special intervention other than addressing the underlying problem. A brief course of sedative-hypnotic medication is occasionally warranted and may reduce the risk of developing long-term insomnia. Travel across time zones brings about a mismatch between the body clock and the day-night cycle that induces transient insomnia known as "jet lag." Combined with fatigue from travel, jet lag can ruin the first few days of a trip. Shift workers may experience the same phenomenon and can suffer severe health and social consequences because of it.

In a large multicenter study, the diagnosis of chronic insomnia accounted for 40–88% of patients in medical, psychiatric, and sleep clinics who presented with a primary complaint of insomnia. Chronic insomnia is a diagnosis of exclusion, and must be differentiated from the many other causes of long-term sleep disruption (see later discussion). Chronic insomnia goes by many names: psychophysiologic insomnia, conditioned insomnia, learned insomnia, and primary insomnia. These terms all imply what is known about this condition: it is a chronic ailment that develops over time in what is conceived as operant conditioning to an arousal state incompatible with deep, sustained, restful sleep. It may develop after a period of sleep disruption from stress, infant care, medical illness, pain, or psychological stress. In rare instances, it may be a lifelong problem caused by biological variation in sleep drive. Despite their severe fatigue, patients with insomnia may not be able to fall asleep for daytime naps, in contrast to people with transient sleep deprivation.

Primary insomnia requires a holistic approach that can include use of medication as well as cognitive-behavioral strategies to reduce anxiety and behavioral changes to improve sleep hygiene (see Table 28-2). Short-term use of sedative-hypnotic medications is appropriate to break the cycle of anxiety, arousal, and insomnia (see "Medical Treatment," below). In some patients, the symptoms suggest another disorder that can be targeted separately (depression, restless legs syndrome [RLS]).

CHRONOBIOLOGICAL DISORDERS OF THE SLEEP–WAKE CYCLE

The timing of sleep is influenced by the hypothalamic circadian pacemaker or "body clock." Disturbances in the circadian timing of sleep may be transient, as in jet lag and shift work syndromes, or chronic, as in DSPS, advanced sleep-phase syndrome, and free-running sleep syndrome. The last is most common in blind persons, who lack the critical input of the light–dark cycle in regulating circadian rhythms. Diagnosis of chronobiological disorders is based on the understanding that except for its timing, sleep is normal in these conditions. Given the freedom to choose sleep times based only on internal cues of sleepiness, persons with chronobiological insomnias usually sleep well on weekends or while on vacation. A mismatch between the body clock and the hours that a person attempts to sleep may cause insomnia.

RESTLESS LEGS SYNDROME

This condition comes on with rest and produces an irresistible need to move, stretch, or rub the lower extremities. Severe dysesthesia may occur, sometimes described as "creepy-crawling sensations," aching, tension, tingling, or prickling. Most people with RLS also have periodic limb movements during sleep, leading to further sleep disruption. RLS can interfere with plane travel, deskwork, reading, and especially sleep onset. The syndrome is common, affecting at least 5% of the population, and may be even more common in periodic or subclinical form. In females it sometimes first appears during pregnancy, but in both genders it can run in families and tends to worsen with age. It is especially common in patients with renal failure and Parkinson disease (PD). Many physicians do not think to ask about this symptom and hence fail to recognize it as a source of discomfort and insomnia for their patients.

The first-line treatment of RLS involves the use of the newer nonergotamine dopamine agonist agents (e.g., pramipexole and ropinirole) Dopamine precursor

---

Table 28-2. Cognitive-behavioral treatment for insomnia.

Essential Cognitive Technique	Essential Behavioral Change
1. Talk about the frustration of not falling asleep and put this into perspective, i.e., decatastrophize being awake	1. Bed or sleep restriction (out of bed if awake more than 30 min, no TV, reading, or eating in bed)
2. Education about sleep requirements (not everyone needs 8 h) and day napping (OK if very sleepy)	2. Stimulus control: go to bed only when sleepy, use bedroom only for sleep and sex, remove stress and clutter from bedroom
3. Confront patient's belief that they are "defective" in sleep and will always be a poor sleeper; instill hope for better sleep but without unrealistic expectations that every night will be filled with sound sleep	3. Improved sleep hygiene: no caffeine, alcohol, or nicotine late in the day, mild-to-moderate exercise in the afternoon, keep naps short and early

treatment levadopa/carbidopa is effective as well, but may be associated with "rebound" or "augmentation" effects, with a tendency for the symptoms to develop earlier in the day. Anticonvulsant and sedative-hypnotic drugs may be helpful. Opiates may be indicated in severe or refractory cases. The syndrome is so distressful for some of its sufferers that there is a national support group and newsletter (see "Resources," below for reference to the RLS Foundation on web-link to the National Sleep Foundation).

PERIODIC LEG MOVEMENTS DURING SLEEP (PLMS)

These are repetitive myoclonic movements of the lower extremities that come in bursts lasting from a few seconds to many minutes; they are more common in, but not limited to, the first half of the night. The movements are usually associated with brief arousals and can lead to nonrestorative sleep and daytime somnolence. The prevalence of PLMS increases with age—5% in people 30–50 years of age, 29% in those 50–65, and 44% in those over 65—and is often seen in metabolic and neurodegenerative diseases. PLMS should be distinguished from nocturnal leg cramps, which are painful, prolonged involuntary contractions of the muscles of the lower legs. Tricyclic antidepressants, lithium carbonate, and withdrawal from benzodiazepines and alcohol can induce or worsen PLMS. It is often asymptomatic, but in severe form patients may have sleep-onset insomnia, nonrestorative sleep, or frequent arousals during the night from more robust myoclonic movements. Not infrequently, the bed partner is the one complaining about the jerking leg movements at night.

Whereas RLS is primarily a symptomatic diagnosis, PLMS is best documented by polysomnography in the home or sleep laboratory. PLMS responds to some of the same treatments as RLS. Sedative-hypnotics can improve sleep continuity in PLMS patients, but not reduce the number of leg movements. Dopaminergic agents may be the treatment of choice, but rebound of symptoms in the second half of the night or during the following day may make dosing a challenge. Opiates, such as a bedtime dose of codeine, work well in PLMS (as in RLS), but should be reserved for patients with severe symptoms.

MENTAL ILLNESS AND INSOMNIA

Sleep disturbances are among the most common symptoms of mental illnesses, particularly mood and anxiety disorders. Major depression should always be considered in patients complaining of frequent nighttime awakenings and early morning arousal, particularly when those arousals are accompanied by anxiety and worry. On the other hand, many depressed patients complain of hypersomnia with fatigue and difficulty getting going in the morning. This symptom is especially characteristic of seasonal affective disorder (SAD) and so-called atypical depression. Both are common in young and middle-aged adults.

Mania is frequently accompanied by a reduced need for sleep, making change in sleep a cardinal diagnostic symptom of the disorder, although patients will not usually complain about this change. Depressed patients, however, find their sleep changes very distressing. Sedating antidepressant medications may help with the insomnia symptom, but can also lead to daytime sedation. Mirtazapine may be prescribed for depressed patients with insomnia, although daytime sleepiness can occur. Older tricyclic antidepressants (e.g., doxepin, amitriptyline, and nortriptyline) may be considered. They combine moderate-to-severe sedation with effective antidepressant activity but must be used with caution due to overdose toxicity and anticholinergic effects. Serotonin reuptake inhibitors generally will not improve sleep immediately, and can even increase leg movements and arousals. A brief course of a sedative-hypnotic agent for help with sleep is a comforting strategy for some patients. The sleep medication can be tapered and discontinued as the depression and secondary insomnia improve.

Anxiety disorders can also present with initial and middle insomnia. Nightmares, particularly in posttraumatic stress disorders, frequently complicate the picture. Antidepressant medication, prazosin, and mood stabilizers, have been reported to be helpful with sleep-related symptoms.

Bereavement is usually accompanied by anxiety and insomnia. Short-term use of sedative-hypnotic medications may help patients who struggle to get through long nights.

ALCOHOL AND DRUGS

Alcohol has variable influence on sleep patterns, but it generally impairs both alertness and sleep. Like other sedatives, alcohol suppresses slow-wave sleep, making sleep lighter. With its short half-life, alcohol also tends to produce a rebound arousal in the second half of the night and can reduce total sleep time.

Other drugs can affect sleep. Amphetamines and cocaine cause marked reduction in sleep during acute intoxication and profound hypersomnia during the withdrawal phase. Opiates have acute tranquilizing effects and improve sleep when nighttime pain contributes to insomnia. Caffeine causes longer sleep latency (time needed to fall asleep) and increased wakefulness during the night. Some people do not perceive the effects of caffeine on sleep even when they are documented on sleep EEG; others are very aware of these effects. Caffeine can even affect sleep when ingested several hours before bedtime.

Both prescription and over-the-counter (OTC) sedative-hypnotic medications can contribute to rebound insomnia when doses are missed. Drugs with short half-lives can lead to rebound insomnia in the second half of the night, whereas drugs with long half-lives can cause daytime sedation. Although they are common geriatric problems, memory impairment and unexplained falls should cue the physician to consider alcohol or sedative-hypnotic abuse in elderly patients. For example, the anti-histamine diphenhydramine, a component of many OTC sleep-promoting products, has potent anticholinergic effects and can cause mild cognitive impairment and rarely, frank delirium in old people.

Education about the effects of these substances on sleep may motivate patients to reduce their intake. Patients with more severe dependency and abuse problems need referral to specific treatment programs for chemical dependency (see Chapter 21).

MEDICAL DISORDERS

Pain, rheumatologic disorders, neuromuscular diseases, cardiac disease, pulmonary diseases, dyspepsia, inflammatory bowel diseases, and nocturia are all common medical causes of insomnia. One of the classic medical syndromes affecting sleep is fibromyalgia, a condition in which sleep is characterized by alpha-wave intrusion into non-REM sleep. This syndrome produces non-restorative sleep, in which patients complain of feeling tired despite sleep duration in the normal range. Improved sleep can produce significant remission in pain. Acquired immunodeficiency syndrome (AIDS) has been associated with daytime sleepiness, decreased total slow-wave sleep with alpha-wave intrusions, increasing arousals, and frequent nightmares. Patients with chronic disease are often desperate for good sleep, making adequate nighttime analgesia and sedative medications very welcome.

Acute illnesses often cause diffuse cerebral dysfunction in the frail elderly. The resulting delirium is almost always accompanied by disruption of sleep and alertness. Medications can also cause insomnia and daytime drowsiness. Bronchodilators, activating antidepressants, and steroids, for example, often interfere with sleep, whereas many psychotropics, opioid analgesics, and clonidine can cause daytime drowsiness.

NEURODEGENERATIVE DISEASE AND SLEEP

There is no localized sleep center in the brain; rather, there are several neuronal circuits that function in maintaining sleep or alertness. Diseases that affect diffuse brain functions invariably affect sleep and alertness; Alzheimer disease (AD) and PD have been studied more than most others. AD causes the same kinds of changes in sleep as normal aging does, but they are more severe: less clear day–night difference with more daytime and less nighttime sleep. Complete day–night reversal is rare, but sleeping nearly as much during the day as at night is common. This is very stressful for

caregivers, who must continue to supervise their charges for safety during these nocturnal wanderings. Sleep disruption is among the most stressful aspects of caring for a person with dementia at home.

PD patients also have severe sleep problems. Akinesia causes physical discomfort over pressure points that normally would be relieved by tossing and turning in sleep. Medications used to treat PD can also impair sleep. Furthermore, the neurodegenerative and neuro-transmitter changes caused by the disease adversely affect sleep quality. Dementia with Lewy bodies, a disease related to PD, is associated both with impaired nighttime sleep, poor daytime alertness, and increased motor activity during REM sleep (see "REM Behavior Disorder," below).

TREATMENT OF INSOMNIA

Reframing the Psychosocial Context of Sleep Disturbance

Sleep problems in children and adolescents usually affect the rest of the family, causing sleep loss in parents and siblings who may in some respects suffer as much as the patient. Because misinformation and inappropriate blaming may confound the problem, the disturbed sleep of such patients needs to be addressed as a problem for the whole family.

Modifying family routines may be helpful. Good sleep hygiene, including well-maintained bedtime rituals such as bathing, storytelling, and rocking a small child can facilitate the winding-down process that is an important prelude to sleep. Occasionally, a child becomes overly dependent on a particular routine (e.g., repeated drinks of water every time he or she wakes up) and the parents must set limits. After an expected period of protest, most children relinquish the need for unnecessary attention. These benign disruptions must be differentiated from the more serious panic that some children experience with separation. For this latter kind of anxiety, parental access through the night may be necessary, at least for a time.

In adolescence, sleep is often shortened at both ends by social demands. In the evening, there is homework, telephone socializing, school athletic events, and family life. In the morning, high school schedules often begin quite early, sometimes preceded by an even earlier bus ride. For many teenagers, the morning includes a formidable grooming ritual. Add to this the increasing tendency for teenagers to take part-time jobs after school, and the result is an epidemic of chronic sleep deprivation that is of increasing societal concern. Weekend sleeping-in may recover some of the lost sleep, but it tends to produce a phase delay that reinforces the tendency to stay up late during the week. In one experiment, high school students increased their

IQ scores by 20 points after a week in which they systematically extended their sleep time.

In counseling teenagers, some flexibility and compromise are usually most effective. Adding naps during the day may improve alertness. A warning about the dangers of driving while sleepy, intoxicated, or both is important. Chronobiological interventions, such as light therapy, may be needed to counteract extremely delayed sleep. Outside the office, informed and politically active physicians may be able to influence public policy to help alleviate the problem, such as adopting sensible work rules for teens and scheduling school activities at reasonable hours.

Adults are not immune to the effects of social and occupational demands on sleep. Many working adults become progressively more sleep deprived as the workweek progresses. Educating patients about appropriate sleep hygiene and cognitive measures helps them regain some sense of control over their symptoms of fatigue (see Table 28-1). New knowledge of the health consequences of sleep deprivation can help motivate people to prioritize sleep as an important health behavior.

Persons with more persistent insomnia or those who appear to have severe emotional distress as a result—or cause—of the sleep disturbance may warrant evaluation by a mental health specialist.

As they do in children, sleep disorders in adults can affect family members. Partners and caregivers of patients with severe sleep disorders may need both emotional support and education about the nature of the sleep disturbance. Understanding the problem can help them to support the patient in following treatment recommendations.

Cognitive Behavioral Therapy

There is now ample evidence that cognitive-behavioral therapy (CBT) for primary insomnia, especially over the long term, is at least as effective as sleep medication. The basic approach is to counsel patients to change critical beliefs that induce anxiety around falling asleep and to motivate them to change bedtime behaviors that may be perpetuating insomnia (see Table 28-1). The National Sleep Foundation web site (www.sleepfoundation. org) has many helpful suggestions for people interested in improving sleep hygiene under "Hot Topics: Can't Sleep."

Medical Treatment

Insomnia has a good prognosis acutely, but can become chronic and recurrent. Acute insomnia should be treated with sedative-hypnotic drugs in conjunction with a sleep-hygiene program to maximize efficacy and reduce the dosage and duration of treatment (see Table 28-1). These medications should not be used in pregnancy.

Cognitive-behavioral therapies will be helpful in these patients. People with secondary insomnia from depression, pain, substance abuse, medications, or circadian rhythm disorders are also at risk for chronic insomnia if the acute symptoms do not resolve and may need specific sleep therapies in addition to treating the underlying cause of sleeplessness.

BENZODIAZEPINES

All benzodiazepines have sleep-promoting effects, although only five are currently marketed as sedative-hypnotics. These drugs work well for short-term treatment of insomnia; tolerance and dependence can develop quickly in some patients. However, many people—especially those with an anxiety component to their insomnia—may benefit from long-term use. Benzodiazepines alter sleep structure, reducing both REM and slow-wave sleep, but the clinical significance of this is uncertain. They are generally safe for younger adults, even in overdose, although combining them with alcohol and other depressants can produce potentially catastrophic synergistic effects. In older individuals, the safety profile is less benign; amnesia, ataxia, confusion, and worsening sleep apnea may develop.

Choosing one benzodiazepine over another for a specific patient is partly based on drug half-life, and this will require prioritizing goals. Short-acting drugs such as triazolam are useful for the treatment of sleep-onset insomnia, but many individuals will have rebound insomnia in the second half of the night or anxiety the following day. Longer-acting drugs such as flurazepam may work better for middle of the night insomnia, but some persons will have morning "hangover" effects. Longer-acting drugs can be particularly troublesome in the elderly, as drug accumulation will lead to ataxia, confusion, and daytime sedation. Temazepam and estazolam are intermediate in half-life and represent reasonable compromises for patients with sleep maintenance insomnia who get hangover effects from the longer-acting drugs.

These drugs should not be prescribed for patients with sleep apnea, severe respiratory disease, gait and balance problems, or alcohol abuse. Doses should be kept low in elderly patients and those with hepatic insufficiency. Rebound insomnia can complicate withdrawal from these drugs, causing patients to return to their use.

BENZODIAZEPINE RECEPTOR AGONISTS (BzRA)

These drugs are structurally unrelated to benzodiazepines, but share some characteristics with them due to the fact that they have agonist activity at more sleep-specific benzodiazepine receptors (GABAα). They have varying half-lives (eszopiclone zolpidem, 1.4–3.8 hours; zaleplon, 1.0 hours), so they are most suitable for patients with sleep-onset or initial sleep maintenance problems. These medications preserve natural sleep architecture, which provides at least a theoretical advantage

Table 28-3. Sedative hypnotic medications.

	Trade Name	Type	Half-life	Dosing Range
Tamazepam	Restoril	Benzodiazepine	8–15 h	7.5–30 mg
Triazolam	Halcion	Benzodiazepine	2–5 h	0.125–0.25 mg
Zolpidem	Ambien	Benzodiazepine agonist	3 h	5–10 mg
Zolpidem CR	Ambien CR	Benzodiazepine agonist	3 h	6.25–12.5 mg
Zaleplon	Sonata	Benzodiazepine agonist	1 h	5–10 mg
Eszopiclone	Lunesta	Benzodiazepine agonist	5–7 h	1–3 mg
Ramelteon	Rozerem	Melatonin agonist	2–5 h	8 mg

over benzodiazepines. Precautions similar to benzodiazepines apply to these medications in terms of dependency, abuse, and adverse effects. Eszopiclone (Lunesta) and zolpidem in continuous-release formulation (Ambien CR) have been shown to retain efficacy over 6 months, and are the only benzodiazepine or BzRA that are FDA approved for chronic insomnia (see Table 28-3).

MELATONIN AGONIST

Ramelteon (rozerem) is a potent melatonin agonist that is the first nonscheduled, prescription sedative-hypnotic. It has the capacity to shorten sleep latency in people with sleep-onset insomnia, but does not help people stay asleep. It has no potential for abuse, tolerance, or physical dependency, and does not cause ataxia, confusion, or worsen sleep-related breathing disorders. In the clinical trials, the drug was associated with an increase in prolactin in a few subjects. Ramelteon is prescribed at 8 mg before bedtime. Higher doses have not been shown to improve response, but there is some evidence that the response improves over several weeks. Combining ramelteon with CBT or sleep hygiene measures seems a benign and potentially effective long-term strategy for many insomnia patients.

SEDATING ANTIDEPRESSANTS

Many clinicians use sedating antidepressants such as trazodone, mirtazapine, doxepin, and amitriptyline for long-term treatment of insomnia, especially when chronic pain, depression, or anxiety are comorbid conditions. Theoretical advantages over benzodiazepines include less cognitive impairment and more slow-wave sleep. Treatment of underlying depression in many insomnia patients provides another advantage. Tolerance to the sedating effects of these drugs develops in some patients. Side effects of these drugs are numerous, and special care must be taken in elderly patients, especially with amitriptyline, because of its potent anticholinergic effects. The other issue with these medications is that there are no large controlled trials for insomnia, and use of antidepressants for insomnia without depression is off label and without a controlled

database for safety and efficacy. However, years of widespread clinical use does at least imply clinical consensus on the utility of these medications in patients with sleep disturbances (see Table 28-3).

ANTIHISTAMINES

Diphenhydramine is sedating and is found in many OTC preparations. It is generally safe and effective for short-term use, although tolerance develops very quickly after nightly ingestion. Diphenhydramine has some anticholinergic properties and can cause confusion and urinary retention in elderly persons.

COMPLIMENTARY AND ALTERNATIVE MEDICINES

The pineal hormone melatonin, sold in this country as a food supplement, has sleep-promoting effects in some people. Melatonin is the best studied of the food supplements and OTC remedies for insomnia and is commonly available at health food stores and pharmacies. Patients should be cautioned that melatonin remains an experimental drug and a naturally occurring hormone with potential neuroendocrine, immunologic, and reproductive effects, although it appears to be quite safe with short-term administration. Results from placebo-controlled trials of melatonin for insomnia in various populations suggest it has only modest efficacy, though some individuals respond quite well. Moreover, when taken at the correct point in the circadian cycle, melatonin can be an effective remedy for jet lag and can help people adapt to shift work (see "Chronobiological Therapies," below). Commercial preparations may contain 0.5–5 mg of melatonin per capsule (sometimes in combination with vitamins). The most effective dose is unknown, and may vary from person to person. Doses in the 1–10 mg range are reasonable.

CHRONOBIOLOGICAL THERAPIES

Sleep–wake cycle disorders can be treated with scheduled exposure to bright natural or artificial light. Patients with advanced sleep-phase syndrome need to have a corrective phase delay with exposure to bright light in the evening. Bright light exposure must be carefully timed so that the circadian pacemaker is phase shifted to move sleep propensity to later hours, allowing these patients to be more alert in the evening. For the more common DSPS, patients need to force themselves awake by receiving appropriately timed light exposure, which should begin around the time they want to wake up. The first few days are very difficult, but after several mornings of 30-minute light exposure, patients can begin falling asleep before midnight and wake up for morning classes or work. For safety and efficacy, patients should use special fixtures marketed to treat seasonal affective disorder ("SAD lights"). Light fixtures are available from numerous commercial vendors. The Society for Bright Light and Biological Rhythms (see "Resources," below) can provide a list of vendors and more details about using bright light exposure in treating sleep disorders and winter depression.

Melatonin may achieve this same goal with greater convenience, although probably with less robustness and with opposite timing. For example, people with DSPS who want to advance the timing of their sleep might take synthetic melatonin (0.5–1 mg) in the evening at 9:00 or 10:00 P.M.—hours before their own phase-delayed melatonin secretion begins and more synchronous with the timing of melatonin onset in people with earlier sleep—to reset their body clock to the desired phase position. There are data suggesting that the melatonin agonist ramelteon (rozerem) can be effective when used in this same way. These treatments may also be of value in helping shift workers, time zone travelers, and some blind individuals adapt to a new sleep-wake schedule. Shift workers should be counseled to try to maintain their workweek sleep schedule on their off work days, although this can be difficult because of family and social demands.

CASE ILLUSTRATION 1

Greg is a 27-year-old man who presents with a complaint of insomnia. He describes having trouble getting up in the morning. He is chronically late for work and his job is in jeopardy. No matter what time he goes to bed, Greg cannot fall asleep until about 2:00 A.M. and then sleeps through the alarm set for 7:00 A.M. His wife has given up trying to wake him, and although he has arranged for an answering service to call him, the ringing telephone does not awaken him either. He is often tired and sleepy during the day, but in the evening gets his second wind just as his wife goes to bed. He craves weekends and vacations when he sleeps until noon and feels alert the rest of the day.

Greg likely has DSPS. Persons with this disorder are extreme night owls and have severe difficulty adjusting their sleep times according to school, work, and social demands.

Origins of DSPS are probably multifactorial. Sleep timing is delayed, there is a surge of energy in the evening, sleep onset is late, and there is severe morning sleepiness.

This syndrome is common in teenagers and young adults, in whom the insomnia complaint is usually prolonged sleep onset, with an inability to fall asleep until several hours past midnight. Parents or spouses may describe their frustration with getting the patient out of bed in the morning. Treatment involves bright light exposure in the morning (to phase-advance the body clock) and short-term use of a sedative-hypnotic medication to facilitate earlier sleep onset and make getting up for bright light exposure manageable. OTC melatonin or the prescription melatonin agonist ramelteon administered 2 hours before desired bedtime will also help with the therapeutic circadian phase advance. Successful management calls for fairly strict adherence to a lifestyle that avoids late-night activity, because deviation from the early-to-bed schedule will result in relapse to a delayed sleep-phase cycle. This last requirement is, of course, especially difficult for teenagers and young adults.

CASE ILLUSTRATION 2

Francine is a 47-year-old woman complaining of anxiety. She feels restless and fidgety during the day, but she is also tired. She cries easily and has trouble concentrating, making decisions, and getting things done, all of which are out of character for her. Although quite fatigued, it can take her an hour to fall asleep. When sleep finally comes, it is restless and interrupted by many awakenings, filled with worried thoughts.

Francine's diagnosis is likely to be major depression, presenting with prominent symptoms of anxiety and insomnia. A primary medical or neurologic disease presenting with comorbid depression also needs to be considered. If depression is the primary disorder, disease education, emotional support, and antidepressant medication are indicated. Short-term CBT can be very helpful both for the depression as well as the insomnia. Short-term use (several days to weeks) of a sedative-hypnotic can be offered if a less-sedating antidepressant is chosen as the primary agent. The antidepressant medication trazodone, although considered to be less effective for depression, is commonly prescribed at bedtime to augment other antidepressants and help patients sleep. This is a widespread clinical practice, but its safety and efficacy have not been studied in randomized, placebo-controlled trials.

The Sleepy Patient: Disorders of Excessive Somnolence

Patients are more likely to complain about insomnia than about excessive daytime sleepiness. They may complain of fatigue or feeling tired, but sleepiness per se may not be acknowledged without specific inquiry by the clinician. Two questions that should be included in every sleep-related "review of systems" are:

- Do you struggle to stay awake while driving, reading, watching television and movies, or listening to lectures during daytime hours?
- Do you feel tired, fatigued, and lacking in energy during the day, especially in the morning?

If the answer is "yes" to either question, follow-up questions should be directed to determine if the problem is inadequate nighttime sleep from insomnia, drowsiness from medications, narcolepsy, or sleep-related breathing problems. The Epworth Sleepiness Scale is a validated instrument used to assess pathologic sleepiness in patients. It is a questionnaire that scores a patient's tendency to fall asleep in seven hypothetical situations. Scores above 10 suggest the need for referral to a sleep disorders specialist. A discussion of driving or operating machinery while sleepy should also be initiated.

Sleep-related Breathing Problems

SNORING

Apart from being a nuisance to bed partners, snoring may herald the development of serious respiratory obstruction during sleep along a continuum of partial to complete airway closure. Males snore more than young females, but after menopause females snore almost as much as men. Aside from male gender, other factors associated with snoring include anatomic narrowing of the airways, body habitus (obese) and sleep position (supine), the use of alcohol and sedative-hypnotics, endocrinopathy (hypothyroidism, acromegaly), smoking, and, possibly, genetic factors. The view of snoring as a mild form of OSA is supported by the transient drop in SaO_2 and rise in pulmonary and systemic pressure that can occur. Weight loss, the avoidance of sedating medications or alcohol, and appliances to prevent back sleeping (tennis ball sewn at the back of nightshirt) are warranted in severe cases. A number of different dental appliances that thrust the tongue or mandible forward during sleep may be helpful. Laser surgery to enlarge the oropharynx is increasingly popular, but the long-term effects are unknown. Because surgery can eliminate the noise of snoring without affecting an associated obstruction, PSG evaluation prior to an operation should be performed to rule out OSA.

OBSTRUCTIVE SLEEP APNEA SYNDROME

OSA is a significant cause of cardiovascular morbidity and daytime somnolence in adults. Originally thought of as a relatively rare disturbance in severely obese patients with the classic "Pickwickian Syndrome" of somnolence, hypoventilation, and polycythemia, OSA is now known to represent a wide range of severity in upper airway narrowing in sleep that begins earlier in life and is more prevalent than previously thought. In midlife, 2% of women and 4% of men have OSA with serious daytime sequelae. Nighttime symptoms of OSA include loud snoring (often beginning early in adulthood and progressively worsening with age and increased weight), snorting and gagging sounds, restlessness, night sweats, abrupt awakenings with a feeling of choking, and profound sleep disruption. The arousals triggered by the apneic episodes cause subjective daytime fatigue and sleepiness in addition to mounting evidence of objective deficits in cognitive processing, attention, and executive functions. In mild cases, insomnia may be the chief complaint. Patients are often unaware of the severity of the sleep disruption and may attribute their sleepiness to some other cause, such as working too hard. The degree of sleepiness is variable, but is a key symptom. People may be so accustomed to living with fatigue that they are not fully aware of how sleepy they are. Questions about dozing while reading or watching television, nodding off at the wheel, or poor concentration need to be posed directly to patients. Assessment with a scale measuring daytime sleepiness (such as the Epworth Sleepiness Scale or Stanford Sleepiness Scale) may be helpful. Untreated OSA may lead to hypertension and is a risk factor for lethal cardiovascular events including myocardial infarction and stroke. Clinical assessment by PSG in a sleep laboratory confirms the diagnosis and helps determine the proper setting for continuous positive airway pressure (CPAP) devices, which are the major form of treatment. Surgical uvuloplasty, tracheostomy, and dental devices designed to keep the tongue from falling back and occluding the airway are other forms of treatment available for milder cases of OSA or for those who cannot tolerate continuous or bilevel positive airway pressure (BIPAP). The correct diagnosis of OSA can help improve quality of life and may prevent serious accidents and cardiovascular disease.

Obstructive apneas also occur in 1–3% of younger children. Tonsil and adenoid hypertrophy are thought to contribute, since resection of these results in relief from OSA in the majority of children. However, the size of these tissues does not correlate with the presence or degree of OSA. OSA should also be considered in children with craniofacial abnormalities, macroglossia, neuromuscular disease, and obesity. As in adults, loud snoring, restless sleep, and witnessed pauses in breathing are symptomatic. Children with OSA may not complain of sleepiness; instead they may manifest daytime irritability, decreased attention, or declining school performance. Some children have even been misidentified as intellectually impaired. Secondary nocturnal enuresis is another important symptom of OSA. Parents should be asked about snoring and breath-holding during sleep. Consultation with an ear, nose, and throat specialist is advised whenever OSA is suspected. Tonsillectomy is curative in up to 90% of cases and should be the first step in treatment. Other causes of OSA can be treated with CPAP, though careful monitoring for midface hypoplasia should be undertaken in children less than 12. Surgical approaches such as tracheostomy or craniofacial reconstruction may be necessary in rare cases.

CENTRAL APNEA

Central apnea is defined as the cessation of airflow for at least 10 seconds with no ventilatory effort. Patients with predominantly central apnea tend to complain more of insomnia than of the hypersomnolence that is so typical of patients with obstructive apnea. Arterial oxygen desaturation usually occurs with central apnea, but serious cardiovascular sequelae are less common than in obstructive apnea. Predisposing factors to central apnea are congestive heart failure (mechanism unknown) and neurodegenerative diseases that affect the central nervous system's (CNS) respiratory control or induce profound hypoventilation from respiratory muscle weakness.

Central apneas are often seen in sleeping neonates, especially premature infants, and may contribute to SIDS. The cause of SIDS remains a mystery, but a wide variety of intrinsic and extrinsic factors are thought to play a role. A public information campaign to encourage mothers to avoid placing infants prone ("Back to Sleep"), has been ongoing since 1995 and subsequent epidemiologic assessments have shown a dramatic decrease in the amount of SIDS cases.

CASE ILLUSTRATION 3

Jim is 64 years old and visits his primary care physician for a follow-up of his hypertension treatment. His wife has accompanied him to the office to ask whether there is any medical explanation for her husband's fatigue. Close questioning reveals that the fatigue predates the antihypertensive medication and is not clearly attributable to the drug. The tiredness is accompanied by true sleepiness; Jim can fall asleep anytime during the day while reading or driving. He minimizes the problem, yet acknowledges having trouble with memory and concentration. He falls asleep easily after getting into bed at night, but his wife describes him as a restless sleeper who snores loudly.

Jim may have OSA. The clues are his snoring, daytime sleepiness, and hypertension. Referral to a sleep disorders specialist should help confirm the diagnosis and provide a review of the best treatment options.

NARCOLEPSY

Narcolepsy is a disorder in which elements of sleep intrude into wakefulness and wakefulness intrudes into sleep. It consists of four primary symptoms: excessive daytime sleepiness, cataplexy, and less frequently, sleep paralysis and hypnagogic hallucinations. It occurs in approximately 1 in 2000 people. Narcolepsy usually begins in the teens or early twenties but onset as old as the eighth decade has been reported. It is more common in males than females and a formal diagnosis is frequently not made until 5 or 10 years after the onset of symptoms. If the syndrome is not diagnosed and treated, people with the disorder may be perceived as lazy and unmotivated. Additional sequelae of a missed diagnosis include poor school and work performance, social stigma, and accidents. Orexin (hypocretin), a neuropeptide secreted by the hypothalamus, is thought to play an important role in this disorder. Projections from the hypothalamus to centers promoting wakefulness (such as the locus ceruleus) are presumably disrupted in some way, leading to decreased orexin and excessive sleepiness. Some combination of infectious, immune, or genetic factors may play a role in narcolepsy, with at least two genes being involved, one of them HLA related. The cardinal symptom is sleepiness that comes on suddenly and irresistibly in what are called "sleep attacks." Low-grade, persistent sleepiness affecting concentration, thinking, and memory may also occur. Sleep episodes may be brief (several minutes to an hour), but the person usually awakens feeling more alert and the next sleep episode usually does not come on for at least an hour. Narcolepsy can impair nighttime sleep with frequent awakenings, vivid nightmares, and intense, realistic hallucinations prior to sleep onset (hypnagogic). The hallucinations are usually visual, but may involve any sensory modality.

Cataplexy, the brief, sudden loss of muscle tone leading to neck muscle weakness, buckling of the knees, or rarely, complete collapse, is triggered by strong emotional reactions such as laughter or anger. **Sleep paralysis** is transient immobility on awakening, often accompanied by the vivid hallucinations of REM dreaming, all while the patient is lying in bed perfectly alert. The spells are brief, lasting several minutes at most.

Confirmation of the diagnosis should be undertaken with overnight PSG followed by a multiple sleep latency test (MSLT). The finding of mean sleep latency less than 5 minutes and REM periods during at least two naps confirms the diagnosis. Care should be taken in the assessment of these patients, however, as patients with narcolepsy may have normal testing on a single day 20–30% of the time. Without the symptoms of cataplexy, the diagnosis is more difficult. In ambiguous cases, it is advisable to refer to a sleep disorders specialist, since diagnosis often means a commitment to long-term medication treatment.

Excessive daytime somnolence may be treated with modafinil (Provigil) at doses of 100–200 mg each morning and midday and can significantly improve daytime function. Sodium oxybate (Xyrem), a relative of gamma-hydroxybutyrate (GHB), is useful in some cases to treat both sleepiness and cataplexy. The older CNS stimulants, dextroamphetamine (5–60 mg/day), methamphetamine (20–25 mg/day), and methylphenidate (10–90 mg/day), are widely used as well. Cataplexy and sleep paralysis are treated with REM suppressant drugs such as tricyclic antidepressants and selective serotonin reuptake inhibitors (SSRIs). Joining a narcolepsy support group will help patients cope with the psychological sequelae, which result from the social and occupational stigma of having little control over sleep onset.

Patients With Abnormal Nighttime Behavior: The Parasomnias

An accurate diagnosis of the underlying causes of bizarre nighttime behavior can be challenging. Possible considerations include seizure disorders, psychosis, delirium, and intoxication, but parasomnias, the least common class of sleep disorders, but perhaps the most dramatic in their presentation, need to be included in the differential.

PAVOR NOCTURNUS

Sleep terrors (pavor nocturnus) are very disconcerting to parents but are usually quite benign. The child (usually aged 3–6) awakens with a scream and appears terrified, with signs of autonomic arousal: eyes bulging, heart racing, sweating. Most episodes last only a few minutes. Attempts at comfort are to no avail and may exacerbate or prolong the episode. In the morning, the child is amnestic for the episode or may have a fragmentary memory of a bad dream. Sleep terrors involve partial arousals from stage 4 (deep) sleep. Reassurance of the parents is the usual treatment; in persistent night terrors, however, benzodiazepines may be justified.

NIGHTMARES

True nightmares occur in REM sleep and involve a narrative story people can often relate once awake. Nightmares are usually a transient problem, presumably triggered by stressful personal events. Persistent nightmares are a serious concern, however, and may require referral to a mental health specialist.

SOMNAMBULISM

Like sleep terrors, sleepwalking is a partial arousal from stage 4 sleep. Occasional sleepwalking is very common in childhood and may follow a period of stress or sleep deprivation. The main concern is accidental injury, and protective measures, such as placing gates in front of a stairwell, may be needed.

REM BEHAVIOR DISORDER (RBD)

In this syndrome, loss of normal REM sleep muscle atonia leads to dream-enactment behavior. The diagnosis is made in patients with sudden bursts of excited, intense, sometimes violent activity during sleep. The syndrome may be subtle, in the form of leg movements and talking, or dramatic, with punching, kicking, grabbing, strangling, running, and moving about the bedroom. Dreams of an intense, violent nature are typical. RBD is seen frequently in toxic or metabolic delirium, but the most persistent forms of the syndrome occur in old age, and are presumed to be idiopathic, ischemic, or neurodegenerative in etiology. The syndrome is especially common in patients with PD and dementia with Lewy bodies.

DIAGNOSTIC EVALUATION & REFERRAL

Most types of insomnia are diagnosed on the basis of history, and PSG evaluation of insomnia is rarely necessary or reimbursed. Clinicians should be able to accurately diagnose and treat transient insomnia without referral or consultation. Referral to a sleep specialist should be considered for patients with persistent symptoms who do not respond to initial treatment. Patients with severe RLS and chronobiological sleep disorders should usually be referred. Sleep-related breathing problems, periodic leg movements, narcolepsy, and the adult parasomnias all require PSG validation and expert management and will require a sleep specialist to validate the diagnosis and initial treatment plans.

RESOURCES

The National Sleep Foundation publishes a newsletter for physicians and health professionals, and has an outstanding web site (www.sleepfoundation.org). The web site offers information on many sleep-related topics, access to educational resources, and direct linkages to other relevant web sites, including those of the American Sleep Apnea Association, Narcolepsy Network, RLS Foundation, and American Academy of Sleep Medicine.

The Society for Light Treatment and Biological Rhythms offers information on treating chronobiological sleep disorders and SAD. Contact information of vendors of bright light fixtures for clinical use is also available. The society has a web site (www.sltbr.org).

The official web site of the National Institutes of Health (www.nih.gov) provides many opportunities to learn about the ongoing research and resources of the National Center for Sleep Disorders Research (NCSDR), a part of the National Heart, Blood and Lung Institute (NHBLI).

SUGGESTED READINGS

Silber MH. Chronic insomnia. *N Engl J Med* 2005;353:803–810.

Doghramji K. Assessment of excessive sleepiness and insomnia as they relate to circadian rhythm sleep disorders. *J Clin Psychiatry* 2004;65(Suppl 16):17–22.

Pearson NJ, Johnson LL, Nahin RL. Insomnia, trouble sleeping, and complementary and alternative medicine. *Arch Intern Med* 2006;166:1775–1782.

Morin CM. Cognitive-behavioral approaches to the treatment of insomnia. *J Clin Psychiatry* 2004;65(Suppl 16):33–40.

Morin AK. Strategies for treating chronic insomnia. *Am J Manag Care* 2006;12:S2230–S2245.

National Institutes of Health State of the Science Conference on Manifestations and Management of Chronic Insomnia in Adults, June 13–15, 2005. *Sleep* 2005;1049–1057.

Roth T. Characteristics and determinants of normal sleep. *J Clin Psychiatry* 2004;65(Suppl 16):8–11.

Spiegel K, Knutson K, Leproult R, et al. Sleep loss: a novel risk factor for insulin resistance and Type 2 diabetes. *J Appl Physiol* 2005;99:2008–2019.

Sexual Problems

David G. Bullard, PhD, Harvey Caplan, MD, & Christine Derzko, MD[1]

Sex is a problem for everyone.... Indeed, for a couple of weeks or a couple of months, or maybe even for a couple of years, if we are lucky, we may feel that we have solved the problem of sex. But then, of course, we change or our partners change, or the whole ball-game changes, and once again we are left trying to scramble over that obstacle with this built-in feeling that we can get over it, when actually we never can. However, in the process of trying to get over it, we learn a great deal about vulnerability and intimacy and love.... (Peck, 1993, Further Along the Road Less Traveled)

INTRODUCTION

Primary care practitioners are in an optimal position to evaluate sexual problems, as they often have the most comprehensive and long-lasting relationship with the patient. In contrast to most other medical diagnoses, however, it is the patient who usually defines when a sexual problem exists. Although referral to medical or mental health specialists (or both) may be indicated in certain situations, many problems can be diagnosed and treated by the primary care practitioner. When questions about sexuality are approached in an open, matter-of-fact manner, most patients are relieved and respond positively. They appreciate the affirmation that these issues are valid and important, whether or not they have current sexual concerns or are sexually active (Table 29-1).

CHALLENGE FOR CLINICIANS

To provide patients with helpful responses to their sexual health concerns health professionals need to have the following:

- A willingness and ability to discuss sexual topics comfortably.
- Awareness of the range and diversity of human sexual practices and concerns, as well as the importance of the circumstances or conditions under which individuals function best.
- The ability to separate their own personal beliefs and values from those of patients. Unless the practitioner encounters information indicating objective harm to someone involved, it is important to maintain a non-judgmental demeanor.
- Skill at taking a sex problem history in appropriate detail.
- Knowledge of simple interventions, such as permission-giving, and the ability to transmit accurate information, make specific suggestions (e.g., for making sex less pressured and more pleasurable), and make referrals to other resources, when appropriate.

Health professionals may have limited sexual experience, as well as questions and problems of their own, and consequently may be uncomfortable in discussing particular sexual material. Time, thought, and experience, however, can build confidence and expertise in talking about sexual problems. Health care providers can increase their comfort level by examining their own attitudes, beliefs, assumptions, and experiences; reading in the literature; discussing these issues with friends and colleagues; and routinely incorporating sexual health questions into the general health assessment of patients.

Of course, no one—patients *or* caregivers—should be forced to talk about sexuality. It is important for everyone to recognize the limits of their own interest, comfort, and competency. Sexual health is an integral part of health care, however, and all who deal with patients should be alert to the possibility of sexual concerns and, at a minimum, be able to respond with non-judgmental listening and reassurance or by referring patients to a colleague who is comfortable and competent in discussing sexual issues.

[1]The authors would like to thank Linda Perlin Alperstein, LCSW, Jean M. Bullard, RN, MS, Lisa Capaldini, MD, Deborah Grady, MD, MPH, & William B. Shore, MD, for reviewing earlier drafts of this chapter. Our appreciation especially goes to the coeditors of this book for their valuable comments and suggestions. Finally, the contributions to the study of sexuality by Raymond C. Rosen, PhD, have been inspiring to us.

Table 29-1. Sexual concerns of patients.

- **Common sexual worries about normalcy**, such as: Am I O.K.? What is a "healthy" sex life? How do I compare? Is my sex life satisfactory?
- **Sexual identity questions** relevant to lifestyle, orientation, and preference.
- **Developmental issues of sexuality** for children, adolescents, parents, and the elderly, including the development of gender identity, masturbation, genital exploration, child sex play, sexuality, and the single life, marriage, divorce, and death of a partner.
- **Reproductive concerns** covering infertility, family planning, contraception, pregnancy, and abortion.
- **Sexual desire, satisfaction, and dysfunctions**, such as a couple's differing levels of desire, and problems with vaginal lubrication, erections, orgasm, and pain.
- **Sexual changes** due to physical disability, medical illness, and treatment.
- **Sexual trauma** resulting from molestation, incest, and rape.
- **Safe sex practices:** AIDS and STDs.
- **Paraphilias and sexual compulsions**.

PERSPECTIVES ON HUMAN SEXUALITY

Although a knowledge base of human sexual response is developing, even the most scholarly sexual research is rarely value free. Sexuality encompasses an enormous range of behaviors, beliefs, desires, experiences, and fantasies that patients may discuss with their health care providers. Sexuality can also have legal, medical, moral, political, and religious aspects. It is difficult to find a more controversial area of human experience!

Motivations for human sexual expression are complex and numerous, existing throughout the life cycle in times of illness as well as health and varying from culture to culture and from individual to individual. Included are the need to express love; the need for physical release, reproduction, and recreation; and the need to increase self-esteem. Conversely, sexuality can also be used to coerce, control, or degrade others, or in the service of addiction or compulsion.

Sexual worries or difficulties are probably experienced by most people at some periods of their lives and may result from developmental growth and changes in life circumstances rather than from pathology alone. Sexual problems are sometimes a blessing, such as when they compel a person to get help for symptoms that indicate underlying medical problems, problems with self-esteem, or problems with a relationship. For some people, seeking help for problems involving erection or orgasm may be more acceptable than seeking help for issues involving self-esteem such as not liking themselves.

Because the language of sex is broad and varied, it is helpful to become familiar and comfortable with the vernacular and to be able to discuss calmly and in detail matters such as masturbation, sexual positions, oral sex, anal sex, penis size, and breast size. The following section discusses a few of the areas in which misconceptions about these subjects can be resolved.

COMMON SEXUAL ISSUES

From a medical viewpoint, **masturbation** is "normal," universal, and physically harmless at all ages. It is highly correlated with self-acceptance and sexual adjustment, and is often used to further sexual self-awareness in sex therapy. Some people freely choose not to masturbate, perhaps following personal or religious tenets. Guilt about masturbation, however, continues to affect many patients. Some may use masturbation compulsively to avoid personal or relationship issues. Sex offenders may reinforce their antisocial fantasies via masturbation. Those who are truly addicted to some sexual behaviors may suffer from a variety of life difficulties common to other addictions.

There is no standard for what constitutes acceptable **sexual frequency**. Individuals who are celibate may still consider themselves sexual beings, whereas others may have sex rarely but find it satisfying and enjoyable when they do. Compulsive, frequent sex can become unrewarding for some, whereas others thrive on a frequent and active sex life. What is "right" for a particular individual or couple must be determined based on the various meanings and expectations they associate with sexuality.

Sexual fantasies are limited only by human imagination and may be enjoyed for their own sake. They may be exciting to a person who would never want to experience them in real life, or they may be yearned for. Obsessive and intrusive images that cause discomfort may need to be addressed with psychotherapy.

The majority of women enjoy and need direct **clitoral stimulation** manually or orally to reach orgasm. Unfortunately, many men assume that their female partners enjoy only intercourse. A result of this overemphasis on intercourse is that many women and men are uncomfortable with genital caressing alone. Couples can benefit from encouragement and permission to learn about and enjoy noncoital sex.

Most gay, lesbian, or bisexual patients do not wish to have their **sexual orientation** changed or challenged and often present the same concerns as heterosexuals about normalcy, dysfunction, and intimacy.

Normal changes in sexual response with **aging** include the following:

1. More direct genital stimulation and more time are needed for arousal (lubrication or erection).
2. Women may experience irritation and pain with intercourse, especially after menopause or periods of abstinence.
3. Erections may become less rigid.

4. Orgasm may not occur with each sexual encounter and the urge to ejaculate may become less intense.

5. The refractory period (the time interval between a man's ejaculation and his next erection) increases.

Many adults in their 70s, 80s, and even later years are willing to experiment in response to changes in their interest, sexual physiology, and partner status. Some older men and women become less focused on intercourse, finding increased enjoyment in petting, oral sex, and masturbation. Others may be happy to have retired from an active sexual life.

Oral medications such as sildenafil (Viagra), tadalafil (Cialis), and vardenafil (Levitra) enhance erectile functioning in many men, and in the future may be found to benefit select groups of women.

DISCUSSING SEXUALITY IN THE GENERAL MEDICAL EXAMINATION

Some patients may be more reluctant to discuss their diet or exercise patterns than the details of their sexual life, whereas others feel they risk disapproval or judgment when talking with a medical authority about sexuality, and particularly about their sexual practices. It is often helpful to introduce the topic of sexuality and acknowledge that the patient might feel some embarrassment. By routinely asking questions about sexual health in an initial history taking, a caregiver shows acceptance of sexual health as an integral part of a person's well-being and removes much of the "charge" around sexuality.

The following is a potential way to initiate a discussion about sexuality:

Doctor: One area of health care that is often neglected is sexual health, yet it can be important to people. Do you have any questions about your sex life that you would like to discuss?

A "no" response can be accepted, without ruling out possible future discussion.

Doctor: If you have any questions later on, I'd be glad to talk with you or help you find someone with whom you would be comfortable talking.

When providers are uncomfortable about a sexual topic, they can make comments such as "I feel somewhat awkward bringing this up," or "I haven't had that experience, but let me find out," or "Can you educate me about that?" These phrases are acceptable to most patients and can extricate the clinician from some difficult situations, as well as foster patient rapport.

As part of the psychosocial component of the general medical examination, a brief sex history should cover the following:

- "Are you sexually active now?" "How many current partners do you have?" If none, "When was the last time you had sex?" "Is that O.K. for you at this point in your life?"

- "Are you sexually active with men, women, both, or neither?" To encourage the confidence of lesbian, gay, or bisexual patients, ask about the patient's "partner" rather than using the gender-specific terms "wife," "husband," "boyfriend," or "girlfriend." And ask about "sexual encounters" rather than "intercourse."

- "How satisfied are you with your sexual experiences and functioning?" (Frequency, variety, who initiates, etc.)

- "Do you experience any problems with lubrication, orgasm, erection, or ejaculation?"

- Before assessing type of contraception and consistency of use, ask "Do you have a need for contraception?" rather than assuming contraception is necessary.

- History of sexually transmitted diseases (STDs) and their treatment. Discussion of human papillomavirus (HPV) vaccine and relevance to cervical cancer prevention.

- "Have you ever been tested for human immunodeficiency virus (HIV), and if so do you know if you are positive?" "Are you aware of safer sex precautions, such as the use of condoms and barrier protection, even when there is no risk of pregnancy or when other contraceptives (e.g., intrauterine device [IUD] or "the pill") are used?"

- "Have you ever had a difficult, disturbing, or abusive sexual experience?"

Use questions that show openness to other than the modal heterosexual preferences. Making assumptions about a person's sexuality based on age, gender, race, ethnicity, marital status, or sexual orientation may be diagnostically misleading and send damaging messages to the individual (e.g., an elderly patient assumed to be sexually inactive may in fact have multiple sexual partners, and important risk factors for STDs and acquired immunodeficiency syndrome [AIDS] may be missed; a monogamous gay male may feel stereotyped or misunderstood if it is assumed that he has multiple partners).

Make sure that the terminology is *mutually understood.* Overly general or euphemistic terms such as "having sex," "getting it on," "making out," "making love," or "losing one's nature" may obscure important details. Terms that are too technical ("coitus," "copulation," "cunnilingus") or too colloquial ("cunt," "cock," "fucking") may be inappropriate for use in the professional relationship.

Avoid words that convey *moral judgments or indicate little* about what an individual is actually experiencing (e.g., "adultery," "frigid," "impotent," "nymphomaniac," "perversion"). Clinicians can help patients discard demeaning labels by substituting behavioral descriptions such as "having sex outside of your primary relationship," "difficulty getting erections or getting aroused," or "trouble learning to have orgasms." Again, time and experience with a variety of patients provide a sense of what terms are most useful in conveying information to a given patient.

Patients may bring up vague or psychosomatic-like complaints (e.g., insomnia, fatigue, musculoskeletal aches, indigestion, headaches, or any specific symptoms of depression or anxiety) as a veiled request to talk about sexual concerns. Others mention a sexual concern at the end of a visit in an offhand manner, when there is little time for the problem to be adequately evaluated. The provider may then choose to assess the problem briefly and validate the importance of investigating this as soon as a new appointment can be scheduled.

Because sexual problems are often the result of a distressing gap between the patient's expectations and experiences, the effective sexual interview aims to elucidate both sides of the equation: if expectations are unrealistic, the treatment is education; if the experience fails to meet realistic expectations, intervention or referral is indicated. Often education and other clinical interventions are combined.

 CASE ILLUSTRATION 1

One couple sought help from a sex therapist because, after 30 years of enjoyable and satisfying sex (involving intercourse that would last less than 5 minutes), they had read an article extolling the virtues of extended intercourse and began to feel inadequate. When encouraged to value their own unique sexual patterns, versus what might be right for someone else, they were relieved and decided they didn't have a problem after all. They then felt freer to build upon what was already satisfying to them in a spirit of exploration, rather than of attempting to be more "normal."

SEX PROBLEM INTERVIEW

As with any other medical problem, five basic areas need to be addressed for the patient presenting with a sex problem (Table 29-2):

1. Explicit symptom or question
2. Onset and course of the symptoms
3. Patient's perception of the cause and maintenance of the problem
4. Medical evaluation, including medical history, past treatment, and outcome
5. Current expectations and goals for treatment

Answers to the preceding inquiries can help guide the clinician to specific interventions.

PHYSICAL EXAMINATION

The detailed examination of the genitourinary system should include checking for signs of androgen or estrogen deficiency or excess, neurologic dysfunction, genital abnormalities, infections, and vascular disease.

For men, the examination should include the penis (to exclude conditions such as Peyronie's disease, penile discharge, and hypospadias); testes and scrotum (for masses, atrophy, hernia, or varicoceles); and skin, prostate, and rectum. Testing should be conducted for evidence of gynecomastia, peripheral vascular disease, and neuropathy. Testicular self-examination should also be taught.

For women, the examination should look for evidence of atrophic vaginitis; skin disorders, for example, lichen sclerosis; cracks/fissures suggestive of chronic yeast infections; labial or hymenal abnormalities; swelling or tenderness of any of the vestibular glands; as well as vulvitis cystitis, vaginitis, or urethritis. Internal examination should assess tonicity of the pelvic muscles, deep tenderness/painful trigger points, pelvic inflammatory disease, and endometriosis. Vaginal estatrophy and atresia should be excluded, and assessment should include evidence of defective vaginal repair, as well as significant prolapse of the uterus including cystocele and rectocele. In situations where the patient is experiencing dyspareunia or is concerned about a perineal lesion or abnormality, she should be encouraged to use a mirror to help identify the specific lesions or painful areas.

The gynecologic examination provides an excellent opportunity for teaching patients breast self-examination.

When pathology can be excluded, patients can be reassured that their genitals look "quite healthy" and are in the normal range. This can help counter the shame that many people feel about these vulnerable areas of the body. Naming specific genital parts, such as the foreskin and glans of the penis and the clitoris and labia as you examine them, may give increased permission for the patient to ask any questions or express any concerns they may have about them. Men concerned about the size of their penis or women with worries that their genitals are somehow abnormal are more likely to voice these concerns after the clinician has comfortably used these words.

LABORATORY TESTS

In general, few laboratory tests are necessary for patients presenting with the most common sexual problems. For complaints of low sexual desire, patients should be screened for depression and fatigue, and also tested for anemia; endocrine, liver, and renal disease; or any other debilitating medical problems suggested by the history

Table 29-2. Sex problem interview.

Description of current symptom in detail

- Signal that you are glad the patient brought up the problem (to give approval, counteract shame, and encourage the patient).
- Help the patient specify exactly what the problem is, being careful to use understandable language—low desire, not getting wet or lubricating, difficulty getting or losing a "hard-on" or erection, difficulty "coming" or having orgasm, "coming too quickly" or rapid ejaculation, and so on.
- *I'd like to ask a few questions to help us sort it out.*
- *Tell me what happens.*
- *How is that a problem for you?*
- *Anything else that has changed?*

Onset and course

- *Does it happen alone with self-pleasuring or masturbation, with a specific partner, or with any partner?*
- *How does your partner respond when the problem occurs?*
- *Was there a time it was more enjoyable and then changed?*
- *Any situations when it's not a problem?*

Patient's perception of cause and maintenance of problem

- *Anything you think might be causing it or that you worry might be causing the problem or keeping it going?*

Medical evaluation, past treatment, and outcome

- *Do you smoke or use prescription or over-the-counter medications, drugs, or alcohol?*
- *Do you have any medical illnesses or treatments, depression, anxiety, or relationship problems?*
- *For women: Are your menses normal, regular? Have you had any children? Were any problems associated with pregnancy, delivery, breast-feeding?*
- *For men: Do you notice morning or nocturnal erections? Are they firm enough for penetration?*
- *Do you have a need for birth control; if so, what methods do you use?*
- *Are you concerned you might have gotten a sexually transmitted disease?*
- *Any history of physical, emotional, or sexual abuse?*
- *What have you already tried to help to change the problem?*
- *Have you ever had psychotherapy, couple or sex therapy? If yes, was this sexual problem addressed in the treatment?*
- *Have you discussed this problem openly with your partner?*

Current expectations and goals for treatment

- *How important is it to you to get help with this problem and are you interested in trying to change it now?*
- *What would be the minimum improvement you would need in order to feel it was worth your time and effort in dealing with this problem?*
- *Mostly, everyone has sexual concerns at one time or another. Talking about them is the most important first step. I'm glad you've felt comfortable talking with me and I suggest ... (or will suggest some things after I've had a chance to review the best resources for you). Many people have been helped with these issues.*

and physical examinations. Negative sexual side effects may be caused by antidepressants (notably the selective serotonin reuptake inhibitors [SSRIs]), gonadotropin-releasing hormone (GnRH) agonists, and narcotics. Recognized underlying endocrine factors might include low thyroid, low estrogen, low androgen, or high prolactin levels. While checking serum levels of thyroid-stimulating hormone (TSH) and prolactin is generally considered appropriate in women with sexual problems, routine measurement of serum estrogen and/or androgen concentrations generally is not recommended, as their measured serum levels do not correlate with sexual function.

Some authorities recommend evaluation of serum testosterone, TSH, and prolactin levels in all male patients with erectile failure or low libido. Elevated prolactin levels can be the result of many medical conditions, including pituitary tumors; renal dysfunction; sarcoidosis; thyroid disease; trauma; pelvic surgery; or use of medications such as cimetidine, haloperidol, and phenothiazine. If any of these tests is abnormal or other endocrine problems are suggested by the history or physical examination, specific, relevant additional tests should be performed as indicated.

In some men with erectile dysfunction (ED), testing by a urologist may be indicated. These may include monitoring of nocturnal penile erections (NPT) in a sleep laboratory or, more commonly and less expensively, with a home monitoring unit or simple snap-gauge.

Increasingly, a trial with a phosphodiesterase (PDE5) inhibitor such as sildenafil (Viagra), vardenafil (Levitra), or tadalafil (Cialis) is recommended for both diagnosis and treatment.

ORGANIC & PSYCHOGENIC FACTORS

Rather than describing sexual problems with a simple differential diagnosis of either organic *or* psychogenic etiology, it is useful to identify *both* categories of causal factors. These can be assessed with the psychosocial history, sex problem interview, physical examination, and laboratory testing. A symptom that is generalized (occurring in all circumstances) may indicate major organic or psychogenic involvement, whereas situational symptoms tend to be psychogenic (Table 29-3).

ORGANIC FACTORS

Organic factors may be suspected when a man reports an absence of nocturnal or morning erections or is unable to get erect with masturbation. For painful intercourse, important situational variables to identify include whether the woman has been adequately stimulated and aroused prior to penetration, whether she feels pain with masturbation or when having sex with another partner, and whether she is able to direct the extent and timing of thrusting or is passive. Also, organic factors should be considered when a patient has not responded to an adequate course of sex therapy.

MEDICAL CONDITIONS & TREATMENTS

Medical conditions and treatments affecting sexuality are listed in Table 29-4.

Table 29-3. Symptom patterns and etiology.

Symptom patterns suggestive of principally organic etiology
• Generalized (especially for absent desire, erectile disorder, secondary premature ejaculation, and painful intercourse. Even when generalized, however, primary rapid ejaculation and primary female orgasmic disorder in otherwise healthy individuals are rarely organic.) • Gradual onset • Rapid onset when associated with certain medications
Symptom patterns suggestive of principally psychological etiology
• Situational • Rapid onset (unless medications are suspected) • Sexual phobia and aversion

Table 29-4. Medical conditions commonly associated with sexual disorders.

- Arthritis/joint disease
- Diabetes mellitus
- Endocrine problems
- Injury to autonomic nervous system by surgery or radiation
- Liver or renal failure
- Mood disorders, including depression, anxiety, and panic
- Multiple sclerosis
- Peripheral neuropathy
- Radical pelvic surgery
- Respiratory disorders (e.g., COPD)
- Spinal cord injury
- Vascular disease

Abbreviation: COPD, chronic obstructive pulmonary disease.

Medications

Medications of many kinds have been implicated in sexual dysfunction (Table 29-5). Older antidepressants such as amitriptyline (Elavil) and doxepin (Sinequan) have anticholinergic properties that undermine sexual arousal. The widely used SSRIs—antidepressants such as fluoxetine (Prozac), sertraline (Zoloft), and paroxetine (Paxil)—may inhibit orgasm for women and ejaculation and orgasm for men, while decreasing sexual desire for both. Strategies to alleviate such dysfunction include

Table 29-5. Medication and drug categories commonly associated with sexual disorders.

- Alcohol
- Anticancer drugs and hormones
- Anticonvulsants
- Antihypertensives, including beta-blockers (at high dosage), excluding ACE inhibitors
- Carbonic anhydrase inhibitors
- Cytotoxic drugs
- Digitalis family
- Diuretics
- H_2 receptor antagonists
- Nonsteroidal anti-inflammatory agents
- Opiates
- Pain medications
- Psychedelic and hallucinogenic drugs
- Psychiatric medications (benzodiazepines, tricyclic antidepressants, monoamine oxidase inhibitors, SSRIs, antipsychotics, lithium carbonate)
- Recreational drugs (tobacco, alcohol, and opiates)
- Sleep medications
- Tranquilizers

Abbreviation: ACE, angiotensin-converting enzyme inhibitors.

(1) reducing the dosage, (2) taking a weekend "holiday" in which the last dose for the week is taken on Thursday morning and the medication is resumed at noon on Sunday, (3) switching to another medication, or (4) coadministering other medications, such as bupropion-SR (Wellbutrin-SR), neostigmine (Prostigmin), cyproheptadine (Periactin), bethanechol (Duvoid), and yohimbine (Yohimex) 1–2 hours prior to sexual activity. It is hoped that antidepressants currently in development will have fewer negative sexual side effects.

PSYCHOLOGICAL FACTORS

Psychological factors often play a causal role in maintaining sexual dysfunction. This possibility should be considered even in cases when a medical condition or use of a medication which is known to cause a problem has been identified as a cause (Table 29-6). For example, a female patient experiencing difficulty reaching orgasm since being treated with an SSRI antidepressant may continue to have this problem even after switching to a lower dosage or different medication, because of a conditioned performance anxiety.

Following hysterectomy, some women report increased sexual enjoyment because of the relief from uncomfortable physical symptoms and bleeding, whereas others find the surgery difficult and have a psychological response to the loss of these organs and to their reproductive capacity. These women may then experience a decrease in sexual desire, arousal, or orgasmic responsiveness. The research is mixed as to the effects of hysterectomy on orgasm in women; it has been proposed that women differ in the extent to which they perceive uterine and cervical contractions during orgasm, with differing sense of loss after the surgery. There is similar variability in men after prostatectomy. For many, orgasm may feel satisfactory even with a "dry" or retrograde ejaculation, with semen going into the bladder, but others may complain of a loss of orgasmic sensation.

CASE ILLUSTRATION 2

Juan, a 38-year-old male patient complaining of ED with a possible organic component (type II diabetes) and performance anxiety, declined treatment with sildenafil (Viagra), saying that he wanted help without more medication. By quitting smoking cigarettes and engaging in noncoital caressing with his partner to decrease his pressure to perform, he was able to experience satisfying erections firm enough for intercourse. In this case, the diabetes by itself was not the determining factor in maintaining the problem.

Table 29-6. Psychological conditions commonly associated with sexual disorders.

I. Immediate causes (of most concern for the general medical practitioner)
  A. Performance anxiety—fear of inadequate performance
  B. Spectatoring—critically monitoring one's own sexual performance
  C. Inadequate communication with partner regarding sex
  D. Fantasy—absence of fantasy, fantasy incompatible with sexual arousal, or distracting thoughts
II. Deeper causes (for referral)
  A. Intrapsychic issues—early conditioning, sexual trauma, depression, anxiety, guilt, fear of intimacy, or separation
  B. Relationship issues—lack of trust, power and control issues, anger at partner
  C. Sociocultural factors—attitudes and values, religious beliefs
  D. Educational and cognitive factors—Sexual myths or expectations (gender roles, age and appearance, proper sexual activity, performance expectations), sexual ignorance

---

Source: Adapted, with permission, from Plaut SM, Lehne GK. Sexual dysfunction, gender identity disorders, and paraphilias. In: Goldman HH, ed. *Review of General Psychiatry*, 5th ed. New York, NY: McGraw-Hill, 2000.

Some medical illnesses and treatments are believed to decrease sexual desire or to cause sexual dysfunction *directly.* Psychosocial adaptations to virtually any medical condition, however, can *indirectly* affect sexual desire or functioning. For example, fears of rejection by a sexual partner because of a stoma or mastectomy or concerns about sexual functioning may lead to a suppression of sexual feelings and avoidance of sexual opportunities. Of course, many medically healthy men and women either choose to be sexually inactive or refrain out of a sense of inadequacy. The capacity to enjoy one's sexuality therefore cannot be predicted on the basis of medical diagnosis alone.

Psychological problems such as depression or anxiety can be either the *cause* or the *effect* of diminished sexual desire or functioning. Both may be true to some degree. In other instances, depression and sexual problems may both be the result of a third underlying factor, such as an endocrine disorder.

Sexual problems might have remote psychological causes, such as childhood trauma or prohibitions about sexual pleasure, but almost all such problems can be seen as having current maintaining variables of anxiety or depression. In general, psychological etiology is primarily suggested when the problem is situational; seems related to performance anxiety, depression, or guilt; or is associated with significant relationship and communication problems.

PSYCHOLOGICAL MANAGEMENT & BRIEF SEX COUNSELING

A paradigm shift occurred in the treatment of sexual dysfunctions with the publication in 1970 of Masters and Johnson's signal work on sex therapy. The previous emphasis on the diagnosis and treatment of individual psychopathology, with somewhat poor treatment results for the sexual dysfunctions, gave way to an understanding of the importance of the **conditions** (internal variables such as attitudes, expectations, and lack of knowledge, as well as external factors related to the partner or the situation) under which people attempt to function sexually.

Education and suggestions for focusing on pleasure rather than on performance were found to lower anxiety and to promote improved sexual functioning and enjoyment.

Anxiety is considered one of the major psychological causes of the sexual dysfunctions, whether stemming from individual or relationship issues. Are patients comfortable, at ease, and feeling close to their partners or are they anxious due to lack of information, strained relationships, unrealistic attitudes about and focus on sexual performance goals, or other conditions? In these cases, modern sex therapy commonly provides anxiety-reduction interventions, many of which can be adapted for use by primary care providers. These include validating that most people at some time experience sexual problems and that such problems are often an understandable response to stress, worry, and concerns about performance; encouraging open communication between partners; dispelling maladaptive beliefs about sex; suggesting ways that patients can increase their level of comfort and safety and their ability to relax during sex; and encouraging the view that noncoital sex can be very satisfying and does not have to be considered "second best."

THE P-LI-SS-IT MODEL

Annon's P-LI-SS-IT model is a useful hierarchical guide to anxiety-reduction approaches to sexual problems and can be used by primary care practitioners. The letters in the acronym stand for different levels of intervention.

P = Permission

The fundamental intervention is to give patients permission to discuss their sexual concerns. Empathic listening, including verbal and nonverbal reassurance, helps give patients permission to talk openly about sexual issues and may encourage and enable them to discuss the problem more directly with a partner. Reassurance and permission can help validate that having a sexual prob-

lem is normal rather than pathologic. Inquire into positive exceptions: patients can describe those areas of sex about which they do feel good; for example, a woman can appreciate her ability to become aroused despite difficulty reaching orgasm, and a man can be a skillful lover despite his erectile disorder. Permission to choose not to be sexually active may be very helpful for patients who feel pressured to have sex or who feel inadequate if they don't care to be sexually active.

LI = Limited Information

Facts can add to the effectiveness of reassurance and can be at the disposal of any clinician who has done basic reading about sexuality and keeps up through the literature or review courses. Keeping responses focused and limited to the expressed concern saves time and does not overwhelm the patient with extraneous information (Table 29-7). Such information gives the patient the choice of maintaining or changing sexual practices or attitudes. A simple explanation of the psychophysiology of sexual arousal and the importance of conditions for relaxation helps "normalize" the symptoms and refocuses attention on conditions that can be changed to alleviate the problem rather than on trying to determine what is wrong with the patient. This can be conveyed by the following "rhinoceros" story about sexuality:

> *Imagine you are lying on a blanket in a secluded meadow with a loving partner after having had a wonderful picnic lunch on a beautiful sunny day. You start kissing and feel arousal in your genitals, when, all of a sudden, a rhinoceros charges out of the jungle straight for you. What happens to your arousal (lubrication or erection)? The fight-or-flight response causes a rapid redirection of blood to the brain and large-muscle groups, with a corresponding loss of erection or genital arousal. The rhinoceros represents worrisome thoughts and anxieties about having erections, arousal, or orgasm, or fears that you won't please your partner or be seen as a good lover. Some simple suggestions can help you keep the rhinoceros out of your bedroom!*

SS = Specific Suggestions

Where permission and limited information do not suffice, the patient may benefit from specific suggestions to help overcome a sexual problem. Most sex counseling interventions are designed to help the patient (and partner, if available) communicate better about sex and enjoy increased sexual pleasure by reducing performance anxiety about attaining the goals of arousal, lubrication, erection, and orgasm. Helpful interventions taken from sex therapy include (1) temporary agreement not to have intercourse; (2) suggestions for focusing on pleasurable touch, genital caressing, Kegel exercises (tensing and

Table 29-7. Maladaptive ideas and therapeutic responses to them.

Maladaptive Idea	Therapeutic Response
My sexual problems are because I'm too old.	For those who are interested and willing to be creative, sex can be an enjoyable part of life in their 70s, 80s, and beyond!
I should be interested only in survival, not sex (for someone with terminal or chronic illness).	If sex was important to you before your illness it can remain so or become so again.
I am *asexual* because I don't have an active sex life.	We are *all* sexual beings. You can be aware of and enjoy your sexual feelings without being sexually active.
Sex equals love.	Many people have very loving relationships without being sexually active, and, of course, some people have sex without having loving feelings.
Sex equals intercourse.	There is no one *right* way to be sexual, and many people enjoy touching and caressing more than intercourse.
Having sex is the same as *enjoying sex*.	Many people have to learn to enjoy their sexuality.
It is not proper to talk about sex, either with your partner or a health care provider.	It is often a great relief when people can talk confidentially about their sexual feelings and concerns.
You shouldn't talk about sex because it will destroy the mystery.	Most people find that talking about their important feelings deepens intimacy, and trust develops when you know you can be vulnerable with another. You can create more mystery from deeper sharing.
You should be interested in having sex with any willing partner.	It is most important to be able to respect yourself. Your sexuality is a gift that you share only with those you truly want to share it with.
You should be able to enjoy sex with a partner even when you are tired, angry, or feel hurt.	We all have our own conditions for what makes a sexual encounter enjoyable, and feeling close to and loved by your partner is important to most of us.
I try not to masturbate and feel guilty when I give in because I have a partner and shouldn't need to do that.	Most married people continue to masturbate and find it does not interfere with the pleasure they have with their partner.
Sex is a performance, and it would be grim and catastrophic to "fail."	Sexual sharing can be playful, with the goals of giving and receiving feelings of pleasure and caring. If things don't go as planned, there is always next time!
A new partner will not like the size of my (breasts/penis).	Most men and women enjoy having sex with a person, not a body part. Most men compare themselves to other men when their penises are soft … size differences are usually not as great when erections are compared. Vaginas accommodate different penis sizes, with the outer third and the clitoris the most responsive areas for many women.
Sex should result in orgasm every time.	Does *not* having dessert ruin a fine meal? Orgasm is only one of the pleasurable aspects of a sexual encounter. Many people find it a relief to not have "should's" in their sex life.
Sex should never be a problem. Experiencing a problem is not normal.	Sex is perfectly natural, but not naturally perfect. Probably everyone has "problems" with sex at some time or another.

relaxing the pubococcygeal [P.C.] muscles), and progressive muscle relaxation methods; (3) correction of cognitive distortions ("self-talk"); and (4) suggestions to improve emotional and sexual communication.

Even for couples who previously enjoyed certain patterns of lovemaking, predictable repetition over time can lead to sexual boredom. Suggesting that a couple agree, for example, to temporarily forego intercourse or otherwise change their usual sexual pattern often helps them focus on moment-to-moment pleasure. Rather than making assumptions about what the other wants, the couple can communicate their likes and dislikes.

Many people remember how arousing and exciting it was when they were younger and were "making out" (sexual petting) without intercourse. If agreeable to both, they can take turns exploring other ways of caressing and pleasuring each other. The **sensate focus** exercise, from Masters and Johnson, is done for the interest of the person doing the touching, rather than for the pleasure of the receiver. To minimize performance anxiety, each is encouraged to take turns "savoring" the experience of touching and exploring the other's body, in contrast to worrying about "turning on" or performing for the partner. For many people, permission for **genital caressing** in this way increases sexual pleasure and satisfaction.

Arranging for follow-up after giving specific suggestions keeps the health care provider informed as to their effectiveness, helps the patient stay focused on problem solving, and informs the clinician about the necessity for further intervention.

IT = Intensive Therapy

This is the last step in the hierarchy and involves referral to an appropriate specialist when the previous three levels of intervention have not been effective (see "Indications for Referral," below).

ADDITIONAL PATIENT EDUCATION

Pamphlets detailing approaches for safe sex for the prevention of AIDS can supplement discussions and should be made readily available for patients. Many good self-help books dealing with common sexual disorders enable patients to move at their own pace. Often people who are reluctant to enter counseling or who are hesitant about discussing their problems in depth are willing to read about the problems in the privacy of their home where they can be relaxed and comfortable. Several books are recommended at the end of this chapter.

INDICATIONS FOR REFERRAL

Refer patients to an appropriate medical specialist if the brief treatment suggestions in this chapter fail to help or if the history and physical examination suggest primarily an organic component. Refer patients to a mental health specialist trained in sex therapy if the problem is situational, occurring only with a certain partner; if functioning is adequate under certain conditions; or if significant emotional distress is present.

Primary care clinicians can develop a resource list of providers for sex-related problems. Colleagues, teachers, friends, and clinical societies can be asked for recommendations. Identify medical and mental health specialists with expertise in treating sexual issues. Practitioners can be licensed in psychiatry, psychology, social work, psychiatric nursing, or marriage and family counseling. Most states do not license "sex therapists" or "sex counselors."

COMMON SEXUAL DISORDERS

Low or Absent Sexual Desire & Sexual Aversion

The range of issues concerning sexual desire is wide (Table 29-8). Some people simply put a low priority on sex, some are inhibited or find sex aversive, and some are clinically phobic. These problems can be of recent origin or reflect a long-standing pattern. Lack of desire may pertain only to certain sexual partners or practices (such as oral sex). Couples with different levels of desire may disagree as to which partner's level is "abnormal." In this situation, each side has valid feelings, and it is important not to stigmatize the patient with the lower level of desire. Most couples occasionally deal with periods of discrepancy in desire or mutually low desire and feel they should have sex more often than they do. Demands of family, career, and friends often take precedence over sex.

Problems with desire or sexual aversion can derive from deeper relational power struggles or reflect childhood sexual, physical, or emotional abuse that requires couple counseling or individual psychotherapy for resolution. The following case example, however, demonstrates how permission and encouragement to talk about sex directly, together with specific suggestions, can have a powerful positive influence.

 CASE ILLUSTRATION 3[2]

Alice, a healthy 33-year-old primary school teacher, reported having lost her desire for sex. Her sex problem history established that although she had enjoyed sexual activity with her husband for the first 2 years of their marriage, in the past year it had become a chore that she never put on her extensive "to do" list. Because sex was seen as a bedtime activity, when she was usually tired, their sexual frequency dropped from weekly to once every several months. They did not address the problem directly, and Alice and her husband's feelings of estrangement from each other continued to grow.

*When asked what steps they had taken to address these problems, Alice disclosed that she and her husband had never had an open discussion about sex. Her primary care physician validated that this was common among couples and that most people have to learn to talk more comfortably about their sexual needs (**P**ermission and **L**imited **I**nformation). The physician also explained that everyone has certain conditions that need to be met to be interested in sexual activity (**P** and **LI**) and encouraged Alice to think about her conditions and then, with her husband, to "set some private time aside outside of the bedroom to let*

---

[2]Cases 3–10 described in this chapter were of actual patients seen in primary care settings as reported in consultation with the first author. Although some identifying characteristics of the patients have been changed to ensure confidentiality, the essential clinical issues presented are accurately portrayed. We thank all the patients and their health providers who helped us gather these examples.

Table 29-8. DSM-IV-TR sexual disorders and treatment approaches.

Disorder	Diagnostic Criteria	Treatment Approach
Hypoactive sexual desire disorder (302.71)	Persistently or recurrently deficient (or absent) sexual fantasies and desire for sexual activity. The judgment of deficiency or absence is made by the clinician, taking into account factors that affect sexual functioning, such as age and the *context of the person's life.*	After organic causes ruled out or if situational: **Permission and limited information:** (a) restate problem in behavioral terms, (b) explore patient conditions for good sex (rhinoceros story), including whether patient receives adequate direct stimulation, (c) validate patient's right to say "no" to sex, (d) may be secondary to depression, anxiety, panic, or phobic disorder (occasionally related to childhood sexual abuse), or (e) may be symptomatic of hidden arousal or orgasmic disorder (if so, treat appropriately). **Specific suggestions:** (f) Listening exercises to increase *communication* with partner, (g) *suggested readings* (Barbach, 2000, 2001; Gottman, 1999; Schnarch, 1998; Zilbergeld, 1999). **Intensive therapy:** Refer to mental health professional trained in sexual therapy.
Sexual aversion disorder (302.79)	Persistent or recurrent extreme aversion to, and avoidance of, all (or almost all) genital sexual contact with a sexual partner.	
Female sexual arousal disorder (302.72); Male erectile disorder (302.72)	Persistent or recurrent inability to attain, or to maintain until completion of the sexual activity, an adequate lubrication-swelling response of sexual excitement (female) or erection (male).	**Permission and limited information:** (a–d) above, (h) give brief explanation of the physiology of arousal and the need for relaxation, (i) is sexual desire present? (if not, treat as desire disorder). **Specific suggestions:** (f–h) above, (j) enough and desired kind of direct stimulation by partner? (k) use of lubricants (Astroglide, K-Y, and so on) or vaginal moisturizers (Replens), (l) suggest temporary intercourse ban, (m) sensate focus, (n) genital caressing, (o) progressive relaxation and Kegel exercises, (p) explore ways other than intercourse of pleasuring partner, (q) hormonal therapy, (r) low-dose beta-blocker (10 mg Inderal) if high performance anxiety, (s) vacuum device, especially if organic and older male, (t) intracorporeal penile injection or intraurethral application of PGE_1, (u) penile implant, (v) sildenafil (50 mg Viagra) for males.
Premature ejaculation disorder (302.75)	Persistent or recurrent ejaculation with minimal sexual stimulation before, on, or shortly after penetration and before the person wishes it. The clinician must take into account factors that affect duration of the excitement phase, such as age, novelty of the sexual partner or situation, and recent frequency of sexual activity.	**Permission and limited information:** As above, and explore masturbation patterns—may have conditioned himself to ejaculate rapidly. Explain connection between rapid ejaculation and anxiety vs. relaxation and longer-lasting erections. **Specific suggestions:** (l–p) above, (w) increase frequency of ejaculation, (x) stop-start exercises (Zilbergeld, 1999), (y) clomipramine (Anafranil 25 mg as needed) or SSRI antidepressant medication, (z) prilocaine-lidocaine cream with condom.

(Continued)

Table 29-8. *DSM-IV-TR* sexual disorders and treatment approaches. *(Continued)*

Disorder	Diagnostic Criteria	Treatment Approach
Female and male orgasmic disorder (302.73)	Persistent or recurrent delay in, or absence of, orgasm following a normal sexual excitement phase. Women exhibit wide variability in the type or intensity of stimulation that triggers orgasm. The diagnosis of female orgasmic disorder should be based on the clinician's judgment that the woman's orgasmic capacity is less than would be reasonable for her age, sexual experience, and the adequacy of sexual stimulation she receives. For the male, the clinician should take into account the person's age, and judge the stimulation to be adequate in focus, intensity, and duration.	**Permission and limited information:** (a–e) above. **Specific suggestions:** For primary preorgasmic woman, recommend Barbach (2001); for male, Zilbergeld (1999). If orgasmic disorder is secondary (at one time patient was orgasmic), then evaluate and treat for desire or arousal disorder or relationship problems. (f), (j), (l–p) above.
Dyspareunia (302.76); Vaginismus (306.51)	Recurrent or persistent genital pain associated with sexual intercourse in either a male or a female (dyspareunia). Recurrent or persistent involuntary spasm of the musculature of the outer third of the vagina that interferes with sexual intercourse (vaginismus).	**Permission and limited information:** (a–e) above. **Specific suggestions:** (f–k), (m–p) above. Encourage explicit communication with patient's partner about her need to have enough stimulation prior to penetration, give control to the woman to choose when penetration occurs and timing of thrusting. **Intensive therapy:** Sex therapy may be necessary for long-standing dyspareunia and vaginismus, due to conditioned expectation of pain.

yourselves have a discussion about this, even if it is awkward" (**S**pecific **S**uggestions).

Doctor: It can be good for relationships when people risk being a little uneasy. You don't have to have the same perspective. You are each entitled to your own separate feelings about the situation, but together you can talk it out, try to understand each other, and see what other choices you have (**P**, **LI**, and **SS**).

The physician also recommended a self-help book (**SS**) and offered to refer them to a therapist who treats couples, should their attempts to communicate falter (**I**ntensive **T**herapy).

 CASE ILLUSTRATION 3 (CONTD.)

At her 1-month follow-up appointment, Alice reported significant progress. When the couple set time aside to discuss their sex life, they had a very meaningful and tender talk. The husband was

relieved to learn about the major sources of Alice's lack of desire and she acknowledged feeling resentful that he seemed unresponsive to her needs. He admitted that he had taken her lack of desire very personally, secretly and painfully interpreting the problem as her lack of desire for him. With these hidden resentments expressed, they could set aside their power struggles and cooperate in addressing these issues. Recognizing how they had both felt lonely and uncared for allowed them to take specific actions, such as planning a regular evening each week just for the two of them to talk and nurture their intimacy.

Management

PERMISSION AND LIMITED INFORMATION

Some couples can learn to accept that low desire may be understandable given their immediate circumstances (e.g., the months prior to and after childbirth) and that their previous levels of desire can be expected to return over time. Validate the patient's right to say "no" to sex.

A "prescription" to go away on a weekend or to arrange a sleepover for children with relatives may help couples "break the ice" and re-experience intimacy. Suggest that patient and partner set time aside to talk about each other's feelings and discuss conditions for more enjoyable sex, with each taking an uninterrupted amount of time for self-expression. Self-help books may also be recommended.

OTHER MEDICAL INTERVENTIONS

Hormonal replacement therapy, especially testosterone, may be helpful for those with low levels, but this is not universally accepted in the medical community. For example, vaginal application of testosterone cream may be considered if not contraindicated for some women who experience a loss of desire following chemotherapy for breast cancer.

FEMALE SEXUAL AROUSAL DISORDER

Symptoms & Signs

Problems with female arousal are primarily manifested as vaginal dryness and may be reported separately from or together with lack of desire, difficulty reaching orgasm, or pain experienced during intercourse. The most common medical cause in older women is estrogen deficiency with resulting signs of vulvar irritation and atrophic vaginitis. Arousal may be inhibited by anxiety and depression; it may also be a side effect of antidepressant medication. These possibilities should be explored (see Table 29-5).

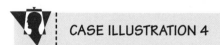

CASE ILLUSTRATION 4

Betty, a 78-year-old patient, had an appointment with her female physician. She brought along her 82-year-old husband because she wanted to discuss what she called her "sexual problems." Betty said she did not care about sex, that her husband was often angry with her lack of enthusiasm, and that this pattern had existed throughout the 50 years of their marriage. She believed she was not "a sexual person" because she had never been very excited by intercourse. She did enjoy kissing and caressing and mentioned that on several occasions she had been able to have orgasm when he stroked her labia and clitoris, but that she had never had orgasm from the "real sex" (intercourse) that he preferred. The physician responded that there really is no one way to be a "sexual person," that many people cherish the sensual and emotional aspects

*of sex, and that Betty did not need to consider herself asexual just because she preferred different aspects of sexual intimacy than her husband (**P** and **LI**). The physician further explained that the majority of women reach orgasm more often from manual caressing than from coitus, and that many couples enjoy bringing each other to orgasm without intercourse (**P** and **LI**). The couple was relieved and admitted to having curiosity about trying this petting more. They were given brief instructions to take turns at home touching and stroking each other without the goal of orgasm (sensate focus), to get reacquainted with each other's body, and to refrain from any attempts at intercourse for 2 weeks (**SS**).*

A follow-up telephone call confirmed that they were enjoying taking turns caressing each other, that orgasm often happened for each, and that they occasionally progressed to intercourse. A 1 ¹/₂-year follow-up was especially poignant—the husband reported that Betty had recently died from a stroke, and, although grieving her loss, he expressed profound appreciation for having gotten help for their sexual conflicts from the physician.

Husband: Settling those old battles over sex made our last year together more loving and caring than ever before in our marriage.

Management

PERMISSION AND LIMITED INFORMATION

Is the patient getting stimulation in the way that works best for her? Feeling distant from or angry with a partner can inhibit sexual arousal, and such relationship concerns need to be addressed.

SPECIFIC SUGGESTIONS

Homework may be suggested for her to identify what stimulation works best. The goal is to experience the pleasure of arousal in that mode—not to reach orgasm. Inquiry should be made into the quality of the patient's relationship. Commercial lubrication (Astroglide, KY Jelly, and so on) and vaginal moisturizers such as Replens can be suggested and, if this is inadequate, a local estrogen preparation may be needed to treat the vaginal atrophy and dryness. Self-help books can be recommended.

INTENSIVE THERAPY

Recommend couple or individual therapy.

MALE ERECTILE DISORDER

Symptoms & Signs

Generally, a man with a significant psychological component is aware of nocturnal or morning erections, is able to maintain his erection for a reasonable time and then ejaculate with masturbation, or has good erections in some situations but not in others. He may be able to get a firm erection but lose it after penetration or may not get an erection with a partner at any time. The original cause of the problem is often distinct from the maintaining variable, which is generally anxiety. Consider possibilities such as performance anxiety, lack of direct physical stimulation of the penis, conscious or unconscious guilt (e.g., "widower's syndrome"), anger at his partner or other relationship issues, or childhood issues such as sexual abuse.

CASE ILLUSTRATION 5

*Carl, a 58-year-old HIV-negative gay male, confided to his physician that he had been "impotent" since the death of his partner of 17 years, with whom he had had an active and monogamous sexual life. Attributing this problem to aging and worries about HIV infection, Carl nonetheless asked for any help the primary care physician could provide. A full session was scheduled for talking only. His partner had died suddenly from cardiac arrest a year before. In the past month, Carl had attempted sex on four occasions with two different men and was unable to get an erection. After a thorough socio-sexual history, Carl was seen to fit the "widowers' syndrome." Clearly, he was still grieving the loss of his partner but attempted to control his tears with statements such as "I should be over this by now" and "Life has to go on; he wanted me to go on." Carl then revealed that he was very afraid of feeling such loss, fearing that he would never be able to come out of the sadness. His grieving was acknowledged and validated (**P**), and it was explained to him that temporary sexual problems were common after such loss because of a number of factors: performance pressure of being with a new partner, continuing feelings of loyalty to a deceased partner, subsequent guilt at having sex with new people, and concerns about HIV infection with a new partner (**LI**). The physician encouraged Carl to join a grief support group or to contact a psychotherapist comfortable with gay sexuality (**SS**). In addition, the doctor referred Carl to a book on male sexuality, with suggestions on how to talk to a potential partner about both safer sex practices and ways they could reduce the pressure to have erections (**LI** and*

*SS**). At a follow-up visit 4 months later, Carl reported he had been able to cry more about his loss and was enjoying sex and intimacy with a new friend who had also lost a partner.*

Management

PERMISSION AND LIMITED INFORMATION

Many patients over 40 years old report previous successful sexual encounters when they were younger in which they became erect without direct physical stimulation of the penis. If their pattern for sexual interaction has rarely or never included direct touching by a partner, it might help them to learn that such touching becomes more necessary as men age, and that it can be an enjoyable part of sex.

SPECIFIC SUGGESTIONS

Institute a temporary ban on penetration and suggest sensate focus, progressive relaxation, and Kegel exercises. The couple should agree *not* to attempt penetration or intercourse even if the patient gets an improved erection.

> **Doctor:** For every minute you are relaxing with your partner and have an erection, your body is remembering just what it needs to do to get and maintain an erection. Your mind can be free to enjoy the pleasurable feelings and sensations of being caressed and kissing your partner. You might even allow your erection to go away. If you stay relaxed, it will likely return again with resumed stimulation.

OTHER MEDICAL INTERVENTIONS

PDE5 inhibitors. Sildenafil (Viagra), vardenafil (Levitra), and tadalafil (Cialis) are three oral medications popularly known to have revolutionized the medical treatment of male ED. Although contraindicated in men taking organic nitrate medication for angina, these medications have been found to have broad-spectrum effectiveness across men of all ages and medical conditions, including diabetes, hypertension, neuropathy, postprostatectomy, and depression.

Testosterone replacement therapy. For men with demonstrated low levels of serum testosterone, hormone replacement therapy may be helpful. This does not benefit men whose serum testosterone is within normal limits. Side effects can be serious, including increase of any existing prostatic cancer, enlargement of the prostate, retention of fluids, and liver damage. Careful monitoring and follow-up prostate-specific antigen (PSA) screening and prostate examinations are necessary.

Antidepressant medication. Antidepressants, especially bupropion-SR (Wellbutrin-SR), can be effective treatment for some, but other patients may find that SSRI antidepressants hinder erection and ejaculation.

Low-dose beta-blocker therapy. For some men whose performance anxiety is very high, 10–20 mg of propranolol (Inderal) as needed has been effective.

External penile vacuum device. With the aid of a vacuum cylinder a tension ring is placed around the base of the penis after it has become erect. This device may work better for men who clearly have a major organic component to their erectile problem, such as severe diabetes, multiple sclerosis, or spinal cord injury. Although this device can create erections functional for intercourse, men with a more psychogenic etiology may be disappointed when the erections are not as firm as they had been expecting. Side effects may include bruising of the penis.

Intracorporeal penile injections or intraurethral delivery of prostaglandin E_1 (PGE$_1$). These methods were originally used diagnostically by urologists. However, patients can now be taught to inject themselves prior to sexual encounters, resulting in firmer erections that often do not disappear at orgasm or ejaculation and last about an hour. Side effects are priapism in less than 3% of patients and pain. In addition, scarring may be a concern with repeated injections over time.

Penile implant surgery. Since the advent of effective oral medications, implants with semirigid silicone rods or inflatable cylinders are less commonly utilized. Total costs are high, ranging from $6,000 to $15,000. Complications include device failure (requiring additional surgery) and infection.

RAPID EJACULATION (PREMATURE EJACULATION)

Symptoms & Signs

Terms such as *rapid* or *early ejaculation* are clinically preferable to the established *premature ejaculation,* as they highlight the subjective nature of the problem and are less pejorative. No absolute measure—either in number of minutes or thrusts—is applicable to the diverse numbers of men presenting with this problem. Factors to be assessed include a patient's subjective evaluation, degree of sexual satisfaction, and sense of control.

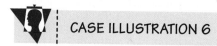

CASE ILLUSTRATION 6

*Donald, a 45-year-old divorced male, reported ejaculating after 1 minute or less of intercourse. This had been his pattern since becoming sexually active in his late teens. He reported proudly that he never masturbated but had a high sex drive, which led him to multiple sexual partners including prostitutes. His primary care physician gave Donald a supportive talk about how he could teach himself to last longer with certain physical exercises (**P, LI,** and **SS**). The patient was willing to do "self-stimulation" or "self-pleasuring" exercises for this "medical reason" and was comforted that as with the physical fitness regimen that he valued, he could tone up his P.C. muscles and learn to relax the pelvic muscles during sexual stimulation. Donald was advised to increase his frequency of ejaculation, was told about the importance of relaxation for maintaining erection, and was encouraged to read Zilbergeld's self-help section on "stop-start" exercises for lasting longer (**P, LI,** and **SS**). As his confidence grew through the solo exercises, and as he increased the frequency of ejaculation, Donald was able to try the stop-start exercises with a partner with increasing success. He said that it also helped him to read about the experiences of other men (getting validation from the universality of sexual concerns) and about how many women enjoy a variety of forms of sexual stimulation in addition to intercourse.*

Management

PERMISSION AND LIMITED INFORMATION

Point out that early ejaculation is a very common problem—one study found 35% of married males reported that they ejaculated too quickly. Tell the patient that men with this problem have a high success rate when they try one or more specific suggestions that will be given to him for this problem. Give a *brief explanation of the psychophysiological mechanism.*

> **Doctor:** Men aren't supposed to be able to have long-lasting erections if they are too nervous or distracted. The fight-or-flight response generally makes men more likely to ejaculate. Most men have trained themselves through rapid masturbation to get erect and ejaculate quickly; so it makes sense that they would continue to ejaculate quickly when they are with a partner.

Assure the patient that men often report more intense orgasms after they have learned to last longer and that it is highly likely that he will gain greater ejaculatory control by following these suggestions.

SPECIFIC SUGGESTIONS

The patient may need to *increase his frequency of ejaculations,* alone or with a partner, perhaps masturbating to orgasm earlier on a day that a sexual encounter with a partner is anticipated. Discuss *other ways he can please his partner,* so he doesn't feel pressure to do it all with an erect penis. Discuss the importance of muscle relaxation in achieving a prolonged erection. Suggest *breathing exercises and progressive muscle relaxation exercises*, targeting the P.C. muscles or those in the buttocks.

In contrast to common attempts by men to diminish sensations in hope of lasting longer, they actually need to *increase their tolerance for the good sensations and feelings* and can best do this by concentrating on their feelings and getting more "turned on." Focusing on these feelings in a relaxed "practice" atmosphere can increase the threshold of enjoyment before ejaculation and orgasm.

He and his partner can read about and practice the "*stop-start technique.*" Encourage the patient to change positions and to go from intercourse to oral or manual stimulation of his partner, and then back to intercourse (following the desires of his partner); changing positions and pleasuring a partner to orgasm without intercourse helps many men last longer.

OTHER MEDICAL INTERVENTIONS

Clomipramine (Anafranil, 25 mg as needed) or SSRI antidepressants help men prolong their erections prior to ejaculation.

Prilocaine-lidocaine cream applied to the penis and then used with a condom has been recommended by some clinicians (although "numbing" of the genitals may detract from enjoyment for both partners).

FEMALE & MALE ORGASMIC DISORDER

Symptoms & Signs

Many women do not learn to have orgasms until they are in their 20s, 30s, or even later. A **primary anorgasmic** or **preorgasmic** woman is not yet able to reach orgasm reliably either with a partner or by herself. A woman with **secondary orgasmic disorder** was previously able to reach orgasm but is no longer able to do so. **Situational orgasmic disorder** refers to a condition in which a woman can have orgasm with masturbation but not with a partner, or with one partner but not with another. She may reach moderate-to-high levels of arousal without experiencing the pleasure and release of climax. If no arousal or interest is present, she should be evaluated for a desire or arousal disorder.

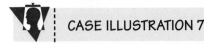

CASE ILLUSTRATION 7

Ethyl's complaint of low sexual desire and difficulty feeling aroused led the physician to do a brief sex problem interview. With this more open discussion, Ethyl revealed that she had never been able to climax, but had been highly aroused in the first year of her 5-year marriage. Their lovemaking style was focused on intercourse, and Ethyl's husband didn't seem to understand why she didn't enjoy it as much as he did. She had not faked orgasm but had never told him about her feelings of frustration about not reaching orgasm. Ethyl had never masturbated and remembered vague attitudes conveyed by her parents and her church that masturbation was not a correct thing to do. The physician then validated that many women first learn about self-pleasuring as adults and that the information she could get about how her own body worked would then be useful in her sexual relationship with her husband. It was suggested that Ethyl read a self-help book for women who want to learn to have orgasms (**P, LI, and SS**). At a visit 3 months later, Ethyl reported that she had proudly experienced her first orgasm by herself and felt so encouraged by this that she was able to talk more openly with her husband, who then agreed to go with her to see a marital/sex therapist to discuss ways they could bring more pleasure into their own lovemaking.*

For males, the equivalent *DSM-IV-TR* category primarily refers to delayed or absent ejaculation despite prolonged intercourse or other stimulation. Some report ejaculation without the sensation of orgasm (see Table 29-8).

CASE ILLUSTRATION 8

*Frank, a 24-year-old man, confided that he had never reached orgasm with a partner. A sex problem history revealed that he had never ejaculated during intercourse and that his partners had never tried to bring him to orgasm manually or orally. Frank was able to ejaculate with masturbation, describing a vivid sexual fantasy (which he did not allow himself to have when with a partner) and a lifelong pattern of stimulation in which he rubbed his penis back and forth against a pillow without using his hands. He was congratulated for bringing this problem to his physician's attention (**P**) and was told that anxiety was often a cause of this problem, together with a masturbation pattern that did not simulate the type of sensations he would have during intercourse (**LI**). The physician encouraged Frank to take a stepwise approach to the problem by enlisting the help of a willing partner and starting with those elements that had been successful for him. He was also encouraged to expand on the kind* *of physical stimulation he received during masturbation by gripping his penis with his hand and stroking it. With his partner, Frank was to focus on the goal of having high arousal while his partner stimulated his penis manually and he was imagining his "tried-and-true" fantasy. The next step was to reach higher levels of arousal in this manner and to stimulate an orgasmic response (**SS**). Frank was also referred to a self-help book (**P, LI, SS**). Follow-up indicated that Frank had successfully reached orgasm with manual stimulation with a partner in 3 weeks and was following suggestions in the book on his goal toward ejaculation during intercourse.*

Management

PERMISSION, LIMITED INFORMATION, AND SPECIFIC SUGGESTIONS

Both men and women may present with difficulties in achieving orgasm because of a repeated pattern of masturbation that does not approximate the stimulation they receive from a partner. Although physical arousal may be apparent (erection or lubrication), these patients may not be feeling excited if they have to forego the fantasies or kinds of stimulation that had worked for them while masturbating. Encouraging them to incorporate the conditions under which they can reach orgasm when alone into their sexual play with a partner is the first step in their expanding their sexual enjoyment. In some instances, use of a vibrator may be recommended to provide the more intense stimulation needed for some people.

OTHER MEDICAL INTERVENTIONS

Whereas the PDE5 inhibitor medications such as sildenafil (Viagra), vardenafil (Levitra), and tadalafil (Cialis) are broadly effective with men, research results have not been as clear for women; efforts are continuing, however, to identify selective subgroups of women who might also benefit from them.

SEXUAL PAIN: DYSPAREUNIA AND VAGINISMUS

Symptoms & Signs

Female dyspareunia—pain associated with penile–vaginal intercourse or other forms of vaginal penetration—may be one of the most common and perhaps most underreported of the female sexual dysfunctions. **Vaginismus,** the involuntary spasm of muscles around the vagina, may cause dyspareunia and is highly curable with psychological and physical interventions. Little if any systematic, controlled research has been conducted

on the etiology of dyspareunia. Manual–visual examination is of course important, but Meana and Binik warn against assuming that observed pathology causes the pain. Also factors that originally caused the pain may not be the maintaining variables. Psychological causes of vaginismus vary and may include fears of penetration because of confusion about genital anatomy and physiology, or fears resulting from other trauma or irrational fears, causing a conditioned response of involuntary spasm of the vaginal muscles.

 CASE ILLUSTRATION 9

*Nineteen-year-old Gina complained to her primary care provider that she had dyspareunia, was losing interest in sex, and was worried that her boyfriend was becoming impatient with her avoidance of sex. The physician then encouraged her to describe this problem behaviorally and in detail (**P**). Gina said that she had enjoyed intercourse since age 17 and always used latex condoms, but on one occasion 6 months ago she suddenly felt as if her vagina "was being rubbed with sandpaper" when her partner penetrated her. Although the physical pain had not actually returned in subsequent lovemaking sessions, Gina's fear of the pain recurring diminished both her interest in and her enjoyment of sex. When asked what she would do if the pain happened again during intercourse, Gina replied that she "would have to ask him to hurry up, but sometimes he lasts longer then." The physician asked how she would feel about telling him to stop all movement immediately and to withdraw when she felt discomfort or pain. Gina expressed concern that an abrupt withdrawal from intercourse might result in her boyfriend having testicular pain. She was reassured that this would create no lasting discomfort for him, and that there were alternatives for reaching ejaculation and orgasm, either with her or alone (**P, LI,** and **SS**). She was also offered some suggestions for reading about how couples learn to increase their enjoyment of sex (**SS**). The physician also praised Gina for having shown the courage to discuss this personal issue and encouraged her to bring up any future concerns (**P, LI**).*

Management

SPECIFIC SUGGESTIONS

These issues can be approached gradually, by encouraging the woman to speak with her partner about her needs and to be a full participant in the sexual encounter. She and her partner should be educated about the need for sufficient stimulation and arousal prior to attempted penetration, and about the importance of her being in control of the sexual movement, so that she can stop it instantly if pain is felt. Instruction in Kegel's P.C. muscle exercises increases the woman's awareness and control of her vaginal muscles. Vaginal self-dilatation can be accomplished with graduated cylinders or with fingers, from the little finger to multiple fingers, while practicing muscle relaxation and calming mental imagery. The patient should be encouraged to be the one in control by bearing down on the finger(s) or penis as if pushing something out of the vagina, then relaxing. It helps for some women to imagine "capturing" the penis or other object in this manner, instead of being "penetrated."

OTHER MEDICAL INTERVENTIONS

Other medical suggestions include the use of artificial lubricants, such as Astroglide, Gyne-Moistrin, or KY Jelly (not good with latex); vaginal moisturizers, such as Replens; vaginal and vulvar application of estrogen creams; surgical repair of the vulvar region; and excision of abnormal growths in the genital area. Diseases thought to cause the pain, such as vaginitis, condylomata, endometriosis, pelvic inflammatory disease, and other gynecologic or pelvic diseases, all may be treated directly. When painful intercourse has been a longstanding problem, however, medical intervention alone is seldom adequate and should be followed by sex therapy directed at the probable fear and expectation of pain that have been conditioned.

SEXUAL DISORDERS DUE TO A GENERAL MEDICAL CONDITION

CASE ILLUSTRATION 10

When Hannah was 22, she was diagnosed with clear cell adenocarcinoma of the vagina and had surgery that removed one ovary, her uterus, tubes, the upper two-thirds of her vagina, and her bilateral pelvic lymph nodes. None of her health care team was able to comfortably discuss sexuality with her. She was completely unprepared for the first attempts at intercourse several months following the surgery and was shocked and distraught to discover how little genital sensation she had left. She sought help from a male psychiatrist who listened as she expressed her grief and fears that she would never find a man because of her sense of diminished sexual self-worth. After rapport was established, he acknowledged her fears by saying that she might never have a "clitoral" orgasm again,

but that there were other routes to orgasm and sexual pleasure. He discussed with her ideas that have been helpful to others who have sustained the loss of genital sensation: that her brain knew how to feel pleasure and have orgasms, that men and women can learn to focus on sensations from other, nongenital parts of the body, such as breasts, neck, ears, and lips, and that with or without accompanying fantasy, one can thus relearn to enjoy a sense of orgasmic release and pleasure. Twelve years after her surgery, Hannah wrote, "The growth in my ideas and experiments with sexuality have increased manyfold since my surgery. What was most helpful was being able to share my experiences with people who could understand and be accepting, and finding people who were trained and had accurate information on how I could help myself. Health professionals don't have to have all the answers, but they should know their own limitations and be able to refer when necessary."

OTHER SEXUAL PROBLEMS NOT OTHERWISE SPECIFIED

Other more serious sex-related human problems may be best dealt with by a psychotherapist trained in sexual issues. A patient with truly **compulsive sexual behavior**—sometimes described as **sexual addiction**—may be suffering from a form of obsessive-compulsive disorder and may require intensive psychotherapy, use of support groups, and medications such as the SSRI antidepressants. Patients with **gender identity disorders**, patients who have experienced **spousal abuse, incest,** and **rape**, and patients troubled by **paraphilias** require referral for specialized treatment.

CONCLUSION

For every human being, sexuality—like health—is a challenge at some point. Feelings of personal vulnerability are inherent in sexual interactions and help to make sexuality a powerful and unique part of life. Problems of sexual desire, arousal, or functioning can lead us to confront and overcome our fears of not being lovable and to seek better communication and increased intimacy with others. The deepest expressions of love often result from just sharing our vulnerabilities or problems.

SUGGESTED READINGS

Annon J. *Behavioral Treatment of Sexual Problems.* New York, NY: Harper & Row, 1976.

Bokhour BG, Clark JA, Inui TS, et al. Sexuality after treatment for early prostate cancer: exploring the meanings of "erectile dysfunction." *J Gen Intern Med* 2001;16:649–655.

DeBusk R, Drory Y, Goldstein I, et al. Management of sexual dysfunction in patients with cardiovascular disease: recommendations of The Princeton Consensus Panel. *Am J Cardiol* 2000;86:175–181.

Finger WW, Lund M, Slagle MA. Medications that may contribute to sexual disorders. A guide to assessment and treatment in family practice. *J Fam Pract* 1997;44:33–43.

Heiman J, ed. Medical advances and human sexuality. *J Sex Res* Special Issue 2000;37:193–305.

Kloner RA, Brown M, Prisant LM, et al. Effect of sildenafil in patients with erectile dysfunction taking antihypertensive therapy. Sildenafil Study Group. *Am J Hypertens* 2001;14:70–73.

Leiblum SR, Rosen RC. *Principles and Practice of Sex Therapy*, 3rd ed. New York, NY: Guilford Press, 2000.

Leiblum SR. What every urologist should know about female sexual dysfunction. *Int J Impot Res* 1999;11(Suppl 1):S39–S40.

Masters WH, Johnson VE. *Human Sexual Inadequacy*. New York, NY: Little, Brown and Company, 1970.

Maurice WL. *Sexual Medicine in Primary Care*. St. Louis, MO: Mosby, 1999.

Meana M, Binik YM. Painful coitus: a review of female dyspareunia. *J Nerv Ment Dis* 1994;182:264–272.

Peck MS. *Further Along the Road Less Traveled*. New York, NY: Touchstone, 1993.

Phillips NA. Female sexual dysfunction: evaluation and treatment. *Am Fam Physician* 2000;62:127–137.

Rosen RC. Prevalence and risk factors of sexual dysfunction in men and women. *Curr Psychiatry Rep* 2000;2:189–195.

Rosen RC. Sexual pharmacology in the 21st century. *J Gend Specif Med* 2000;3:45–57.

Seidman SN, Roose SP, Menza MA, et al. Treatment of erectile dysfunction in men with depressive symptoms: results of a placebo-controlled trial with sildenafil citrate. *Am J Psychiatry* 2001;158:1623–1630.

Shifren JL, Braunstein GD, Simon JA, et al. Transdermal testosterone treatment in women with impaired sexual function after oophorectomy. *N Engl J Med* 2000;343:682–688.

Sipski ML, Alexander CJ, Rosen RC, et al. Sildenafil effects on sexual and cardiovascular responses in women with spinal cord injury. *Urology* 2000;55:812–815.

BIBLIOGRAPHY

Barbach L. *For Each Other*. New York, NY: Signet, 2001. (Encouragement and suggestions for couples wanting to enhance their sexuality and intimacy.)

Barbach L. *For Yourself—Revised*. New York, NY: Signet, 2000. (A revised classic that empowers women to enjoy their own sexuality, with suggestions for women who want to learn to become orgasmic.)

Butler RN, Lewis MI. *Love and Sex After 60* (revised). New York, NY: Ballantine, 1996.

Carnes P, et al. *In the Shadows of the Net: Breaking Free of Compulsive Online Sexual Behavior*. New York, NY: Hazelden, 2001.

Carnes P. *Out of the Shadows: Understanding Sexual Addiction*. New York, NY: Hazelden, 2001.

Ellison CR. *Women's Sexualities*. Oakland, CA: New Harbinger, 2000. (Respectful and helpful exploration of female sexuality from women of all ages.)

Gottman J, Silver N: *The Seven Principles for Making Marriage Work*. Pittsburgh, PA: Three Rivers, 1999. (Results of over 20 years of research pointing out the danger signals for troubled marriages, with helpful suggestions.)

Holstein L. *How to Have Magnificent Sex: The 7 Dimensions of a Vital Sexual Connection*. New York, NY: Harmony Books, 2001.

Kydd S, Rowett D. *Intimacy After Cancer: A Woman's Guide*. (Based on the personal stories shared by cancer survivors and nurses, oncologist and psychiatrist treating cancer patient; for more information, see www.intimacyaftercancer.com).

Leiblum SR, Sachs J. *Getting the Sex You Want: Becoming the Sexual Woman You Want to Be*. New York, NY: Crown, 2002. (Great insights and suggestions from some of the most experienced sex therapist/educators.)

Mellody P, et al. *Facing Love Addiction: Giving Yourself the Power to Change the Way You Love*. New York, NY: HarperCollins, 1992.

Ogden G.: *The Heart & Soul of Sex*. New York, NY: Trumpeter Books, 2006. (Discussion of national survey of ethnically diverse women ages 21–85 years in expanding the view of sexuality, intimacy, spirituality, and religion. Suggests various strategies to enhance and explore women's sexuality.)

Perel E. *Mating in Captivity: Reconciling the Erotic and the Domestic*. New York, NY: HarperCollins, 2006. (Fresh, provocative, and intelligent exploration of the erotic imagination vs. the sexless marriage.)

Person E. *Dreams of Love and Fateful Encounters*. New York, NY: Penguin (USA), 1989. (Literate and wise exploration of romantic love.)

Schnarch DM. *Passionate Marriage: Sex, Love, and Intimacy in Emotionally Committed Relationships*. New York, NY: Holt, 1998.

Schover LR. *Overcoming Male Infertility: Understanding Its Causes and Treatments*. New York, NY: Wiley & Sons, 2000.

Schover LR. *Sexuality and Fertility After Cancer*. New York, NY: Wiley & Sons, 1997. (Compassionate and hopeful resource for women and men who have had cancer.)

Weinberg M, Williams C, Pryor D. *Dual Attraction: Understanding Bisexuality*. New York, NY: Oxford University Press, 1995.

Zilbergeld B. *The New Male Sexuality—Revised*. New York, NY: Bantam, 1999. (A common-sense, practical, and sane antidote to media pressures on males to be sexual superstars. Excellent discussion of the fantasy model of sex and myths of male sexuality, the importance of an individual's conditions for good sex, and specific self-help chapters dealing with common male sexual problems.)

WEB SITES

Sexuality Organizations

American Association of Sex Educators, Counselors and Therapists Web site. www.aasect.org. Accessed October, 2007.

Kinsey Institute Web site. www.kinseyinstitute.org. Accessed October, 2007.

Sex Information and Education Council of the United States Web site. www.siecus.org. Accessed October, 2007.

Society for the Scientific Study of Sexuality Web site. www.sexscience.org. Accessed October, 2007.

Sexuality Education

CDC (Centers for Disease Control) National Prevention Information Network Web site. www.cdcnpin.org. Accessed October, 2007.

Sexual Health Network Web site. www.sexualhealth.com. Accessed October, 2007.

Electronic Journals

Electronic Journal of Human Sexuality Web site. www.ejhs.org. Accessed October, 2007.

International Journal of Transgenderism Web site. www.haworthpress.com/store/product.asp?sku=j485. Accessed October, 2007.

SECTION V
Special Topics

Complementary & Alternative Medicine

30

Ellen Hughes, MD, PhD & Susan Folkman, PhD[1]

DEFINITIONS

Various terms have been used to describe a broad range of healing approaches that are not widely taught in medical schools, not generally available in hospitals, and not routinely reimbursed by medical insurance. Many of these approaches have their roots in nonwestern cultures. Others have developed within the west, but outside what is considered conventional medical practice. Complementary and alternative medicine (CAM) is the name chosen by the National Institutes of Health for these healing approaches.

Classification of CAM Modalities

The National Institutes of Health National Center for Complementary and Alternative Medicine (NCCAM) classifies CAM modalities under five domains (see Table 30-1).

EPIDEMIOLOGY OF CAM

Who Seeks CAM & Why?

Nearly half the U.S. population turns to complementary and alternative practices to maintain or improve their health. The total number of visits to CAM practitioners actually exceeds the total number of visits to primary care

physicians each year. CAM is attractive to many people because it treats the "whole person" (body, mind, and spirit), emphasizes health promotion/prevention, and values the uniqueness of each individual. Independent predictors of CAM use in one survey included higher level of education, poorer health status, and a "holistic" interest in health, personal growth, and spirituality. People with conditions such as anxiety and chronic pain were also more likely to have used CAM in the previous year. Dissatisfaction with conventional medicine is not an independent predictor of greater use, so it appears that patients are more "pulled toward" CAM rather than "pushed away" from conventional medicine.

Epidemiology of Herbal Medicine Use

More than 39 million Americans take dietary supplements on a weekly basis. Twenty-five percent of patients who take prescription medicines also take at least one nonvitamin dietary supplement. Many are drawn to herbal products because they appear "safe and natural." Regular users hold strong beliefs about what they take. In one survey, more than 70% reported that they would continue to take their favorite supplement, even if there were government research data that indicated it was not effective!

REGULATION OF HERBAL MEDICINE

In 1994, Congress passed the Dietary Supplement Health and Education Act (DSHEA), which limited regulatory control over botanicals. DSHEA classifies herbs, vitamins, minerals, and amino acids as nutritional

---

[1]The authors gratefully acknowledge Dr. Bernard Lo for his valuable input in the preparation of this manuscript.

Table 30-1. NCCAM classification of CAM.

Domain	Example
Alternative medicine systems	Traditional oriental medicine, acupuncture, ayurveda, naturopathy, homeopathy
Mind–body interventions	Meditation, hypnosis, guided imagery, dance, art, and music therapy, spiritual healing
Biological-based therapies	Herbal medicines and dietary supplements, special diets
Manipulative and body-based methods	Chiropractic, osteopathic manual medicine, massage, other "body-work" systems
Energy therapies	Reiki, therapeutic touch, magnets, methods that affect the body's "bioelectric" field

or dietary supplements. It allows these products to be marketed without proof of efficacy, safety, or quality, as long as no claims to diagnose, treat, cure, or prevent disease are made. As a result, consumers taking herbal medicines have no guarantee that the plant was accurately identified, another plant part/species was not substituted, the herb is pure (i.e., no microbial, pesticide, or heavy metal contamination), safe, and effective, or that the next bottle will contain the same ingredients at the same dose. In addition, in contrast to prescription drugs, the Federal Food and Drug Administration must first prove that an herbal preparation is unsafe before it can be taken off the market. Examples of some of the potential risks associated with botanical products are summarized in Table 30-2.

COMMUNICATING WITH PATIENTS ABOUT CAM

Despite the growing numbers of patients seeking CAM, less than 40% of alternative therapies used are disclosed to physicians, even though the majority of people who use CAM do so along with conventional medicine because they perceive the combination to be superior to either alone. The absence of disclosure is alarming, at the very least, because some CAM therapies can interact adversely with conventional treatments. Further, discussions about CAM offer valuable opportunities for the practitioner to explore a patient's health care beliefs and concerns.

This chapter will focus primarily on communicating with patients about their use of herbal medicines, because these are among the most popular CAM modalities and because of the potential for interaction of botanicals with conventional drug therapies.

Barriers to Disclosure

Patients may be reluctant to disclose their use of CAM practices for a variety of reasons. In a study of CAM use among breast cancer patients, the most frequently cited reason was the belief that the physician was not interested in the patient's use of CAM. Even when patients attempted to disclose CAM use, the physician was

Table 30-2. Potential risks of botanical products.

Lack of quality assurance	Variable quality and quantity of herb in the product Lack of batch-to-batch consistency
Misidentification of herb	Renal failure when *Aristolochia*, a renal toxic herb, misidentified as *Stefania* in a diet preparation
Adverse effect of herb itself	Hepatitis/liver failure with germander, comfrey, kava Stroke, myocardial infarct, death with *ephedra*
Contamination of herb	Heavy metals in Asian patent medicines
Adulteration of product	Undeclared prescription medicines (benzodiazepines, nonsteroidal anti-inflammatory drugs, steroids) in Asian patent medicines
Herb–drug interactions: herb decreases level of prescription drug	St. John's wort with indinavir, cyclosporin, digoxin, warfarin, ethinyl estradiol
Herb increases potential for bleeding	Ginkgo, ginger, garlic, feverfew
Herb may interact with anesthetics	Some anesthesiologists recommend discontinuation of herbs 2–3 weeks before surgery
Herb has additive effect with prescription medications	St. John's wort and selective serotonin reuptake inhibitors, kava and benzodiazepines, ginkgo and warfarin

often unresponsive, which prevented further discussion. Patients say, "I did tell the doctor . . . and he didn't say "Good," or "Not good," or "Okay," or anything. It's like, "We're looking at the platelets here, and the white count—let's not get too far afield!" Many patients believe that disclosure will not yield any benefit because their physician has inadequate training in or knowledge of CAM or may be biased against alternative health systems. Physicians may also communicate a reluctance or unwillingness to work with an alternative practitioner. Without such consultation, patients may feel that disclosing their interest in CAM will not be fruitful. Some patients believe that their physicians will actively disapprove of their use of CAM. Disapproval can be interpreted as disrespect for the CAM practice, and even worse, as disrespect for patients because they sought nonconventional care.

Not all barriers to disclosure have to do with negative expectations about how physicians will respond. Some patients believe that their CAM use is not relevant to medical decision making. They may be using an herb, for example, to help regulate anxiety, which is not the problem for which they are seeing their physicians. This is borne out in a recent survey of patients who sought care from both a conventional and a CAM practitioner. Sixty percent of these patients did not reveal their use of CAM to their physician, giving the following reasons for their nondisclosure: "It wasn't important for the doctor to know" (61%), "The doctor never asked" (60%), "It was none of the doctor's business" (31%), "The doctor wouldn't understand" (20%), "The doctor would disapprove" (14%), and "The doctor wouldn't continue to take care of me" (2%). Similarly, 70% of people aged 50 or older who used CAM, but didn't tell their doctor, said they didn't because the MD never asked, they didn't know they should and/or there was not enough time.

Facilitating Disclosure

It is important for physicians to recognize that CAM practices are not limited to specific demographic groups. CAM practices are widespread, and all patients have the potential to be interested in or use a wide variety of treatments.

Patients are more likely to disclose their CAM practices if they anticipate that their physicians will be respectful, open-minded, and willing to listen. Behavior that conveys respect and open-mindedness includes asking questions nonjudgmentally or initiating a dialogue with patients' alternative practitioners. Lack of respect and closed-mindedness can be conveyed subtly through nonverbal behavior such as frowning or cutting off a response. If patients perceive that physicians disapprove of CAM, they may be reluctant to discuss other issues, such as noncompliance or substance use, of which the physician may disapprove. It is also easier for patients to disclose CAM use if they perceive that their physicians expect such use to be common and routine. This expectation can be conveyed by physicians through the use of questions about CAM practices. For example, "People use a variety of different methods to maintain or improve their health. What kinds of things are you doing to take care of [your health/this problem]?" Preoperative evaluations provide another opportunity to ask about CAM. Up to 50% of patients may not reveal that they are taking herbal medicines during presurgical evaluations, so it may be helpful to prompt them with examples of specific CAM therapies. "Many patients take herbal medicines like gingko or use acupuncture for their health. Have you found any of these useful?" Finally, patients' comfort with disclosure is also facilitated by honest acknowledgment by physicians of the limitations of their own knowledge. "I'm not familiar with this specific therapy, but will try to find out more about it before our next visit." "Even though there may not be a lot of data available, I want to work together with you to come up with a good plan." Patients can be encouraged to contribute knowledge to the discussion and thereby strengthen the therapeutic relationship. "Why don't you bring in the information you've gathered about this therapy, so we can go over it together?" Ways in which physicians can facilitate disclosure are summarized in Table 30-3.

Communicating With Patients Interested in Herbal Medicines

In the following case, a patient asks her physician about an herbal remedy she is interested in trying. It presents a typical conversation that might occur when there is uncertainty on the part of the physician regarding the effectiveness and safety of an herbal medicine. Although the physician is acting in the patient's best interests, her responses have the effect of constraining rather than facilitating communication that could lead to more satisfactory outcomes.

 CASE ILLUSTRATION 1

Near the end of her annual check-up, a 57- year-old teacher with well-controlled type 2 diabetes mentions that she's considering taking an herbal supplement she found at the health food store.

Patient: A friend of mine told me about this new supplement that gives her more energy and boosts her immune system. I'm thinking about trying it.

Table 30-3. Suggestions for talking with patients about CAM.

1. Ask if the patient is considering or using CAM, using specific examples.
   "Many patients use a variety of alternative medicines for their health. Are you taking any herbs such as ginkgo, or seeing a practitioner such as an acupuncturist?"
2. Explore patients' concerns and wishes that led them to be interested in CAM.
   "Tell me more about this therapy."
   "Can you share with me how you hope this therapy will help?"
   "You mentioned that this medicine helps people feel more energy. Have you been feeling less energetic lately?"
3. Establish a connection with the patient. Help identify, validate, and reflect back underlying emotions/concerns to the patient.
   "It's clear that you're interested in improving your health."
   "I sense that using something 'natural' is important to you. Is that right?"
   "It sounds like you're experiencing some difficulty with this prescription and might prefer something with fewer side effects. Is that true?"
4. Acknowledge that there is often inadequate information about safety and efficacy to guide clinical decision making.
   "Why don't you bring in the information you have gathered about this therapy, so we can go over it together?"
   "Even though there aren't a lot of data available, we can work to make a plan together."
5. Identify good resources (see "Suggested Reading," above).
6. Explore potential risks and benefits of CAM with the patient (to the extent that they are known) as well as how CAM might interface with their ongoing care.
   "From what we found out about this supplement, it looks like it will be safe for you to add into your program of a low fat diet and exercise."
7. Encourage the patient to keep a diary of symptoms and schedule follow-up for ongoing assessment of safety and efficacy.
   "If you're willing to keep track of your blood pressures at home as you start this new supplement, we can see if it has any effect. If your pressure starts to go up before our next appointment, I'd recommend you stop the supplement and give me a call."
8. Be clear when you are concerned that a CAM intervention may be harmful.
   "I care about your well-being and understand your desire to stop your prescription medication and start this herbal therapy. This is a difficult situation, though, because I feel there are some dangers associated with this."
   "I want to support you in your desire to lose weight, but I'm worried that this medicine could be harmful to your health. How do you think we could best work together on this?"

Doctor: Oh. What is it?

Patient: Here, I brought the bottle in for you to see.

Doctor: Hmm. Unfortunately, I don't recognize the ingredients that are listed here, so I can't tell if they're safe or if they might affect your diabetes. As you may be aware, many claims made about these kinds of products are not backed up with scientific data, so I'm not sure that it's a good idea for you to take this.

Patient: I've actually been feeling a little bit better since starting it and my blood sugars have been fine.

Doctor: So, you're already taking the supplement. It's important for me to know everything you're taking, because of possible interactions with your prescription medications. I am happy to hear that your sugars haven't been affected by this medicine, but given that I don't know if it's safe or even what it does, I still don't feel comfortable with you taking it.

Patient: When I checked out the manufacturer's web site, I saw that many people who take it find it to be very safe. They feel better, have more energy, and catch fewer colds. My friend feels great after taking it for just 2 weeks.

Doctor: Commercial web sites often contain testimonials, but rarely mention potential side effects. I don't think you can trust these kinds of sites on the Internet. It's certainly your choice, but I don't feel comfortable with you continuing to take this product.

Patient: OK. I guess I'll stop it then, even though I think it's safe and would like to have given it a chance.

In this interaction, the physician does most of the talking. At no time does she ask any exploratory questions to determine her patient's needs and concerns. She sees herself as an expert whose responsibility it is to communicate information and give clear recommendations. The doctor is legitimately concerned about the lack of reliable product information and the potential risks of taking the supplement for her diabetic patient. She responds to this uncertainty by deciding that it's not a good idea for her patient to take the herbal medicine, although she admits to not being familiar with its ingredients. By focusing exclusively on issues of safety, the doctor misses several opportunities to explore and validate her patient's underlying concerns. No doors are left open for further discussion, so this patient may be less likely to ask questions about CAM or other potentially sensitive issues in the future. Further, the patient may continue to use the product "in secret," and not tell the physician.

CASE ILLUSTRATION 2

This case presents the same patient interacting with a physician whose style of communication is very different.

Patient: A friend of mine told me about this new herbal supplement that gives her more energy and boosts her immune system. I'm thinking about trying it.

Doctor: Many of my patients take herbal supplements for their health. How do you think this one might help you?

Patient: Well, for the past 2 months I don't seem to have any energy, so I was hoping this could make me feel better.

Doctor: Can you tell me more about what it means when you say you don't have any energy?

Patient: I'm sleeping OK, but get up each morning feeling tired. I keep catching colds. I can't afford to feel run down like this all the time.

Doctor: Do you have any idea what might be causing you to feel run down?

Patient: My sugars have been fine, so I know it's not my diabetes. I'm worried that with all the stress I've been under at work, my immune system isn't working. I'm not feeling depressed, just run down. That's why I started taking the herbal medicine. Do you think it will help?

Doctor: I understand better now why you're interested in taking something to boost your energy and immunity. Truthfully, I'm not familiar with the ingredients in this supplement, but I'm happy to try to find out more about this remedy before our next visit. More importantly, I'd like to understand better what's been going on for you. Is there anything else that's concerning you?

Patient: Well, I guess I'm worried that my being run down may be a sign that something more serious is wrong. My mother's cancer was first diagnosed when she went to the doctor with low energy.

Doctor: I can imagine how this might be scary for you. The good news is that your examination today and all your recent tests have been normal. And there are things you can do to help manage your stress. I'd like us to be able to talk more about this, but we don't have time now. Let's schedule another appointment as soon as possible. How does that sound?

By focusing on the patient and not on the herbal supplement, this physician was able to uncover important concerns that were completely missed by the first physician. She listened more than she talked, asked open-ended questions, validated her patient's concerns, and responded with empathy. From the onset, this doctor helped create a "safe" and respectful environment for her patient. She normalized the patient's interest in supplements by mentioning that many of her patients used herbal therapies. She was genuinely interested and attentive each time the patient spoke. Her goal was to help identify and explore her patient's concerns and needs, rather than to serve as an expert conveyer of information and advice.

Like the first physician, she was unfamiliar with the ingredients in the supplement. She dealt with her lack of knowledge in a different way, however. Instead of immediately concluding that the supplement wasn't a good idea, she kept the door open by offering to learn more about it. She also reacted empathetically, rather than defensively, when the patient admitted she had already started taking the supplement ("I understand better now why you'd want to take something that boosts your energy and your immunity" rather than "So, you've already started taking it.")

Lack of time in a busy clinical practice can be a significant barrier to discussing CAM. Some physicians fear that asking patients about "one more thing" will result in a conversation that cannot be completed in the limited time available to them. This is a legitimate concern, but using a patient-centered communication style may not always take more time. The second doctor–patient interaction takes approximately 15 seconds longer than the first. Discussions of CAM with patients who are less insightful and articulate certainly might take more time. As well, an additional follow-up appointment was generated in the second case. Some would argue, though, that an additional visit to deal with a patient's concerns and fears would be worth the investment, particularly when the patient will be working with the physician on a long-term basis.

Communicating with Patients when CAM may be Potentially Harmful

Physicians regularly help their patients assess the risks and benefits of different therapies. Their responsibility to "first, do no harm" applies to CAM as well as to conventional medical interventions. In the previous case, the physician and patient were discussing a supplement for which there was no clear information about its safety and efficacy. The conversation would be more challenging if the supplement had known toxicity and the patient wanted to continue using it. The same strategies that allowed the second physician to identify and address the patient's concerns would hopefully forge an alliance with the patient strong enough to allow them to negotiate a mutually acceptable plan. Openly acknowledging that the situation is difficult or challenging may be helpful.

Doctor: I care about your well-being and understand your desire to stop taking your prescription medication and start this herbal therapy. This is a difficult situation, though, because I feel there are some dangers associated with this.

Doctor: I want to support you in your desire to lose weight, but I'm worried that this medicine could be dangerous for your health. How do you think we could best work together on this?

Helping Patients Inform Themselves about Herbal Medicines

One of the principles of integrative medicine is the concept of self-care. Patients are encouraged to become knowledgeable participants in their treatment programs. Table 30-4 provides some practical advice for patients with respect to herbal medicines.

Communication Regarding Other CAM Modalities

Exploratory questions about CAM use may reveal that the patient is using other CAM practices, such as acupuncture, massage, or energy therapy. As with the use of botanicals, asking why the patient is turning to these practices can elicit additional information about the patient's total situation that can be helpful in treatment. The physician may be concerned about the safety of the alternative treatment, in which case the physician can offer to contact the CAM practitioner to learn more about the treatment and its potential risks and benefits. Although this clearly takes additional time and effort, it shows a respect for the patient's concerns, and could strengthen the relationship between the patient and the physician. The physician can also offer to discuss what is learned in a subsequent appointment.

CONCLUSION

Approximately half of the U.S. population is using some form of CAM, most often in combination with the conventional medical care they receive from their health care providers. It is important for physicians to

Table 30-4. Practical advice for patients taking herbal medicines.

Communication
Discuss use of all therapies with your medical and CAM providers, especially if you are pregnant or taking any prescription medications.
Talk with your physician to reevaluate efficacy and safety on a regular basis.
Report any adverse reactions to the FDA MedWatch.

Product selection
Choose products that have the following information on the label:
Common and scientific names of the herb(s)
Part(s) of the plant used
Indication
Dose and frequency
Potential side effects and interactions
Name and address of the manufacturer
Lot number
Date of expiration
Use products that are standardized to specific marker compound(s).
Select formulations that have been studied in clinical trials, when available.
Select products that have undergone independent quality testing.

facilitate rather than constrain discussions about CAM so they can understand how it impacts care that they are providing. By taking the time to discuss a patient's interest in CAM, the physician may uncover important concerns and needs that impact ongoing care and medical decision making. Exploring and responding to these concerns can also significantly strengthen the provider–patient relationship.

SUGGESTED READINGS

General Reference Books

Ernst E, Max H Pittler and Barbara Wider, eds. *The Desktop Guide to Complementary and Alternative Medicine: An Evidence-based Approach*, 2nd ed. St. Louis, MO: Mosby, 2006.

Kliger B, Lee R, eds. *Integrative Medicine: Principles for Practice.* New York, NY: McGraw Hill, 2004.

Rakel D, ed. *Integrative Medicine*, 2nd ed. Philadelphia, PA: Saunders Elsevier, 2007.

Ulbricht C, Basch E, eds. *Natural Standard Herb and Supplement Reference: Evidence-based Clinical Reviews*. London: Elsevier, 2005.

General Reference Articles

Adler SR, Fosket JR. Disclosing complementary and alternative medicine use in the medical encounter: a qualitative study in women with breast cancer. *J Fam Pract* 1999;48:453–458. PMID: 10386489.

Barnes P, Powell-Griner E, McFann K, et al. Complementary and alternative medicine use among adults: United States 2002. *Adv Data* 2004;343:1–19. PMID: 15188733.

Eisenberg DM. Advising patients who seek alternative therapies. *Ann Intern Med* 1997;127:61–69. PMID: 9214254.

Eisenberg DM, Kessler RC, Van Rompay MI, Kaptchuk TJ, Wilkey SA, Appel S, Davis RB, et al. Perceptions about complementary therapies relative to conventional therapies among adults who use both: results from a national survey. *Ann Intern Med* 2001;135: 344–351. PMID: 11529698.

Gariner P, Graham RE, Legedza AT, Eisenberg DM, Phillips RS. Factors associated with dietary supplement use among prescription drug users. *Arch Intern Med* 2006;166: 1968–1974. PMID: 17030829.

WEB SITES

Food and Drug Administration. Center for Food Safety & Applied Nutrition Web site. http://www.cfsan.fda.gov. Accessed October, 2007.

Food and Drug Administration. MedWatch Web site. http://www.fda.gov/medwatch. Accessed October, 2007.

National Institutes of Health. National Center for Complementary and Alternative Medicine Web site. http://nccam.nih.gov. Accessed October, 2007.

NIH Office of Dietary Supplements Web site. http://dietary-supplements.info.nih.gov. Accessed October, 2007.

The Longwood Herbal Task Force Web site. http://www.longwood-herbal.org. Accessed October, 2007.

U.S. Pharmacopoeia Web site. http://www.usp.org. Accessed October, 2007.

DATABASES

CAM on PubMed: Developed jointly by the National Library of Medicine and the National Center for Complementary and Alternative Medicine. Contains 220,000 citations with links to text. Available at: http://www.ncbi.nlm.nih.gov/entrez/query.fcgi?CMD=Limits&DB=PubMed. Accessed October, 2007.

Cochrane Registry of Randomized Controlled Trials in CAM: Cochrane Complementary Medicine Field. Available at: http://www.compmed.umm.edu/cochrane.asp. Accessed October, 2007.

Stress & Disease

31

John F. Christensen, PhD

INTRODUCTION

Human history is replete with stories of the connection between stress and disease. A story about John Hunter (1728–1793), a surgeon and medical educator at St. George's Hospital in London, is that he stated publicly, "My life is at the mercy of any rogue who chooses to provoke me," and soon afterward died following a contentious meeting with hospital administrators. A review of coroner's records in Los Angeles in 1994 revealed a marked increase in deaths, including sudden death, related to atherosclerotic cardiovascular disease on the day of the 1994 Northridge earthquake. In 1999 during a 7.3 earthquake in Taiwan, patients on Holter monitors showed heart rate variability derangement due to withdrawal of parasympathetic activity and increase in sympathetic arousal. In the quarterfinal of the 1996 European football championships between the French and Dutch teams a draw at the end of overtime resulted in a sudden death penalty shoot out, which was won by the French. An analysis of mortality in the total population of Dutch men and women aged 45 or more revealed a relative risk of death from acute myocardial infarction (MI) or stroke of 1.51 among the men on the day of the match, compared with the 5 days on either side. There was no such effect on French men.

The psychological sequelae of exposure to life-threatening stressors are also problematic and disruptive to people's lives. The terrorist attacks on the World Trade Center and the Pentagon on September 11, 2001, were witnessed directly by an estimated 100,000 people and vicariously by millions of Americans and others worldwide. In the period of time between October 16 and November 15, 2001, it is estimated that 7.5% of Manhattan residents south of 110th street were suffering from posttraumatic stress disorder (PTSD) and 9.7% were suffering from depression. In a representative

sample of the American population surveyed 3–5 days following the attacks, 44% reported one or more substantial symptoms consistent with acute stress disorder (ASD), and 90% had one or more symptoms to some degree. Refugees and prisoners of war who have been exposed to torture are also likely to develop symptoms of PTSD, anxiety, and depression. Chronic stress has also been implicated in the so-called Central-Eastern European health paradox, which involves a crisis of morbidity and mortality in these transforming societies.

Less dramatically, research since the late 1960s has demonstrated correlations between significant changes in individuals' lives and the subsequent onset of various types of physical and psychological illness. A consistent relationship has even been found between daily hassles and the onset of illness.

The interrelationship between mental stress and physical disease is complex and multifactorial. As a result, the study of stress and disease embraces a wide range of behavioral, emotional, cognitive, physiological, hormonal, biochemical, cellular, environmental, and even spiritual interconnections not easily understood or encapsulated in the controlled clinical trial.

It has been estimated that up to 70% of visits to primary care physicians are for problems related to stress and lifestyle. Most clinicians, however, have not been trained to extend their diagnostic workup and treatment interventions into the psychosocial context of these illnesses. Yet adequate treatment and prevention require that providers regard their patients' illnesses and suffering in the context of their life struggles. This perspective allows the clinician to intervene at multiple points along the continuum from mind to molecule. The ***biopsychosocial model*** of medicine, originally proposed by Engel, regards illness as multidetermined—by biochemical alterations on the molecular level and by psychological and social events on the molar level. This model encourages clinicians to move conceptually up and down the hierarchy from patients' genetic susceptibilities and pathophysiologic processes to their unique life circumstances, stressors, and psychological meanings by which

Previous editions of this chapter were authored by John F. Christensen, Ph.D. and Jeffrey L. Boone, MD, MS.

they construct their reality in order to understand fully the origins of disease and the most appropriate therapies.

This chapter offers a framework for clinicians to think broadly and clinically about the stress–illness connection and suggests some approaches to assessing and treating stress-related illness. It offers a brief background of the research base for this new perspective; provides a conceptual framework to guide diagnosis and treatment; suggests methods for communicating with patients about stress; and offers some options for stress assessment, prevention, and intervention.

DEFINITIONS

The concept of stress was borrowed by physiology and psychology from physics, where it generally refers to a force acting against some resistance. Hooke's law of elasticity states that "stress $= K \times$ strain," where K is a constant (the modulus of elasticity) that depends on the nature of the material and type of stress used to produce the strain. This constant K (i.e., the stress–strain ratio) is called Young's modulus. In materials science, stress is what is imposed on a material by the outer world; strain is the reaction of the material to the stress.

Hans Selye is generally credited with introducing the concept of stress into physiology. He defined stress loosely as "the rate of wear and tear in the body" and more rigorously as "the state manifested by a specific syndrome which consists of all the nonspecifically induced changes within a biological system." In this specific syndrome, termed by Selye the **general adaptation syndrome** (GAS), glucocorticoids are secreted by the adrenal cortex in response to adaptational demands placed on the organism by such disparate stressors as heat, cold, starvation, and other environmental insults—hence the expression "nonspecifically induced changes."

Various other definitions of stress have been offered by researchers. Some, like Selye's, refer to a state of the organism; others refer to the stressful stimuli; and still others refer to a combination that includes stimuli, organismic responses, and intervening variables. Currently, a distinction is usually made between stress and stressors. Although **stress** is sometimes loosely used to refer to the environmental sources of threat to the organism, the term **stressor** is more appropriate in reference to these agents.

More recent definitions of stress in humans emanate from a transactional model that takes into account the interactions between persons and their environment. In this view, stress occurs when a situational demand presents a call for action that the individual perceives as exceeding available resources. I have proposed the following working definition: "Stress is a process of interchange between an organism and its environment that involves self-generated or environmentally induced changes that, once they are perceived by the organism as exceeding available resources (internal or external), disrupt homeostatic processes in the organism–environment system." This definition includes the traditional notion of stress as originating with an external demand (environmentally induced change) that exceeds the coping resources of the organism. It also includes, however, those expectations of events that arise from within, that are seen as essential to one's life project, and that cannot be accommodated by the environment (exceeding external resources). The disruption of homeostasis in the organism–environment system can have its primary manifestation as a pathologic end-state in the organism (illness or tissue damage) or as a destructive alteration of the environment (domestic violence as a stress response).

RESEARCH BACKGROUND

Stressful Life Events

In the 1930s, Adolf Meyer advocated the use of a life chart in medical diagnosis. Data were entered on date of birth, periods of disorders of various organs, and various life situations and the patient's reactions to them. In 1954, a program of studies in life changes and illness patterns was initiated at Cornell University. These studies found that illnesses appeared to be associated with definite periods of life change, although illness patterns varied among those who had been through major life changes. In 1967, Holmes and Rahe published a scale of 43 life events, along with a method of quantifying life changes according to the amount of readjustment they require for the average person. This scale allowed greater quantitative precision in life change and illness studies and provided a pivotal methodological leap that broke through the circularity in which the stressful life changes had been measured in terms of illness outcome, rather than in terms of the inherent magnitude of the stressor. Questionnaires based on this and similar scales have gathered data on several populations globally. Retrospective studies have shown a relationship between recent life change and a host of pathologic outcomes, such as sudden cardiac death, onset of MI, occurrence of fractures, pregnancy and birth complications, aggravation of chronic illness, tuberculosis, multiple sclerosis, diabetes, onset of leukemia in children, and onset of mental disorders such as depression and schizophrenia. Prospective studies, particularly those conducted on U.S. Navy populations while deployed at sea, predicted future illness based on life change scores prior to deployment and subsequently verified the accuracy of those predictions by inspection of medical records.

Although a consistent relationship has been found between stressful life events and illness patterns, this does not account for why some individuals who undergo significant change develop illnesses but others undergoing equally intense changes remain healthy. Recent attention has focused on individual and situational variables that may mediate the relationship between life change and illness. Among the psychological variables that seem to mediate the stress response are locus of control (including the extent to which individuals prefer control in their lives and how much control they perceive they have over specific life events), need for stimulation, openness to change, stimulus screening, self-actualization, the use of denial, the presence of social supports, and emotional self-disclosure. In one study of Illinois Bell executives during the divestiture of AT&T, those executives who experienced high stress while remaining healthy differed from those with high stress and high illness on a dimension of "hardiness." This personal characteristic consists of "the 3 C's": a strong *commitment* to self, work, family, and other important values; a sense of *control* over one's life; and the ability to see change as a *challenge* rather than a threat. More recently researchers suggest a "fourth C": *coherence*, a belief that one's internal and external environments are predictable and that things will work out as well as can be expected.

Work-related Stress & Burnout

The demands of the workplace in industrialized societies are a persistent and intense stressor. Job strain is defined as a combination of high job demands and low perceived control. In a prospective study of healthy young adults (Cardiovascular Risk in Young Finns study), job strain was associated with increased carotid atherosclerosis among the men, but not the women. In another prospective study, the degree of job stress over time increased the risk of the metabolic syndrome in a linear fashion. Subjects with lower grades of employment suffered disproportionately from the effects of stress as a risk factor for the metabolic syndrome, with men showing more susceptibility than women. Burnout is a syndrome associated with unrelenting stress and has been studied extensively as a phenomenon in a variety of work settings and professions, including physicians. It includes symptoms of emotional exhaustion, depersonalization, and a decreased sense of personal accomplishment. In a prospective study, burnout was associated with an increased risk of type 2 diabetes in apparently healthy individuals.

Timing of Cardiac Events

Data from the Framingham study, the Massachusetts Death Certificate Study, and other large epidemiologic studies provide information regarding the timing of cardiovascular events such as angina and sudden cardiac death.

Such events tend to occur with a greater frequency during the morning hours before noon with a second peak in the early evening hours. From the perspective of stress medicine, this circadian frequency data may be an objective description of the stress response as it affects the presentation of serious cardiovascular events. A closer look at the data reveals that the death rate during the daytime work hours plummets over the noon hour to less than half the rate seen at 9:00 A.M. The stress model suggests this may be more than coincidence. The peak death rates occur in the early hours of the workday and in the early evening hours when workers return home. These peaks are substantially blunted during the corresponding hours of the weekend days when people are moving toward recreation. Furthermore, circadian peaks in cardiac events are steeper and more deadly on Monday than on other days of the week. Employed workers die more frequently on Monday, whereas age-matched unemployed workers die on random days of the week.

Cardiac death also tends to occur on days that are more psychologically stressful than others. One study that examined death certificates in the United States found that among Chinese and Japanese, who are more likely to consider the number "4" unlucky, a peak of cardiac-related mortality occurred on the fourth day of the month, in contrast with white controls who showed no such peak. This was consistent with the hypothesis that cardiac-related mortality tends to increase on psychologically stressful occasions.

Behavioral & Emotional Triggers of Acute Coronary Syndromes

Several behavioral and emotional events have been implicated as probable triggers of acute coronary syndromes (MI and sudden cardiac death) in vulnerable individuals. Recent research has focused on events within a 1- to 2-hour period before the onset of symptoms. Behavioral triggers include physical exertion (more common in men than women), sexual activity, sleep disturbance, and heavy consumption of alcohol. Well-studied emotional triggers include earthquakes, sporting events, war, high-pressure deadlines at work, and anger. In one study, the relative risk of acute MI in the 2 hours following an anger episode was 2.3, and in comparison with a control period 24 hours earlier it was 4.0. This effect was independent of age, sex, cardiovascular risk factors, and use of beta-blockers. The risk of anger triggering an MI was inversely related to socioeconomic status. In a large-scale study, the relative risk of anger triggering an MI was 9.0 compared to usual levels of anger, but when limiting the analysis to patients who had no premonitory symptoms the relative risk increased to 15.7.

Personality Influences on Cardiovascular Disease

In the 1950s, Friedman and Rosenman began studying the relationship between coronary heart disease and a personality style they labeled "Type A"—hard driving, time urgent, and hostile. This was contrasted to a personality style they labeled "Type B," which was defined as the absence of Type A characteristics, that is, easygoing, patient, and soft-spoken. Their initial findings were that Type As were more than twice as likely as Type Bs to develop heart disease in the form of angina, silent heart attacks, overt heart attacks, and coronary death. Although subsequent large-scale studies failed to show this relationship, more recent research has isolated a "toxic core" of Type A that includes hostility, anger, cynicism, suspiciousness, and excessive self-involvement. Hostility is conceptualized as comprising three elements: the emotion of anger, its expression, and cognitions of cynical mistrust. Using well-validated measures of the cognitive aspect of hostility, recent research has linked higher hostility scores with subsequent coronary events like hospitalizations for angina, nonfatal MI, stroke, and congestive heart failure. Higher hostility has also been associated with coronary risk factors, such as increased plasma homocysteine levels, triglycerides, body mass index, waist-to-hip ratio, glucose levels, alcohol consumption, and smoking. In a study of middle-aged women each one-point increase in hostility scores predicted a significantly higher intimal-medial thickening in the carotid arteries.

Psychoneuroimmunology

Psychoneuroimmunology (PNI) involves the study of the interactions of consciousness, the central nervous system (CNS), and the immune system (involving the body's defense against infection and aberrant cell division). The compelling evidence of these studies is that the CNS influences immune function and that, conversely, the immune system can influence the CNS. It is likely that the brain is normally part of the immunoregulatory network. Specifically, stimulation of the hypothalamic–pituitary–adrenal (HPA) axis leads to down regulation of immune system function in response to stress. Stressful thoughts and emotions may reach the hypothalamus by axons projecting from the limbic system or from the forebrain. Corticotropin-releasing factor (CRF), produced in the hypothalamus under conditions of stress, acts on the anterior pituitary to form adrenocorticotropin hormone (ACTH), which in turn stimulates the production of corticosteroids in the adrenal cortex. Under conditions of acute stress, corticosteroids have immunosuppressive effects on the lymphoreticular system and marked antiallergic and anti-inflammatory effects.

In addition, CRF leads to release of catecholamines, which themselves may produce changes in lymphocyte, monocyte, and leukocyte functions. Opiates are also elevated with stress, and they are generally reported to be immunosuppressive. Finally, growth hormone and prolactin, which are immuno-enhancing factors, are initially elevated at the onset of acute stress, but under conditions of prolonged stress their secretion is inhibited.

Thus, the combined effect of elevated corticosteroids, catecholamines, and opiates, along with inhibition of growth hormone and prolactin, is to dysregulate the immune system.

Recent evidence indicates that chronic psychological stress can lead to increased production of proinflammatory cytokines, particularly interleukin (IL)-6, which is also triggered by infection and trauma. Proinflammatory cytokines have been implicated in a range of diseases in older adults that can be traced to inflammation, including cardiovascular disease, osteoporosis, arthritis, type 2 diabetes, certain lymphoproliferative diseases or cancers (including multiple myeloma, non-Hodgkin's lymphoma, and chronic lymphocytic leukemia), Alzheimer's disease, and periodontal disease. IL-6 promotes the production of C-reactive protein, which is an important risk factor for MI. Depression and anxiety also enhance the production of proinflammatory cytokines, which is a possible mediator of the association of these disorders with increased morbidity and mortality (see Chapters 22 & 23). A recent study has shown that depressed subjects, compared to nondepressed controls, showed an impaired ability to regulate inflammation triggered by acute stress.

Another recent development in stress research involves the concept of "allostatic load," which is the wear and tear on organisms that result from chronic overactivity or underactivity of allostatic systems. These systems, which include the autonomic nervous system, HPA axis, and the cardiovascular, metabolic, and immune systems, protect the body by responding to internal and external stress in an attempt to achieve stability through change. Activation of allostatic systems in response to a stressor includes the release of catecholamines from nerves and the adrenal medulla, as well as the stimulation of cortisol release from the adrenal cortex via the HPA system described above. Four types of allostatic load can result from prolonged stress: (1) Repeated elevations of blood pressure over weeks or months accelerates atherosclerosis, increasing the risk of MI. (2) When adaptation to repeated stressors is lacking, there may be prolonged exposure to stress hormones. (3) There may be an inability to shut off allostatic responses after stress is terminated, leading to conditions such as hypertension or decreased bone mineral density. (4) Inadequate responses in some allostatic systems, such as cortisol secretion, may lead to compensatory increases in other systems, such as proinflammatory cytokines (which are down regulated by cortisol).

Effect of Psychological Interventions on the Immune System

In a series of studies on asymptomatic men following notification of HIV seropositivity, a 10-week program of cognitive-behavioral stress management and aerobic-exercise training programs buffered distress responses and immune alterations. The same intervention had positive effects on mood and immune function in gay men whose disease had become symptomatic. Recent meta-analyses of the placebo effect have shown positive effects in various inflammatory and immune-related diseases, including asthma, cancer symptoms (pain and appetite), Crohn's disease, chronic fatigue, duodenal ulcer, irritable bowel syndrome (IBS), and multiple sclerosis (relapse frequency). A meta-analytic review showed that three classes of interventions could reliably alter immune function. ***Hypnosis with immune suggestions*** showed a positive influence on total salivary immunoglobulin A (IgA) concentration and neutrophil adherence, along with a modest suppression of intermediate-type hypersensitivity erythema. These effects were mediated through relaxation. Some studies have shown differential delayed skin sensitivity reactions on the right and left arm of subjects depending on which arm was suggested under hypnosis to show no changes. ***Conditioning interventions***, in which a neutral stimulus is initially paired with an immune-modulating stimulus and later elicits the immune changes on its own, were able to enhance natural killer (NK) cell cytotoxicity. ***Disclosure interventions***, which encourage patients to write essays about previously inhibited stressful experiences, have shown some success in reducing antibody titers to Epstein-Barr virus and enhancing the body's control over latent herpes simplex virus production.

Expressive Writing about Stressful Experiences

Recent research has demonstrated the effectiveness of expressive writing about stressful events in improving the health status of patients with asthma (improved lung function) or rheumatoid arthritis (reduction in disease severity). These improvements were assessed 4 months after the intervention and were beyond those attributable to standard medical care.

Gender Differences

Females have been noted to respond to stress with a "tend-and-befriend" way of coping, in contrast with the "fight-or-flight" model that may be more characteristic of males. When confronted with stress females tend to engage in nurturing activities that protect themselves and their offspring and that enhance social support, which has been identified as a powerful stress buffer. In particular, there may be links between estrogen and a blunting of oxytocin, which is implicated in the fight-or-flight response. The "tend-and-befriend" response may also lower blood pressure.

Positive Cognitive Styles

Evidence is accumulating from a variety of studies that optimism, perceptions of personal control, and a sense of meaning are protective of physical health. These cognitive resources assume special significance in helping people cope with intensely stressful events. Even unrealistically optimistic expectations appear to slow down the progression of disease in men infected with HIV. In a study of healthy older adults, a sense of coherence (one indicator of resilience) moderated the association between anticipation of moving and reduced NK cell lysis, with a low sense of coherence associated with poorest levels of NK cell lysis.

Religion & Spirituality

Several studies have shown a relationship between religious or spiritual practice and health outcomes. "Religion" can be considered a collection of beliefs and practices that are external expressions of spiritual experience. These expressions can be organizationally based or private, but are usually grounded in a collective tradition. "Spirituality" can be considered an orientation toward or experiences with the transcendent, existential, or sacred dimensions of life. That which is transcendent or sacred is considered as something beyond oneself, whether it be conceptualized as a divine being, higher power, nature, spirit, or the ultimate ground of being. It is possible for people to engage in religious activities independent of having spiritual experiences, just as some people consider themselves intensely spiritual without being religious. Some consider their religious practice to be a pathway toward spirituality.

Types of studies on the religion–health connection have included cross-sectional as well as prospective and retrospective studies where participation in religious or spiritual practice is correlated with some health outcome measure, as well as intervention studies in which subjects were randomized into treatment and control groups. Correlational studies of religious or spiritual involvement and health outcomes have shown a positive association with longer life; less cardiovascular disease; less hypertension; more engagement in health-promoting behaviors; decreased risk of depression, anxiety, substance abuse, and suicide; better coping with illness; and better health-related quality of life. Among the intervention studies the best evidence for efficacy with health outcomes has been with religiously oriented cognitive therapy, meditation, 12-step fellowships, forgiveness therapy, and intercessory prayer. These studies need further replication with better designed controls.

Both religion and spirituality represent a heterogeneous group of belief systems, religious practices, and spiritual experiences. Most of the research linking religious or spiritual practice to health outcomes does not account for this heterogeneity, and thus the generalizability of results is limited. Nevertheless, the growing accumulation of evidence of positive health correlates of religion and spirituality warrants not only more sophisticated research but also the attention of clinicians seeking to improve the health of patients.

A STRESS MODEL FOR MEDICAL CARE

The etiology of illness and its waxing and waning course are multifactorial. Any given illness episode is determined by many circumstances. The complex pathway by which stress influences the outcome of illness is subject to the ongoing accumulation of data and elaboration of heuristic and clinical models. A model of stress that can aid diagnosis, prevention, and intervention is shown in Figure 31-1. Adapted from an optical model first proposed by Rahe and Arthur (1978), it depicts stressors as light rays filtered through successive lenses representing the individual's perception (threat appraisal), coping, physiologic processes, and arousal reduction activities, and then projected onto illness outcome screens. Each lens either augments or diminishes the intensity of light (heavy bold lines or dotted lines, respectively) on its pathway to illness outcome, and represents a potential focal point for the clinician's diagnosis of a stress influence or risk factor for patient illness. Each lens also represents a potential focus of preventive health care or intervention.

Perception refers to the person's appraisal of the threat involved in various stressors. Several personal variables that may affect the degree of perceived threat are shown in Figure 31-1. For example, the degree of a person's openness to change or the extent to which he or she values change influences whether a particular life change, such as a child leaving home, is perceived as a threat to the self or an opportunity for growth. The degree of control individuals prefer to have in their lives, as well as the amount of control they perceive they have over specific stressors, also influence their perception of threat. Thus, a parent with a high need to control an adolescent child's outside activities experiences more stress when the child struggles toward emancipation than does a parent who has less of a need for control and who trusts the child's judgment.

Coping refers to methods an individual uses to mitigate the influence of stressors perceived as threatening. One approach to coping is "exposure management," or attempts to increase or decrease the amount and intensity of stressors encountered. Thus, an overworked, overcommitted manager might attempt to mitigate stress by withdrawing from some commitments and by reducing work hours by delegating more responsibility to subordinates. Social supports are an important stress buffer, and successful coping with stressors may involve both developing confiding relationships and increasing the amount of one's self-disclosure about the effect of stressors in one's life. There is some research evidence that emotional self-disclosure about stressors enhances immune functioning. In the aftermath of the September 11, 2001, attacks, it is estimated that 98% of Americans coped by talking with others, 90% by turning to religious or spiritual practices, 60% by participating in group activities to memorialize the events, and 36% by making donations. "Stimulus screening" involves techniques to focus attention on relevant stimuli and to regulate the overall flow of stimulation to one's optimal level of functioning.

Two major classes of **physiologic response** to stressors that lead to target organ pathology are autonomic hyperreactivity and immunosuppression. Both are cortically mediated through the individual's perceptions and methods of coping. **Hyperreactivity** in the presence of stress, sometimes called the **defense reaction,** has been shown to be a factor in disease processes specific to vulnerable organ systems in persons with established disease. Thus, exaggerated pressor responses in hypertensives, increased electromyelogram responses in those suffering from tension headaches and chronic back pain, disturbances in glucose metabolism in insulin-dependent diabetics, and bronchoconstrictive responses in asthmatics are all examples of hyperreactivity in the presence of a definable stressor. In the case of hypertension, hyperreactivity is present in normotensives at risk for the disorder and in some studies has predicted future blood pressure levels. Other examples are increased levels of serum cholesterol seen in studies of tax accountants in the 2 weeks prior to April 15 and of fighter pilots landing on aircraft carriers compared with pilots on long commercial airline flights.

One of the adaptive functions of sympathetic activation is to prepare the organism for large-muscle movement to either attack or flee a threat. In twenty-first century human society, these somatomotor responses are often voluntarily suppressed or sublimated, leading to delayed elimination of released glucose and fatty acids and often bringing more powerful and prolonged increases in blood pressure. In addition, the relative absence of skeletal muscle exertion in affluent societies (without compensatory aerobic exercise) prevents the activation of endorphins that normally accompanies muscle exertion. Because these endorphins dampen mental arousal and sympathetic activity, in the absence of skeletal muscle exertion these arousal and activation states are prolonged.

Immunosuppression, as discussed previously, occurs through the mechanisms of increased levels of circulating corticosteriods, catecholamines, and opioids and decreased levels of growth hormone and prolactin under conditions of prolonged stress. Sometimes referred to as the **defeat reaction,** this response pattern occurs when patients are exposed to long-term stressful situations that tend to overwhelm ordinary coping mechanisms, thus leading to despair or deep sorrow in situations that appear to be beyond all hope and rescue. Rather than working directly on target organ systems as in the case of hyperreactivity, downregulation of the immune system

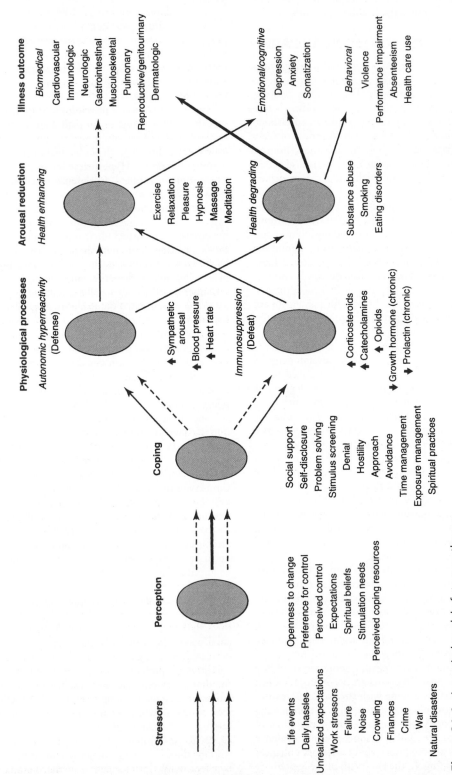

Figure 31-1. An optical model of stress pathways.

in the defeat reaction increases vulnerability to external invasive organisms and endogenous neoplasms.

Several **arousal reduction** strategies are available to individuals to mitigate physiologic activation and disruption of homeostatic processes in conditions of stress. These include both **health-enhancing** and **health-degrading** activities. Among the health-enhancing arousal-reduction strategies are exercise, which expends accumulated corticosteroids and dampens sympathetic activation through the release of endorphins, and various approaches to stimulating the parasympathetic nervous system. This includes relaxation exercises, abdominal breathing, self-hypnosis, meditation, listening to soothing music, massage, and contact with nature.

Health-degrading activities, which may be attempts at physiologic arousal reduction but that actually magnify the stress response and lead to target organ disease, include substance abuse, tobacco use, and eating disorders. Intensification of all of these behaviors may coincide with stressful life episodes. An example is the mediating role of increased alcohol intake in the relationship between occupational stress and hypertension seen in studies of air traffic controllers.

Various **illness outcomes** of stress include **biomedical disease** manifested in specific organ systems, such as cardiovascular, immune, and neurologic disorders; **emotional and cognitive disorders**, such as depression, anxiety, and somatization; and **behavioral disorders**, such as violence, performance impairment, absenteeism, and overuse of health care resources. These stress outcomes are the usual focus of medical and mental health intervention, but the larger model of the stress pathway provides primary care clinicians with potent opportunities for comprehensive preventive health care.

HEALTH OUTCOMES OF STRESS

Each organ system has a unique susceptibility to stress. The following is a brief overview of some of the stress implications in specific diseases.

Cardiovascular

Cardiovascular disease is the leading cause of mortality in the United States. Stress contributes to all expressions of heart disease, including coronary artery disease, congestive heart failure, and sudden cardiac death. Because fully a third of sudden cardiac deaths and MIs cannot be explained by the severity of the standard cardiac risk factors—family history, hypertension, dyslipidemia, diabetes, or tobacco use—stress may explain some of this variance. As mentioned above, there is a connection between hostility and cardiac disease. It has been shown that hostility contributes independently of other risk factors to the pathogenesis of heart disease through lipid accumulation, increased blood pressure, and heart rate and platelet physiology.

Immune

Clinical expressions of immune deficiencies are in part the result of stress. They range from the common cold to some forms of cancer. Although research on the relationship between stress and cancer is still inconclusive, there is some evidence that stress and surgical excision of the primary tumor can promote tumor metastasis by suppression of cell-mediated immunity. The perioperative period is a particularly important window during which psychological or pharmacological interventions to prevent or reduce stress may offer a reduced risk of metastasis. Other immune-mediated diseases such as rheumatoid arthritis and systemic lupus erythematosus may show a pattern of exacerbation brought on by stress.

HIV

More rapid disease progression in people infected with HIV has been associated with greater concealment of homosexual identity, more cumulative stressful life events, and less cumulative social support over a 5-year period. Alternatively, more deliberate cognitive processing about the death of a close friend or partner has been associated with greater likelihood of finding positive meaning in the loss, less rapid decline in CD4+ cell levels, and lower rates of AIDS-related mortality over a 9-year period in HIV-seropositive men.

Neurologic

All forms of stroke show a circadian expression in their presentation, with peaks during the early morning hours when catecholamines are highest. Dizziness, vertigo, and other balance disorders often have stress as a causative or contributing factor. One of the most common neurologic expressions of stress in clinical practice is headache. Both tension headache and migraine headache are substantially influenced by patient stressors.

Gastrointestinal

Peptic ulcer disease may have an association with stress. Gastric hyperacidity and excess pepsin production are hallmarks of the sympathetic arousal that occurs during stress. IBS, which is characterized by abdominal pain with altered bowel habits (constipation or diarrhea) in the absence of a definable lesion or structural abnormality, frequently correlates with periods of emotional stress. The human "defense reaction" (fight-or-flight response) promotes activation of the cardiovascular system along with inhibition of gastric motility.

Musculoskeletal

Some forms of arthritis show stress-related exacerbations. Complex syndromes such as fibromyalgia seem to have a psychosocial trigger. Temporomandibular joint (TMJ) dysfunction and its related pain syndrome are frequently associated with mental stress. Chronic pain tends to correlate with stress in a person's life. Persistent pain and psychological symptoms frequently seen after motor vehicle accidents (MVA) may involve the impact of acute stress interacting with past experience, post-MVA behavior, and cognitive/psychological consequences to alter activity in brain pathways which process pain.

Pulmonary

Asthma and chronic obstructive pulmonary disease appear to be worsened by stress. Conversely, one of the more powerful self-regulatory stress-control techniques is relaxed abdominal breathing. Asthmatics who participate in stress reduction programs have shown improved physical activity and decreased medical visits. Hypnosis has helped some asthmatics decrease their use of bronchodilators (see Chapter 5).

Reproductive & Genitourinary

The neurohormonal, vascular, and immunologic effects of stress significantly impact the reproductive and genitourinary systems. Changes in estrogen and testosterone levels can show marked association with environmental and psychological stressors. Amenorrhea frequently occurs during stressful times in the lives of women. Fertility also can be affected by stress. Dysmenorrhea, dyspareunia, endometriosis, and impotence all have substantial stress and strain connections.

Dermatologic

A variety of skin lesions and rashes have been associated with the stress response. Stress-induced vasomotor changes may aggravate inflammatory dermatoses. Vasodilation is considered to be responsible for the thermal aggravation often expressed as pruritus. This lowering of the itch threshold by vasodilation may account for the pruritus seen with many dermatologic syndromes. Emotional stress, fear, and pain are all accompanied by substantial drops in skin temperature of the fingers.

Wound Healing

Psychological stress has measurable negative consequences for production of proinflammatory cytokines, and stress-related delays in wound healing have ranged from 24% to 40% with effect sizes between .30 and .74. These effects on wound healing are consistent with other studies that have shown that greater fear or distress prior to surgery is associated with poorer outcomes, including longer hospital stays, more postoperative complications, and higher rates of rehospitalization.

Frailty in the Elderly

Elevated serum levels of the proinflammatory cytokine IL-6 have predicted future disability in older adults. These cytokines slow muscle repair after injury and accelerate muscle wasting. IL-6 and C-reactive protein play a pathogenic role in several diseases associated with disability among the elderly, including osteoporosis, arthritis, and congestive heart failure.

DIAGNOSIS

Given the multivariate, multiple-pathway nature of the stress response, clinical diagnosis of stress assumes a multifactorial approach. Traditional medical diagnosis and treatment occur at the point of illness manifestation in target organ systems. From the broader perspective of stress medicine, however, each of the lenses in the optical model (see Figure 31-1) is a potential focus of diagnosis.

The Medical Interview

The richest source of data concerning stressors, perception, coping, and arousal reduction strategies is the medical interview (see Chapter 1). Having the stress model in mind allows the primary care clinician to inquire about current and recent life stressors and to make note of significant clusterings of stressors that precede illness onset. A careful history should uncover whether life stressors are temporally related to the onset of chronic disease and to periods of disease exacerbation.

During the interview, the clinician can ask patients about their beliefs, expectations, self-perceptions, and needs that influence how stressors are perceived. For example, asking patients how much control they prefer in their lives and how much control they perceive that they have over specific life events can determine whether there is congruence or incongruence between preferred control and perceived control. Incongruence tends to amplify the effect of stressors. It is also helpful to ask patients how they view their own resources (internal and external) for coping with stressors, since the more the perceived threats exceed the perceived personal resources, the greater the stress involved.

Patients' approaches to coping with stressors should also be probed in the interview. The presence or absence of social supports as well as the ability of patients to access these supports through self-disclosure are critical data for facilitating stress management. The perceptual and coping styles uncovered in the interview have implications for primary care management of the patient's health, both in prevention and intervention.

It is also important to assess patients' approaches to arousal reduction and to ascertain the balance of health-enhancing and health-degrading strategies. The following questions can be helpful in this regard: "What are

Figure 31-2. Life stress inventory.

In the blanks below list the major events, changes, or stressors that have happened to you within the last year. Also list those events that you expected but that failed to occur. In the next column place a check next to those stressors that are current, ongoing problems. In the last column opposite each stressor, indicate the degree to which this event has been under your control by writing a number corresponding to the scale at the top.

Life Event or Stressor	Current Problem	Within Your Control	Outside Your Control
		1 2 3 4 5 6 7 8 9 10	
1._____	_____		_____
2._____	_____		_____
3._____	_____		_____
4._____	_____		_____
5._____	_____		_____
6._____	_____		_____
7._____	_____		_____
8._____	_____		_____
9._____	_____		_____
10._____	_____		_____
		Control score _____ (mean of ratings)	

John F. Christensen, PhD.

the signs indicating that you are experiencing stress?" "What are the physical symptoms?" "What happens in your emotional life?" "How do you act differently when you are stressed?" Methods used to mitigate this arousal can then be ascertained: "When you notice these signs of stress, what do you do to reduce the intensity of the physical symptoms?" It is also important to elicit the short- and long-term outcomes of these strategies: "How does this strategy work for you?" "How does it affect the way you feel immediately? Several hours later? The next day?" Sometimes it is helpful to ask about specific arousal reduction techniques: "Do you practice a form of meditation or relaxation exercise?" "Do you get regular physical exercise?" When questioning patients about substance use or tobacco use, it is helpful to ask whether their use is associated with periods of stress.

Self-report Questionnaire

A multitude of self-report questionnaires and inventories have been developed for research purposes that measure stressors and many of the variables listed in Figure 31-1 related to perception and coping. Given the limitations of physician and support staff time in primary care settings, it is recommended that any questionnaire be simple, brief, and provide data that can be used by the provider in counseling patients in the area of stress management. An example of such an instrument is the Life Stress Inventory shown in Figure 31-2. Borrowing from the life event scaling studies and the critical role that perceived control plays in mediating stress, this inventory asks patients in an open-ended way to list the major events (and expected

nonevents), changes, and stressors that have occurred during the previous year. They are asked to check those stressors that are current, ongoing problems. In addition, patients are asked to rate each stressor on a scale of 1 to 10, indicating the extent of perceived control they had over these events. The provider can take the mean of the control ratings and place that number (1 to 10) in the "control score" blank. This instrument provides both qualitative and quantitative data on the nature of patients' stressors, those that are a current source of struggle, and patients' perceived control over these events. The higher the external control score, the more at risk the patient is for adverse consequences of stress. Examining with patients those stressors that seem under their control can allow the clinician to suggest lifestyle changes in those areas. In some instances, patients can be counseled to adjust their perceptions of no control in the direction of greater control. For example, a patient who perceives that she has no control over her work hours can be helped to see areas in which limits can actually be set. In other cases, patients can be led to consider changing their expectations and accepting areas that are truly beyond their control.

MANAGEMENT: PREVENTION & INTERVENTION

Stress Management in the Intensive Care Unit

The immune system of many patients in the intensive care unit (ICU) is suppressed due to trauma, sepsis, or profound physiological and psychological stress. Increases in cortisol levels have been found to correlate with severity of injury in minor and moderate trauma immediately after injury and hours later. Sepsis often begins as a local process of inflammation involving cytokine upregulation. These cytokines eventually, however, may move into systemic circulation, leading to inflammatory processes systemically. Psychological stressors reported by ICU patients include pain, sleep deprivation (due to noise, disturbances by health care staff, and pain), and fear or anxiety (which may manifest in the extreme as delirium, confusion, and other unreal experiences), each of which is associated with decreased immune functioning. The implications for the ICU team are that intervening to reduce these psychosocial stressors may help prevent nosocomial infection. Feelings of anxiety and isolation can be buffered by a nurse providing a nurturing presence. Anxiety can be decreased through the use of benzodiazepines, which may also aid sleep. Nurses can attempt to minimize noise levels as much as possible and decrease the number of times patients are disturbed. Although many analgesic drugs used in the ICU can suppress immune function, alternative approaches to reducing pain should be attempted, since pain itself is immunosuppressive.

CASE ILLUSTRATION 1

Deborah Jones, an ICU nurse with 10 years' experience in critical care, joined a process improvement team (PIT) to examine an increased trend in nosocomial infections among ICU patients over the previous 12 months. Having recently completed a continuing education course in psychoneuroimmunology she was sensitized to the effect of stressors in the ICU environment on patients' immune functioning. Deborah shared this information with the team, and the group (including a physician critical care specialist, a pharmacist, the ICU nurse manager, a pulmonologist, and the chief medical resident) came up with some suggested modifications in the environment and administration of care. Staff entering the ICU were reminded verbally and with a posted sign to speak softly near patient beds. A review of all mechanical noise sources was conducted, and it was determined that a few changes could reduce ambient noise by 30%. Rounding on patients was coordinated to cluster around certain times of the day, and an attempt was made to have greater predictability to staff disturbance of patients when resting. Different staff members, regardless of discipline, were assigned to specific patients for brief visits of a nonmedical

nature to provide support and nurturance, either verbally or through appropriate touch. A palliative care specialist was consulted to develop a menu of pain medications and doses to minimize the risk of immunosuppression, and alternative procedures such as acupuncture were sometimes ordered in collaboration with the patient. Within 3 months, it was noted that the rate of infection in the ICU had dropped 40%. In the face of that data, Deborah was delegated by the PIT to make a formal presentation to hospital administration, and the changes became hospital policy.

Stress Management in Primary Care

The model of stress shown in Figure 31-1 offers the clinician various foci for illness prevention and intervention, just as it does for diagnosis. The clinician familiar with this model should be able to tailor specific psychological, social, behavioral, and pharmacological strategies to the unique needs of individual patients. This is preferable to referring the patient for "stress management," since this generic term does not address the multiplicity of stress-related variables and pathways discussed earlier.

Communicating With Patients about Stress

A primary component of stress prevention and treatment involves the way stress is discussed with patients. Avoiding the implication that "it's all in your head" is of great importance. Equally important is avoiding the message that "you are responsible for your illness," which implies greater personal control over somatic processes than is realistic. Here the risk is inducing guilt in patients who become ill and who feel they have failed at being a "better person." Avoiding negative emphases, for example, "Your hectic pace is going to kill you," in favor of a positive framing of the health benefits of stress management is more likely to have a positive influence (see Chapter 5). For example, the clinician can express optimism about the patient's ability to influence health as follows: "Fortunately, there are many avenues available for examining and changing your habits of thought and ways of responding to life challenges. I'd like to give you an overview of some strategies that we can discuss now and in future appointments." Showing the patient a model such as that in Figure 31-1 can be helpful as part of this discussion.

It is also important to frame beneficial lifestyle changes as the patient's choice. Rather than using the stress model to assume more responsibility for patients' lives, the primary care provider can act as a consultant and coach, clearly giving feedback to patients about the patterns of stress revealed by the diagnostic workup and offering concrete strategies for health promotion along with likely consequences for adherence and nonadherence (see Chapters 16 and 17).

Counseling About Perception & Coping

The perception and coping variables listed in Figure 31-1 represent potential topics for primary care counseling with patients. Depending on the clinician's expertise, inclination, and time, this could be done during a portion of several primary care visits. For example, a parent who is feeling stressed because of a teenager's oppositional behavior could be invited to reflect on how much parental control is needed and coached on ways of setting realistic limits. With an accountant feeling overwhelmed about a recent promotion to senior management, the clinician could elicit his recollections of previous adaptations to challenging life changes in order to help him become cognizant of his own resources.

Referring a parent of a child with recently diagnosed leukemia to a support group of other parents is an example of a coping strategy. Encouraging a widower to confide feelings of sadness to close friends is an example of helping a patient improve his use of social supports. Referring a teacher with a chronically explosive temper for short-term anger management therapy would potentially reduce a cardiac risk factor.

Counseling patients about time management offers a rich opportunity for clinicians to raise questions concerning the patients' values and missed opportunities for personal renewal. For example, the clinician can ask the patient to reflect on those important but nonurgent activities that can contribute to personal well-being (e.g., time spent playing with a child), but which are consistently postponed in favor of more urgent but less important tasks (e.g., keeping track of the performance of stocks). A list of potential nonpharmacologic strategies related to perception and coping that can be suggested to patients is shown in Table 31-1.

Nonpharmacologic Strategies for Improving Physiologic Processes

Once identified in clinical practice, sympathetic hyperreactors may benefit from both nonpharmacologic and pharmacologic treatment interventions. The nonpharmacologic treatment of elevations in blood pressure related to stress is outlined in Table 31-2. Included are strategies for exercise, diet, and weight control.

Arousal Reduction Strategies

For patients showing a high degree of autonomic hyperreactivity, the clinician can provide or suggest several arousal reduction strategies that can work synergistically with perception and coping skills, as well as with pharmacologic interventions. These strategies are listed in

Table 31-1. Nonpharmacologic interventions related to perception and coping.

1. Improve time management
2. Improve sense of humor
3. Pursue personal and vocational activities consistent with life values
4. Explore the meaning and purpose of life
5. Cultivate spiritual and transcendent activities:
   a. Prayer
   b. Communal religious observances
   c. Spiritual retreat
   d. Seasonal ritual celebrations
6. Increase emotional self-disclosure
7. Pursue short-term psychotherapy
8. Clarify values
9. Cultivate social support network
10. Increase assertiveness
11. Reduce exposure to unnecessary stressors
12. Monitor sensory input
13. Help others

Table 31-3. Mindfulness meditation in particular is an effective method of stress reduction that not only activates the parasympathetic response, but also builds a mental habit of staying present to the task at hand while assuming a nonjudgmental stance toward the progression of one's thoughts and emotions (see Chapter 7). Referring patients to introductory books on mindfulness meditation, such as those listed at the end of this chapter, or encouraging them to take a meditation class, can provide them with a powerful stress management resource. A recent study has shown that 16 weeks of transcendental meditation improved components of the metabolic syndrome (blood pressure, insulin resistance, and heart rate variability) among patients with stable coronary heart disease.

Table 31-2. The nonpharmacologic treatment of blood pressure elevations related to stress.

Exercise
1. Pursue daily aerobic exercise
2. Improve physical fitness and stamina

Diet and weight control
1. Reduce excess body weight and fat
2. Reduce alcohol intake to less than 1 oz/day
3. Reduce dietary sodium
4. Increase dietary potassium
5. Increase dietary calcium
6. Increase dietary omega-3-fatty acids

Table 31-3. Health-enhancing arousal reduction techniques.

1. Meditation
2. Self-hypnosis
3. Relaxation exercises
4. Time in nature
5. Massage
6. Abdominal breathing
7. Singing
8. Tai chi
9. Listening to soothing music

Referral for Psychotherapy

The clinician may choose to refer patients for psychotherapy or to educational groups to achieve some of the desired outcomes in the areas of perception, coping, and arousal reduction techniques. These referrals are more effectively targeted to the unique needs of patients if the clinician uses the multifactorial model in Figure 31-1. This model can also aid the primary care clinician in communicating with the psychotherapist about possible foci for treatment. Psychotherapy may be more effective than primary care counseling for altering dysfunctional belief systems (e.g., no control of one's life) or coping habits (e.g., excessive need for achievement) that amplify stress. In addition, it may offer focused training in the acquisition of arousal reduction skills such as meditation and self-hypnosis.

 CASE ILLUSTRATION 2*

History: *A 54-year-old female with a history of chronic migraine headaches, hypertension, hypercholesterolemia, mild obesity, and smoking presented to a new primary care physician. She was treated by her previous physician with Tylenol #3, one tablet twice a day, for the migraines, and she routinely called in halfway through the month for extra refills. Other medications included atenolol 25 mg a day for blood pressure elevation and migraine prophylaxis, as well as over-the-counter antacids for occasional heartburn.*

Patient interview: *The patient appeared angry and complained that the medication was not helping her pain. The new physician listened to her complaints and agreed at the end of the visit to refill her medications, but told her he would not prescribe*

more than the previous doctor. He asked her to return for her annual Pap smear, at which time he would take a history and do a physical examination.

Social history: *At the follow-up appointment the physician took a social history, which revealed that the patient had been smoking a pack of cigarettes every day for the last 35 years but did not use alcohol or street drugs. Although never married, she had been involved in a 10-year relationship with her boyfriend, who suffered from severe emphysema and was dependent on oxygen. Three years previously this man had assumed responsibility for raising his two granddaughters (ages 8 and 11) because his daughter, the girls' mother, was a drug addict serving time in prison. The patient was not consulted about this custody decision. She accepted the stressor out of love for her partner, who was also dependent on her. The oldest granddaughter was now 14 and had become unruly, rebellious, sexually active, and aggressive. She had asked the patient for help obtaining birth control. Although the patient wanted to leave this demanding social situation, she saw it as her responsibility to care for her partner and the two children. The history correlated these recent life events with increased frequency of migraines and initiation of daily use of Tylenol #3.*

Physician facilitation of emotional self-disclosure: *The physician actively listened to the patient's self-disclosure, which was accompanied by crying. At the end of the interview the patient thanked the physician, who noted that she had not complained of migraines during that visit.*

Brief counseling and referral for family therapy: *In the follow-up visit the physician counseled the patient to realize that she was not isolated. He validated her efforts to work with the situation, even though she had the real option of leaving. He recommended family therapy, to which the patient agreed. Further medical treatment was deferred until after the family had engaged in therapy. The patient made no mention of pain medication during this visit.*

Change of medication and of lifestyle: *Prior to the next visit there were no further calls for pain medication refills. At that visit the patient stated that the migraines, although still present, were not as disabling. The focus of the visit was on improving management of hypertension, high cholesterol, and migraines. They discussed starting an exercise program, initiating a low-fat diet and weight loss, and quitting smoking. The physician remarked that the patient appeared to be gaining control over the life events involving her family.*

Disposition: *After several months of family therapy the patient had established a primary care relationship with a pediatrician to help her with the medical and hormonal issues of the grandchildren. Her boyfriend had increased his level of help. She had lost 8 lb over 4 months, started walking 4 days a week for*

---

*I am grateful to Kerry Kuehl, MD, for sharing this case.

30 minutes, and began a low-fat diet, all without pain medication. She agreed to start a smoking cessation program. The patient demonstrated a marked change in attitude and treatment of office staff, and the primary care provider developed a changed perception of her and an appreciation of the healing potential in "drug-seeking patients."

CONCLUSION

The relationship between stress and disease is well established, although the specific pathways are complex and multifactorial. Clinicians increasingly are asked to examine the cost-effectiveness of the time spent with their patients with a view to improving outcomes within the constraints of available financial and human resources. Attention to the function of stress in patients' illnesses creates the potential for improving treatment outcomes and preventing or delaying the onset of costly target organ disease or the exacerbation of chronic illness. Applying a multidimensional stress model that includes patients' perceptions, coping strategies, physiologic arousal mechanisms, and arousal reduction strategies offers the health care professional multiple opportunities for influencing the ecology of disease.

SUGGESTED READINGS

Beaton R, Murphy S. Psychosocial responses to biological and chemical terrorist threats and events. *AAOHN J* 2002;50: 182–189.

Ben-Eliyahu S. The promotion of tumor metastasis by surgery and stress: immunological basis and implications for psychoneuroimmunology. *Brain Behav Immun* 2003;17:S27–S36.

Borrell-Carrio F, Suchman AL, Epstein RM. The biopsychosocial model 25 years later: principles, practices, and scientific inquiry. *Ann Fam Med* 2004;2:576–582.

Christensen JF. The assessment of stress: environmental, intrapersonal, and outcome issues. In: McReynolds P(editor): *Advances in Psychological Assessment*, Vol 5. Jossey-Bass, 1981.

DeKeyser F. Psychoneuroimmunology in critically ill patients. *AACN Clin Issues* 2003;14:25–32.

Engel GL. The need for a new medical model. *Science* 1977;196: 129–136.

Holmes TH, Rahe RH. The Social Readjustment Rating Scale. *J Psychosom Res* 1967;11:213–218.

Kiecolt-Glaser JK, McGuire L, Robles TF et al. Psychoneuroimmunology: psychological influences on immune function and health. *J Consulting & Clinical Psychol* 2002;70:537–547.

Kobasa SC. Stressful life events, personality and health: an inquiry into hardiness. *J Pers Soc Psychol* 1979;37:1–11.

McEwen BS. Protective and damaging effects of stress mediators. *N Engl J Med* 1998;338:171–179.

Miller GE, Rohleder N, Stetler C, et al. Clinical depression and regulation of the inflammatory response during acute stress. *Psychosom Med* 2005;67:679–687.

Rahe RH, Arthur RJ. Life change and illness studies: past history and future directions. *J Hum Stress* 1978;4:3–15.

Schuster MA, Stein BD, Jaycox LH, et al. A national survey of stress reactions after the September 11, 2001, terrorist attacks. *N Engl J Med* 2001;345:1507–1512.

Seyle H. *Stress in Health and Disease.* Boston: Butterworth, 1976.

Shrestha NM, Sharma B, Van Ommeren M et al. Impact of torture on refugees displaced within the developing world: symptomatology among Bhutanese refugees in Nepal. *JAMA* 1998; 280:443–448.

Smyth JM, Stone AA, Hurewitz A, et al. Effects of writing about stressful experiences on symptom reduction in patients with asthma or rheumatoid arthritis. *JAMA* 1999;281:1304–1309.

Spickard A, Gabbe SG, Christensen JF. Mid-career burnout in generalist and specialist physicians. *JAMA* 2002;288:1447–1450.

Strike PC, Steptoe A. Behavioral and emotional triggers of acute coronary syndromes: a systematic review and critique. *Psychosom Med* 2005;67:179–186.

Taylor SE, Klein LC, Lewis BP et al. Biobehavioral responses to stress in females: tend-and-befriend, not fight-or-flight. *Psychol Rev* 2000;107:411–429.

SUGGESTED READING FOR PATIENTS

Hanh TN. *The Miracle of Mindfulness: A Manual on Meditation.* Beacon Press, 1987.

Kabat-Zinn J. *Wherever You Go There You Are: Mindfulness Meditation in Everyday Life.* New York: Hyperion, 1994.

WEB SITES

American Institute of Stress Web site. http//www.stress.org. Accessed October, 2007.

Center for Mindfulness in Medicine, Health Care, and Society Web site. http://www.umassmed.edu/cfm/index.aspx. Accessed October, 2007.

University of Pennsylvania Authentic Happiness Center Web site. http://www.authentichappiness.sas.upenn.edu/. Accessed October, 2007.

Pain

32

Gregory T. Smith, PhD

> *"There are among us those who haply please to think our business is to treat disease. And all unknowingly lack this lesson still 'tis not the body, but the man is ill.'"* S. Weir Mitchell (cited in Turk, Meichenbaum, and Genest, 1983).

INTRODUCTION

Pain is a common symptom of an underlying disease process or injury. Acute pain arises from a known disease or injury, while chronic pain arises from a known disease or injury or from unknown etiology. Pain is modulated, increased, or decreased, by arousal (central nervous system [CNS] activity) caused by physical movement, psychological status (such as depression and anxiety), environmental factors (such as stressors or reinforcers), and conditioning history.

Although a number of pain scales exist, pain is not measurable directly like blood pressure or body temperature; instead the clinician must rely on pain behavior (verbal and nonverbal patient expressions; see Table 32-1) together with known modulating variables, to assess the level of pain. Acute pain is primarily a symptom of a pathologic process or injury, and treating the illness or injury often will reduce or eliminate the pain symptoms. Pain medications are often used for comfort during the healing process. Chronic pain is pain that has usually not responded to the treatment for acute pain, and the modulating variables mentioned above can become the primary etiologies of the pain complaint. Comorbid psychiatric conditions can and often do occur with both acute and chronic pain. The goal of treatment, both acute and chronic, is to improve function and return the patient to as normal a lifestyle as possible, which in many cases includes return to work. Pain relief alone typically will not achieve this goal.

The objectives of this chapter are:

- To provide practical strategies for assessment of pain.
- To provide information about treatment strategies and patient education.
- To provide for safe and ethical pain management practice.

CLINICIAN–PATIENT RELATIONSHIP

Establishing a good clinician–patient relationship is the key to treating pain. The effectiveness of this relationship is defined largely by the clinician's ability to acknowledge the patient's problem, address the patient's goals, and establish a collaborative approach on which both clinician and patient can agree. Because the primary concerns of clinician and patient can differ, there is potential for miscommunication.

Patients who are in pain come to medical attention with a number of possible feelings and goals:

1. They may simply want to discover the cause of the pain to allay their fears about serious disease.
2. They may be interested only in relief from the pain.
3. They may want to regain impaired function in order to return to normal work or recreational activities.
4. They may want medical and social acknowledgment that the pain is preventing or interfering with normal activities.

Pain is a symptom not perceivable to the observer. Pain behaviors are the functional medium for observing pain. Moreover, pain behaviors are often embedded in family interactions and dynamics that can lead unintentionally to reinforcing a sick role or to family dysfunction, which can promote increased pain behavior.

Pain can be the central complaint in somatization disorder and psychophysiologic reactions. It is often accompanied by a sleeping disorder. Depression, anxiety, and fear are common comorbid reactions to pain. Pain associated with a somatization disorder or psychophysiologic reaction may not derive initially from

---

Gregory T. Smith and Douglas Beers were authors of the first and second editions of this chapter.

Table 32-1. Pain behaviors.

Pain behaviors can be separated into 4 categories:
1. *Pain complaints*: verbalized in the presence of pain, complaining, moaning, grimacing.
2. *Posturing*: the nonverbal expression of pain; limping, leaning, use of a cane.
3. *Impaired functioning*: reduction of activities, avoidance of certain activities, impaired personal and sexual relationships.
4. *Somatic interventions*: taking medications or seeking treatment.

---

injury or illness, but may instead be an expression of the psychological conflicts that define that disorder.

The "three-function model of the medical interview" (see Chapter 1) can be utilized for ongoing evaluation and re-evaluation while treating patients for pain (see Table 32-2).

Pain treatment is based on a number of strategies:

1. Obtain a description of the pain and the meaning or impact of the pain on the patient and others around the patient.
2. Assess for comorbid psychiatric conditions.
3. Take a pain-related history and compare with physical examination findings.
4. Review or obtain diagnostic studies that might rule in treatable physical pathology.
5. Provide relief and comfort through medication and reassurance.
6. Use multiple treatment modalities.
7. Assess for change in pain behavior and function.
8. Reinforce improvement in function or reduced pain, and discontinue ineffective treatments.

Table 32-2. The three-function model of the medical interview.

---

1. *Data gathering*: elucidate the etiology (physical and psychological) of pain. Arrive at a tentative working diagnosis even while considering alternative hypotheses.
2. *Relationship building*: elicit the meaning of the pain in the patient's life and develop an understanding of "pain behaviors" and pain dysfunction, both physical and social.
3. *Management*: explain the role of pain medications, including the duration of their use, the importance of time contingency, and an expectation of the degree of relief.
   a. Plan the use of physical and other therapies designed to improve function.
   b. Acknowledge the roles and limitations of rest periods.
   c. Establish the value of return to normal work and recreational activity to overcome pain behavior and dysfunction.

TREATMENT MODALITIES

Pharmacotherapy and injection therapy: Medications commonly used in the treatment of pain include nonopioid medications such as nonsteroidal anti-inflammatory drugs (NSAIDs), tricyclic antidepressants, anticonvulsants, opioid analgesics (Table 32-3), and adjuvant analgesics (Table 32-4).

Injections include trigger-point injections, epidural injections, and nerve blocks. Trigger-points are localized areas of muscle tenderness and pain, often injected in the treatment of myofascial complaints for temporary short-term relief. Epidural injections insert local anesthetics or steroids into the epidural space and can be used for both diagnostic purposes as well as to provide short-term relief. Trigger-point and epidural injections should not be used in the treatment of chronic pain. Nerve blocks are typically used for peripheral neuropathy for short-term temporary relief of pain. Nerve blocks are often provided in a series of three to five injections over a period of 2 or 3 weeks.

Physical and occupational therapy: Physical therapy treatment for acute pain is typically passive at first (hot packs, ultrasound, myofascial techniques, and so on) and leading to active physical therapy (stretching, strengthening, and endurance techniques, and so on) over a 6- to 12-week period. Physical therapy is most useful for musculoskeletal pain complaints. Active physical therapy has been shown in combination with other behavioral approaches and education to be most effective in the treatment of chronic low back and upper back pain. Occupational therapists often evaluate and treat activities of daily living and daily functioning, both at home and in the work setting. Work site and home modifications and use of adaptive equipment can be established by an occupational therapist to improve independent functioning.

Behavior therapy and psychotherapy: When patients present with comorbid psychiatric conditions, such as depression or anxiety, a referral to a clinical psychologist or psychiatrist who works with chronic pain patients should be considered. In addition, cognitive-behavioral therapy (CBT) has been shown to assist patients to reduce pain and suffering and improve function and coping skills. CBT can be provided in collaboration with other rehabilitative and medical techniques.

Stress management: Relaxation and stress management have been shown to be useful in reducing comorbid anxiety and report of pain. Hypnosis can also be utilized through imagery and relaxation to focus attention and assist with reduced pain and improved sense of well-being (see Chapter 5).

Biofeedback: Biofeedback is a computerized audio and visual feedback system correlated with various physiologic measures, including muscle contraction (electromyography [EMG]), arousal, skin temperature change, heart rate, and electroencephalogram (EEG).

Table 32-3. Drugs for relief of pain.

Generic Name	Dose, mg	Interval	Comments
Nonnarcotic Analgesics: Usual Doses and Intervals			
Acetylsalicylic acid	650 PO	q 4 h	Enteric-coated preparations available
Acetaminophen	650 PO	q 4 h	Side effects uncommon
Ibuprofen	400 PO	q 4–6 h	Available without prescription
Naproxen	250–500 PO	q 12 h	Delayed effects may be due to long half-life
Fenoprofen	200 PO	q 4–6 h	Contraindicated in renal disease
Indomethacin	25–50 PO	q 8 h	Gastrointestinal side effects common
Ketorolac	15–60 IM	q 4–6 h	Available for parenteral use (IM)
Celecoxib	100–200 PO	q 12–24 h	Useful for arthritis

Generic Name	Parenteral Dose, mg	PO Dose, mg	Comments
Narcotic Analgesics: Usual Doses and Intervals			
Codeine	30–60 q 4 h	30–60 q 4 h	Nausea common
Oxycodone	—	5–10 q 4–6 h	Usually available with acetaminophen or aspirin
Morphine	10 q 4 h	60 q 4 h	
Morphine sustained release	—	30–200 bid to tid	Oral slow-release preparation
Hydromorphone	1–2 q 4 h	2–4 q 4 h	Shorter acting than morphine sulfate
Levorphanol	2 q 6–8 h	4 q 6–8 h	Longer acting than morphine sulfate; absorbed well PO
Methadone	10 q 6–8 h	20 q 6–8 h	Delayed sedation due to long half-life
Meperidine	75–100 q 3–4 h	300 q 4 h	Poorly absorbed PO; normeperidine a toxic metabolite
Butorphanol	—	1–2 q 4 h	Intranasal spray
Fentanyl	25–100 μg/h	—	72 h Transdermal patch
Tramadol	—	50–100 q 4–6 h	Mixed opioid/adrenergic action

Generic Name	Uptake Blockade 5-HT	NE	Sedative Potency	Anticholinergic Potency	Orthostatic Hypotension	Cardiac Arrhythmia	Ave. Dose, mg/d	Range, mg/d
Antidepressants[a]								
Doxepin	++	+	High	Moderate	Moderate	Less	200	75–400
Amitriptyline	++++	++	High	Highest	Moderate	Yes	150	25–300
Imipramine	++++	++	Moderate	Moderate	High	Yes	200	75–400
Nortriptyline	+++	++	Moderate	Moderate	Low	Yes	100	40–150
Despiramine	+++	++++	Low	Low	Low	Yes	150	50–300
Venflafaxine	+++	++	Low	None	None	No	150	75–400

Generic Name	PO Dose, mg	Interval	Generic Name	PO Dose, mg	Interval
Anticonvulsants and Antiarrhythmics[a]					
Phenytoin	300	daily/qhs	Clonazepam	1	q 6 h
Carbamazepine	200–300	q 6 h	Mexiletine	150–300	q 6–12 h
Oxcarbazine	300	bid	Gabapentin[b]	600–1200	q 8 h

[a]Antidepressants, anticonvulsants, and antiarrhythmics have not been approved by the U.S. Food and Drug Administration (FDA) for the treatment of pain.
[b]Gabapentin in doses up to 1800 mg/d is FDA approved for postherpetic neuralgia.
Note: 5-HT, serotonin; NE, norepinephrine.
Source: Reprinted from Fields HL, Martin JB. Pain: pathophysiology and management. In: Kasper DL, Braunwald E, Fauci AS, et al., eds. *Harrison's Principles of Internal Medicine*, 16th ed. New York, NY: McGraw-Hill, 2004, p. 74.

Biofeedback has been shown to be effective in the treatment of headache and musculoskeletal back pain, in conjunction with active physical therapy. It is also useful to assist with stress management training.

Multidisciplinary pain rehabilitation programs: Multidisciplinary pain rehabilitation programs utilize the services of pain physicians, pain psychologists, physical and occupational therapists, nurses, biofeedback

Table 32-4. Adjuvant analgesics.

Medication	Indication	Comment
Baclofen	Spasticity or pain from multiple sclerosis.	May impair renal function. Can cause seizures with abrupt withdrawal.
Carisoprodol (Soma)	Acute pain from musculoskeletal conditions. Does not directly relax tense skeletal muscles.	Caution with patients with diminished kidney or liver function. Potential for abuse.
Chlorzoxazone (Parafon Forte)	Acute painful musculoskeletal conditions but does not directly relax tense skeletal muscles.	May impair renal function, may enhance the effects of alcohol or other CNS depressants.
Cyclobenzaprine (Flexeril)	Muscle spasms associated with acute musculoskeletal conditions.	Is contraindicated in combination with heart disorders. May enhance the effect of alcohol, barbiturates, and other CNS depressants.
Orphenadrine citrate (Norflex)	Mild-to-moderate acute musculoskeletal pain.	Safety and efficacy is not established in children.
Tizanidine (Zanaflex)	Acute and intermittent pain associated with spasticity.	Risk of liver injury, hypotension, sedation.
Gabapentin (Neurontin)	Neuralgia.	Can cause dizziness, somnolence and other CNS effects.
Pregabalin (Lyrica)	Painful diabetic neuropathy and postlymphatic neuralgia.	Can cause dizziness, somnolence, other CNS effects.
Topiramate (Topamax)	Migraine prophylaxis.	
Amitriptyline (Elavil)	Neuropathic pain.	Caution with persons with history of seizures, urinary retention, glaucoma.
Duloxetine (Cymbalta)	Diabetic neuropathy.	Do not combine with monoamine oxidase (MAOIs). Can cause seizures, confusion, mania, or hypomania.
Nortriptyline (Pamelor)	Neuropathic pain.	Given at bedtime because of sedative side effect.
Venlafaxine (Effexor)	Diabetic neuropathy.	Do not use with MAOIs. Can cause seizures, confusion, mania, or hypomania.

Source: Adapted, with permission, from American Pain Society: *Pain Control in the Primary Care Setting.* Glennview, IL: American Pain Society, 2006.

specialists, and hypnotherapists, who work together on teams to provide coordinated and collaborative work. These programs often involve primary behavior change and rehabilitative strategies while adjusting medications and improving function. The efficacy for the use of these programs with chronic pain conditions is well documented.

Multidisciplinary pain procedure programs: Multidisciplinary pain procedure programs utilizing injection therapies, medications, implantable pumps and stimulators, together with physical therapy and psychological treatment, work collaboratively to provide pain relief and to assist with improved mobility and coping skills.

Implantable pumps: Intraspinal infusion of opioid analgesics into the intrathecal area through an implanted pump is available. Small levels of opiate are introduced into the intrathecal area, lowering the dose required to provide relief.

Spinal cord stimulator: Neurostimulation is provided by an implanted pulse generator through electrodes that are targeted to the spinal cord with the intent of blocking the pain signal. There is some evidence for the use of spinal cord stimulators for complex regional pain syndrome; however, the efficacy for the use of this procedure is yet to be shown for other pain conditions.

Transcutaneous electrical nerve stimulation (TENS): The TENS unit provides an electrical current topically and is commonly used for pain relief. The efficacy for the use of a TENS unit independent of other therapies has yet to be established.

Complementary and alternative therapies: Alternative medicine techniques, including acupuncture and chiropractic manipulation, have been shown in specific cases to be useful to reduce pain on a long-term basis when provided in conjunction with other treatment modalities (see Chapter 30).

CHRONIC HEADACHE PAIN

CASE ILLUSTRATION 1

Lisa is a 39-year-old woman who sought care for her long-standing headaches. These headaches first appeared at the age of 18, at which time they were characterized by severe left orbital and temporal pain associated with nausea, nasal stuffiness, and photophobia. They were often preceded by a scintillating scotoma in the right temporal/visual field. Her workup included a normal lumbar puncture, several normal EEGs, computed tomography (CT) scans, and blood chemistry. She was virtually headache-free for 1 year following a pregnancy in her early 20s. Headaches gradually recurred but remitted again for a year after a hysterectomy for endometriosis in her early 30s. She now reports that the headaches have increased in frequency, duration, and severity over the past 2 years with more photophobia, nausea, and vomiting.

Treatment modalities have included analgesia (aspirin, acetaminophen, NSAIDs, narcotics), abortive agents (sumatriptan and topiramate), prophylactic medications (amitriptyline, cyproheptadine, phenytoin, valproic acid, propranolol), and vitamins that have had only transient benefit. Dietary and activity prescriptions have also been of minimal success. Her main source or relief over the past year has been repeated emergency room visits for intramuscular narcotics. She has seen multiple internists, neurologists, anesthesiologists (for trigger-point injections and nerve block), allergists and emergency room physicians.

Long-standing, recurrent, incapacitating, nonmalignant pain provides a number of management traps:

1. "doctor shopping" or seeking assistance from a series of caregivers without resolution;
2. a clear fluctuation in the frequency and intensity of the headache seemingly due to physiologic changes, but without an exploration of the possible behavioral or social changes associated with these fluctuations;
3. failure to explore the impact the headache has had on the patient's life.

CASE ILLUSTRATION 1 (CONTD.)

A pain history revealed that Lisa's headaches in early adulthood were infrequent (several per year)

and were managed conservatively. Her single severe attack resulted in a hospitalization that was a source of embarrassment to her and her husband. During the early years of her marriage she continued to have infrequent but more severe headaches. During a period of 6 months of treatment with oral contraceptives she suffered a transient exacerbation. As her daughter grew older and her job responsibilities increased, the frequency and severity of the headaches grew. She further reported that she was best able to control her pain by being alone in a quiet room, reading or listening to quiet music.

The patient is now identifying what may be a clear relationship between marital or social stress and her headache complaint. Whereas the headache can provide "time-out" from the conflicts at hand, it does not interfere with other activities such as listening to music or reading. She further indicates that the headaches did not have a significant impact in her early life.

CASE ILLUSTRATION 1 (CONTD.)

The headache pattern remained unchanged until 1½ years ago. At that time Lisa and her husband relocated as a result of her husband's work and they moved into a home that required major remodeling, the responsibility of which was largely the patient's. She had difficulty replacing her former employment and considered a new career. Although she reported enthusiasm for the remodeling and the relocation, Lisa also reported a marked increase in the frequency of the headaches. She was unable to work around the house remodeling or participate in family discussions when she had the headache, but was otherwise able to prepare meals, do housework, and drive as far as 30 miles one way for social and medical visits. She reported that when she retreated to her room with a headache, her husband and children attended to her until she started to improve. She also indicated that her husband returned home early from work during times of a severe headache. She had seen a cascade of physicians in various specialties with a variety of unremarkable diagnostic tests and specialty workups. Her average length of treatment with any one physician was five visits. She reported with embarrassment that she had been unable to keep up with her diet and exercise program and was increasingly overweight. Otherwise, she was in good health with no other medical problems.

Although the headache event is likely to have muscle contraction, endocrinologic and vascular components, there appear to be a number of clear situations or conditions that accompany its onset and severity. Moreover, it is clear that in early adulthood the headache was manageable with minimal medications and with minimal medical attention. The primary behavioral reinforcing events for the headache complaint appear to be (1) avoidance of stressful marital or environmental situations and (2) increased attention from others. A possible secondary reinforcer may be the conditioned use of opiates in a failed effort to control the headache.

CASE ILLUSTRATION 1 (CONTD.)

The following course of treatment was undertaken:

1. *It was agreed that the best approach was to use as little opiate medication as possible. Even though opiates were found to be useful by the patient, she recognized their addictive potential and agreed to use them only with the direction of the primary care physician. Patient and physician medication management responsibilities were outlined in the medication agreement, which specified the number and frequency of opiate doses.*

2. *It was agreed that the patient would not seek additional medical evaluation or treatment without discussing it with her primary care physician first.*

3. *The primary care physician or her designee agreed to be available within a 24-hour period of being contacted about a headache to discuss the headache and the possible situation surrounding it. It was agreed that these conversations were to be no longer than 5–10 minutes.*

4. *An effort was made to encourage active patient participation. A course of biofeedback training was initiated together with physical therapy for neck exercises.*

5. *A family conference affirmed to all that the headaches were to be treated as both a symptom of stress and as a problem in itself. A referral for CBT was provided to the patient.*

6. *If this plan did not show significant reduction in headaches within 3 months, referral to a multidisciplinary pain rehabilitation program would be considered.*

7. *Finally, the physician would be available for treatment of other medical complaints as needed.*

In this way, the primary care physician redefined treatment for the headache complaint: (1) it does not need immediate or intensive medical care; (2) it does not need further diagnostic evaluation; and (3) it does not need multiple/different medical trials. By creating a meaningful relationship with the patient, acknowledging the severity of her complaint, setting expectations for how to respond to symptoms, and securing the patient's commitment to work within these limitations, the physician involved the patient in establishing a framework for pain management.

Treatment Guidelines

Pain description:	Long-standing unilateral headache with nausea, nasal stuffiness, and photophobia.
Pain impact:	Avoidance of stressful, marital, and environmental situations. Increased attention from family and others.
Pain history and examination findings:	Adolescent onset, minimal impact in adolescent and early adulthood. Decrease in headache with pregnancy, hysterectomy, increase with contraceptives and increased environmental and marital stressors. Incidents of increased family attention with headache episodes.
Diagnostics:	Unremarkable for invasive process, disease process, or endocrinologic or allergic abnormalities.
Primary diagnosis:	Chronic unilateral headache.
Comorbid diagnosis:	Rule out depression.
Treatment recommendations:	*Medical*: Medication agreement, treatment with primary care physician only, availability and frequency defined, minimal use of opiates. *Physical*: Neck exercises with physical therapy and musculoskeletal biofeedback. *Behavioral*: CBT evaluation. *Alternative*: None.

CHRONIC INTRACTIBLE PAIN: CHRONIC LOW BACK PAIN

CASE ILLUSTRATION 2

Michael is a 45-year-old man with known controlled hypertension who presented with low back pain. He reported that while working on a farm 2 years ago he experienced a motor vehicle accident that resulted in a herniated disc in his lumbar spine. A lumbar laminectomy and discectomy followed with some recovery for approximately 3 months. Since that time he had been seen twice a week for 6 weeks for passive physical therapy (hot packs, ultrasound, massage, gentle stretching) and he was provided with additional pain medication, including oral opiate and NSAIDs by his surgeon. He had not returned to work since the day of the injury and was currently involved in a vocational rehabilitation plan.

On physical examination, the patient was tender to palpation across his low back bilaterally. Passive straight leg raising was normal. Sharp, dull, and light touch sensations were intact throughout, with symmetric reflexes in both lower extremities. Imaging studies revealed old surgical repair of a herniated disc without other abnormalities. Recent nerve conduction studies were unremarkable for nerve slowing. The patient's surgeon who had "nothing more to offer" referred him back to his primary care physician for continued treatment. The primary care physician referred for a series of three epidural injections. The first injection resulted in partial relief for 2 weeks. The last 2 injections produced no relief of pain.

Chronic low back pain often has the following characteristics:

1. subjective complaint of pain with minimal objective findings;
2. prominent pain behaviors which may have secondary gain features (e.g., avoidance of work);
3. use of "passive" instead of "active" physical therapy; and
4. continuous use of opiate medication in escalating dose to manage the pain.

 CASE ILLUSTRATION 2 (CONTD.)

The patient went on to report that he spent much of the day sitting in his reclining chair, either watching television or reading. He moved from the chair two or three times each day, primarily for meals. He frequently napped during the day and reported disrupted sleep at night, averaging 5–6 hours sleep. He felt depressed and hopeless about his recovery and believed that unless his pain was relieved he would be unable to return to work. He acknowledged that his spouse and children were angry with him and about his inability to return to work.

On further questioning, it is discovered that the social "cost" of the pain is high. Michael's daily activities are greatly impaired. His self-esteem and affect have plummeted, and he is further emotionally isolated from his family. In a circumstance in which a patient's chronic pain is associated with the belief that pain relief is necessary to return to a degree of normal living, the doctor must accurately establish expectations for recovery and the probable outcomes of treatment. Because the patient is usually still focused on the pain as a continuation of the original precipitating injury, it becomes necessary to identify and deal with the patient's pain beliefs while treating to reduce pain behaviors.

Although Michael reported feelings of depression, it is inaccurate to say that the pain is caused by the depression, but rather it is comorbid to the pain. It has been shown, however, that the intensity of pain and depression often diminishes with a trial of antidepressant medication which can improve sleep as well (see Table 32-4).

The goals of treatment for chronic low back pain are primarily focused on improving patients' activity levels, diminishing their reliance on medications, and reducing pain behaviors (e.g., changing the focus of treatment from decreasing pain/enhancing activities to increasing activity level for meaningful tasks). In this way, the clinician assists in "managing" the pain behavior.

At the same time the doctor should challenge the commonly held belief that increased opiate medication is necessary for increased activity. While this is often the case for acute pain conditions the same is not true for chronic benign pain conditions. The doctor also should encourage the patient to recognize that increased pain with activity does not indicate a worsening condition. Furthermore, the clinician should reinforce the patient's use of nonpharmacologic behavioral and physical methods of pain control while increasing functional activity levels.

 CASE ILLUSTRATION 2 (CONTD.)

After a careful explanation by the doctor of the anatomy, physiology, and possible/probable causes of Michael's low back pain, a collaborative discussion followed, leading to an agreement on the following treatment plan:

1. *A course of physical therapy using primarily active exercises (e.g., aerobic exercise, walking, strengthening, and stretching) would be started. In addition, the patient agreed to take progressively longer walks each day. It was expected that with increased activity there would be an initial increase in pain. For that reason it was agreed that the patient could continue to use his opiate medication at the same dose for a short time.*

Table 32-5. Behavioral treatment methods for pain.

1.	Cognitive-Behavioral Therapy	This approach often involves the monitoring of automatic thoughts that are negative; recognizing the connections between thoughts, affect, and behavior; and alternatively replacing dysfunctional thoughts with more reality-oriented interpretations. Recent advances in CBT for the treatment of chronic pain have resulted in behavioral and cognitive methods to challenge dysfunctional beliefs about pain and the impact pain has on normal functioning and replace them with more accurate reality based beliefs.
2.	Biofeedback	Computer-assisted measurement of physiologic changes previously thought to be involuntary, for the purposes of training the patient to bring them into voluntary control. Measurements often include surface electromyelography, skin temperature, galvanic skin response, respiration, heart rate, pulse time, distal polysomnography, and EEG.
3.	Autogenic and relaxation training	A series of mental exercises designed to produce relaxation imagery that may be guided by a practitioner through suggestion or can be coupled with relaxation and exercise.
4.	Progressive muscle relaxation	A systematic approach to relaxation with exercises involving the tensing and relaxing of muscle groups from head to foot.
5.	Hypnosis	A state of enhanced focus or awareness that can lead to increased levels of suggestibility. This can be helpful in the blocking of painful sensations (hypnoanalgesia).

2. *Oral opiate medication was placed on a time contingent basis, gradually extending the number of hours between pills without increasing the dose. This regimen avoided linking the patient's pain perception with the timing and amount of dosing. This was managed through bimonthly dispensing of medications through the pharmacy. It was agreed that any request for change in his medication regime would be directed only to the primary care doctor and not to emergency rooms or other physicians. This was outlined and signed in a patient medication agreement.*

3. *The patient would be seen once monthly by the doctor. It was agreed that after the first 4 weeks of physical therapy a reduction of medication, as described above, would begin. A primary focus of future visits would be discussion about daily activities or return to work goals if appropriate rather than pain interferences with life.*

4. *Progress toward increased functional activities and reduced reliance on medications was monitored monthly through a brief activity-oriented questionnaire filled out at each doctor's visit.*

The doctor has now, in collaboration with the patient, established the parameters of treatment, clarified the expected outcomes in terms of function, reduced or discontinued the use of opiate medications, and progressed toward meaningful employment goals if appropriate. These steps define the treatment effort to reduce pain perception and pain behaviors while changing beliefs about pain impact. In this way the doctor becomes a

"change agent." Patients who respond favorably to this treatment of chronic pain usually report either that the pain is significantly reduced or that it does not bother them as much as it used to. When pain behavior is more entrenched (the patient is unresponsive to treatment due in part to beliefs about pain impact or secondary gain or both), referral to a multidisciplinary pain rehabilitation facility is recommended (see "Treatment Modalities," p347).

CBT and other behavioral approaches (see Table 32-5) are often useful therapies independent of the multidisciplinary pain rehabilitation programs.

Treatment Guidelines

Pain description:	Constant low backache with bilateral radiation secondary to walking/standing, lifting, and carrying. Pain temporarily reduced with reclining, massage, and opiate medication.
Pain impact:	Unable to work since date of injury. Report of depression. Spouse and family angry with his inability to return to work.
Pain history and examination findings:	No history of previous injury or low back pain. On examination, found to be tender to palpation across the low back. Passive straight leg raising is normal. Sensation intact. Reflexes are symmetrical.

Diagnostics: MRI reveals old surgical repair with no new abnormalities. Nerve conduction studies unremarkable for nerve compromise.

Primary diagnosis: Chronic low back pain with mechanical lower extremity radiation.

Comorbid diagnosis: Situational depression.

Treatment recommendations: *Medical:* Medication agreement to treat with the primary care doctor only. Medications are to be prescribed on a time contingent basis and gradually withdrawn by increasing the length of time between doses. Doctor–patient communication progressively focuses on function and return to life goals and activities and less on pain impact or interference with life. For patients who are unresponsive to treatment referral to a multidisciplinary pain rehabilitation program should be considered.
Physical: Active physical therapy initially with a gradual decrease to a home exercise program.
Behavioral: CBT could be considered if marital/family problems not resolving.
Alternatives: Acupuncture can provide for temporary pain relief for some individuals while in treatment as an alternative to opiates. Nutrition counseling can be a useful adjunctive therapy in conjunction with improved dieting for weight loss in the treatment of low back pain.

FIBROMYALGIA

CASE ILLUSTRATION 3

Kim is a 46-year-old female with a known history of gastroesophageal reflux disease (GERD) who presented with total body pain. She reported that while lifting some baked goods in her kitchen she felt an acute snap coming from her right shoulder. Thereafter, she complained of persistent weakness in her right upper extremity, was later diagnosed with thoracic outlet syndrome, and underwent removal of her first rib. She experienced pain relief for approximately 8 months with a recurrence of symptoms followed by an additional supraclavicular surgery. She continued to report having neck and shoulder pain, was then diagnosed with cervical spondylosis, and had a cervical laminectomy 5 years later with good benefit. Thereafter, she was tapered from her pain medications and returned to normal life, including work as a baker. For approximately 10 years following her surgery she reported essentially no recurring symptoms. She then had an onset of pain in her shoulders and upper extremities bilaterally.

Kim now presented with pain in all four quadrants of her body and was positive for increased sensitivity for 16 of 18 tender points when applying 9 lbs of pressure. Kim also reported having an increased sensitivity to pain with increased symptoms in her neck and shoulder.

Fibromyalgia is a syndrome or cluster of symptoms for which there is little agreement as to cause or etiology. Complaints of total bodyache in all four quadrants of the body, plus tenderness in 11–18 tender points when applying 9 lbs of pressure, are sufficient to make diagnosis. Report of symptoms of fibromyalgia can occur with no known traumatic event or illness.

CASE ILLUSTRATION 3 (CONTD.)

On physical examination, sensation was intact throughout with symmetric reflexes without evidence of clubbing, cyanosis, or edema. She had full range of motion in the bilateral upper and lower extremities with no motor deficits identified. MRI of the cervical spine reveals old cervical repair with no abnormalities. Kim was then referred to a pain relief specialist (anesthesiologist) at a multidisciplinary pain procedure program.

Evaluation at the multidisciplinary pain procedure program described pain symptoms, together with chronic fatigue, sleep disturbance, intermittent headaches, loss of weight, subjective feelings of weakness, an intermittent report of irritable bowel, and anxiety. The multidisciplinary evaluation included a psychological evaluation, which diagnosed comorbid depression and anxiety with an above normal arousal response to stress.

The multidisciplinary evaluation identifies a number of other symptoms which are commonly found with fibromyalgia, including report of fatigue, sleep disturbance, intermittent headaches, weight loss or weight gain, weakness, irritable bowel, and anxiety and depression. Not uncommon with fibromyalgia is an abnormal startle response as well as decreased coping in the presence of increased stress or stimulation.

CASE ILLUSTRATION 3 (CONTD.)

Kim reported that she was a single mother of three teenage daughters, two of whom were living at home. She reported her ex-husband to be estranged from her and her children. He had not provided child support, requiring that Kim work full time as the sole support of the family. As her daughters grew to their midteen years, an increasing number of conflicts occurred between them. Kim reported that she was most worried about her eldest 17-year-old daughter, who had recently dropped out of school. She was living with a boy and may have been involved in street drug use. Kim reported having missed several days at work due to her pain, and she had been warned by her employer on two occasions that further absences might lead to disciplinary action. Finally, she reported that she was involved romantically with a man who seemed to like her daughters and had been responsive to her needs for support as her pain problems seemed to worsen.

While it is unknown if stress is one of the causes of the onset of fibromyalgia, it is not uncommon to find comorbid environmental or personal situations which can promote symptoms of anxiety and depression.

CASE ILLUSTRATION 3 (CONTD.)

Treatment initiated at the multidisciplinary pain procedure clinic included selective serotonin reuptake inhibitor (SSRI) antidepressant medication, Gabapentin, a trial of muscle relaxant medication, and a series of myofascial trigger-point injections. She was also seen for a course of CBT designed to improve problem-solving capabilities and teach stress management techniques. In addition, she was treated with passive physical therapy modalities (such as ultrasound, massage, and gentle stretching). Kim reported improved mood with the antidepressant medication, no recognizable benefit from the Gabapentin, and improved relaxation in response to the passive physical therapy techniques and muscle relaxant medications. There was no reported benefit from the trigger-point injections. Finally, it was reported by the psychologist that her decision making about her 17-year-old daughter was improving, with evidence of improved coping skills. Kim also had scheduled relaxation into her daily routine. She had begun a course of oral, short-acting opiate medications, and she decided to take a leave of absence from her employer on short-term disability.

In the absence of a true etiology, the tendency is to treat the symptoms of pain. The symptoms are often vague and transient and do not respond well to standard treatments for acute pain. While Kim does benefit from treatments that are designed to reduce arousal and improve coping skills, she continues to report the symptoms of pain leading to increased disability.

CASE ILLUSTRATION 3 (CONTD.)

Kim was discharged from the multidisciplinary pain procedure program and returned to the care of her primary care physician. In collaboration with her doctor, Kim agreed to continue with her use of the antidepressant medication and to gradually reduce and discontinue her use of muscle relaxant and opioid medications. Consideration was given to use of low-dose NSAIDs. In addition, a physical therapy regime was initiated that included walking in the swimming pool three times a week for 1 month, followed by light aerobic exercises three times a week and, finally, active physical therapy for muscle fitness. It was agreed that hot packs and massage could be used for temporary relief in lieu of the opioid or muscle relaxant medication. She was to continue her relaxation practice throughout the day and agreed to continue CBT to assist with coping.

After 6 months of treatment Kim was able to improve her function and daily activity sufficiently to return to work on a full-time basis. She was able to plan for her future wedding with her now fiancé and reported that her total body pain had reduced substantially, but "waxed and waned" intermittently.

In the absence of a known etiology and in the presence of known social or behavioral stressful life events that are likely participating in the physical symptoms, the doctor works as a "change agent" to help the patient return to as normal a life as possible, minimizing medicines and medical procedures, while maximizing therapies that invite patient participation in an effort to return as much normal function as possible.

Treatment Guidelines

Pain description:	Reported total body pain in all four quadrants of her body with increased sensitivity for 16 of 18 tender points with 9 lbs of pressure.
Pain impact:	Discontinued work and compromised her ability to support her family.
Pain history and examination findings:	History is positive for GERDs, two thoracic procedures with diagnosis of thoracic outlet syndrome and cervical spondylosis and cervical laminectomy. Patient was asymptomatic for 10 years following surgeries before onset of total body pain.
Diagnostics:	MRI revealed old cervical repair with no abnormalities.
Primary diagnosis:	Fibromyalgia.
Comorbid diagnosis:	Depression with agitation.
Treatment recommendations:	*Medical*: Continue antidepressant medication. Taper and eliminate muscle relaxant opioid medication. Initiate treatment with low-dose NSAIDs. Establish a Patient Medication Agreement, where patient keeps written records of her medications and exercise schedule, and doctor agrees to be responsive to patient by telephone within 24 hours, should she experience a flare-up in-between monthly visits.
	Physical: Walking in the swimming pool three times a week for 1 month followed by light aerobic exercise three times a week followed by active physical therapy for muscle fitness.
	Behavioral: Continue CBT for problem solving and improved coping. Biofeedback could be considered.

CANCER PAIN FROM ACUTE TO CHRONIC

 CASE ILLUSTRATION 4

Jorge is a 58-year-old Hispanic man who presented to the emergency room with complaint of severe right upper quadrant pain. Jorge was admitted to the hospital for observation, evaluation, and diagnostics. Initially, Jorge was treated with oral short-acting opiates for pain control but during the night Jorge's report of pain increased. It was decided to initiate the use of a PCA (patient-controlled analgesia) pump so that Jorge could exercise a degree of control over the use of opiates for his own pain relief and remove the nurses from the role of being "drug cops." Jorge was able to find an appropriate level of pain relief, and the nursing staff could function as "behavioral coaches," that is, encouraging relaxation and providing reassurance to reduce fear while the medical evaluations and diagnostics were being scheduled. Jorge's wife as the primary caregiver was allowed to be present throughout his hospital course and involved in all levels of decision making. Jorge was later diagnosed with colon cancer.

In acute stages of pain, allowing the patient as much control as possible, including medications for pain relief, as well as reducing fear and anxiety about being in a foreign environment such as a hospital, can inject some degree of normalcy into the situation and can lead to enhanced pain relief at the time and later on.

 CASE ILLUSTRATION 4 (CONTD.)

Jorge returned 18 months later with progressive weight loss and right upper quadrant pain. Chemistries and imaging studies confirmed multiple metastases in the liver. He was increasingly fatigued and was forced to leave his job as an electronics technician. He now reported that his pain now included the entire abdomen, present constantly, but worse in the evening and with any activities. He is married, has five children, and his spouse is employed. A schedule was arranged to allow at least one of his children to be present to help him and his wife each day. Despite this help, he was becoming increasingly incapacitated and complained of pain with minor tasks. His family was concerned that he was "always in pain and losing the will to live."

Cancer pain represents a physical and psychological challenge to both providers and patients. Often pain is an outgrowth of simple tissue destruction by advancing tumor mass. Accompanying this, however, is the progressive loss of "hardiness" (strength, independence, and social identity) that accompanies the cancer. Patients often believe that cancer is a painful condition; for example, it has been shown by verbal report that sciatic pain hurts more and requires more analgesia after a malignant diagnosis is made. In addition, the patient suffers changes in a number of key roles in the face of the disease. As Jorge gives up the roles of parent, spouse, and worker, his pain behavior increases to match his new dependency. Finally, anxiety about both deteriorating health and family responses increases the pain.

CASE ILLUSTRATION 4 (CONTD.)

A meeting with the patient and family was scheduled specifically to address the issue of pain. Cancer pain treatment was reviewed, with an explanation of the importance of identifying and dealing with biological, social, and psychological issues that affect the pain. At the time of this examination, only abdominal pain with radiation to the back was identified as a limiting pain.

Although cancer has a devastating and lasting effect on family function, involving the family in treatment decisions and planning is crucial. An early discussion of the effect of the pain on the patient and his family is the key to the collaborative treatment of pain. If the patient and family do not understand how the physician needs to integrate treatment as an aspect of daily life, they often feel that reports of pain are being discounted or diminished. Similarly, soliciting and supporting the use of home and cultural remedies can further this communication and collaboration. Medications to control cancer pain must be used effectively, regularly, and in adequate doses. Opiates should be used with time contingent dosing around the clock in long-acting form rather than on an as-needed basis. As-needed medications encourage both patient and family to gauge the pain, thus providing an unnecessary focus on the pain. The use of inadequate pain medication may also lead to distrust and resentment between patient and physician. Specific adjunctive medications can be used to afford more relief with less sedation (NSAIDs for bone pain, steroids for pain associated with local inflammation and edema, Baclofen for muscle spasm, and sedatives for insomnia).

Cognitive-behavioral interventions can be tailored to the specific family and cultural circumstances of the patient. In the case of Jorge, his family expects him to yield his traditional roles and to need help as his disease and pain behavior increases. Therapy can thus be directed to both patient and family with the goal of increasing the patient's independence and decreasing the family's tendency to respond to all of his pain behaviors with fear. In addition, Jorge believes that cancer is painful and disabling, neither of which is to be tolerated. This attitude engenders helplessness and suffering. Behavior therapy should address this belief with techniques to provide control over his pain, such as single-symptom autogenic training, relaxation, hypnosis, or CBT. For example, the patient can be trained to interpret sensations as routine rather than threatening. In this way, he and his family can learn to accept rather than potentially distort his disease and pain.

Treatment Guidelines

Pain description:	Right upper quadrant pain, progressive weight loss, and fatigue.
Pain impact:	Jorge takes on the sick role, relinquishes role of parent and spouse, and is forced to leave work. Psychologically, there is a loss of hardiness (strength, independence, and social identity).
Pain history and examination findings:	18 months of progressive weight loss, upper quadrant pain, fatigue, and distended abdomen. No previous history of abdominal pain or cancer.
Diagnostics:	Chemistries and imaging studies confirm colon cancer with metastases to the liver.
Primary diagnosis: Comorbid diagnosis:	Colon cancer, Duke's stage C. Situational anxiety with symptoms of depression.
Treatment recommendations:	*Medical:* Time contingent adequate dosing of opiate to maximize pain relief; use adjuvants to manage symptoms and establish a collaborative approach to patient care. *Physical:* Encourage return to as normal as possible physical functioning around the house. *Behavioral:* CBT to assist with attitude changes and improve pain control. *Alternatives:* Cultural remedies should be considered.

SUMMARY

In this chapter, we presented several approaches to the treatment of persons suffering various types of pain that emphasize the evaluation and treatment of not only the biological but also the psychological and social implications of the problem. Clinicians are encouraged to use the three-function model for interviewing and ongoing communication with their patients (see Chapter 1). The following key principles should guide the treatment of pain:

- **Identifying pain as an issue:** Address pain directly and comprehensively (including medical, social, and psychological factors) at the onset, instead of when it becomes a problem.
- **Pain behaviors:** Whereas the patient may be quick to understand the pain largely as derived from the precipitating event or factors, the treating clinician must always attend to the social causes and consequences of the pain and its implications in the patient's behavior at work, home, and in play.
- **Meaning and impact of pain:** Cultural influences may dictate differing attitudes and roles in the expression of pain. Changes in lifestyle or work can have a profound effect on quality of life.
- **Clinician as "change agent":** In addition to providing direct treatment and advice, the clinician can influence adherence to treatment by maintaining a quality relationship with the patient.
- **Improved function is the goal of treatment:** The clinician's attention and focus can influence the patient's thoughts and behaviors. By commenting on improving function as an indicator of healing, the clinician can redirect the patient's attention away from the pain and toward increased functioning.

SUGGESTED READINGS

American Pain Society: *Pain Control in the Primary Care Setting.* Glennview, IL: American Pain Society, 2006.

American Pain Society: *Principles of Analgesic Use in the Treatment of Acute Pain and Cancer Pain*, 5th ed. Glennview, IL: American Pain Society, 2003.

Anderson VC, Burchiel KJ. A prospective study of long-term intrathecal morphine in the management of chronic non-malignant pain. *Neurosurgery* 1999:44(2):289–300.

Benedetti C, Brock C, Cleeland C, et al. NCCN practice guidelines for cancer pain. *Oncology* 2000;14:135–150.

Catalano E, Hardin KN, eds. *The Chronic Pain Control Workbook: A Step-by-Step Guide for Coping With and Overcoming Pain*, 2nd ed. Oakland, CA: New Harbinger Publications, 1999.

Caudill M. *Managing Pain Before it Manages You.* New York, NY: Guilford Press, 2002.

Gatchel RJ, Okifuji A. Evidenced-based scientific data documenting the treatment and cost effectiveness of comprehensive pain programs for chronic nonmalignant pain. *J Pain* 2006;7(11): 779–793.

Hay EM, Mullis R, Lewis M, et al. Comparison of physical treatments vs. a brief pain management program for back pain in primary care: a randomized clinical trial in physiotherapy practice. *Lancet* 2005;365:2024–2030.

Kobasa SC. Stressful life events, personality and health: an inquiry into hardiness. *J Pers Soc Psychol* 1979;37:1–11.

McCracken LM, Turk DC. Behavioral and cognitive-behavioral treatment for chronic pain, outcome, predictors of outcome and treatment process. *Spine* 2002;27:2564–2573.

Olsen Y, Daumit GL. Opioid prescribing for chronic nonmalignant pain in primary care: challenges and solutions. *Adv Psychosom Med* 2004;25:138–150.

Rakel B, Barr JO. Physical modalities in chronic pain management. *Nurs Clin North Am* 2003;38:477–494.

Turk DC. Clinical effectiveness and cost effectiveness of treatment for patients with chronic pain. *Clin J Pain* 2002;18:355–365.

Winterow C, Beck A, Gruener D. *Cognitive Therapy With Chronic Pain Patients.* New York, NY: Springer, 2003.

PATIENT SELF-HELP RESOURCES

American Pain Foundation. www.painfoundation.org. Accessed October, 2007.

Catalano E, Hardin KN, eds. *The Chronic Pain Control Workbook: A Step-by-Step Guide for Coping With and Overcoming Pain*, 2nd ed. Oakland, CA: New Harbinger Publications, 1999.

Caudill M. *Managing Pain Before it Manages You*, revised edition. New York, NY: Guilford Press, 2002.

Chronic Pain Support Group. www.chronicpainsupport.org. Accessed October, 2007.

HIV/AIDS

Lisa Capaldini, MD, MPH & Mitchell D. Feldman, MD, M.Phil

INTRODUCTION

Infection with the human immunodeficiency virus (HIV) is associated with a range of social, emotional, and neuropsychiatric complications. While HIV/AIDS has become a potentially manageable chronic disease, living with HIV/AIDS continues to be a practical and psychospiritual challenge. Persons at highest risk for HIV/AIDS (we use the term HIV/acquired immunodeficiency syndrome [AIDS] to designate the entire spectrum of clinical manifestations of HIV disease, from asymptomatic infection through advanced AIDS) are disproportionately likely to suffer behavioral and mood disorders and to be socially disenfranchised and economically disadvantaged. Once infected, they must contend with a stigmatized, contagious, and if untreated, a relentlessly progressive medical condition. In addition, many people with HIV have other significant comorbid conditions, such as chronic hepatitis, psychiatric problems, and/or substance use that may make adhering to HIV treatment more difficult. Although undiagnosed and untreated patients with HIV/AIDS can present with life-threatening neuropsychiatric sequalae of HIV (central nervous system [CNS], opportunistic infections, HIV dementia), most patients' behavioral concerns will be focused on maintaining medication adherence, maximizing quality of life, and managing lifestyle issues.

EPIDEMIOLOGY & PREVENTION

Human immunodeficiency virus is primarily transmitted through sexual exposure or shared injection drug paraphernalia (sharing needles). Initially, an epidemic concentrated among gay men in cities, new cases of HIV infection now are disproportionately seen in socioeconomically disadvantaged populations, especially women and men of color. Some patients do not fit "classic" risk factor profiles. For example, a monogamous woman may be infected through her husband who is bisexually active. Although past HIV prevention programs successfully reduced rates of new HIV infections in gay men, incidence of new HIV infection in multiple patient populations is significant. These patient groups include men who have sex with men but who do not self-identify as "gay," speed users who share straws for intranasal use, teenagers, elders, and women. In the United States, almost one-third of the approximately 1 million HIV-positive persons have never been tested and are not being treated. In spite of the great advances in prognosis with antiviral therapy, HIV/AIDS remains underdiagnosed and undertreated in the United States and worldwide.

In 2006, the Centers for Disease Control (CDC) formally modified its HIV screening recommendations from that of focused testing in high-risk groups and in high prevalence settings to universal testing. In this paradigm, *all* patients are encouraged to be tested as part of routine preventative care, and detailed consent procedures modified to opting in or out of HIV testing as part of routine care. Newer rapid testing procedures allow for patients to receive their results at the time of testing, improving the number of patients who receive their results and facilitating triage for medical follow-up. Importantly, these simplified tests—involving oral swabs or finger sticks—are as sensitive as the enzyme-linked immunosorbent assay (ELISA)/Western blot tests, which require phlebotomy and more time to be processed.

Integrating HIV screening and HIV prevention counseling into routine health care maintenance activities can facilitate this discussion in primary care settings. For example, following discussion of other lifestyle/health-related issues like cigarette smoking and exercise, sexual practice, and substance use questions a practical context. As in all patient interviews, open-ended questions with the use of specific and understandable language is most likely to put the patient at ease and generate accurate information. For example:

- Are you sexually active with men, women, both, or neither? How about in the past?
- What, if any, street drugs do you use, for example, speed, pot, etc? How about in the past?

The purpose of these screening questions is not only to identify which patients to test but to identify high-risk behaviors that may be modified, for example, through condom use or needle exchange. Thus, HIV testing is paired with HIV prevention counseling, pairing screening with harm reduction education. Harm reduction programs like needle exchange clearly reduce the spread of HIV infection but have not been implemented in most communities due to political and social concerns about promoting drug use; these concerns are not supported by research. Substance use, including alcohol, is highly correlated with unsafe sex behaviors, and all patients need to be educated about the risk of combining recreational substances and sexual activity.

Because HIV/AIDS is a significant under-recognised and undertreated public health problem in the United States, generalist practitioners in both the outpatient and inpatient settings must become competent in its screening and prevention.

THE PSYCHOSOCIAL IMPACT OF HIV/AIDS

Overview

Although the course of HIV/AIDS is different for every patient, some common clinical and life events are associated with psychological distress, ranging from mild anxiety and discouragement to feelings of despair and suicide.

Later in the course of illness there may be loss of employment or a reduction in responsibilities, consequent financial hardships compounded by heavy medical expenses, and dislocation or alienation from established social networks. Fatigue, pain, and other symptoms may diminish quality of life. Weight loss and disfiguring body composition changes (e.g., lipodystrophy) may lead to loss of pride and bodily integrity as well as privacy concerns (patients initially who chose not to disclose their HIV diagnosis may be forced to do so). Although persons with HIV undergoing treatment are unlikely to suffer from life-threatening opportunistic infections, they may remain or become disabled, often from the side effects of medication or from residual fatigue and cognitive dysfunction. For most patients, the challenge is learning to live with the hardships and limitations imposed by chronic HIV disease. Importantly, some patients with HIV may be relatively asymptomatic, and with the exception of taking daily medication and having periodic medical monitoring, have lives relatively unaltered by their HIV disease. Clinicians should periodically reassess the impact of HIV on each patient's life and use supportive services as appropriate.

Women and men with HIV benefit from empathic relationships with their medical providers and from connections with other HIV-positive people. For example, in adherence studies of adult women with HIV, a robust predictor of medication compliance is the patient's perception of her relationship with the clinician. In addition, women who meet other women with HIV (through retreats, support groups, newsletters) are more likely to be medication adherent and keep medical appointments.

In many urban areas, support groups exist for HIV patients from diverse risk groups (e.g., patients in recovery, gay men with HIV, and so on). In more rural and underserved areas, public health departments may offer case-management services for people with HIV. In some cases, these case managers may be the only local source of information, clinician referral, and psychosocial support for patients.

COUNSELING PATIENTS WHO TEST POSITIVE FOR HIV

For most patients, getting an HIV diagnosis is traumatic. In some cases, patients may be unaware that use of highly active antiretroviral therapy (HAART) has transformed HIV disease from a relentlessly fatal to a potentially manageable chronic condition. For other patients, the distress attendant to an HIV diagnosis is about identity and life choices: Will I be able to date or marry? Can I have children? Can I continue to do the work I do? Will I be able to get health insurance? Practitioners must anticipate this distress and counsel patients with up-to-date information, and arrange referrals to appropriate HIV care sources, including medical providers and support groups. Web sites can be excellent resources and are best complemented by local support services.

Patients who test positive for the presence of HIV may experience and express a variety of emotional responses (see Chapter 3). In general, the practitioner should allow the patient to express his or her feelings, and should actively listen to the expressed emotions in a nonjudgmental manner. Effective use of empathic statements such as: "I can understand how difficult this must be for you" and "We can work on this together" can help the patient to feel a little less overwhelmed and helpless when informed of a positive test result.

Clinicians should be alert to the potentially wide range of emotional responses expressed by patients and then check their understanding with a reflective statement such as "You seem quite suddened by this news." Often, the emotion that unexpectedly wells up in the physician (e.g., sadness, anger, panic) is indicative of what the patient also feels. Physicians can use their own emotions as diagnostic information to help gain insight into the patient's feelings (see Chapter 2).

Paradoxically, although many persons seek testing to relieve the uncertainty of not knowing their status, testing positive for HIV can create additional uncertainty. This can be quite unsettling for patients, especially those for whom maintaining tight control over their lives has been highly valued. Suddenly, they are confronted with not knowing how long they will remain well, who will care for them if they become ill or debilitated, how they will support themselves, and many other unknowns. The physician can help the patient cope with this sudden uncertainty by providing both information and emotional support. It may be helpful to say: "Many people who test positive are concerned because they do not know what to expect—is this true for you?" Some patients are comforted by the physician's acknowledgment that they are the same person they were before the test, but now they possess new information about their health that can be addressed. For example, the clinician can say: "You are the same person today as you were yesterday, only now you *know* that you are HIV-positive. It is important that you have this information so that we can now work on keeping you healthy." Patients should be given up-to-date information about treatment, prognosis, and other medical data, especially if they request it. It has been shown that distress can be decreased if patients are informed about their disease and the treatment options.

Physicians should also remember that informing patients of their HIV status is different from informing them of other medical illnesses because of the stigma still associated with HIV. This may be especially true for gay men who, in addition, have to deal with the social and personal consequences of being gay, such as discrimination, homophobia, and at times, feelings of shame and isolation. It may be important to address these issues of social stigma and shame to help patients cope with their seropositive status. Referral for individual counseling is often helpful.

Other emotions that the seropositive patient may express include anger, fear, denial, and depression. Patients may feel angry for many reasons: about having an incurable illness, about perceived loss of control, about current or future discrimination. Some patients are angry at themselves for having become infected or at the partner who may have transmitted the virus to them. Allow patients to express their anger and frustration; often the anger dissipates with empathic listening.

Fear is often a less evident emotion and may need to be elicited with questions such as: "What are your major fears about HIV?" and "From your experience with other people with HIV, what kinds of things are most frightening for you?" Seropositive persons may fear loss of job, friends, or health insurance or have more global fears of declining health, increasing pain, or becoming a burden on family or friends.

These fears should be acknowledged as legitimate, and when possible, the physician can help the patient to deal concretely with those problems that can be anticipated and ameliorated. It may be helpful to have the patient make two lists dividing the current or anticipated problems into those that are to some extent controllable and those that are basically uncontrollable. The controllable problems can be addressed through specific **problem-solving** strategies, but the clinician should focus on **emotion-handling skills** for the basically uncontrollable problems and emotions that arise (see Chapters 1 and 2).

Denial is a common response to the news of a positive HIV test. For some patients this initially may be a healthy way of not allowing themselves to be overwhelmed by potentially devastating information. In fact, some people need several months to a year to come to terms with the diagnosis. If, however, denial leads patients to harm themselves (e.g., by refusing potentially life-enhancing or life-extending treatment) or to harm others by exposing them to HIV, the physician should challenge the denial. This can be done gently, for example, by saying: "I can understand why you would wish that you were not infected, but you are, and we need to deal with it." Such statements may need to be repeated at subsequent visits until the patient is ready to accept the fact and consequences of seropositive status.

Depression and anxiety are also common responses in persons who test positive for HIV. The clinician should assess the severity and duration of these symptoms to determine the appropriate treatment. Some studies have found that the risk of suicide is substantially increased in the 3–6 months following a serologic diagnosis, so all patients should be screened for *reactive depression and suicidal ideation.* It is best to use direct, open-ended questions such as: "How are you handling your HIV diagnosis?" and "What fears or concerns do you have?"

In the weeks and months following a positive test, the clinician can assist patients in coping more effectively by assessing their social support system. This can be done by asking: "Who are you talking to about your concerns and issues?" If patients are isolated, provide them with phone numbers of local AIDS service organizations. Family members can also provide valuable support, but often HIV-infected people avoid seeking their help, or the family has previously rejected them because of their lifestyle. Clinicians can help patients by offering to have family or significant others attend medical appointments, and by integrating supportive others into the treatment team.

The Lazarus Phenomenon

Some adults diagnosed with HIV/AIDS, particularly those diagnosed prior to 1996, expected to die from their disease. For those patients who now benefit from HAART, surviving with HIV can be a paradoxical burden—having planned to die, soon, these patients may have spent their savings, stopped school, left jobs, and made other decisions that make their living with HIV pragmatically and spiritually difficult.

In the gay male population, many of these "Lazarus" survivors, in addition to HIV-negative gay men, may feel bewildered, guilty, and angry that they survived while scores of friends and lovers died. These spiritual struggles may result in substance use, HIV medication adherence problems, depression, or unsafe sex. Empathic acknowledgement by the clinician of the paradoxes of living with HIV disease can validate these patients' feelings and struggles. Patients with persistent symptoms should be referred for group and/or individual therapy.

Managing Substance Use

Active substance use is a risk factor for HIV acquisition, for medical nonadherence, and for re-exposure to HIV through unsafe sex and needle sharing. Many cases of new HIV infection are correlated with unsafe sex during alcohol or drug binges, even in cases where patients clearly understood the how's and why's of safer sex. Patients in drug and alcohol recovery have been shown to be able to achieve good adherence. All patients with current or past drug or alcohol problems should be screened for comorbid psychiatric disorders.

Methadone has significant interactions with nonnucleoside reverse transcriptase inhibitors (NNRTIs) and protease inhibitors (PIs). These interactions are not always predictable (e.g., one agent, nevirapine, can both raise and lower methadone levels). When antiviral drugs are changed, patients should be monitored for both methadone intoxication and withdrawal, and their methadone treatment center informed of the need to adjust the methadone closage.

Many street drugs, for example, heroin and ecstasy, are metabolized by cytochrome P450 3A4 and 2D6 enzymes, enzymes which may be downregulated by a PI booster, ritonavir. Inadvertent drug overdoses have occurred due to these interactions. Patients who continue to use street drugs and who are on HAART should be counseled in a harm reduction model about these potentially fatal interactions.

WORKING WITH ASYMPTOMATIC & SYMPTOMATIC PATIENTS

CASE ILLUSTRATION 1

Juan, a 27-year-old Hispanic man with HIV infection is admitted with shortness of breath and fever, and diagnosed with PCP (Pneumocystis carinii pneumonia). He was started on HAART (efavirenz, FTC, tenofovir) 6 months ago when his T cells were 210 but he did not keep his follow-up appointment. Once interviewed, he reported that his

antivirals made him "dizzy" and "sleepy" and that he stopped them because he was unable to work while taking them. He was unaware that he needed to take this regimen at bedtime to avoid these symptoms. An HIV genotype test showed no resistance and a plan was made to reinitiate these antivirals once his PCP treatment was completed. While hospitalized, he was visited by an adherence counselor and a case manager who helped review his regimen and identify adherence barriers, as well as help with scheduling his clinic follow-up.

Without treatment, many persons will remain asymptomatic for several years after infection with HIV. During this stage, regular preventive medical care includes periodic testing of surrogate markers of disease progression including CD4 lymphocyte counts ("T cell counts") and HIV viral load. Waiting for and receiving these results can be intensely stressful for patients. Physicians must counsel patients prior to testing about the clinical variability in the test, about the limited clinical significance of a one-time change in counts, and about plans for repeat testing and other follow-up in the event of specific results. Nevertheless, the clinician must anticipate that, despite reassurances, any decline in CD4 count may be deeply discouraging. This is particularly true when the CD4 count drops below one of the current staging thresholds, which, although serving only as rules of thumb to experienced HIV clinicians, still represent important clinical benchmarks in the course of HIV/AIDS.

Clinicians use trends in CD4 cells, viral load, and the presence of significant symptoms (fever, weight loss) to determine when antiviral treatment should be initiated. For many patients, especially those familiar with potential medication side effects, needing to start antiviral medication in and of itself may feel like "the beginning of the end" and reduce the patient's sense of health and integrity. Involving patients in the timing and choice of antiviral medications may reduce their anxiety and improve long-term adherence with antiviral medications. When patients know what side effects are possible with each medication, and what the demands are of different HAART regimens, they can assist the clinician in selecting the most workable antiviral combination. Adherence to a medication regimen is a challenge for all patients with chronic illness (see Chapter 17) and adherence to HIV medications is an especially crucial skill for HIV-positive patients. Depending on the "backbone" of the regimen, up to 95% adherence is necessary to suppress HIV replication and prevent drug resistance from emerging. Newer HIV treatment paradigms underline that HAART regimens differ in how "forgiving" they are of nonadherence—with NRRTIs being the least resilient and with boosted protease inhibitors being the most "forgiving." Skilled clinicians take these differences into account when selecting and reformulating HAART regimens.

Ironically, while HAART adherence is critical to success, it is difficult to predict or measure. Multiple studies have revealed that even skilled HIV/AIDS practitioners are often inaccurate at assessing or predicting any individual patient's medication compliance. Across studies, active substance use, untreated psychiatric and disorders, isolation, transportation problems, health system barriers (to visits or to pick up medications), and changes in routine are risk factors for nonadherence. On the positive side, patients who experience their clinicians as knowledgeable, trustworthy, and approachable are more likely to comply with their medications, reinforcing the importance of the clinician–patient relationship.

Clinicians should assess and address adherence initially and on an ongoing basis. Open-ended and supportive questions are useful: "How are you doing with remembering your meds?" "How many doses did you miss yesterday? Last week?" "Are you having any side effects that cause you to skip doses?" This assessment provides important clinical information and reinforces the critical importance of medication adherence for the patient.

For most patients, linking doses to routine activities (walking the dog, brushing teeth, waking the children) is helpful. Medisets, beepers, periodic adherence checks by case managers may also be helpful. Clinicians can regularly reassess each patient's regimen, considering off-label but studied dosing schedules that may be more user-friendly than on label dosing. During periods when the patient is at high risk of nonadherence, temporarily suspending antivirals (a structured treatment interruption) may be preferable to poor adherence.

SPECIAL ISSUES & POPULATIONS

Hepatitis B & C Coinfection

All patients with HIV should be offered screening for chronic hepatitis B and C. For some patients learning they have chronic viral hepatitis, in addition to HIV, can be overwhelming. In addition, evaluation for treatment of hepatitis B and C may involve liver biopsy, and currently available treatments for hepatitis C (interferon, ribavirin) can cause severe flu-like symptoms, major depression, and cytopenias.

The clinician should assess each patient's ability to cope with another diagnosis and plan diagnostic studies accordingly. Patients on an interferon-containing regimen should be closely monitored for depression. Noting the high incidence of interferon-associated depression and its role in treatment discontinuation, some

investigators have advocated prophylactic antidepressant therapy.

Women

Isolation and stigma are especially common in women with HIV. Irrespective of how they acquired HIV, women fear being judged "a whore or an addict." Women may be especially fearful about disclosing their HIV status for fear of domestic abuse, loss of child custody, or loss of employment. Referral to local and national organizations is often helpful (see "Web Sites," at the end of chapter).

Pregnant women with HIV benefit from multidisciplinary care teams that can both optimize their HIV care and provide appropriate perinatal care to mother and baby. They should be advised about the risks and appropriate management of perinatal transmission of HIV, and that with HAART the risk of vertical transmission can be reduced to 1%.

Chronic Pain

Chronic pain is a common complication of HIV disease that is often underdiagnosed and undertreated. Specific causes of chronic pain include postherpetic neuralgia, peripheral neuropathy, avascular necrosis (AVN), and HIV myelopathy (spinal cord dysfunction). In 10% of HIV patients with chronic pain a specific etiology is not found.

Untreated pain can cause insomnia, depression, substance use, and medication nonadherence. Patients at highest risk of undertreatment are women, minority patients, and patients with prior or active substance use. General pain management principles (see Chapter 32) are used in treating HIV-associated pain: attempt to make a specific diagnosis to target treatment, but do not forego treating pain in the absence of a firm etiologic diagnosis.

Many analgesic and adjunctive medications (e.g., tricyclic antidepressants [TCAs], carbamazepine, methadone) are metabolized through cytochrome P450 and may interact with NNRTIs and PIs. Gabapentin (Neurontin), Lamictal (lamotrigine), Lyrica (pregabalin), nonsteroidal anti-inflammatory drugs (NSAIDs), acetaminophen, and aspirin have no significant interactions, but their use may be complicated by rash, sedation, renal dysfunction, and other side effects. In patients requiring narcotic therapy, longer-acting agents supplemented by fast-acting narcotics as needed for breakthrough are generally most effective.

While formal studies have failed to demonstrate that acupuncture is effective for HIV-associated pain syndromes, many patients and clinicians have observed significant benefits both for reducing pain itself and helping patients cope with pain.

Fatigue

Many patients with HIV, even those successfully treated with antivirals, suffer from disabling HIV-related fatigue. Typically, patients wake with a good deal of energy only to develop severe fatigue with minor activities. Many patients will need to nap and sleep longer than is usual for them. Researchers have speculated that this fatigue may be due to cytokine effects in the brain, neuroendocrine dysregulation, and/or autonomic/circadian rhythm dysregulation.

Before ascribing fatigue to idiopathic HIV-associated fatigue, an extensive differential diagnosis should be considered including depression, anemia, testosterone, deficiency, sleep apnea, chronic hepatitis, hypothyroidism, chronic pain, and medication side effects. Idiopathic HIV-related fatigue may respond to bupropion (Wellbutrin) or stimulants. Patients who are otherwise well and wish to resume a full life need validation that their fatigue is real and need to be informed that even with aggressive treatment their stamina may remain limited.

NEUROPSYCHIATRIC COMPLICATIONS

Management of Neuropsychiatric Complications of HIV/AIDS

Clinicians caring for HIV infected patients must be able to identify specific syndromes (e.g., depression, psychosis), formulate preliminary differential diagnoses, and make appropriate psychotherapy and psychopharmacologic referrals. HIV-related neuropsychiatric syndromes are evaluated and treated with the following guidelines:

1. HIV-associated opportunistic infections, which may present as behavioral disorders, are very uncommon in patients with >200 CD4 cells or in patients with <200 CD4 cells and low or undetectable viral loads.
2. Side effects of prescription or over-the-counter medication commonly cause neuropsychiatric symptoms.
3. Drug interactions (both with prescription and recreational drugs) are of special concern in patients receiving potent suppressors of cytochrome P450 3A4 and 2D6, particularly ritonavir.
4. Recreational drug use and withdrawal can cause symptoms directly or exacerbate preexisting disorders (e.g., bipolar affective disorder).
5. With a few exceptions, HIV-associated neuropsychiatric symptoms are guided by the same treatment principles as for the general population; most psychiatric medications are used at the same dosages and for the same indications.

DRUG EFFECTS

Some of the medications used to treat HIV/AIDS and its complications have common neuropsychiatric side effects. Side effects may be related to cumulative dose or to peak levels but may be unpredictable and idiosyncratic. Furthermore, in patients with advanced HIV disease, the homeostatic mechanisms responsible for maintaining therapeutic drug levels may be disrupted by end-organ involvement, such as decreased renal excretion, hepatic metabolism, or cardiac output; diminished body fat; immunologic dysregulation; and a predisposition toward dehydration. These patients with HIV are therefore also more susceptible to side effects from more commonly used medications. The rule of thumb for prescribing to persons with advanced HIV is "say no, start low, and go slow," that is, avoid unnecessary medications, use reduced dosages of those that are necessary, and increase doses slowly and cautiously. Most patients, however, *will* require conventional doses of medications used to treat psychiatric disorders, so the edict "go slow" includes reaching therapeutic doses eventually.

Drug effects and toxicities must always be considered in the initial differential diagnosis of any neuropsychiatric abnormality. Table 33-1 describes the adverse reactions associated with some drugs commonly used in the treatment of HIV/AIDS. A few general principles should be kept in mind. First, use agents with favorable side effect profiles. Second, use caution in the coadministration of medications with similar side effect profiles or those that significantly affect one another's pharmacodynamics. An example of the first situation is the simultaneous use of any combination of antidepressants, antihistamines, neuroleptics, or antimotility agents, all of which have substantial anticholinergic effects.

The second concern arises in the use of agents such as rifampin or rifabutin, which induces the hepatic cytochrome P450 enzyme system and thereby accelerates metabolism of many other drugs or conversely, agents such as ritonavir or delavirdine which inhibit the P450 enzyme.

A third concern is that adherence to complex medication regimens is often unreliable. Incorrect dosing may result in undertreatment for some conditions, but confusion may also result in inadvertent overdosing. Always simplify the regimen and use the lowest dose of the fewest drugs likely to be effective. The assistance of a pharmacist is invaluable in addressing these concerns. If possible, the regimens of patients with advanced HIV/AIDS or on multiple medications should be periodically reviewed by a pharmacist.

Persons with HIV/AIDS on average have higher levels of substance use, in part because of the association between preexisting drug use and the risk of acquiring HIV/AIDS, and perhaps because of self-medication for depression or anxiety. Stimulant drugs such as cocaine or amphetamines can cause agitation, psychosis, or delirium, as can withdrawal from sedating drugs such as benzodiazepines and alcohol. Sedatives and narcotics can of course cause somnolence, confusion, and psychomotor slowing but

Table 33-1. Psychiatric side effects of drugs used to treat HIV infection.

Drugs	Adverse Reaction	Comment
Antiretroviral		
Zidovudine (AZT)	Mania, anxiety, auditory hallucinations, confusion	Idiosyncratic reaction; resolves within 24 h after stopping drug (rare).
Didanosine (ddI)	Anxiety, irritability, insomnia	Idiosyncratic reaction; self-limiting, does not require drug discontinuation (rare).
Efavirenz	Confusion, abnormal thinking, impaired concentration, abnormal dreams, insomnia, amnesia, hallucinations, euphoria	Up to 50% of patients experience symptoms that may start on day 1 and last 2–4 weeks; only 2–5% require discontinuation of the drug.
Antivirals		
Acyclovir	Lethargy, delirium, hallucinations, agitation, paranoia	Dose-related reaction, more common after high-dose oral or parenteral therapy, or in patients with renal impairment. Uncommon with dihydroxyphenylglycol (DHPG).
Ganciclovir (DHPG) Foscarnet	Hallucinations, confusion	Association uncertain. Alterations in calcium and magnesium levels are contributory.
Antimicrobial		
Amphotericin B	Delirium, confusion	Rare reports; might be related to hyperthermia and irreversible leukoencephalopathy.
β-Lactam antibiotics	Confusion, paranoia, hallucinations, mania, coma	Dose-related; high doses in patients with renal dysfunction; increased risk with procaine penicillin.
Quinolones	Psychosis, delirium, seizures, anxiety, insomnia, depression	Dose-related; high doses in patients with renal dysfunction
Sulfonamides	Psychosis, delirium, confusion, depression, hallucinations	Dose-related; high doses in patients with renal dysfunction and the elderly. Direct neurotoxic effect.
Isoniazid (INH)	Paranoia, confusion, anxiety, hallucinations	Doses exceeding 17 mg/kg/day. Intravenous pyridoxine recommended.
Dapsone	Mania, psychosis, anxiety	Several reports in patients with overdosages; resolves within 24 h after discontinuation.
Anabolic steroids	Mania, psychosis, depression, aggressiveness	Anecdotal reports in patients receiving 10–100 times the recommended doses; abrupt withdrawal after prolonged usage.
Dronabinol (Marinol)	Anxiety, confusion, psychosis, mania, depression, hallucinations	Dose-related; self-limited, usually resolves within 12 h after acute usage; abrupt withdrawal produces similar symptoms.
Opiates	Delirium, psychosis, depression, nightmares, hallucinations	Dose-related; might be more frequent with tincture of opium and long-acting narcotics; responds to dose reduction.
Corticosteroids	Mania, "steroid psychosis," depression, euphoria	Dose-related >40 mg/daily of prednisone; resolves with dosage reduction.
TCAs, neuroleptics, and other anticholinergics	Confusion, hallucinations, delirium, psychosis, mania, anxiety	Dose-related; resolves within 24–72 h after stopping the drug. Physostigmine 1–2 mg intramuscularly or intravenously can reverse toxicity.
Fluoxetine	Anxiety, insomnia, mania	Administer in morning; can inhibit metabolism of TCAs and phenytoin and increase their toxicity.
Benzodiazepines	Confusion, disorientation, paradoxical agitation, paranoia and rage; rebound anxiety and insomnia	Related to abuse and abrupt withdrawal after prolonged therapy. Increased risk with short-acting agents.

can also cause paradoxical reactions, including agitation, paranoia, and rage. This may be especially true of the short-acting benzodiazepines.

With regards to specific antiviral agents, two specific points need emphasizing. Firstly, delavirdine or ritonavir-containing regimens, through inhibition of cytochrome P450 enzymes, *may* dramatically raise the level of many prescribed and recreational drugs. These substrates include many anticonvulsants (carbamazepine, valproic acid, phenytoin), narcotics (meperidine, methadone), recreational drugs (3,4-methylenedioxymethamphetamine [MDMA] or Ecstasy), and other agents (warfarin, digoxin, estrogen). Patients receiving these cytochrome P450 inhibiting antivirals should be monitored carefully for these potential interactions (see Table 33-2 for a list of psychotropic medications that interact with the cytochrome P450 system).

Secondly, the first 2 weeks after starting efavirenz, patients may experience disrupted sleep, depression, agitation, and exacerbation of previously stable psychiatric disease. While anecdotal reports of delayed or persisting neuropsychiatric symptoms due to efavirenz have also been reported, a prospective double-blinded study failed to show any lingering or delayed CNS side effects attributable to the medication. Patients with stable psychiatric disorders may be prescribed efavirenz but should be monitored for drug-associated agitation or depression. All patients who are starting efavirenz should be provided with sleeping medication for the first 2 weeks,

either a standard benzodiazepine, or if substance misuse is a concern, a low-dose atypical antipsychotic.

Depression

 CASE ILLUSTRATION 2

Marjorie, a 36-year-old ex-intravenous drug user with a 5-year history of stable HIV disease (undetectable viral load, T cells 500 on HAART), is noted to have a viral load of 14,000. On interview, she reports missing "a few" doses due to "spacing out," "just forgot." She has maintained her sobriety but is not attending Narcotics Anonymous (NA) meetings— "too tired." On further questioning, she reports morning fatigue, insomnia, anhedonia, and hopelessness. A diagnosis of depression is made and she is offered initial treatment with therapy or medication. After attending a support group she recognizes that she has been "depressed a long time" and agrees to both counseling and psychopharmacologic treatment. Because she also has chronic pain from peripheral neuropathy, a dual-active/ serotonin norepinephrine reuptake inhibitor (SNRI) medication is initiated with the hope of decreasing pain, improving sleep, and treating her depression.

Table 33–2. Clinically important cytochrome P-450 psychotropic interactions in the treatment of patients with HIV/AIDS.

Psychotropic Medication	Key Enzyme	Clinical HIV Implications
Fluoxetine, paroxetine	2D6, 3A4	May raise PI levels, but not to a clinically significant extent; increased TCA levels
Steraline	2D6, 3A4	Milder effects, not significant
Citalopram	3A4, 2C19	Not clinically significant
Venlafaxine	3A4, 2D6	Few drug–drug interactions
Mitrazapine	3A4, 2D6, 1A2	Not clinically significant
Bupropion	2B6, 3A4	Levels raised with PIs; sezure risk
Nefazodone	3A4	Significant inhibitor; caution with PIs or NNRTIs
Lithium	None	Renally excreted ion
Valproate	2D6	Ritonavir interactions
Alprazolam, triazolam, zolpidem, zaleplon	3A4	Increased sedation with PIs
Risperidone	2D6	Avoid with ritonavir
Olanzapine	1A2, 2D6	Cigarettes will decrease levels
Seroquel	3A4	No reported PI or NNRTI interactions
Ziprasidone	Not significant	Check QTc duration
St. John's wort	3A4	May lower levels of PIs

Reproduced from Levine JM: Psychiatric aspects of HIV care. AIDS Clin Care 2001;13:106.

Major depression is the most common psychiatric disorder in persons with HIV/AIDS. The lifetime incidence is unknown but rises dramatically as the disease progresses. As with non-HIV-infected depressed patients, the cardinal symptoms include depressed mood, anhedonia, feelings of worthlessness and hopelessness, disturbances in sleep and appetite, weight loss or gain, fatigue, psychomotor slowing, agitation, and preoccupation with morbid thoughts (see Chapter 22). A family history of an affective disorder or alcoholism may be present. Depression may be more difficult to diagnose in the presence of HIV/AIDS, however, for several reasons. First, its manifestations, and particularly the vegetative symptoms commonly (fatigue, weakness, weight loss, and loss of libido), overlap with the constitutional symptoms commonly attributable to HIV infection or its complications. Second, the multiple losses that many persons with HIV/AIDS often experience may result in a chronic grieving state that shares many of the affective aspects of depression. Third, thoughts of death and suicide may be viewed as appropriate or rational as disease progresses. Fourth, organic impairment due to the HIV-associated dementia complex may have affective manifestations. Fifth, HIV-associated hypogonadism (low testosterone) may cause fatigue, impaired libido, and other depressive symptoms. For some patients, testosterone supplementation has been shown to reverse depressive symptoms. Finally, some medications and the use of or withdrawal from other psychoactive substances, can have mood-altering effects as described previously. Nevertheless, depressive disorders including major depression and dysthymia are diagnosed by the same criteria for HIV-infected as for non-HIV-infected persons and should never be treated as a normal finding. Indeed, recent surveys have documented that untreated depression is a major correlate of poor quality of life in people with HIV disease, and is an important risk factor for HAART non-compliance.

The clinician should screen for depression with open-ended questions such as: "How have things been going for you lately?" or "How are you coping with all of this?" Certain clues may help to distinguish depressive from constitutional symptomatology. For example, progressive fatigue that worsens with exertion and over the course of the day is characteristic of somatic disease (e.g., anemia), whereas an inability to get going in the morning, which improves with activity, may suggest depression. Similarly, nondepressed patients may report that nausea or dysgeusia (an abnormal sense of taste) interferes with their appetite, whereas depressed patients often report simply no interest in eating. Nondepressed patients often report their symptoms and limitations with frustration and concern, whereas apathy and resignation are more characteristic of major depression. Anhedonia and a sense of worthlessness are rarely symptoms of a somatic condition, and should

therefore be directly investigated as specific indicators of depression. Depressed patients may appear more anxious or preoccupied than sad. Patients with depression and anxiety may self-medicate with recreational drugs or alcohol; patients with substance use should be screened carefully for depression and anxiety disorders.

The treatment of depression in HIV/AIDS does not differ from the non-HIV-infected population. Regular, empathic listening and short-term psychotherapeutic techniques may be very effective. Explicit recognition and validation of the patient's losses and fears help to establish a trusting therapeutic relationship and may permit developing joint strategies to cope with them. Emphasizing that depression is a common ailment in the setting of HIV/AIDS and is amenable to treatment is important. All nonmonoamine oxidase inhibitor (MAOI) antidepressants (selective serotonin reuptake inhibitors [SSRIs], SNRIs, TCAs, bupropion) can be used to treat depression in patients with HIV disease. As with other patients, choosing among the many available agents should be largely a matter of selecting the most desirable or tolerable side effect profile. While most antidepressants have drug interactions with HAART regimens, most are not clinically significant.

The clinician must be alert to how the activity and toxicity profile of particular agents may help in simultaneously addressing other concerns of the patient. For example, appetite and sleep-stimulating medications such as mirtazapine may be effective in patients who suffer from insomnia. A TCA such as nortriptyline may be an ideal choice in a patient with neuropathic pain, who may also benefit from the drug's pain-modulating effects. The risk of cardiac arrhythmias associated with tricyclic drugs may be increased in persons taking the antivirals ritonavir and delavirdine. Bupropion is especially useful in patients with fatigue, and along with mirtazapine are unlikely to cause sexual dysfunction. SSRIs are especially useful in patients with anxious depression or comorbid anxiety disorders.

Stimulants may be used with other antidepressants in patients with severe refractory fatigue, and can also be used to palliate narcotic-associated fatigue and sedation. Because of their abuse potential, these agents must be used selectively, and their efficacy varies considerably from patient-to-patient.

Tearfulness, anhedonia, preoccupation, agitation, and insomnia may characterize an acute grief reaction, which can be expected in the wake of bereavement or at any of the life transition points or disease progression benchmarks mentioned previously. Grieving persons often benefit from emotional and social support and spiritual counseling, and group or individual psychotherapy may be effective in encouraging adaptation. It is appropriate to treat short-term insomnia or agitation with limited courses of benzodiazepines. If vegetative symptoms persist or normal social functioning remains significantly impaired beyond 1 month after the acute loss, treatment for depression should be considered.

Major depression dramatically increases the risk of suicide, which is no more the result of a "rational" choice in persons with HIV than it is in the depressed non-HIV-infected population. Attempting suicide is correlated with a history of psychiatric treatment, substance abuse, persistently high levels of psychological distress, HIV-related interpersonal and occupational problems, poor perceived social support, and recent evidence of disease progression. Physicians should be prepared to intervene under such circumstances with crisis counseling, social support, and psychiatric hospitalization.

Occasionally for patients with advanced HIV suicide may indeed appear to be an attractive and rational alternative to continued deterioration. Perhaps most importantly, the idea that suicide is eventually an option is a comfort to many persons with HIV/AIDS and other chronic degenerative diseases, for whom it represents ultimate control over their condition, and a hedge against the fear of complete dependence and debilitation. Physicians must walk a fine line, detecting and intervening to prevent depression-associated suicide, but remaining careful not to take away the comfort and hope that ultimate control over one's fate confers. Regardless of physicians' own ethical or religious positions on physician assisted aid in dying, they must be willing to openly and honestly probe and discuss the patient's suicidal thoughts and, most importantly, the fears and concerns that have led to them. As with requests for aid in dying, a discussion of suicide with one's physician is often a disguised cry for help. It may reflect exasperation or exhaustion over symptoms inadequately treated, fear of uncontrollable future pain or suffering, anxiety over burdening caregivers, or the desperate need to be reassured that one will not be abandoned by care providers in one's time of greatest need. What begins as a discussion about suicidal thoughts often ends in the discovery of previously unsuspected or unarticulated fears and needs, a situation that permits physician and patient to work together to chart a clear, practical course to address them.

Anxiety

As with some depressive symptoms, anxiety may be a normal response to many of the stressors associated with living with HIV. Symptoms of anxiety may include poor concentration, restlessness, preoccupation or intrusive thoughts, insomnia (particularly trouble falling asleep), and fatigue. Persons with poor coping skills may be particularly prone to periods of uncontrollable anxiety. Withdrawal from nicotine, alcohol, or illicit drugs, or overuse of caffeine may cause symptoms of anxiety. Some medications used adjunctively in HIV/AIDS, particularly corticosteroids and decongestants, can produce anxiety or agitation, and, rarely, agitation may be the presenting manifestation of underlying CNS disease.

Treatment is indicated if anxiety impairs social or occupational functioning, or is persistently uncomfortable. Pharmacotherapy generally involves the use of SSRIs and other serotonergic antidepressants or benzodiazepines. For episodic and unpredictable bouts of anxiety, short- to medium-acting benzodiazepines, such as lorazepam (Ativan) or alprazolam (Xanax) are generally more effective, due to their more rapid onset of action. The physician should carefully monitor the frequency of refilling of anxiolytic prescriptions; a pattern of escalating use may suggest that a longer-acting agent or antidepressant therapy is preferable. For chronic disabling anxiety, longer-acting benzodiazepines such as clonazepam (Klonopin), which maintain more stable blood levels, may be more effective and better tolerated. SSRIs are useful maintenance agents in the treatment of anxiety syndromes like panic disorder, obsessive-compulsive disorder (OCD), and posttraumatic stress disorder (PTSD).

Patients with anxiety symptoms should be screened for PTSD. PTSD symptoms include easy startling, flashbacks or nightmares, and dissociative symptoms. For some patients, the trauma of living with HIV rekindles memories of prior traumas (abuse, rape, accidents). Studies of incarcerated women with HIV have demonstrated a high rate of PTSD. PTSD is best treated with focused counseling although SSRIs have been shown to help alleviate some of its symptoms.

PRIMARY CNS DISEASE—THE HIV-ASSOCIATED DEMENTIA COMPLEX

Human immunodeficiency virus-associated dementia is a subcortical dementia characterized initially by cognitive and behavioral dysfunction and in its most advanced stages by motor dysfunction. Advanced HIV dementia is rarely seen in patients with more than 200 CD4 cells or who are on HAART. Although antivirals differ in their penetration of cerebrospinal fluid (CSF), all combinations of antivirals that suppress serum viral load are likely to prevent HIV dementia. Rarely, genotypic analysis of CSF and blood reveals the presence of different HIV strains. In these rare cases, some experts recommend that antiviral medication may need to be adjusted to treat the CSF strains.

All patients with HIV dementia should be evaluated for comorbid depression, as depressive symptoms can easily be misattributed to dementia. A trial of antidepressants may result in gratifying functional improvement in these patients. As in all patients with organic brain disease, sedating agents like antihistamines and benzodiazepines should be used with great caution and in general avoided.

Anticholinesterase inhibitors, used to treat Alzheimer disease, have not been studied in patients with HIV dementia. These agents are unlikely to be useful in HIV dementia, however, as they have shown utility only in cortical dementia, and theoretically could exacerbate a subcortical dementia such as HIV.

HIV-associated Minor Cognitive Disorders

Although HIV dementia is rare in HIV patients undergoing treatment and in patients with more than 200 CD4 cells, minor cognitive problems can persist and even progress in patients with good surrogate markers (e.g., adequate CD4 cells and/or suppressed viral load). HIV-associated minor cognitive disorders are characterized by word-finding problems, difficulty sequencing complex tasks, and immediate memory dysfunction. Patients may note pauses in conversations while searching for words, difficulty performing clerical tasks and functional forgetfulness (e.g., misplacing keys, forgetting medicines).

Minor cognitive disorders may persist or progress in patients who are otherwise responding well to antiviral therapy. While minor cognitive disorders tend not to progress, they are often disabling, despite patients appearing "normal." These cognitive symptoms need to be carefully recorded in patients charts should disability status need to be assessed. Formal neuropsychiatric testing can document subtle cognitive dysfunction but is rarely more clinically useful than a thorough history. Neuroimaging studies performed in research settings have correlated loss of both frontal lobe volume and frontal metabolic activity in patients with these symptoms.

Delirium

Delirium is an acute confusional state that includes disorientation, inattention, and an altered sensorium or disorganized thinking. It is *never* simply a manifestation of HIV/AIDS and should always be considered to reflect a potentially life-threatening acute disorder that has affected the CNS. Patients with cognitive impairment due to the HIV-associated dementia complex or other underlying brain pathology are at particular risk for having delirium precipitated by a metabolic insult, but the dementia itself is never the sole cause of delirium. The list of possible complications of HIV/AIDS that may cause delirium essentially overlaps the differential diagnosis of delirium, with the specific addition of opportunistic infections in patients with CD4 counts under 200. Delirium is generally of abrupt onset and is marked by fluctuating consciousness, poor attention, disorganized thought and speech, and perceptual abnormalities such as visual or auditory hallucinations. It may also be accompanied by either extreme agitation or apathetic withdrawal.

The search for and correction of the underlying abnormalities must be undertaken emergently, in a closely supervised setting such as an intensive care unit. Depending on patients' level of consciousness, frequent attempts may be made to keep them oriented, with careful attention paid to lighting and noise so that sensory stimulation is adequate but not overwhelming. Mechanical restraints should be avoided if possible but are sometimes necessary to prevent patients from injuring themselves or from pulling out lines and catheters. Agitation commonly complicates delirium and can be managed with escalating doses of atypical antipsychotics (e.g., olanzapine, risperdal) or haloperidol, and if necessary, with short-acting parenteral anxiolytics. Delirium should be aggressively treated with these agents while diagnostic studies are in progress.

Mania

Mania can be a terrifying and dangerous complication of HIV/AIDS. As in non-HIV-infected persons, mania is characterized by hyperactivity and psychomotor restlessness, euphoric or irritable mood, insomnia and perceived decreased need for sleep, pressured or rapid speech, grandiosity or paranoia, racing thoughts, distractibility, hypersexuality, and reckless or disinhibited hedonistic behavior. Mania in HIV/AIDS can be due to a preexisting bipolar diathesis precipitated by substance use, stress, or intercurrent illness. Less frequently, mania may be an initial manifestation of HIV-associated organic brain disease like opportunistic infections or dementia. Medications reported to cause mania include high-dose corticosteroids, antidepressants, zidovudine, efavirenz, and stimulant drugs such as cocaine and amphetamine derivatives.

Treatment involves first discontinuing any potential pharmacologic precipitant and ensuring a safe social environment. No specific antimania drug is best for HIV-associated mania—pragmatically, agents should be selected with the goal of calming the patient without undue sedation. Lithium, a mainstay of treatment for bipolar affective disorder in non-HIV-infected patients, is risky for patients with advanced AIDS in whom levels appear to fluctuate unpredictably. Dehydration, due to diarrhea, fever, or poor intake can quickly result in toxic lithium levels, further complicating management. However, lithium can be used safely in medically healthy HIV patients.

Psychosis

As with mania, psychotic symptoms are generally due to underlying psychiatric disease (schizophrenia) or drug (prescription, recreational) side effects. Psychotic symptoms include hallucinations, typically auditory rather than visual; delusions, which tend to be paranoid in content; looseness of association; and flight of ideas.

Personal care and hygiene may be neglected, and medication adherence is poor. Use of or withdrawal from many illicit drugs, including amphetamines, phencyclidine, cocaine, alcohol, marijuana, and opiates, may cause a transient psychosis, and psychosis caused by methamphetamine in particular may last for days or weeks. Psychosis may complicate administration of the anticytomegalovirus drugs ganciclovir and foscarnet, anabolic or corticosteroids, zidovudine, efavirenz, opiates, other psychoactive pharmaceuticals including sedatives and antidepressants, and, very rarely, many ordinary antimicrobial agents (Table 33-1). Psychosis is a rare manifestation of underlying secondary CNS infection or neoplasm.

Treatment of HIV/AIDS-associated psychosis involves identification and removal of precipitating drugs and treatment as appropriate of underlying disease. Psychiatric consultation is essential to confirm the diagnosis, identify possible secondary causes, and optimize management. Atypical antipsychotic agents are effective in acute and maintenance treatment of psychosis. These atypical agents are less likely to cause tardive dyskinesia and are less sedating than older agents.

Many patients with schizophrenia and HIV are "triply diagnosed," that is, they also use recreational substances. These patients often benefit from day treatment programs where medical treatment is integrated with their mental health care, and where medication adherence can be facilitated through directly observed therapy.

CONCLUSION

Like all chronic medical disorders, HIV disease can be complicated by a myriad of psychiatric and spiritual challenges—isolation from one's family or community, re-emergence of previously stable psychiatric disease, the transition from planning to die of HIV disease to learning to live with it—and many others. Some patients acquire HIV as a result of their psychiatric disorders; other people with HIV face psychospiritual challenges as they attempt to not only survive, but also thrive, with HIV.

Although all patients benefit from accurate psychiatric assessment, patients also benefit from an ongoing relationship with a clinician they perceive as knowledgeable, caring, and trustworthy. In the authors' experience, no other area of medicine requires such a skillful integration of the science and the art of medicine, nor offers such rewards for doing so.

SUGGESTED READINGS

Kalichman HC, Heckman T, Kochman A, et al. Depression and thoughts of suicide among middle-aged and older persons living with HIV-AIDS. *Psychiatr Serv* 2000;51(7):903–907.

Low-Beer S, Chan K, Benita Y, et al. Depressive symptoms decline among persons on HIV protease inhibitors. *J Acquir Immune Defic Syndr* 2000;23(4):295–301.

Treisman GJ, Angelino AF. *The Psychiatry of AIDS: A Guide to Diagnosis and Treatment.* Baltimore, MD: John Hopkins University Press, 2004.

WEB SITES

ACTIS (AIDS Clinical Trials Information Service) Web site. http://www.actis.org/. A central resource for federally and privately funded HIV/AIDS clinical trials information. Accessed October, 2007.

HIV Insite Web site. http://hivinsite.ucsf.edu/InSite. Provides comprehensive up-to-date information on HIV/AIDS treatment, prevention, and policy with links for clinicians and patients. Accessed October, 2007.

Project Inform Web site. http://www.projinf.org. An HIV advocacy organization that issues up-to-date information about HIV research. Accessed October, 2007.

WORLD Web site. http://www.womenhiv.org/. A national support group for women with HIV. Accessed October, 2007.

Mistakes in Medical Practice

34

Albert W. Wu, MD, MPH, Stephen J. McPhee, MD, & John F. Christensen, PhD

INTRODUCTION

Mistakes are inevitable in the practice of medicine. The most obvious causes are failures in individual performance, such as attention, memory, knowledge, judgment, skill, and motivation. However, they also result, in part, from the nature of medical work, such as the complexity of medical knowledge, the uncertainty of clinical predictions, and the need to make timely treatment decisions in spite of limited or uncertain knowledge. And importantly, mistakes are caused by system factors that influence working conditions. Although much attention has been focused on the effects of errors on patients, it must be understood that medical mistakes are correspondingly distressing for physicians, evoking shock and feelings of remorse, guilt, anger, and fear.

If dealt with effectively, mistakes can provide powerful learning experiences for physicians; however, difficulty in dealing with mistakes may impede both learning and efforts to prevent future errors. Professional norms that assume physician infallibility and treat mistakes as anomalies also pose significant barriers to learning. Judgmental institutional responses and fear of litigation are further disincentives to the open discussion of mistakes. Although some individuals may learn from their own mistakes and make appropriate changes in practice, others are less likely to benefit from these lessons.

Definitions

It is useful to define a number of terms related to what are commonly referred to as "mistakes" or "errors." The Institute of Medicine (IOM) defines an **error** as "the failure of a planned action to be completed as intended (i.e., error of execution), or the use of a wrong plan to achieve an aim (i.e., error of planning). An error may be an act of commission or an act of omission." An **adverse event** is an injury due to health care (IOM, 2000). **Errors** differ from negligence or malpractice in that an error is not necessarily a proximate cause of harm to a patient. It is also clear that not all judgments that precede bad outcomes are necessarily wrong.

Prevalence

Most studies of medical error have focused on the hospital setting and on adverse events rather than mistakes. Although the overall prevalence of medical mistakes is difficult to ascertain, it appears that they are common. One of the earliest studies examined hospitals in New York State in 1984, and found that injuries occurred in nearly 4% of admissions, with one quarter of these judged to have been due to negligence. A study using the same methodology on hospitals in Colorado and Utah in the 1990s found that adverse events occurred in 3.5% of admissions.

In 2004, the Canadian Adverse Events Study reported on the incidence of adverse events among hospital patients in Canada. The authors randomly selected 4 hospitals (1 teaching, 1 large community, and 2 small community hospitals) in each of 5 Canadian provinces and reviewed a random sample of charts for nonpsychiatric, nonobstetric adult patients hospitalized in each hospital during 2000. Trained reviewers screened all eligible charts, and physicians reviewed the positively screened charts to identify adverse events and to determine whether they were preventable. After adjustment for sampling, the adverse event rate was 7.5 per 100 hospital admissions (7.5%). Among the patients with adverse events, events judged to be preventable occurred in 36.9% and death in 20.8% (95% CI 7.8–33.8%). According to the physician reviewers, the adverse events were associated with an estimated 1521 additional hospital days. Although men and women experienced equal rates of adverse events, older patients had significantly more adverse events than younger patients.

From the physician's viewpoint, in a 1991 study of 254 medical residents by the authors, 114 (45%) responded and reported a significant mistake made during the prior year. In a cohort of internal medicine residents followed between 2003 and 2006, 34% reported making at least one major mistake, with 14.7% reporting making an error each quarter.

The prevalence of mistakes in outpatient practice is just beginning to be studied, but one investigator has documented a prescription error rate of 7.6%, and another suggests errors in at least one quarter of encounters. Some studies of ambulatory specialty clinics suggest prescription errors in the majority of patients.

Types

Mistakes occur in every aspect of medical practice—in diagnosis, in decision making (often because of ignorance of facts), in the pace of evaluation or its timing, in prescribing medications, and in performing tests and procedures (Table 34-1). The Harvard Medical Practice Study found that among 1133 patients with disabling injuries caused by medical treatment, 28% of the injuries were judged to be due to negligence. The most common adverse event involved performance of or follow-up of a procedure or operation (35%). Failure to take preventive measures (e.g., failure to guard against accidental injury) was the next most common error (22%), followed by diagnostic errors (e.g., failure to use indicated tests, act on test results, or avoid delays in response) (14%), errors involving drug treatment (9%), and system errors (2%). A critical subset of diagnostic errors arises through cognitive errors, especially those associated with failures in perception, failed heuristics, and biases. Errors also occur elsewhere in the system, such as in the clinical diagnostic laboratories, the pharmacy, and the preparation and maintenance of medical devices.

Medication errors are very common, in part because of the ubiquity of the use of medications. In the United States, more than four out of five adults take at least one medication in a given week, and almost a third of adults take at least five different medications. The goal of safe and effective medication use is referred to as "the five rights:" the right drug, right dose, right route, right time, and right patient. However, errors can occur with any drug product at any point in the medication use process. It is estimated that over 1.5 million people are injured by medication errors each year and that, on average, hospitalized patients are subjected to an average of one medication error per day.

Causes

A combination of individual and system-related factors can lead to adverse events. Human error occurs close to the patient and includes deficits in skill (attention, memory, and execution), knowledge, decision making, and following of rules. Systems errors occur at multiple levels, including at the levels of patient, task, individual provider, team, unit environment, department, and institution (Vincent, 1998). Examples of specific factors include uncooperative patients, use of handwritten prescriptions, team members who are unfamiliar with one another, understaffed units, inadequate equipment, long work hours, and production pressures. It should be kept in mind that individuals are part of and function within the system of health care delivery.

Individual physicians report a variety of reasons for their mistakes and frequently attribute the mistakes to more than one cause. In one study, house officers most often reported that mistakes were caused in part because they did not possess specific essential knowledge (e.g., being unaware of the significance of a prolonged episode of ventricular tachycardia). Almost as often, they cited "too many tasks" (one resident neglected to continue a required medication because he was "too busy with other sick patients, and supervising interns and students"). Fatigue was a significant factor (after inadvertently ordering potassium replacement as a bolus, one resident commented, "It was 3:00 A.M., and I'm not sure I was completely awake").

A systems-oriented view acknowledges that errors are expected even in the best organizations. Many errors are caused by conditions in the workplace and organizational processes largely independent of clinician attributes. Studies of system factors demonstrate the predictive power of these characteristics independent of physician identity.

One study of an inpatient medical service found cross-coverage to be a significant predictor of preventable adverse events. Recent studies suggest that staffing ratios tend to be related to patient outcomes. The pressures of practicing medicine in a managed care setting, especially in capitated systems with higher demands for productivity, may increase the risk that a hurried physician will overlook important diagnostic information or make an error in prescription. Similarly, the incentives offered by third-party payers to order fewer diagnostic tests and to limit the number of referrals to subspecialists can lead to errors of omission.

Circumstances

Mistakes seem to occur frequently during residency training, possibly because interns and residents are learning new

Table 34-1. Types of medical mistakes.

Error	Example
Diagnosis or evaluation	Missed diagnosis
Medical decision making	Inappropriate or premature discharge
Treatment	Waiting when treatment is indicated
Medication	Incorrect dosage
Procedural complications	Faulty technique
Faulty communication	Failure to convey information during sign-out
Inadequate supervision	Failure to review treatment plan

Source: Adapted, with permission, from Wu AW, Folkman S, McPhee SJ, LoB. Do house officers learn from their mistakes? *JAMA* 1991;265: 2089–2094.

skills, honing their clinical judgment, and accepting new responsibilities. Additionally, they are caring for patients who are acutely ill. However, although first-year residents made the highest proportion of prescription errors (4.25 per 1000 orders) according to one study, even more experienced physicians have reported making serious medical mistakes.

Many mistakes happen in the inpatient or emergency department setting. The surgical specialties and intensive care units have also been identified as areas of high risk for patient safety. Severely ill patients require rapid assessment of a complex clinical picture as well as multiple procedures, evaluations, and decisions, thus affording many opportunities for mistakes to occur. One study found that patients in intensive care units had on average 178 activities performed on them, with 1.7 errors observed per day.

Patient characteristics can also increase the risk of mistakes. The risk of iatrogenic events increases with increased age, severity of illness, length of hospital stay, and number of drugs prescribed. Older patients, for example, are likely to have advanced disease and comorbid conditions and are more likely to be taking numerous medications. These factors increase both the risk of errors and the likelihood that complications of treatment will make these errors consequential.

Serious medical mistakes also occur in office practice. Some practicing physicians contend that the probability of making a serious error increases with more years in practice and particularly with greater pressures to increase productivity.

THE OUTCOMES OF MEDICAL MISTAKES

Consequences for Patient & Family

Errors, if recognized and corrected, may have no major consequences. In such cases, clinicians may not even acknowledge that a mistake has occurred. Often, however, errors have significant consequences for the patients involved, such as physical discomfort, emotional distress, need for additional therapy or procedures, increased and prolonged hospital stay, worsening of disease, permanent disability, or death. Mistakes can also cause distress for family members, including worry, anger, and guilt, particularly if they were involved in making treatment decisions.

Consequences for Physicians

Physicians also experience emotional distress in reaction to a medical mistake, often reporting a variety of emotional responses from remorse, anger, guilt, and feelings of inadequacy to shame and fear—particularly the fear of negative repercussions, such as malpractice suits. After a fatal mistake involving a young patient, one

house officer wrote, "This event has been the greatest challenge to me in my training."

Self-perceived errors have been associated with decreased quality of life, depression, and burnout among physicians. Some physicians report persistent negative psychological effects from mistakes. After a mistake caused the death of a patient, one house officer commented, "This case has made me very nervous about clinical medicine. I worry now about all febrile patients, since they may be on the verge of sepsis." For another house officer, a missed diagnosis made him reject a career in subspecialties that would involve "a lot of data collection and uncertainty."

Consequences for the Physician–Patient Relationship

In some cases, depending on the severity of the outcome for the patient and the quality of communication between physician and patient, the physician–patient relationship may be harmed by a mistake. For the physician, feelings of guilt and shame or shaken confidence may lead to avoidance of the patient or to a diminution of open and frank discussion. One physician, for example, reported that his guilt from the death of a patient led him to act like an indentured servant to the patient's family, attempting to expiate his "crime" over a prolonged period of time by spending more time with the family and reducing his fees.

For the patient, learning about a mistake may cause alarm and anxiety, destroying the patient's faith and confidence in the physician's ability to help. There may be anger, erosion of trust, decreased respect, or feelings of betrayal that diminish openness. Patients may become disillusioned with the medical profession in general, causing them to reduce their adherence to beneficial treatments or habits.

To the extent that the doctor and patient can discuss their emotions directly and with mutual understanding and acceptance, the relationship is likely to endure; it may even deepen with time. The negative effect of a mistake on the doctor–patient relationship may also be mitigated if there is a history of shared decision making, which diffuses the responsibility of the physician, especially when there has been uncertainty about treatment.

Mistakes that are nationally—or even locally—reported in the press can damage public trust in the medical profession. Any loss of credibility can be harmful to the public health by creating cynicism about medical care and research, and discouraging individuals from seeking care or adopting healthful behaviors.

RESPONDING TO MEDICAL MISTAKES

The way in which physicians respond to mistakes can turn these experiences into powerful opportunities for learning and for personal growth. Figure 34-1 outlines a

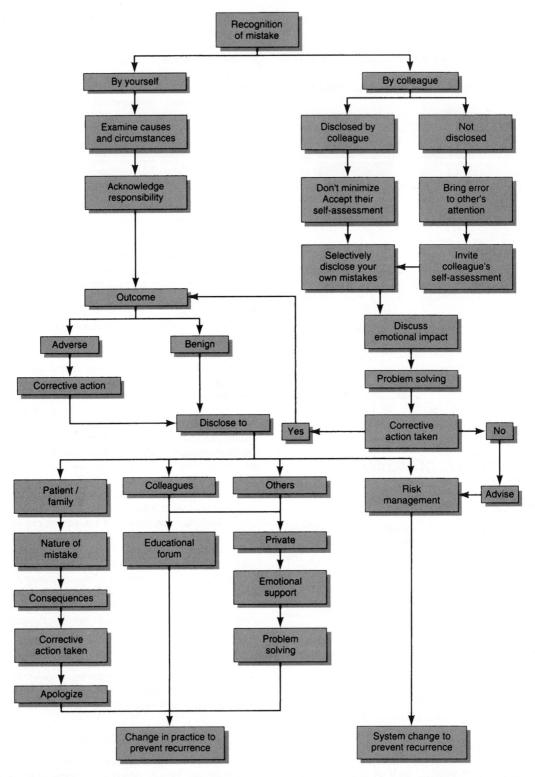

Figure 34-1. Process of responding to a mistake.

strategy for handling a mistake, whether made by oneself or by a colleague.

Individual Responses

After recognizing that a mistake has occurred, the first step is to take any corrective action possible, followed by beginning to cope, disclosure to the patient, disclosure to colleagues and Risk Management (sooner if there is a serious adverse outcome), and attempting to learn from the incident.

Coping With Mistakes

Two major modes of coping are *problem focused*, in which coping is directed at the problem causing the distress, and *emotion focused*, in which coping is directed at managing the emotional distress caused by the problem (Table 34-2). Effective coping can prevent unhealthy responses such as denial, cynicism, and excessive concern. The use of effective coping strategies can also play a role in modulating physician stress and increasing physician work satisfaction.

Table 34-2 briefly summarizes some of the many possible strategies for coping with medical mistakes. Among these, accepting responsibility and problem-solving techniques may be those most often used. As an example, "accepting responsibility" would include statements such as "I made a promise to myself that things would be different next time;" "I criticized or lectured myself;" and "I apologized or did something to make it up." Seeking

Table 34-2. Potential strategies for coping with medical mistakes.

Approach	Strategy
Problem focused	Acceptance of responsibility
	Consultation to understand nature of mistake
	Consultation to correct mistake
	Planned problem solving (e.g., obtaining extra training)
Emotion focused	Pursuance of social support
	Reframing of mistake (e.g., recognizing it as inherent in practicing medicine)
	Disclosure to colleague, friend, or spouse
	Disclosure to patient
	Emotional self-control (e.g., repressing one's emotional response)
	Escape/avoidance
	Distancing

Source: Adapted, with permission, from Wu AW, Folkman S, McPhee SJ, et al. How house officers cope with their mistakes: doing better but feeling worse? *West J Med* 1993;159:565–569; Christensen JF, Levinson W, Dunn PM. The heart of darkness: the impact of perceived mistakes on physicians. *J Gen Intern Med* 1992;7:424.

social support and controlling emotions may be somewhat less frequently employed, and escape/avoidance and distancing are used even more rarely.

Accepting responsibility is a prerequisite to an individual learning from a mistake, and physicians who cope by accepting responsibility for their mistakes seem to be more likely to make constructive changes in practice. They may also be more likely to experience emotional distress, however, as in the case of the resident who described persistent feelings of guilt and shame after realizing that inappropriate management of a diabetic patient's foot ulcer led to an amputation.

Disclosure to Patients & Families

It is difficult to disclose mistakes to patients or their families, and several reports suggest that physicians are reluctant to tell patients about mistakes. Studies suggest that physicians and trainees have conflicting feelings of responsibility to the patient, colleagues, institution, and themselves, complicated by fears and anxieties, and an uncertain self-efficacy and outcome expectancy. There are many barriers to disclosure, include fear for one's reputation, as well as fear of disciplinary action and litigation. Even the National Practitioner Databank, designed to improve quality of care, provokes fear and resentment among physicians. In one study, disclosure of mistakes to patients or families was reported by less than 25% of house officers.

Professional societies, including the American Medical Association and American College of Physicians, as well as legal and ethical experts suggest that in general physicians should disclose errors to those involved. In 2001, the Joint Commission on Accreditation of Healthcare Organizations stated that clinicians are obliged to disclose errors to the patient. Disclosure of a mistake also fosters learning by compelling the physician to acknowledge the error truthfully. In addition, when there are serious adverse consequences, disclosing a mistake to the patient may be the only way for the physician to achieve a sense of absolution. Lazare has suggested a framework for the use of apologies that includes four parts: (1) acknowledgement of the offense; (2) explanation for committing the offense; (3) expression of remorse, shame, and humility; and (4) reparation. In his article he suggests how these various aspects of an apology have the potential to heal.

Until recently, there have been no guidelines on how to tell a patient about a mistake that has been made. Therefore, physicians have developed their own approach to each case. Disclosure and discussion of an error with the patient or family can be made easier by several techniques. Physicians should first try to acknowledge their own emotions. Before approaching the patient or family, it may be helpful for physicians to perform a simple relaxation exercise and to remind themselves that the event and present feelings do not define them as either a healer or as a person. Rehearsing a few simple, direct statements ahead of time can provide a road map in this awkward moment. When meeting the patient or family, the physician should make a brief, direct statement, accompanied by a genuine apology. Such directness may help avoid the kind of long and rambling discussion that often increases anxiety for both physician and patient.

The physician who has mistakenly prescribed a medication without checking the patient's allergies, for example, might tell the patient: "Mr. Jones, I've discovered what made you sick last week. I regret to say that I failed to check whether you were allergic to the antibiotic before I prescribed it. You are allergic to it, and that information is clearly written in your chart. I feel awful that my not checking has caused you so much distress. I am truly sorry." It would then be appropriate to pause and allow the patient to respond. Reflecting and accepting the patient's feelings can help to heal the relationship more effectively than overwhelming the patient with information. The doctor–patient relationship can be enhanced by honesty and empathy in this difficult and sensitive moment (see Chapter 3).

It is possible that disclosure of an error of which the patient had been unaware may lead to a lawsuit, particularly if there was serious harm. However, it is certain that the risk of a lawsuit is multiplied if there is an attempt at covering up the mistake. Risk may be reduced if disclosure is made promptly, if the patient appreciates the physician's honesty, if it is part of an ongoing dialogue about the patient's care, and if there is a sincere apology. In the event of serious injury, a prompt and fair settlement may be the most helpful measure. There is little research on this topic. One recent study that modeled the potential litigation consequences of disclosure found that an increase in litigation volume and costs was highly likely. However, the favorable experience of the Lexington Kentucky VA Medical Center, which instituted a proactive policy of full disclosure and assistance for the patient in filing claims, as well as a reduction in claims experienced at the University of Michigan, suggests that this strategy may decrease the institution's losses.

Empirical research on the disclosure of medical errors to patients and their families has been limited. Published studies have focused primarily on the decision stage of disclosure. Fewer have considered the disclosure process, consequences of disclosure, or relationship between the two. More research is needed to understand how disclosure decisions are made, to provide physicians guidance on the process of disclosure, and to help all involved anticipate the consequences of disclosure.

Many publications have examined why patients sue their doctors. While they suggest that some lawsuits may be averted by disclosure of medical errors, these publications do not allow us to estimate the additional lawsuits that could be created by disclosure. More studies are needed of the effect of disclosure on physicians' malpractice liability. One recent study using video vignettes suggests that full disclosure is likely to have a positive or no effect on how patients respond to medical errors.

Disclosure to Colleagues & the Institution

It may be very important for colleagues to know about a mistake, particularly if they are also participating in the care of the patient as a supervisor or other member of the team. Knowing about a mistake can also benefit the institution, enabling it to provide assistance in handling the mistake, to help individuals appreciate the causes or significance of the incident and learn from the incident, and to prevent future occurrences. However, physicians also seem to be reluctant to tell their colleagues about mistakes. Some physicians report that they find this kind of discussion both threatening, because of the fear of judgment by colleagues, and unhelpful, because of the tendency of colleagues to minimize the event. Most often, discussing mistakes with colleagues serves the purpose of problem-focused coping: correcting the situation that led to the mistake. Sharing mistakes with colleagues can also prevent isolation and start the necessary healing process of remorse and learning. The authors have had positive responses from physicians who participate in a workshop on mistakes, in which participants first write a narrative account about a mistake they have made, then share the story of this mistake in small groups, emphasizing the emotional impact of the mistake and how they coped with it.

Changes in Practice

Table 34-3 summarizes changes in practice that often follow medical mistakes. These changes can either be constructive or they can be defensive—and maladaptive—in nature. Constructive changes cited by physicians include paying more attention to detail, confirming clinical data personally, changing protocols for diagnosis and treatment, increasing self-care, changing methods of communication with staff, and being willing to seek advice. Additional constructive action includes attempting to effect institutional change to prevent future incidents.

Physicians also report making defensive changes. These include an unwillingness to discuss the mistake, avoidance of similar patients, and—in some circumstances—ordering additional tests. Defensive changes in practice are more likely to occur if the institutional response to a mistake is punitive or judgmental.

Learning from Mistakes

Several factors may determine the extent to which physicians learn from mistakes. When negative emotions such as shame, guilt, or humiliation follow from the mistake,

Table 34-3. Common changes in practice following mistakes.

Constructive Change	Defensive Change
Increasing information seeking	Being unwilling to discuss the error
• Asking advice	Avoiding patients with similar problems
• Reading	Ordering additional but unnecessary tests
Increasing vigilance	
• Paying more attention to detail	
• Confirming data personally	
• Changing data organization	
• Ordering additional tests as appropriate	
• Improving screening for disease	
Improving communication with patients	
Improving self-pacing	
Improving communication with staff	
Supervising others more closely	

the physician's energy may focus on the emotional aspects of coping. Addressing these negative emotions directly can enhance the physician's ability to learn new information or new approaches to the problem. Failure to appreciate these emotions can lead to denial. The cause to which the physician attributes the mistake can also affect learning. Physicians in one study were more likely to report constructive changes if the mistake was caused by inexperience or faulty judgment in a complex case; they were less likely to do so if they believed that the mistake was caused by job overload. Physicians who responded to the mistake with greater acceptance of responsibility and more discussion were also more likely to report constructive changes.

Responding to Colleagues Who Make Mistakes

When responding to a colleague who discloses a mistake, it is important to try to elicit or accept the colleague's self-assessment and to not minimize the importance of the mistake. At this point, a selective and discreet disclosure of one's own mistakes can reduce the colleague's sense of isolation and legitimize the discussion. It is then appropriate to inquire about the emotional effect of the mistake and how the colleague is coping with it. An important consideration here is that

negative emotions are not necessarily problems to be solved, and they can often be mitigated by acknowledging them. The clinician should return to the content of the mistake and help the colleague to correct it with problem-solving techniques, making the necessary changes in practice and incorporating the new lessons that have been learned.

Witnessing Mistakes by Others

A physician who sees a mistake made by another physician has several options: passively waiting for the physician to disclose the mistake, advising the physician to disclose the mistake, actively telling the patient oneself, or arranging a joint meeting to discuss the mistake. Although some physicians may feel an obligation to report mistakes they have seen, most are reluctant to say anything. Here again, there are many barriers to discussion, including fear of eliciting anger and threatening relationships with colleagues or interference with sources of referrals.

The simplest option, of course, is to wait for the physician who made the mistake to report it. There is no assurance, however, that the patient will actually be informed. Telling the patient directly may be awkward, particularly if the observing physician does not know the patient, and may interfere with the existing doctor–patient relationship. Advising the physician who made the error to tell the patient may fulfill the observing physician's responsibility for disclosure, but the patient may still not be informed. Simultaneously advising the physician and the hospital or clinic quality-assurance or risk-management personnel increases the likelihood that the patient will be told. Arranging a joint conference can satisfy the observer that appropriate disclosure is made while preserving the primacy of the relationship between the patient and the treating physician (Figure 34-1).

INSTITUTIONAL RESPONSES

Hospitals

A goal for institutions is to develop a "safety culture" that allows learning from adverse events. A safety culture encourages clinicians to be aware of the potential for error and to include system thinking in their everyday practices, and it provides adequate data regarding errors to managers. Physicians sometimes feel that the hospital's atmosphere inhibits them from talking about their mistakes and that its administration is judgmental about mistakes. To avoid a vicious circle of blame, denial, and repeated problems, it is crucial for senior leadership in hospitals to assume a blame-free attitude that encourages the reporting and handling of errors. Some institutions have formal settings for discussing mistakes, such as morbidity and mortality conferences.

However, important issues such as a discussion of the physician's feelings about the mistake and disclosure by colleagues of how they coped with their own mistakes are commonly avoided in these conferences. The risk-management departments of hospitals could take a leading role in this area—promoting comprehensive, supportive forums for discussing mistakes and using emotion-focused coping to maximize problem-focused learning and to minimize future errors.

Graduate Medical Education

In spite of fears of public disclosure of mistakes, there is growing consensus that patient safety, physician fallibility, and methods of handling medical errors are appropriate topics for medical school, residency, and fellowship training. Although they may experience initial reluctance, physicians sometimes find that discussing a mistake is a positive experience: "Presenting this case at interns' report was difficult—I felt under a lot of scrutiny from my peers. In the end, I felt as though I had gotten more respect from presenting this kind of case rather than one in which I had made a great diagnosis."

Mistakes can be discussed in attending rounds, at morning report, or at morbidity and mortality conferences. When mistakes are discussed in these conferences, it is important to address issues such as overwork, shared responsibility with other physicians (e.g., consultants, attending physicians), and appropriate protocols for communicating with staff. These discussions also present a good opportunity to expose cognitive biases and explain strategies to reduce them. In addition, although ensuring that everyone involved learns from the mistake, care should be taken that errors are seen as an unfortunate inevitability in the practice of medicine and that there are appropriate ways of coping with them and of responding to colleagues who make them. A few institutions have begun to organize regular "fallibility rounds," interdisciplinary conferences focused on promoting patient safety that recognize the many factors that contribute to errors. To address variability in faculty response and local culture, institutions can disseminate clear, accessible algorithms to guide behavior when medical errors occur. Educators can develop longitudinal curricula that utilize actual cases and model faculty disclosure. Future work could focus on identified themes such as learning from errors and near misses, learning and teaching in emotionally charged situations, and balance between individual and systems responsibility.

Primary Care Practice Groups

As group practice becomes the norm in managed care settings, it is important that such groups implement procedures for responding to mistakes. Collegial support should be an explicit rule, providing a safe and confidential setting for discussion of the mistake (see the guidelines discussed earlier for responding to a colleague's mistake). It would also be wise for the practice group to formalize—and thus legitimize—periodic discussions about mistakes; these could broaden the scope of the emotion-focused support, allow members to learn from colleagues' mistakes, and address system flaws that contribute to the mistakes. A bonus of this approach is the gain in personal well-being of the group members—a nonspecific, yet significant, contribution to the practice climate.

PREVENTING MISTAKES

Reducing the frequency and severity of mistakes is the highest priority. There are several ways to help physicians learn from their mistakes and to make constructive changes in practice.

Physician Responsibility

As noted earlier, physicians should be encouraged to accept responsibility for their mistakes. Although those who do so seem more likely than those who do not to make constructive changes in practice, accepting responsibility for mistakes can engender emotional distress. It is therefore important for colleagues and supervising physicians to respond with sensitivity to the distress of practitioners acknowledging their mistakes. The probability of future mistakes can be reduced if the current error can be reviewed in a way that decreases emotional distress, invites disclosure of uncertainty in diagnosis and management, and leads to a discussion of appropriate changes in practice.

Many medication errors are caused by poor communication or misunderstandings about the use of medication. Therefore, the IOM recommends that patients maintain lists of their own medications and allergies, and that they take every opportunity to share these with their clinicians. Physicians should place greater emphasis on reconciling their own lists with the patients, and informing patients about appropriate medication use.

Simple, easily implemented safety strategies to prevent errors should not be overlooked. These include consistent use of a reliable method to verify patient identity, use of metric measurements, and adequate workplace illumination and organization. An interim step is for all drug orders to be in plain English, rather than in arcane Latin, apothecary script, with shorthand abbreviations that are subject to misinterpretation. Other strategies include elimination of abbreviations and acronyms, provision of up-to-date information at the point of care, and partnering with patients regarding their own safety.

Administration & Supervision

Efforts to forestall errors must begin at the highest administrative levels. Leadership acknowledgment of the inevitability of errors and making patient safety an explicit priority are crucial in helping institutions learn from mistakes. Clinically, more active supervision may prevent some mistakes or mitigate their adverse effects. Senior physicians should be more available to their less experienced colleagues for help in making critical decisions about patient care, especially in complex cases that require more mature clinical judgment. Group practice administrators and training-program directors should address problems in staffing, scheduling, and nature of work—which may all contribute to mistakes. Serious attention must be paid to the workload. Sleep deprivation has been shown to be a source of errors; job overload and fatigue can also lead to mistakes. Working under these conditions may teach house officers to tolerate and rationalize errors; in addition, it may make them less likely to seek the corrective information that could help prevent future mistakes. At the same time, using protocols, standardizing procedures, and employing checklists can help physicians do the right thing. For example, a "Sign Your Site" protocol for surgeons can help to eliminate the risk of wrong-site surgery, a "central line cart" providing needed supplies can help reduce catheter-related bloodstream infections, and a simple checklist can improve medication reconciliation as patients move from surgical recovery room to the ward.

Identifying & Reporting Errors

Delineating the cause of a mistake often suggests specific strategies for preventing future mistakes. Routine mechanisms to identify adverse events, such as anonymous reporting by physicians and nurses or computerized feedback about adverse drug reactions, are beginning to prove useful in providing information about the frequency and nature of mistakes. Developing routine methods of conveying information, such as computerized cross-coverage templates that standardize the type and amount of information exchanged between covering physicians, can also reduce errors.

It is important to take special care with newer medications, "look-alike/sound-alike" medications, and "high alert" medications that should be handled with deliberation, particularly in the high acuity settings of emergency department, operating room, and intensive care unit.

Workplace Design

A "human factors" approach seeks to "optimize the relationship between humans and systems by studying human behavior, abilities, and limitations and using this knowledge to design systems for safe and effective human use. Assuming that the human component of any system will inevitably produce errors, human factors engineers design human/machine interfaces and systems that are tough enough to reduce both the rate of errors and the effects of the inevitable error within the system.

Computerized Systems

Computerized systems can detect and avert medication errors, including overdoses, incorrect routes of administration, drug interactions, and allergies. Computerized order entry systems, automated medication-dispensing machines, and bar coding of medications, blood products, and patients have been shown to reduce the incidence of adverse events.

As part of a comprehensive set of recommendations, a 2006 report from the IOM suggested the elimination of handwritten prescriptions by 2010, with the adoption of computerized prescription writing that would also allow enabling clinical decision support systems.

It is essential, however, that new technology be introduced in a way that acknowledges the risks as well as benefits of such change. Health care workers must receive sufficient preparation and training so that technologies are not disruptive or that they themselves become inadvertent sources of error. There are risks entailed in an overreliance on automation in which vigilance becomes dulled, as was the case in the Chernobyl nuclear disaster.

Managed Care

The demands of practicing in a managed care setting may increase a busy physician's susceptibility to making mistakes. Fatigue, information overload, and increased pressure to be a more productive member of the practice by seeing more patients in less time can lead the physician to overlook important information. In addition, the role of the physician as the gatekeeper of referrals to specialists, along with financial incentives for holding down the number of referrals, tests, hospital admissions, and hospital days, has the potential for increasing errors of omission. Ironically, the risk of malpractice litigation may counter this tendency by inducing physicians to practice defensively by ordering more tests. Within the extremes of these incentives and disincentives, there is a need for continuing education of physicians on standards of practice with regard to tests, referrals, and further treatment.

At its best, managed care has the resources to make a positive system influence on patient safety through quality improvement programs, dissemination of best practices, consumer education, and integration of health services.

SUMMARY

Both physicians and institutions should make whatever changes in practice are warranted to prevent new mistakes and to prevent the recurrence of similar events. Recognizing and dealing with mistakes honestly and directly can improve the quality of patient care and lead to more rewarding practice.

SUGGESTED READINGS

Baker GR, Norton PG, Flintoft V, et al. The Canadian Adverse Events Study: the incidence of adverse events among hospital patients in Canada. *CMAJ* 2004;170:1678–1686.

Bates DW, Cohen M, Leape LL, et al. Reducing the frequency of errors in medicine using information technology. *J Am Med Inform Assoc* 2001;8:299–308.

Benjamin DM. Reducing medication errors and increasing patient safety: case studies in clinical pharmacology. *J Clin Pharmacol* 2003;43:768–783.

Berlinger N, Wu AW. Subtracting insult from injury: addressing cultural expectations in the disclosure of medical error. *J Med Ethics* 2005;31:106–108.

Borrel-Carrio F, Epstein RM. Preventing errors in clinical practice: a call for self-awareness. *Ann Fam Med* 2004;2:310–316.

Boyle D, O'Connell D, Platt FW, et al. Disclosing errors and adverse events in the intensive care unit. *Crit Care Med* 2006;34: 1532–1537.

Brennan TA, Leape LL, Laird N, et al. Incidence of adverse events and negligence in hospitalized patients: results of the Harvard Medical Practice Study I. *N Engl J Med* 1991;324:370–376.

Christensen JF, Levinson W, Dunn PM. The heart of darkness: the impact of perceived mistakes on physicians. *J Gen Intern Med* 1992;7:424–431.

Colford JM, McPhee SJ. The ravelled sleeve of care: managing the stresses of residency training. *JAMA* 1989;261:889–893.

Croskerry P. The importance of cognitive errors in diagnosis and strategies to minimize them. *Acad Med* 2003;78:775–780.

Elder NC, Vonder Meulen M, Cassidy A, et al. The identification of medical errors by family physicians during outpatient visits. *Ann Fam Med* 2004;2:125–129.

Fischer MA, Mazor KM, Baril J, et al. Learning from mistakes: factors that influence how students and residents learn from medical errors. *J Gen Intern Med* 2006;21:419–423.

Folkman S, Lazarus RS. *The Ways of Coping.* Palo Alto, CA: Consulting Psychologist Press, 1988.

Gallagher TH, Garbutt JM, Waterman AD, et al. Choosing your words carefully: how physicians would disclose harmful medical errors to patients. *Arch Intern Med* 2006;166:1585–1593.

Gallagher TH, Waterman AD, Ebers AG, et al. Patients' and physicians' attitudes regarding the disclosure of medical errors. *JAMA* 2003;289:1001–1007.

Gallagher TH, Waterman AD, Garbutt JM, et al. US and Canadian physicians' attitudes and experiences regarding disclosing errors to patients. *Arch Intern Med* 2006;166:1605–1611.

Gander PH, Merry A, Millar MM, et al. Hours of work and fatigue-related error: a survey of New Zealand anaesthetists. *Anaesth Intensive Care* 2000;28:178–183.

Gandhi TK, et al. Missed and delayed diagnoses in the ambulatory setting: a study of closed malpractice claims. *Ann Intern Med* 2006;145:488.

Gandhi TK, Weingart SN, Seger AC, et al. Outpatient prescribing errors and the impact of computerized prescribing. *J Gen Intern Med* 2005;20:837–841.

Gawron VJ, Drury CG, Fairbanks RJ, et al. Medical error and human factors engineering: where are we now? *Am J Med Qual* 2006; 21:57–67.

Hilfiker D. Facing our mistakes. *N Engl J Med* 1984;310:118–122.

Hobgood C, Hevia A, Tamayo-Sarver JH, et al. The influence of the causes and contexts of medical errors on emergency medicine residents' responses to their errors: an exploration. *Acad Med* 2005;80:758–764.

Institute of Medicine. *Preventing Medication Errors.* Washington, DC: National Academies Press. 2006.

Kachalia A, Shojania KG, Hofer TP, et al. Does full disclosure of medical errors affect malpractice liability? The jury is still out. *Jt Comm J Qual Saf* 2003;29:503–511.

Kalra J. Medical errors: overcoming the challenges. *Clin Biochem* 2004; 37:1063–1071.

Kaushal R. Effects of computerized physician order entry and clinical decision support systems on medication safety: a systematic review. *Arch Intern Med* 2003;163:1409–1416.

Kohn LT, Corrigan JM, Donaldson MS, et al., eds. Committee on Quality of Health Care in America, Institute of Medicine. *To Err is Human. Building a Safer Health Care System.* Washington, DC: National Academy Press, 2000.

Kraman SS, Hamm G. Risk management: extreme honesty may be the best policy. *Ann Intern Med* 1999;131:963–967.

Kraman SS. A risk management program based on full disclosure and trust: does everyone win? *Compr Ther* 2001;27:253–257.

Landrigan CP, Rothschild JM, Cronin JW, et al. Effect of reducing interns' work hours on serious medical errors in intensive care units. *N Engl J Med* 2004;351:1838–1848.

Lazare A. Apology in medical practice: an emerging clinical skill. *JAMA* 2006;296:1401–1404.

Levinson W, Dunn PM. Coping with fallibility. *JAMA* 1989;261: 2252.

Lo B. Disclosing mistakes. In: Lo B, ed. *Problems in Ethics.* Philadelphia, PA: Williams & Wilkins, 1994.

Mazor KM, Simon SR, Gurwitz JH. Communicating with patients about medical errors: a review of the literature. *Arch Intern Med* 2004;164:1690–1697.

Mazor KM, Reed GW, Yood RA, et al. Disclosure of medical errors: what factors influence how patients respond? *J Gen Intern Med* 2006;21:704–710.

Pawlson L, O'Kane ME. Malpractice prevention, patient safety, and quality of care: a critical linkage. *Am J Manag Care* 2004;10: 281–284.

Pollack C, Bayley C, Mendiola M, et al. The clinician's role in finding resolution after a medical error. *Camb Q Healthc Ethics* 2003; 12:203–207.

Pronovost P, Holzmueller CG, Needham DM, et al. How will we know patients are safer? An organization-wide approach to measuring and improving safety. *Crit Care Med* 2006;34:1988–1995.

Ralston JD, Larson EB. Crossing to safety: transforming healthcare organizations for patient safety. *J Postgrad Med* 2005;51: 61–67.

Roulson J, Benbow EW, Hasleton PS. Discrepancies between clinical and autopsy diagnosis and the value of post mortem histology; a meta-analysis and review. *Histopathology* 2005;47:551–559.

Schulmeister L. Ten simple strategies to prevent chemotherapy errors. *Clin J Oncol Nurs* 2005;9:201–205.

Studdert DM, Mello MM, Gawande AA, et al. Disclosure of medical injury to patients: an improbable risk management strategy. *Health Affairs* 2007; 26:215.

Thomas EJ, Studdert DM, Burstin HR, et al. Incidence and types of adverse events and negligent care in Utah and Colorado. *Med Care* 2000; 38:261–271.

Tipton DJ, Giannetti. VJ, Kristofik JM. Managing the aftermath of medication errors: managed care's role. *J Am Pharm Assoc* 2003; 43:622–629.

Unruh L, Lugo NR, White SV, et al. Managed care and patient safety: risks and opportunities. *Health Care Manag* 2005;24: 245–255.

Vincent C, Taylor-Adams S, Stanhope N. Framework for analysing risk and safety in clinical medicine. *BMJ* 1998;316:1154–1157.

West CP, Huschka MM, Novotny PJ, et al. Association of perceived medical errors with resident distress and empathy: a prospective longitudinal study. *JAMA* 2006;296:1071–1078.

Wilson J, McCaffrey R. Disclosure of medical errors to patients. *Medsurg Nurs* 2005;14:319–323.

Wu AW, Folkman S, McPhee SJ, LoB. Do house officers learn from their mistakes? *JAMA* 1991;265:2089–2094.

Wu AW, Folkman S, McPhee SJ, et al. How house officers cope with their mistakes: doing better but feeling worse? *West J Med* 1993; 159:565–569.

Wu AW, Cavanaugh TA, McPhee SJ, et al. To tell the truth: ethical and practical issues in disclosing medical mistakes to patients. *J Gen Intern Med* 1997;12:770–775.

Intimate Partner Violence

Mitchell D. Feldman, MD, MPhil

INTRODUCTION

Intimate partner violence (IPV), is defined as any intentional, controlling behavior consisting of physical, sexual, or psychological assaults in the context of an intimate relationship. The data on IPV underscore the magnitude of the problem. In a landmark study, 28% of a random nationwide sample of couples reported violence at some point in their history; almost 4% of the women reported severe violence. If these figures are extrapolated to the general population, it is estimated that about 4 million women are subjected to violence each year in the United States with about 500,000 women requiring medical treatment. Women visiting outpatient medical and obstetric/gynecologic clinics as well as the emergency department (ED) are often there for complaints directly attributable to IPV. Because their complaints are frequently misdiagnosed, they may return time and time again, often with increasingly severe trauma.

Despite its magnitude in society and in medical settings, until recently IPV could be described as a "silent epidemic." Considered a private, family problem by the government, and a social problem by the medical establishment, victims often had nowhere to turn. This predicament has gradually improved. IPV is now acknowledged to be an important public health problem, and medical practitioners have a variety of diagnostic and treatment guidelines available to them (see "Suggested Readings," at the end of the chapter). All practitioners must be knowledgeable about and comfortable with the evaluation and care of patients who are subjected to IPV.

EPIDEMIOLOGY

Research conducted in a variety of medical settings has reported on the prevalence of IPV. Cross-sectional studies from outpatient primary care clinics and ED settings have found the prevalence of IPV among women to be from 6 to 28%; lifetime prevalence rates up to 50% have been reported. Similar rates have been reported by studies conducted in obstetric/gynecologic outpatient clinics. In fact, pregnancy may double the risk of IPV. Differences in prevalence of IPV among various studies can be explained, in part, by their use of different definitions of IPV.

Most studies ask about violence exclusively in the context of heterosexual relationships. However, a similar prevalence of IPV appears to exist in gay and lesbian relationships, with the same physical and emotional consequences. Primary care providers should be aware that it may be more difficult for gay and lesbian patients to disclose that they are in an abusive relationship. In addition, the commonly held bias that violence does not occur in these relationships ("women can't hurt women") further lowers detection rates.

Men report being physically abused by their female partners at rates just below those reported by women. The injuries inflicted by women on men, however, are generally insignificant when compared with same-sex or male-on-female violence.

DIAGNOSIS

Many battered women seek medical care both for the direct and indirect consequences of IPV. Yet only a small percentage of them are diagnosed and treated appropriately. The following case is illustrative of the type of patient commonly seen in medical settings.

 CASE ILLUSTRATION 1

A 40-year-old nurse presents to the ED with a chief complaint of a headache. She reports having been in a motor vehicle accident 3 days earlier and striking her head on the dashboard. She says that her friends encouraged her to come in, and she is accompanied to the ED (but not the office) by her partner. On physical examination, she appears tense and sad, with bilateral, periorbital ecchymoses.

History

A thorough history is the cornerstone of the diagnosis of IPV. Because the presentation is often subtle, with few dramatic injuries, detection requires a high index of suspicion. There are many clues in the medical history, as shown by the case illustration that should prompt the physician to evaluate the patient for IPV (Table 35-1). Clues that should prompt further inquiry include:

- Delay in seeking care
- Illogical explanation of injury
- Multiple somatic complaints
- Depression, anxiety, and other mental disorders
- Pregnancy
- Substance use
- Recent diagnosis of human immunodeficiency virus (HIV)
- Family history of IPV
- Overbearing partner

DELAY IN SEEKING CARE

Patients who have been assaulted often delay seeking medical attention, in contrast to accident victims who generally seek out medical attention immediately.

ILLOGICAL EXPLANATION OF INJURY

Injuries that are attributed to a mechanism that seems illogical should always raise concern. For example, periorbital ecchymoses ("black eyes") generally are not caused by a motor vehicle accident, a "doorknob," or anything other than a fist.

MULTIPLE SOMATIC COMPLAINTS

Some women may present with vague somatic complaints as their only symptom of IPV. Fatigue, sleep disturbance, headache, gastrointestinal complaints, abdominal and pelvic pain, genitourinary problems such as frequent urinary tract and genital infections, chest pain, palpitations, and dizziness are just some of the complaints with which women present. IPV should be considered as a sole or contributing cause of these problems.

Table 35-1. When to screen for IPV.

- Delay in seeking care
- Illogical explanation of injury
- Multiple somatic complaints
- Depression, anxiety, and other mental disorders
- Pregnancy
- Substance use
- Recent diagnosis of HIV
- Family history of IPV
- Overbearing partner

DEPRESSION, ANXIETY, AND OTHER MENTAL DISORDERS

Depression, eating disorders, and anxiety disorders such as posttraumatic stress disorder and panic disorder are more common among victims of IPV than among the general population. If present, the medical practitioner should always screen for IPV. These mental and behavioral disturbances should be thought of as a consequence, not a cause, of the IPV. Some patients may feel hopeless and turn toward suicide as a way out. One of every 10 battered women attempts suicide. Of those, 50% try more than once.

PREGNANCY

Many studies have demonstrated that women are at increased risk of physical and sexual abuse during pregnancy. Clues to be alert for include delay in seeking prenatal care, depressed or anxious mood, injuries to breasts or abdomen, frequent spontaneous abortions, and preterm labor. In addition to the physical and emotional trauma to the pregnant woman, these assaults can result in placental separation, fetal fractures, and fetal demise.

SUBSTANCE ABUSE

Although violence and substance abuse often coexist, it is inaccurate and generally not helpful to frame IPV as secondary to the substance abuse. Although the perpetrator, and at times the woman herself, often assert that the violence was a consequence of altered behavior from drugs or alcohol, in fact, the violent behavior must be addressed as a separate issue and is unlikely to end even if the substance abuse does.

Conversely, some studies have found an increased rate of substance use in victims of IPV. At times, this may take the form of increased use of pain medications or anxiolytics in an effort to cope with the assaults. It is even more imperative in this instance that physicians do not attribute the IPV to the substance use; it is precisely this mentality of "blaming the victim" that has often prevented the appropriate evaluation and treatment of IPV in all medical settings.

RECENT DIAGNOSIS OF HIV

Some women report an initiation or escalation of IPV after informing their partner of their HIV seropositive status. Although every attempt should be made to notify sexual partners of HIV-positive results, practitioners should assess their patient's risk of violence while discussing the issues surrounding notification. Discussion of IPV and review of a safety plan should always be part of posttest counseling.

FAMILY HISTORY OF IPV

Patients who report a family history of IPV, particularly those who witnessed parental violence as a child or adolescent, are at increased risk themselves even if they are not presently in an abusive relationship. Such women should therefore be educated and screened more carefully.

OVERBEARING PARTNER

An overbearing partner who, for example, insists on accompanying the patient into the examining room, acts overly solicitous or concerned (sometimes to the point of knocking on the examining room door to inquire about her well-being), or is hostile to the health care team may be a clue to the presence of IPV. Never probe about IPV if the perpetrator is in the examining room as this may unintentionally escalate the violence and put the patient in extreme danger.

NOT SOCIOECONOMIC OR ETHNIC STATUS

Many health care providers mistakenly believe that IPV disproportionately affects persons from particular ethnic or socioeconomic groups; in fact, it cuts across all ethnic groups and all economic strata. Although some studies have found that women who are uninsured or on medical assistance are at increased risk of IPV, this is most likely due to selection bias in the studies. Women from lower socioeconomic status (SES) groups may be over-represented in some statistics because those from higher SES groups have more resources available to them and the abuse is therefore more likely to remain hidden. Women with fewer resources are forced to take refuge in shelters or county hospital EDs, for example, whereas their middle-class counterparts may flee to a hotel or their offices and are therefore underrepresented by some of the surveys.

CASE ILLUSTRATION 2

A 28-year-old postdoctoral fellow presents to her primary care practitioner (PCP) complaining of new-onset insomnia and headache. On physical examination, the PCP discovers bruising on her chest and back and inquires about IPV. The patient breaks down and reports that her partner, a professor at the university, has been emotionally and physically abusing her for years, and that only one friend was aware of this history. When the abuse escalated, the patient would seek refuge in her lab, sometimes conducting experiments all night.

Physical Examination

The physical examination may provide the first clues of the presence of IPV (Table 35-2), including:

- Inappropriate behavior
- Multiple injuries
- Central pattern of injury
- Injuries at different stages of healing

Table 35-2. Physical examination clues to the presence of IPV.

- Inappropriate behavior
- Multiple injuries
- Central pattern of injury
- Injuries at different stages of healing

INAPPROPRIATE BEHAVIOR

Behavior that appears to be inappropriate at the time of the physical examination may be a sign of IPV. Fright, inappropriate embarrassment or laughter, anxiety, passivity, shyness, and avoidance of eye contact may all be clues that the patient has been battered.

MULTIPLE INJURIES

IPV victims are more likely to have multiple injuries than are ordinary accident victims. Women who have been subjected to IPV, for example, typically have injuries to the head, neck, abdomen, and chest, whereas accident victims often present with less widespread trauma. The common emotional reaction to an IPV assault of denial, confusion, and withdrawal may also lead to more extensive injuries.

CENTRAL PATTERN OF INJURY

Victims of IPV often experience injuries such as bruises, lacerations, burns, bites, and more severe injuries secondary to assaults with a deadly weapon or repeated beatings that cause massive internal injuries and fractures. Injuries are most commonly seen in the central areas of the body—the head, neck, chest, abdomen, breasts—and occasionally upper arms from fending off blows.

INJURIES AT DIFFERENT STAGES OF HEALING

As with child abuse, multiple injuries at different stages of healing should always prompt an inquiry about IPV.

In summary, medical providers must be alert to the signs and symptoms of IPV. It is important to remember that most IPV victims do not present with injuries that require emergency treatment or lead to hospitalization. In fact, for many patients, even in EDs, the presenting complaint is often medical or psychological, rather than an actual physical injury. For this reason, detection of IPV will increase only if practitioners include it on the differential diagnosis and actively screen for it during the medical encounter.

Screening for IPV

While research has not yet demonstrated improved health outcomes of screening for IPV by health care providers or organizations, many experts and national groups such as the American Medical Association advocate universal screening and improved provider education. Since the

Table 35-3. Screening questions.

- We all fight at home sometimes. What happens when you or your partner fight or disagree?
- Do you feel safe in your home and in your relationship?
- Do you ever feel afraid of your partner?
- Because abuse and violence are so common in women's lives, I've begun to ask about it routinely. At any time, has a partner hit or otherwise hurt or threatened you?
- Does your partner ever force you to engage in sex that makes you feel uncomfortable?
- Does your partner threaten, hit, or abuse your children?

Table 35-4. After detection: five tasks to accomplish.

1. Validate the problem.
2. Assess the patient's safety, and review an emergency escape plan.
3. Document clearly and completely.
4. Provide information and appropriate referral.
5. Be aware of reporting and other legal requirements.

potential benefits of screening would appear to outweigh the potential harms, and since research has demonstrated that most women favor routine screening by their health care practitioners, questions about IPV should be incorporated into the routine history and physical examination for all female patients. Some practitioners also screen men, particularly men in intimate relationships with other men. The optimal method of screening, whether by including questions about abuse on the electronic medical record (EMR) or intake medical history questionnaire, or verbally as a part of the social or past medical history, or both, is a subject of ongoing research. The HITS questions ("Have you been **h**it, **i**nsulted, **t**hreatened, or **s**creamed at?) are recommended by some experts. It may help some patients to feel more comfortable revealing IPV by screening with the following questions that seek to normalize the problem:

> Doctor: "We all fight at home. What happens when you or your partner fight or disagree?"

> Doctor: "Because abuse and violence are so common in women's lives, I've begun to ask about it routinely. At any time, has a partner hit or otherwise hurt or threatened you?" (See Table 35-3 for suggested screening questions.)

If the answers are vague or evasive, more direct questions must be asked to determine if abuse is taking place. If this is done in a supportive, nonjudgmental manner, most patients will feel comfortable and respond honestly.

TREATMENT

When IPV is detected, five basic tasks must be accomplished (Table 35-4). First, **validate the problem** by making a clear statement to the patient that violent behavior is unacceptable and illegal, and that nobody has the right to abuse her. The physician's acknowledgment of the IPV as a real issue may be the first step in helping to free her from the abuse. Under all circumstances, avoid language that could be interpreted as blaming the victim for the violence.

Because the majority of women are not ready to leave the relationship when the IPV is detected, a main task for the primary care provider is to build the relationship with the patient. Statements that express empathy can be an effective way to accomplish this task, for example: "I really respect the way you have been dealing with this" and "we can work on this problem together." It is important to help the patient set short-term goals (e.g., to obtain the skills required for a particular job) so that she is not distressed when it takes time to realize her long-term goal of ending the abuse and/or the relationship. Above all, avoid recapitulating the power and control dynamics that so often characterize the patient's abusive relationship. Never insist that she leave the relationship and always allow her the autonomy to make her own decisions.

Second, it is essential to **assess the patient's safety**. Is it safe for her to go home? Other options (such as friends, shelters, and so on) should be explored and an emergency escape plan reviewed if she chooses to return home. For women not returning home, advise them to inform one or two coworkers about the situation as the perpetrator may attempt to find her at work. It is important to ask if there are children who are potentially at risk. Risk factors for escalating violence such as an increase in the frequency and severity of assaults, an escalation in threats, and the availability of a firearm should be carefully assessed.

Third, it is imperative that practitioners **document clearly and completely** when they uncover IPV. The medical record should include a complete description of the assault with quotes, if possible, from the patient's own account. Include relevant details in the past medical history and social history. Be sure to write legibly; successful prosecution should never be compromised by sloppy recordkeeping. Injuries should be described and visually documented, either with a body chart or with photographs, if the patient consents (include the patient's face in at least one photograph). If the police are called, always include the name of and any actions taken by the investigating police officer.

Fourth, the patient must be provided with **information and appropriate referral**. Health care providers should be familiar with the social and legal services available for battered women in their area. Information about shelters should be offered even if the woman intends to return home (though it is important to understand that discovery of such information by the perpetrator may lead to an escalation of the abuse). All patients should be assessed for the presence of psychiatric or substance abuse problems that would benefit from treatment or referral. Practitioners should have a basic understanding of legal options, such as restraining orders, so that they can help advise women who wish to take immediate action to ensure their safety.

Finally, understand the IPV **reporting requirements**, if any, in your state. For example, in California, health practitioners are required to report to the police all incidents of IPV that result in an injury. The usual doctor–patient privileged communication is explicitly preempted by this law. Providers should work with their ED, hospital, or clinics to be sure that information about reporting requirements as well as other patient education literature is freely available and in multiple languages.

CASE ILLUSTRATION 3

A 32-year-old man was admitted to the hospital for treatment of injuries and bleeding after reporting that he "fell through a glass door." He required an emergency operation to repair lacerations to internal organs and 2 units of packed red blood cells. Five days postoperatively, he was visited in the hospital by his male partner who became belligerent when the surgical residents attempted to obtain additional history. Later that day, the patient revealed that he had been in a long-term abusive relationship, that the abuse had been escalating over the past 6 months, and in fact he had been pushed through the door by his partner. The hospital social worker was called to speak with the patient and told him that she would report his case to the domestic violence hotline. The patient said that he had finally made the decision to leave the relationship and was intending to press charges and was grateful for the support of the hospital doctors and staff.

What to Avoid

There are four pitfalls to avoid when caring for victims of IPV:

1. Do not insist that the patient terminate the relationship, even if you believe that this is the most appropriate action. Only she can make that decision. Trying to control her behavior, albeit subtly, recapitulates the same negative dynamic that is taking place in the abusive relationship.

2. Recommend couple counseling *only* when the perpetrator acknowledges the problem, wants to change his behavior, and both partners want to preserve the relationship.

3. Do not use the word *alleged* in the medical record. It implies that you do not believe the patient's story, and you may inadvertently impede her ability to bring her case to court.

4. Do not ask what the victim did to bring on the violence.

BARRIERS

Physician Barriers to Detection

Many studies have revealed that physicians and other health care practitioners do a poor job of detecting IPV, with detection rates rarely exceeding 10%. Several factors are responsible for this dismal record. First, many practitioners lack the appropriate knowledge and training to effectively detect and treat victims of IPV. The first step in improving their ability to do so is to disseminate information more widely about its prevalence and consequences and to include IPV in medical school, residency, and continuing medical education curricula.

Lack of institutional support is another important barrier. Despite the enormity of the problem and the increasing requirements that all health care institutions have IPV protocols in place, most hospitals and clinics have few, if any, adequately trained support staff, accessible guidelines for practitioners, or information for patients. In addition, with growing pressure to see more patients and use fewer resources, issues such as IPV may be overlooked. Many of the physicians interviewed in one study identified time constraints as the major deterrent to opening the "Pandora's box" of IPV.

It should be noted, however, that the total annual health care costs from IPV exceed $50 million, plus indirect costs such as lost days from paid work. In addition, the diagnostic and treatment strategies outlined here are not particularly time intensive. Inquiry about IPV adds less than 1 minute to the typical new patient evaluation; if widely employed, it could yield potentially enormous savings through prevention of injury and decreased health care usage.

The third barrier to detection of IPV arises from practitioner discomfort. Many practitioners feel uncomfortable addressing issues that do not fit neatly into the traditional medical model. Numerous studies have shown that many do a poor job discussing issues with their patients having to do with sex, violence, mental disorders, and substance use. Delving into the cause of a suspicious injury may make them uneasy: it is often not amenable to a straightforward solution and may raise embarrassing or uncomfortable feelings. All practitioners must reflect on the feelings that IPV raises in them to be effective in caring for these vulnerable patients.

Patient Barriers to Terminating an Abusive Relationship

Providers often have difficulty understanding why more patients do not terminate their abusive relationship. Why they remain in these relationships is complex. Some of the reasons include the following:

1. *Fear.* Fear for their own safety or for their children. One-third of women are not at home when the assault takes place, so it is clear that leaving is no guarantee of safety.
2. *Economic.* Many battered women lack employment skills or experience and would find it very difficult to support themselves and/or their children outside of the relationship.
3. *Psychological.* Some may find it difficult to leave because of the "psychological dependence" the years of repetitive abuse have created. Battered women are told overtly and covertly that they are "worthless"; some eventually internalize this and come to believe that they are incapable of surviving on their own.
4. *Social support—or the lack thereof.* Women are often encouraged by well-meaning friends and family members to "try to work things out," or they are advised to stay "for the children's sake."
5. *Lack of other options.* Shelters are often full, friends and family unavailable, and legal counsel not accessible.
6. Not all women want the relationship to end, just the battering.

CONCLUSION

Along with the criminal justice system, physicians and other health care providers are most likely to come into contact with victims of IPV. They have a professional and ethical obligation to recognize IPV and intervene appropriately as well as to exert their influence on a broader level. This may be to lobby for more funding for shelters or to advocate for teaching about IPV at all levels of medical education. Screening for and treating IPV should be a routine part of the practice and training of medicine. We all have the obligation to confront the epidemic of IPV and strive to lessen its impact as one of the most important public health issues of our time.

SUGGESTED READINGS

Baig A, Shadigan E, Heisler M. Hidden from plain sight: residents's domestic violence screening attitudes and reported practices. *J Gen Intern Med* 2006;21:949–954.

Campbell JC. Health consequences of intimate partner violence. *Lancet* 2002;359(9314):1331–1336.

MacMillan HL, Wathen CN, Jamieson E, et al. Approaches to screening for intimate partner violence in health care settings. *JAMA* 2006;295(5):530–536.

Stark E, Flitcraft A. *Women at Risk: IPV and Women's Health.* London: Sage Publications, 1996.

WEB SITES

American Bar Association Commission on Domestic Violence Web site. http://www.abanet.org/domviol/. Accessed September, 2007.

Family Violence Prevention Fund Web site. http://www.endabuse.org/. Accessed September, 2007.

Minnesota Center Against Violence and Abuse Web site. http://www.mincava.umn.edu/. Accessed September, 2007.

Same-Sex IPV Web site. http://www.cuav.org/index.php. Accessed September, 2007.

Chronic Illness & Patient Self-management

36

Susan L. Janson, DNSc, RN, NP, FAAN & Roberta Oka, DNSc, RN, NP

INTRODUCTION

Chronic illnesses impose a significant burden on individuals, families, communities, and the health care system. Diseases, such as asthma, chronic lung disease, coronary artery disease, heart failure, diabetes, hypertension, HIV, and chronic depression result in disabling symptoms, loss of functional ability and productivity. Chronic illnesses cost billions of dollars each year in both direct medical costs and indirect impact on work productivity, drain family and community resources, and overburden the health care system. The ability of the U.S. health care system to respond to the crisis of the rising prevalence of chronic diseases is limited by its current focus on acute illness, with care delivered in response to illness in crisis rather than proactive management. This reactive mode of health care delivery has been called the "tyranny of the acute" with few resources devoted to proactively managing chronic illness and preventing exacerbations.

Since many chronic diseases are directly linked to behaviors (e.g., tobacco use, sedentary lifestyle, and unsafe sexual behaviors) and environmental exposures, the course of illness can be modified with planned interventions. A model for chronic illness management, implemented at the system level, was proposed by Wagner et al. and is described in detail in two articles which provide insight into how chronic illness can be effectively managed in primary care (see "Suggested Readings," below). The Chronic Care Model (CCM) incorporates the community, health care system, health care team of providers, and patients in a unified model designed to improve patient outcomes for those with chronic illnesses. The model includes six components or dimensions of care within the health care system that are necessary to maximize effective use of resources and coordinate care. Briefly, the six components include: (1) community resources and policies, (2) the health care organization, (3) self-management support, (4) delivery system design, (5) decision support, and (6) clinical information systems. The last four components exist within the health care organization in an integrated systems model of care. Implementation of this system of care, with linkages to community resources, provides a network of support for a knowledgeable, prepared health care team to work with patients in partnership to manage and control chronic diseases. The CCM suggests a complete redesign of primary care practice to accomplish the goals of chronic illness management.

KEY COMPONENTS OF THE CHRONIC CARE MODEL

The Community: Resources & Policies

The health care organization exists within a local community where individuals with chronic illnesses live. An integral component of the CCM is the cultivation and maintenance of relationships with community resources and agencies. Many organizations in the community provide additional resources and support for individuals with chronic illnesses, such as patient education classes, exercise classes, smoking cessation programs, and home health services. Identifying the relevant resources in the community and facilitating referrals are valuable actions for optimal patient care because they can fill gaps in needed services.

Health Care Organization

The foundation of the CCM rests on the attitudes and values that govern the health care provider's organization and sets the tone for attitudes toward patients with chronic illnesses. If the leadership within the organization supports the importance of chronic care management, innovations are likely to be instituted. Such buy-in and support require commitment to the goals of controlling chronic illness and willingness to fund innovations that will ultimately reduce the cost of chronic illness care by reducing hospital and urgent care visits and allow for appropriate handling of errors. Reimbursement and financial designs are also key to the initiation and sustainability of chronic disease management programs. Most chronic illness is managed in primary care settings with strong links to specialty care for support. Innovations in primary care cannot occur without considerable buy-in and support from the administrative senior leaders of the health care organizations.

Delivery System Design

In order to provide more efficient and proactive health care, the delivery system must change from care delivered by one provider to an expanded primary care team in which roles and responsibilities are clearly delineated. For patients with chronic illness, planned visits are a key component of practice redesign for health care delivery because they provide opportunities for patients to work with the health care team to address self-management goals and disease control in advance rather than only during acute exacerbations of illness. The planned visits are focused on controlling chronic problems and preventing exacerbations and complications. A series of planned visits with mutually decided goals will enable adequate time for teaching and reinforcing patient education in self-management. This approach is enhanced by regular visits with interdisciplinary health care team professionals who can provide support and guidance, such as nurses, pharmacists, educators, nutritionists, social workers, as well as physicians and nurse practitioners. When acute exacerbations occur, they are handled within the context of an ongoing chronic care plan, individualized for each patient. The success of this component depends on the patients' clear understanding and agreement to the partnership in proactive chronic care management, which requires active participation and commitment to keeping appointments. The health care delivery system should be designed to ensure patient access to appointments for regular follow-up care that fits with the patient's cultural background. Clinical case management by trained nurses will be needed for complex patients with multiple concurrent illnesses. Nurse case management has been demonstrated to be an effective strategy to improve patient outcomes in depression and other chronic illnesses. Case managers can monitor patients more closely, provide patient education, and intervene directly if the patient's condition does not improve or worsens.

Decision Support

Decision support for the health care provider team is critical to ensure best practices in chronic illness management. It includes the provision of current clinical education and national guidelines. Ready access to individual patient clinical data and aggregated registry data must be provided so that adherence of the health care team to national practice guidelines is tracked and made available. Guidelines from national organizations can be implemented more easily if they are embedded in electronic data monitoring systems so that key decisions are supported in daily practice. Access to specialist expertise should be integrated with primary care and facilitated. Evidence-based guidelines and goals of treatment should be shared with patients to encourage their agreement and their participation in care.

Clinical Information Systems

Clinical data about individual patients must be available and accurate within short time windows. This information is most easily provided through electronic information systems that track clinical data by patient over time and are programmed to alert providers to values outside normal ranges. The best system will allow development of clinical registries comprised of all the patients with a specific chronic illness served by a health care organization. This approach allows the health care team to identify subpopulations that need improved proactive care and monitoring to improve clinical outcomes. Health care for groups of patients is improved overall by focusing improvement efforts on population-based outcomes. A well-designed clinical information system also allows monitoring of the performance of the practice team and the health care system in meeting national guidelines for processes of care and clinical outcomes by creating a feedback system for selected quality performance measures. Sharing clinical information with patients as well as providers helps to coordinate care and support the patient–clinician relationship.

Self-management Support

The final component of the CCM is self-management support for patients with chronic illnesses. It involves assisting patients and their families in developing the knowledge, skills, and confidence to effectively manage problems, set goals, and receive the support of an active partnership with clinicians and the health care team. The efforts put forth by the health care team with support from the health care organization and the community resources produce activated patients who are motivated to participate in their own chronic care. The goal is for patients to come to each planned visit prepared and willing to work on controlling the disease to ensure the best outcomes.

Implementation of these six model components within an organized health care system for chronic care improvement proactively supports a knowledgeable, prepared health care team to work with activated, motivated patients in partnerships to effectively manage and control chronic conditions. In addition to strong leadership by the health care organization, health care providers may need specific support and incentives to participate actively in the implementation of this system model of chronic illness care.

SELF-MANAGEMENT & PATIENT-CENTERED CARE

Overall, the success of chronic disease management lies in fostering a patient-centered partnership between the patient and health care team. This is particularly important when caring for patients with behavioral health problems. The key features include well-informed patients who are active participants in their care and a well-prepared, proactive health care team that understands and supports the concept of patient-centered care. Emphasis is placed on guiding clinicians to apply the principles of chronic care management to enhance the patient–clinician relationship with a patient-centered care approach. The ultimate goal of this approach is to empower patients to develop the skills and behaviors that will help them self-manage their diseases to achieve better health outcomes. For example, several clinical trials and systematic reviews have concluded that collaborative care models that use a system-based approach with clinical care managers who assist in patient education and self-management are significantly more effective than usual care in recognition and treatment of depression.

Patient-centered Care for the Clinician

Patient-centered care is a critical concept for effective management of chronic illnesses. The concept includes engaging patients in care planning as well as giving patients tools, skills, and knowledge. It means the health care team and primary clinician elicits and accepts the patient's beliefs and concerns about illness, teaches key information and self-management skills in the context of the patient's family, community, and culture, taking into consideration individual needs. The patient's concerns are identified and addressed first (Table 36-1). The team and primary clinician then involve the patient directly in negotiating and implementing the treatment plan, mak-

Table 36-1. Self-management support.

Self-management support is what providers do to assist and encourage patients to be empowered and able to manage their illness. This paradigm shift requires building a partnership with shared responsibility for making and implementing health-related decision between the provider(s) or care management team and the patient.

Table 36-2. Lessons learned from dialog.

- The provider allows the patient to set the agenda.
- The provider assesses the level of importance and confidence and explores what it would take to improve confidence in behavior change. This information also allows the provider to explore the activities patients are interested in pursuing.

ing adjustments and providing options that will meet the goals of controlling the chronic disease. Ask: "What do you want to do this week to improve your health?" Working in collaboration with the patient, the primary clinician and health care team design a treatment program that fits within the context of the patient's life (Table 36-2). Potential solutions and feasible options are offered and patients are invited to choose those they are willing to accept and pursue or modify. The keyword in this context is "collaboration" to work toward mutually acceptable goals. Additionally, primary care providers should be aware of patients' culturally based understanding of the disease and its treatment. Every effort should be made to deliver critical information and self-management instruction in the patient's native language. A patient-centered partnership means that health care providers collaborate with patients to design a treatment program that takes into consideration the patient's attitudes, beliefs, lifestyle, and culture to promote positive treatment outcomes (Table 36-3).

Provider behaviors may contribute to better patient self-management particularly in subpopulations with specific needs. A survey of an ethnically diverse, low income sample of 956 adult patients with diabetes or asthma in 17 academic outpatient practices revealed a strong relationship between higher patient assessments of provider support and patient self-efficacy for self-care. Within the diabetes subgroup, patients who gave high ratings of provider support were significantly more likely to perform self-management tasks than those with low ratings. The findings provide support for the belief that health care providers can successfully promote patient self-management of chronic illnesses (Piatt et al., 2006).

Problems of Living with a Chronic Illness

Living with a chronic illness presents the patient with a number of medical, social, emotional, and physical

Table 36-3. Key element to goal setting/action plans.

- Collaborative between patient and provider, using tools of motivational interviewing.
- Actions are highly specific

challenges that include adjusting to the natural course or progression of the disease, preventing social isolation, normalizing activities and communication within the boundaries of the illness, preventing exacerbations, controlling chronic symptoms, following complex treatment regimens, and finding the necessary financial and tangible resources to pay for treatments and potential loss of employment. To manage these key problems, patients must develop a set of strategies for self-managing the disease and for coping with the problems. Teaching, facilitating, and supporting the patient's attempts at self-management of the chronic condition is at the core of the patient–clinician relationship. Self-management is augmented and enhanced by state-of-the-art, appropriate medical care by an informed health care team that has access to the guidelines-based information for decision support and an accurate clinical information system for tracking patient data. In the CCM, these system features are used to support the health care providers. Equally important is the informed, activated patient, educated in the skills of self-management. Ongoing support for self-management is required in order to ensure the effectiveness of the partnership.

The partnership paradigm is based on acknowledging the expertise of both the provider in understanding the disease, its psychological and physical impact on patients, and therapeutic interventions; and the patients' expertise about their own lives. The new paradigm of provider–patient partnership supports interactions that are primarily based on the patient's agenda, not the providers. It purports a belief that increased self-efficacy for self-care tasks facilitates behavior change that education alone cannot accomplish. In the patient-centered approach, enhanced self-efficacy is the goal rather than adherence to provider advice. Finally, mutually agreed upon decisions are made together by the patient and clinician. Self-management support encourages patients to become more actively engaged to adopt health behaviors and develop necessary skills.

Self-management Support Strategies

The goal of self-management support is to assist the patient to become informed and activated in the management of their health care. The underlying assumption is that patients who are activated are more likely to adopt healthy behaviors thus having a positive impact on clinical outcomes. Several strategies that have been described in the literature are discussed below.

SETTING AN AGENDA

In traditional clinical encounters, the visit is guided by the chief complaint provided by the patient and the agenda is established by the provider. In this paradigm, the agenda is established by the patient and negotiated between provider and the patient.

INFORMATION GIVING USING ASK-TELL-ASK

One technique that has been used in providing patients with information is based upon the "elicit-respond-elicit" motivational interviewing technique first described by Miller and Rollnick (see Chapter 16). This strategy is based on the principle that adult learning is self-directed in which information is selected by the individual. The desired information is provided to the patient and the health care provider then asks if the patient understood and if additional information is desired.

INFORMATION GIVING: CLOSING THE LOOP

A simple but much overlooked strategy is asking the patient to restate instructions provided by the practitioner. "Closing the loop" or "checking" assesses a patient's understanding of the information provided by the practitioner. Closing the loop is a relatively simple strategy that requires further investigation but has promise in improving patient comprehension.

COLLABORATIVE DECISION MAKING

Establishing an agenda and goal setting are based on the spirit of motivational interviewing that include collaboration, autonomy, and a nonjudgmental partnership. The role of the clinician is to first stimulate the patient to reflect on his or her feelings of change, using interviewing techniques to increase their motivation to change then assist with developing an action plan and concrete goals.

Keys to motivational interviewing technique include: (1) assessing readiness to change by determining the relationship between level of importance and level of confidence for change and (2) encouraging discussion of change with the patient and identifying the benefits for change in health behavior. To assess level of confidence and importance, a 0–10 scale or a picture graph can be used. Once the individual is motivated to change a behavior, an action plan is developed by collaboration between the provider and patient. The action plan is very specific with identified behaviors, a start date, and frequency. For example, a patient may wish to walk 3 days per week (Monday, Wednesday, and Friday) at lunchtime, for 20 minutes, beginning Monday. Another example may include reducing candy bar consumption to 1 per day from 3 per day and eating one piece of fruit daily.

The primary goal of action plans is to achieve behavior change through a series of successes. Self-efficacy is defined as an individual's level of confidence in performing a specific behavior or activity. If self-efficacy is high, the behavior is likely to be performed. Thus, enhancing self-efficacy is of primary importance in achieving long-term behavior change. Therefore, the action plan should be simple and achievable. If the patient's efficacy is low for the action plan, the clinician can suggest a more achievable goal to insure success.

THE CYCLE OF CHRONIC ILLNESS EXPERIENCE FOR PATIENTS

Even with a well-planned, patient self-management support and the best intentions of the providers, chronic illnesses go out of control, exacerbations occur, and life events happen that may compromise patients' coping abilities. Psychosocial stress, new symptoms, progressive disease, and increased disability place additional burdens on patients with chronic illnesses. Increasing stress in an individual's life, such as greater work demands, might lead to an increase in activity level, greater fatigue, muscle tension, increased or new symptoms, and the psychological experience of feeling overwhelmed. These developments may contribute to high levels of pain or dyspnea or depressive symptoms, which in turn can lead to a decline in daily functioning, immobility, and the perception of heightened disease activity. These symptoms, perceptions, and loss of control may make the individual aware of the debilitating aspects of the chronic illness and negatively affect self-esteem, contributing to depression. Ongoing problems add to this cycle, characterized by poor coping responses, poor adherence, and an inability to adapt.

People with chronic illness may benefit from being educated about this downward spiral and being provided with strategies to overcome the setbacks and get back on track with self-management. Clinicians can empower patients to be alert to the interplay of these factors in their lives. Once aware, patients can employ actions, such as short-term goals and plans that interrupt the cycle of chronic disease. The ultimate goal is decreased stress and symptoms, increased psychological well-being, and control of the illness.

The natural history of chronic disease can be discouraging for patients and their families and for clinicians, which is why development of an effective health care team approach directed at supporting patients and their families is essential. In the end, chronic care management requires concentric circles of surveillance and care management supported by the health care system and endorsed by the community.

PSYCHOLOGICAL IMPACT OF CHRONIC DISEASE

Patients with chronic illness encounter a number of challenges that impact every aspect of their lives. Therefore, in order to facilitate an engaged and activated patient, clinicians must be able to understand their patients' internal experiences and outward expressions of their emotions and intervene in ways that promote adaptive coping. Adaptive coping means having available a repertoire of responses that can be used to deal with and modulate the ebb and flow of experience.

The goal of coping is to respond cognitively or behaviorally; to manage, tolerate, or reduce the effect of a stressful acute or chronic event. The two major methods of coping are problem-focused and emotion-focused. Problem-focused coping consists of active efforts to change something about oneself or the environment. Emotion-focused coping involves efforts to regulate emotional distress. Most often, people tend to take action to solve problems, but when a stressful experience is uncontrollable, problem-focused coping can be counterproductive. In these situations, efforts at emotional regulation or minimizing emotional distress may be more successful at providing relief.

The problem-focused/emotion-focused distinction in coping is useful, not only in understanding people's coping efforts, but in providing guidelines to primary care practitioners about how to facilitate patients' active involvement in their care and adaptation to chronic disease. Asking questions about patients' concerns and helping them to develop coping solutions are integral to developing a patient-centered partnership that will maximize the potential for positive treatment outcomes.

 CASE ILLUSTRATION 1

Ellen is a 33-year-old African American woman with severe asthma. She also has a 6-year-old child with asthma. Ellen has had numerous asthma exacerbations requiring urgent care visits over the last year. She admits to fear of taking inhaled corticosteroid medications on a consistent basis because she feels the medication is too powerful and will damage her lungs. She uses the steroid inhaler regularly only during asthma exacerbations and for 2–4 weeks after. When her daughter's asthma flares, Ellen focuses her care and attention on the child and neglects her own self-care, resulting in uncontrolled asthma in both parent and child.

During a visit with her primary clinician, Ellen's fears about her asthma medication are explored and current information is given. The clinician tells Ellen that she is worried about her and that the inhaled corticosteroid that she has prescribed is the safest and most effective treatment available. They negotiate a treatment plan that Ellen is willing to try with more frequent visits to review her progress. Ellen is taught how to monitor her peak flow to evaluate her response to the medication on a daily basis. They agree that the goal of her treatment is to stay healthy so she can take care of her child.

Ellen returns 2 weeks later with several days of peak flow values and the report that she has used her medication regularly every day but not always twice daily as it was prescribed. She notes that she feels better, breathing is easier, and her peak flow readings are steadily improving. Although she is still afraid of the long-term effects of the inhaled steroid, she acknowledges that the inhaled medication "seems safer than having to take prednisone" for acute exacerbations. They continue to adjust the plan so that Ellen can keep her asthma under control and care for her daughter. The peak flow monitoring is revised to measurements 3 days per week in the mornings and when symptoms worsen. The clinician provides Ellen with an Asthma Action Plan that guides Ellen to use inhaled albuterol, a short-acting bronchodilator, when symptoms increase and peak flow drops. Subsequent visits are rescheduled to once per month with a plan to revise these planned visits as needed to keep the asthma under control.

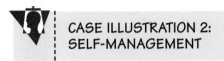

CASE ILLUSTRATION 2: SELF-MANAGEMENT

Maria is a 68-year-old Spanish-speaking woman with adult-onset diabetes and depression. She also has been told that she has high blood pressure (BP) and high cholesterol. She takes several oral medications for these conditions but doesn't know what they are and has not brought them with her to her appointments. She has a glucometer at home but has not checked her blood glucose for several months. She is out of glucometer strips and has not been able to figure out how to obtain them through her new Medicare Part D plan. She is currently living with her husband and daughter. Her meals consist of beans, rice, chicken, and tortillas. Her BP is 150/100.

Key aspects to consider for Maria include:

- Facilitating effective communication between provider and health care team and the patient by scheduling her with a team member who is bilingual.
- Assessing her depression with regular checks of the Patient Health Questionnaire (PHQ-9).
- Performing a fingerstick to check her hemoglobin A1c, which is currently 8.5.

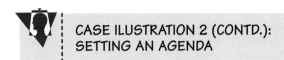

CASE ILUSTRATION 2 (CONTD.): SETTING AN AGENDA

Provider: I just checked your hemoglobin A1c and it is 8.5.

Maria: It seems high, I remember that it should it be lower, like about 7?

Provider: Yes, that is correct. What would you like to do about this?

Maria: I have been taking my medicines. I don't have time for anything else. I don't know what else to do.

Provider: We could talk about a number of different things, for example, medications, diet, exercise, or something else that you would prefer?

Maria: I would be interested to hear about exercise.

Provider: OK, now using a scale "0" to "10," how confident are you that you can make a change in your activity level or exercise? A "0" means you aren't sure you can make a change in your activity level and a "10" means you are 100% sure you can change your activity level (see Figure 36-1).

Maria: It is a "4," I don't have a lot of time and I am not sure what to do.

Provider: Why did you say a 4 and not a "1"?

Maria: It might be nice to take a walk with my husband or daughter, they walk together sometimes.

Provider: What would it take to improve your confidence to around a 7 that you can exercise more?

Maria: Maybe if I could walk with my husband, I would enjoy that and it would encourage me to do it.

Provider: Great! Do you want to set a short-term goal about your exercise? We could come up with an action plan together.

Collaborative Decision Making: Goal Setting/Action Plans

Patients who rate their confidence level at less than 7 are unlikely to maintain a change in that behavior. Here the provider is working with Maria to identify a patient-centered and achievable behavior change that

0	1	2	3	4	5	6	7	8	9	10
Not sure									Very sure	

Figure 36-1. Scale indicating confidence in ability of making a change in one's activity level or exercise.

will contribute to her goal of improving her diabetes management. Goal setting is performed on behaviors that the patient feels they are ready to attempt and it is important to establish realistic, concrete short-term achievable goals. In Maria's case, it may include walking with her husband or daughter beginning the next day for about 20 minutes and then at least once a week on a day that she selects or 2 days per week.

Other key elements to consider for this case as it relates to the chronic care model:

- Matching of language in verbal and written communication.
- Goal setting and action planning can be performed by other key members of the care management team. This can take place after the visit with the primary care provider.
- While not discussed in this illustration, closing the loop is key in this case: closing the loop can also be performed by other team members and should include:
  - Assessing the patients' understanding of the visit. Instructions for medications, what, how, and when to take the medications.
  - System navigation is important and should be incorporated into the latter part of the visit. Do the patients know where to go to get their labs drawn and understand if tests need to be fasting? Where should they go to fill the medications? How does she do her fingersticks?
- Follow-up visits should be scheduled (planned visits) to assess progress with action plans, revise and update goals, and to address management of other chronic conditions. These visits do not need to be with the primary care provider but may be more appropriate for other team members. Follow-up can also be conducted by telephone.
- Community resources: Maria may have access to other community resources such as a park, community center, or church that organizes walking groups or other health-related activities. Referrals can be made to these organizations and may be more convenient for her than returning to the clinic at regular intervals.

- Assessment and treatment of comorbid behavioral health problems: Like many patients with diabetes mellitus, Maria is also being treated for depression. The provider knows that inadequately treated depression can contribute to worsening glycemic control and that conversely, assessing, and managing depression is a key component of the overall management of Maria's diabetes.

Final points are as follows:

- After Maria's visit is complete her information will be entered into a computerized system that will then allow the care management team to follow her BP, hemoglobin A1c, PHQ-9, weight, and so on. This information will be pulled and collated prior to her next visit as a cue to optimal management. Additionally, her health maintenance activities will be recorded and the clinician will be prompted to review her health maintenance needs at the next visit.

SUGGESTED READINGS

Bodenheimer T, Wagner EH, Grumbach K. Improving primary care for patients with chronic illness. *JAMA* 2002;288(14):1775–1759.

Bodenheimer T, Wagner EH, Grumbach K. Improving primary care for patients with chronic illness: the chronic care model, Part 2. *JAMA* 2002;288(15):811–817.

Piatt GA, Orchard TJ, Emerson S, et al. Translating the chronic care model into the community: results from a randomized controlled trial of a multifaceted diabetes care intervention. *Diabetes Care* 2006;29(4):811–817.

Wagner EH, Glasgow RE, Davis C, et al. Quality improvement in chronic illness care: a collaborative approach. *Jt Comm J Qual Improv* 2001;27(2):63–80.

WEB SITES

Chronic Care Model Web site. www.improvingchroniccare.org. Accessed October, 2007.

Group Visits for Chronic Illness Care Web site. http://www.aafp.org/fpm/20060100/37grou.html. Accessed October, 2007.

Patient-centered Care Web site. http://www.ahrq.gov/QUAL/ptcareria.htm. Accessed October, 2007.

Palliative Care, Hospice, & Care of the Dying

Michael Eisman, MD & Timothy E. Quill, MD

37

INTRODUCTION

Clinicians need to ask themselves how they want to be treated if they become seriously ill and are potentially dying. Answering this question helps them discover and clarify their own beliefs and values concerning the care of their very ill patients. The goals of medical practice based exclusively on cure and restoration of function are frequently called into question when patients are irreversibly ill and potentially dying. Goals of pain and symptom management, enhancing quality of life, and finding meaning in the face of death may take precedence, or at least be an important part of the treatment plan. Is death something to be fought at all costs, or is relieving suffering a central part of our responsibility as clinicians? Enhancing quality of life for those afflicted with serious chronic illness is the cornerstone of the rapidly developing specialty of palliative care. As illustrated in Figure 37-1 below, palliative care can be provided alongside aggressive treatment of a patient's underlying disease, but as the patient becomes sicker and closer to death, palliation often becomes the primary objective.

CASE ILLUSTRATION 1

Ella, a 71-year-old woman, develops pains in her lower chest for a month before visiting her personal physician. When a chest film shows several nodular masses suggestive of widespread lung cancer, the physician phones Ella and tells her there is a problem, making an office appointment for the next day. At this visit, the doctor discusses the results of the chest film with the patient and her son. Ella, having long suspected she might get lung cancer from smoking heavily, weeps openly upon hearing the results. Bronchoscopy is recommended, and she is referred to a pulmonologist. Bronchoscopic biopsies show a small-cell lung cancer. The pulmonologist refers Ella to an oncologist who recommends chemotherapy.

The patient and her son return to her primary care doctor to discuss her options. Ella says she would like to proceed with chemotherapy but wants to stop it if she becomes too ill from the treatments. A Roman Catholic, she has discussed with her priest the morality of refusing extraordinary care, including feeding tubes, if she were to have a terminal condition. She has appointed her son as her health care proxy, and discusses her desire not to undergo cardiopulmonary resuscitation (CPR). The physician gives Ella a living will and a do-not-resuscitate (DNR) document; she and her son complete them together. She wants to try all other potentially effective disease-directed treatments, and she also agrees to have her pain and shortness of breath treated aggressively as well. She also knows that cure is very unlikely with this treatment, so she begins to work with a financial planner to get her affairs in order.

Ella undergoes chemotherapy for several months, but gradually grows thinner and weaker. She and her son visit her doctor, and are told that treatment is not controlling the disease, and that the only options left for cancer treatment are experimental. She is referred to a home hospice program, and agrees to a plan that is now directed exclusively at relieving her suffering. Ella lives alone and does not want to die in her apartment. Neither does she want her son to have to provide home care for her when she becomes too dependent to live alone. She also wants to know whether she could move to a hospice house or a nursing home for the very last phase of her illness when she is unable to care for herself at home. Her doctor and her son agree to find other placement when the need arises.

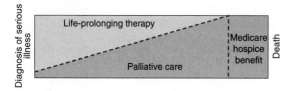

Figure 37-1. The place of palliative care in the course of illness. (Adapted from Clinical Practice Guidelines for Quality Palliative Care. Available at: www.nationalconsensusproject.org.)

When she becomes confused 1 month later and is unable to stay at home, she is admitted to a comfort care floor at a local nursing home. An intensive palliative treatment regimen is initiated, and she dies 2 weeks later with her son at her bedside, 6 months after the initial diagnosis.

Early after this patient's initial diagnosis, she received palliative care alongside aggressive treatment of her disease. Withholding aggressive pain and symptom management until hospice referral is misguided and unfair, depriving patients of optimal treatment of their suffering from the beginning of their illness. This "both/and" approach has been one of the most important conceptual breakthroughs for palliative care, for it allows quality-of-life issues to be addressed for all seriously ill patients, not just those who are referred to hospice. It also allows patients simultaneously to "hope for the best" (that even improbable or experimental treatment will affect their disease and prolong their life) and "prepare for the worst" (make sure that financial affairs are settled and consider religious or existential issues should they wish to do so). It may be easier for some patients to make the transition to hospice when aggressive treatment stops controlling their disease if they have this "both/and" conversation with their physician throughout their illness.

Nonabandonment

When a patient is informed of a life-threatening illness, a wide spectrum of feelings may emerge: denial, intense anxiety, fear, sadness, and anger. If the practitioner is inexperienced in palliative care or is extremely discomfited by death, there may be a tendency to withdraw from the patient's care or to minimize the meaning and impact of the diagnosis. The commitment not to abandon the patient requires that clinicians learn to work through their own feelings, become knowledgeable about palliative care, and recognize that the process of

dying can be a unique spiritual and personal experience for both doctor and patient. The goal is to form a partnership that will help the patient face the future with courage and dignity.

The goals of partnership and shared decision making are sometimes limited by strong emotional reactions as well as long-standing personality traits that can isolate the patient from the clinician, friends, and family. In addition, physicians may be unable to commit the time and energy needed to develop close personal contact with the seriously ill, potentially dying patient. Clinicians need to realize that extraordinary effort is sometimes required to be a partner with patients and their families through what initially may be a vigorous fight against disease, but eventually may end in the patients' death.

The goal of palliative care is to provide the best possible quality of life for the patient and family. Palliative care addresses the biological, psychosocial, and spiritual dimensions of suffering of seriously ill patients, emphasizing state-of-the-art pain and symptom management, and a fresh look at goals and prognosis. Unlike Medicare-sponsored hospice programs, palliative care does not require patients to give up on aggressive treatment of their underlying disease, to accept a prognosis of 6 months or less, or to accept palliation as the central goal of therapy. Thus, it allows "hospice-like" treatments to be made available to those seriously ill patients who want to continue some or all disease-directed treatments. Thus, a patient who is highly likely to die, but wants to try improbable experimental therapy in hopes that it might prolong his or her life, could receive palliative care, but would not qualify for a Medicare-sponsored hospice program. Similarly, a patient with advanced emphysema or Alzheimer disease who has a 40% chance of dying in the next 6 months, but might live several years, could receive palliative care. Such patients, however, probably would not qualify for hospice—even if their primary goals were palliation and comfort—until their functional status declined enough so they were more likely to die in the next 6 months. Thus, palliative care allows better pain and symptom management, careful attention to quality of life, an examination of the goals of treatment, and an opportunity to consider issues of life closure to be provided to a much broader range of patients. Unfortunately, the medical infrastructure that supports the patient and family receiving palliative care at home is much less comprehensive that the medical infrastructure supporting hospice.

Patients confronting a severe potentially terminal illness may opt for all-out, aggressive, disease-oriented medical treatment, or a trial of aggressive medical care with set limits (such as a DNR order). Of course, in both of these situations palliative care should also be initiated simultaneously with this more disease-oriented care. When undergoing limited trials of aggressive care, the patient has the opportunity to gauge whether the suffering engendered by the treatment, given the odds of success, is worth it. When treatments begin to fail, or if supposedly curative treatments become too burdensome, the patient can stop at any time and consider a transition to an approach that emphasizes pure palliation. This would be the time to consider referring to hospice, where relieving symptoms and alleviating suffering then take precedence over attempts to treat the underlying disease.

HOSPICE

Hospice programs provide comprehensive care to dying patients, with a multidisciplinary team of nurses, physicians, social workers, volunteers, and clergy. These programs accept only patients who have a life expectancy of less than 6 months and are willing to forgo disease-directed therapies and hospitalizations. In the United States, only about 30% of deaths occur in hospice programs, and many of these patients are referred to a hospice too late in the course of their illness to take full advantage of the resources and supports available. The palliative care philosophy underlying hospice can be applied in a range of settings from acute-care hospitals to nursing homes to the patient's home. The advantage of hospice programs is the expertise brought to techniques of palliative care by the multidisciplinary staff, as well as the added support for patient and family at home, including payment for palliative medications and medical supplies. In most outpatient programs, the primary care physician and the hospice team form a partnership to care for the patient. The primary care provider, with whom the patient may have a long-term relationship, should be intimately involved in both the decision for hospice referral and the patient's ongoing care. Once distressing symptoms are controlled, the hospice team may then help the patient find avenues to hope, meaning, and ways of saying good-bye.

CASE ILLUSTRATION 2

Carlos, a 70-year-old man, has been diagnosed with an advanced hepatocellular carcinoma. In exploring the treatment options with his physician, he is clear about wanting only palliative measures, and referral to a home hospice program is initiated. Carlos is not a verbal man, and discussions about death and dying meet with little response.

At first, periodic nursing visits are all that is needed. He has an antique tool collection and spends countless hours labeling and ordering the tools. His nurse talks to him about this process, which has come to symbolize his anticipatory grief.

As he deteriorates, nursing visits become more frequent, and home health aides come to help with his personal care. Carlos gradually becomes bed bound. Although his family initially feels uncomfortable with his dying at home, a family meeting with the physician and hospice nurse sets up a rotation of visits to provide for both company and supervision. Children who had been estranged are in the rotation, and it becomes a time of family healing. Although little is explicitly said about his approaching death, the presence of family and talk about the tools provide a vehicle for saying good-bye. Carlos dies quietly at home with his family present.

Hospice care, with its supportive team of physicians, nurses, and other caregivers, helps patients and their families live as fully as possible until their inevitable death by providing quality palliative care.

Dealing with Grief

At times it may be difficult to distinguish normal grief reactions to the dying process from pathologic states that may require consultation and special treatment. There is a natural sadness that human beings experience in regard to death. This sadness, which may be a way of preparing for death, has been called **preparatory** or **anticipatory grief**. Grieving over the loss of physical abilities, social position, and contact with pleasurable routines—whether one's own or those of a loved one—is a natural reaction. The absence of grief over these losses may indicate denial and emotional numbing. Sharing and exploring the grief help both patient and clinician enter a relationship that acknowledges one another's humanity. Having the courage to explore these feelings assists the patient in coming to terms with death and may prevent the isolation and subsequent clinical depression to which some patients are prone.

Depression

Distinguishing clinical depression from the natural grieving process that accompanies a terminal illness may be difficult, as they share many common symptoms (see Chapter 22). The vegetative symptoms of depression—fatigue, changes in appetite, sleep disorders, decreased sexual drive—are all common in serious illness. The affective and cognitive signs of depression, such as loss of interest, withdrawal, sadness, inability to concentrate, and hopelessness may be realistic assessments in the face of severe suffering, fear of a loss of dignity, and the expectation of death. When the cognitive symptoms of dysphoria, shame, guilt, isolation, or suicidal ideation seem out of proportion to the patient's situation, major depression should be considered. Depression in the terminally ill may be very responsive to pharmacotherapy and/or counseling. Depending on the expertise of the physician and other members of the multidisciplinary team, more difficult or dangerous problems with depression and/or anxiety should be referred to a mental health professional. Psychotherapists who are familiar with the dying process and are experienced with medically ill patients can provide an invaluable resource, both diagnostically and therapeutically, in the care of the terminally ill.

TRANSITIONS

Each transition—each diminishment of health—at the end of life includes loss, as well as the potential for personal growth and the acceptance of death. These transitions initially may be treated as another form of bad news, but they provide the opportunity for enhanced meaning and control in the dying process. Physicians caring for terminally ill patients must explore and work through these transitions with their patients. Questions that clinicians can ask their patients in exploring their views on end-of-life issues are listed in Table 37-1. These can be asked as hypothetical questions to explore the patient's beliefs about life and death. In patients with more advanced illness, the questions and their answers may be highly relevant to immediate treatment decisions.

Patients' and their families' willingness and ability to enter into deep discussions about death and dying vary

considerably; clinicians need to be flexible in their expectations about how much exploration is desirable or even possible. It is unusual for a life-long pattern of behavior to be altered by the dying process. Although for some people dying may be a time for personal growth, reflection, and meaning, for others personal factors and emotional reactions block an acceptance of death. The most frequently encountered of these reactions are denial, anger, depression, fear, and anxiety. These reactions may be present in different degrees and at different times in the dying process. Clinicians need to acknowledge, explore, and eventually understand what function the reaction is serving for the patient. Empathy, rather than withdrawal, is the way to deepen the patient–clinician relationship and create an atmosphere in which personal growth is more likely to occur (see Chapter 2).

 CASE ILLUSTRATION 3

At 68 years old, Albert has severe end-stage emphysema, complicated by mitral regurgitation, congestive heart failure, cardiac arrhythmias, alcoholism, and years of smoking. He lives with his wife, whom he has bullied and dominated throughout their 40-year marriage. He has been on home oxygen and has had multiple hospital admissions for shortness of breath.

Table 37-1. End-of-life issues to be discussed with patients.

Life support

- Do you have an advance directive (a living will or health care proxy)?
- Do you know what CPR is? It doesn't work very well for people in your condition, and it is very harsh. I would recommend that you forego CPR, and that we focus our treatments on anything that has a good chance of helping you without harming you.
- In the event an illness led to your being unable to eat or drink on a permanent basis, would you want to be fed with feeding tubes?
- Do you want your medical care primarily geared to prolonging your life, or is improving or maintaining your quality of life more important?

Personal beliefs

- What life experiences have you had around death and dying?
- How have these experiences affected your own attitudes about death?
- What are your worst fears about dying? What are your biggest hopes?
- What would be a "good death" for you?
- What do you believe happens to you when you die?
- If you were to die sooner rather than later, what would be left undone?

Long-term care and support systems

- If you become too ill to take care of yourself, who will take care of you?
- Who would you want to make health care decisions for you if you became unable to do so?
- If you were dying, would you prefer to be at home or in an institution such as a hospital or nursing home?
- Do you know what hospice care is? Would you want that kind of care if you were terminally ill?
- Who would you want to be present at the time of your dying and death?
- Is there anything you need to get done before you die?

Admitted to the emergency room with severe shortness of breath, Albert is found to have pneumonia and heart failure. He had previously decided not to have CPR and wanted "no part of any of those damned machines." He is admitted to the hospital and treated with aggressive medical means but is not put on a respirator. Albert regularly yells and curses at the respiratory therapists, nursing staff, physicians, and his family for not taking care of him, for making him suffer, and for not being prompt enough with meals, medicines, and treatments. He insists that the only thing wrong with him is that the medicines are making him sick.

Efforts to engage Albert in a dialogue that explores his feelings meet first with an unwillingness to talk and then a life history of feeling abandoned, powerless, betrayed by employers, and subject to bad luck. He describes himself as an "ornery son of a bitch." He fears lingering and suffering in the hospital, and although he hopes he will die quickly, he is also afraid to die. One of Albert's fears is of being buried alive, a phobia fed by a television program he had seen about the difficulty of determining when someone was dead and the possibility of being sent to the undertaker while still alive. The anxiety of being trapped in a "tight" place is overwhelming to him.

Albert's physicians had initially resisted placing him on anxiolytic drugs or narcotics out of fear they would compromise his breathing. The palliative care consultant recommended that both be started, and reassured both the treating physicians as well as the patient and family of the safety and effectiveness of these treatments as long as they are started at low doses. Low-dose opioids and anxiolytic medications are eventually started around the clock, and his dyspnea and anxiety are dramatically improved. Placed in a room with a large picture window to the outside, he spends long periods of time staring out the window. His complaints diminish and he seems much more relaxed. He allows the hospital chaplain to visit and to pray with him, though he does not otherwise want to talk about the nearness of death or any regrets he has about his life. He eventually tells his wife he has suffered enough, and does not want to live any longer. He gradually becomes more confused as a result of the rising carbon dioxide levels and dies several nights later.

Patients who are in the dying process, and who have personality and behavioral traits that make their care more difficult are especially challenging to care givers. The use of multidisciplinary specialties—often represented on palliative care teams—to brainstorm potential approaches and to share expertise may facilitate our commitment not to abandon these particularly challenging patients and families.

Information, Prognosis, Alternatives

Clinicians need to provide the patient with information about the disease, the prognosis, the treatment options, and the anticipated course of the illness. Most patients and their families want to know how much time is left when a terminal diagnosis is made. Providing ranges of survival times, allowing for outliers on either end, is better than predicting an exact amount of time. Refusing to give time estimates or withholding other grim information to protect the patient is usually not productive and may not allow the patient and family to prepare for death. The possibility of miracles or rare exceptions to the usual course of the illness allows a glimmer of hope for some patients. On the other hand, clinicians giving prognostic information must discipline themselves to discuss the possibility that death may come sooner than expected, so that patients are not unprepared for this possibility as well. In general, the physician should be guided by patients and their families in determining how detailed the information about the course of the illness should be.

Alternative healing methods sometimes offer hope to some patients when traditional methods are not working, have proven too burdensome, or are not consistent with the patient's preferences. Patients who are interested in pursuing alternative methods of treatment should be supported in doing so, particularly if those treatments are noninvasive, and are therefore unlikely to harm. There is nothing to preclude combining nontraditional treatments with traditional treatments as part of an individually tailored plan. Some patients turn to alternative treatments because they have been told their case is "hopeless" and there is "nothing left to be done." However, selecting such therapies because of a sense of futility, desperation, and abandonment is very different from choosing them because they are consistent with a person's goals and values. Aggressive if unconventional therapeutic alternatives offer some patients a degree of hope. However, clinician and patient together should explore the validity of this type of hope. Examining the risks and benefits of both traditional and nontraditional therapies is frequently enough to begin the dialogue, which can then continue by exploring the possibilities and probabilities of improvement and by distinguishing false hope from a meaningful alternative (see Chapter 30).

 CASE ILLUSTRATION 4

Max, a 63-year-old, recently retired, and previously healthy man, develops abdominal pains and is found to have widely metastasized colon cancer. He goes to a physician and is advised that no treatment would be beneficial and that he has approximately 6–12 months to live. He is given acetaminophen and

codeine for pain and told to come back when the combination no longer relieves the discomfort. Max and his wife cannot bear the thought of just waiting for him to die and decide to cast a wider net in seeking a cure—or at least some kind of treatment. They hear of a cancer-treatment clinic out of the country and go there for a 6-week program of intensive vitamin and herbal treatments, coffee enemas, a variety of teas, and dietary supplements. Max is also given a long list of treatments to follow when he returns home; this keeps him busy trying to "beat" the cancer. The clinic is supposed to provide follow-up by mail or telephone; however, several months go by and there is no contact from the clinic.

Discouraged, Max and his wife go to another physician in their hometown when the pains in his liver intensify and ascites and jaundice set in. The physician and the couple discuss the available options and agree on purely palliative care measures. Max is referred to a home hospice program and dies 4 weeks later, approximately 9 months from the time of diagnosis. His family feels he received superb care for his last 4 weeks, however they feel abandoned and betrayed with regard to his prior treatment. His wife never receives any follow-up information from the overseas clinic, nor does anyone from the original physician's office call to offer condolences on her husband's death.

This patient has been abandoned twice. The first treating physician failed to explore all treatment alternatives (second opinion, experimental therapy, guidance in exploring nontraditional treatments) and then offered inadequate follow-up (come back when these pain pills stop working). The alternative clinic offered the patient an active treatment approach (which he and his wife desperately sought), but then deserted him by failing to follow through after the treatment was completed. The third physician finally helped the patient and family come to grips with the reality of his condition, and arranged for a program that provided caring and follow-up for his final weeks. Nonabandonment is always a key element in the care of the dying patient.

HOPE & MEANING

Throughout the dying process, the search for hope and meaning is always in the background. Hopelessness and despair are disturbing emotions. Hope helps patients and their loved ones endure suffering when faced with a terminal illness. It comes in many forms, not simply through cure or recovery. To hope for a peaceful death, to have a little more time to finish business, to find new meaning and the possibility of personal growth in our

dying, or to become emotionally closer to loved ones or to God are all hopes and wishes not dependent on cure of the body.

CASE ILLUSTRATION 5

Rhea, a 64-year-old woman with metastatic breast cancer, is on high-dose long-acting morphine because of bone pain. She has fractures of the clavicle and both femurs and has requested no resuscitation in the event of cardiac or pulmonary arrest. She hopes to be able to die at home, where she has very close family support, without more painful episodes or fractures. She is enrolled in a home hospice program, and her sister moves in with her to serve the role as primary care provider.

Rhea eventually shows signs of increasing confusion and dehydration. She expresses the strong wish not to die yet, because her children and their families are arriving in 2 weeks. She wants not only to see them, but also to be as alert and pain free as possible while they visit. Bloodwork is done to see if she has anything that might be easily reversed, and hypercalcemia is found. Because she wishes to die at home with only palliative measures taken, she remains at home for another day. She knows that she will likely die from the effects of the untreated hypercalcemia, but that she then would likely not get to see her daughters. Despite attempts at oral treatment she becomes progressively less alert, and is brought to an acute hospice unit when her oral intake stops.

In hope of having her alert for her family's upcoming visit, treatment is initiated with intravenous fluids, diuretics and bisphosphonates. The hypercalcemia is corrected, her confusion clears, and she is able to go home after a week. By the time her children arrive, Rhea is alert and able to communicate coherently. She is quite elated that she can have last words with them and her grandchildren. Despite the need for increased doses of morphine and multiple other medications to control her symptoms, she is not readmitted to the acute hospice unit when her hypercalcemia and the associated confusion recur. She dies quietly at home several days later.

The hope for more time fortunately in this case could be achieved, because the patient was willing to endure relatively aggressive treatment, and the hospice program was able to be flexible in allowing her to meet her short-term goals. Invasive interventions that exceed the usual boundaries of hospice care but that extend meaningful life and improve quality of life are sometimes appropriate even within a hospice approach, as long as the patient consents. Remaining flexible in the face of changing, difficult situations and letting the patient's goals guide the treatment permit the clinician to hope, along with the patient, for a death with as little meaningless suffering as possible.

Trying to find and maintain hope when the patient's goal of recovery is futile calls for personal and spiritual exploration. It may be necessary to probe in depth the patient's feeling of hopelessness before possible new avenues for hope and meaning can be examined. It is important not to provide false hope through simple or formulaic solutions to complex problems; hopeful solutions are often uniquely personal and may be discovered through continuing exploration by the patient with family, friends, health care providers, and clergy.

PLANNING FOR THE FUTURE

Advance Directives

Advance directives are formal documents that direct health care decisions if patients lose the capacity to speak for themselves. There are two types of advance directives: living wills and health care proxies (also called durable powers of attorney).

A living will allows a patient to direct the kinds of treatments wanted if the capacity to make decisions is lost. Some living wills focus on general goals, whereas others specify exact treatments (CPR, artificial ventilation, artificial hydration, and nutrition) and explicit circumstances (terminal illness, persistent vegetative state, unable to make decisions for oneself). Living wills become operative only when patients are unable to communicate for themselves, and when the circumstances specified in the document are realized.

A **health care proxy**, or **durable power of attorney**, allows patients to designate a person to make decisions on their behalf should they become unable to do so. These directives allow much more flexibility than do living wills, as it is difficult to anticipate all possible medical conditions and treatment options that might be in question for a particular patient.

Many people complete both documents: a living will to present an overarching philosophy and a health care proxy to designate a person to help interpret that philosophy when the patient can no longer do so. For healthy persons, discussing a living will or a health care proxy may be the first time they have had to face their own mortality. For those with terminal illness, completing an advance directive may be seen as another indication of their inevitable deterioration.

Involving family members in the discussions of advance directives is useful. A proxy who is uninformed about the values and wishes of the patient has an arduous job when difficult care decisions must be made. Although they cannot cover every situation, living wills with clear statements about goals, values, and directions help the clinician and the designated proxy formulate a care plan. In addition, having a form to fill out helps many patients and their families discuss death and disability-related issues. For severely ill patients, the advance directive decisions can provide a starting point for discussions about the limits of care and the burdens of suffering as well as orders not to resuscitate.

DO NOT RESUSCITATE

The "do-not-resuscitate" order refers to the withholding of CPR, specifically closed-chest cardiac massage, defibrillation, and artificially supplied respiratory support. For most patients with a terminal disease, CPR is ineffective, and its harshness makes it a cruel, expensive, technological death ritual. Many studies have shown that CPR provides no increase in out-of-hospital survival for patients with multisystem disease, particularly patients with advanced cancers and renal failure.

Unfortunately, many patients and their families equate DNR with abandonment or giving up, and agonize over its issuance. This is in part due to the way medical personnel emphasize what will be withheld rather than what will be done. When alternative treatment strategies are not explained, patients and families think that a DNR order means nothing will be done to treat potentially reversible conditions or to relieve uncomfortable symptoms. They sense that second-class treatment will be given—which may indeed happen if clinicians and the institutions they work in are not knowledgeable about the narrow focus on a DNR directive. It should be understood that agreement to a DNR order in no way limits other treatment options. A way of articulating this is to say: *"We want to do everything possible to help you, but we also do not want to harm you. CPR would not work given your condition, and it is very harsh. I would recommend that you set that limit while we continue to provide any and all treatments that will help you."*

DNR orders do, however, signal that things are different. The notion that being resuscitated from cardiopulmonary arrest will not add appreciably to the quality and or quantity of life is an open acknowledgment that death might be near—and that reversing the dying process is not within the power of medicine. Although some patients are initially frightened by this discussion, many feel relieved and appreciate the opportunity to avoid treatment that would not help them.

Emergency rescue crews are obligated to attempt resuscitation unless they have specific instructions not to proceed. DNR orders that are valid in the inpatient setting may not be valid in the outpatient setting unless special forms, which vary by locality, are completed. These issues should be addressed with terminally ill patients who want to remain at home, as resuscitation may be carried out in times of crisis if the proper documentation is not on hand. In Oregon and a few other states, the Physician Orders for Life Sustaining Treatment (POLST) has been accepted as a legal document that must be honored by emergency medical technicians (EMTs) and first responders. This ensures a portability to other settings of the patient's explicit wishes recorded in physicians' orders.

Restricted Interventions

Patients at the end of life, or patients with a high degree of suffering, may elect through their advance directives not to undergo treatments that may be considered routine under other circumstances. Patients have the right to forego therapies such as intravenous fluids, nasogastric feeding, supplemental oxygen, and others. Documentation of these choices is vital if the patient does not wish to undergo treatments. Restricted intervention forms are now available in some states to augment the advance directives.

PAIN AND SYMPTOM RELIEF

An important goal in palliative care is to keep patients as pain free as possible. Long-acting opioid preparations, when given in sufficient quantity in a regular dosing schedule around the clock, with proportionate supplemental doses as needed, are effective in alleviating most chronic pain without significantly compromising quality of life. Knowing that they can control their own pain is reassuring to patients, especially those who have seen painful deaths. Unrealistic concerns about addiction or about respiratory depression from patients, families, and caregivers should be anticipated and addressed, as these worries often present a major obstacle to adequate pain relief. Withholding narcotics in the seriously ill because of unrealistic fears is unwarranted and cruel.

Delirium & Coma

Many patients die in profoundly altered states of sensorium. There is also an increasing number of patients with dementing illnesses in whom cognitive and affective life may have diminished significantly prior to the terminal episode (see Chapter 27). Terminally ill patients with delirium present the physician and the patient's family with a dilemma. Delirium may be due to reversible factors that, if treated, could extend life. The extent to which reversible causes of delirium are searched for and treated depends on the patient's current goals, previous directives, and concurrent discussions with the family. The prior degree of suffering and the patient's wishes should largely determine what should be done.

The internal, subjective experience of a person dying with altered mental status may vary significantly from the outside perception. Patients who recover from delirium and coma sometimes report nightmarish, terrifying visions, out-of-body travel, or visions of light and angelic

beings, or they may not be able to remember anything about the experience. Occasionally, the disorientation becomes profound and the sense of the world is lost.

CASE ILLUSTRATION 6

Caleb, a 101-year-old rugged dairy farmer, has become partly deaf and then blind in the last 5 years of his life but remains alert and communicative. He develops a cough and fever, and despite treatment for pneumonia, becomes progressively more dyspneic. He tells his physician that he does not wish to be resuscitated. Because his elderly wife cannot care for him at home, Caleb is hospitalized. He becomes progressively more confused and withdrawn, and his deafness and blindness further confound communication. He lies still in bed for long periods of time. Efforts by physicians and nurses to engage him in conversation are usually met with short responses such as yes, no, or okay. His physician asks him one morning what experiences he is having, and he replies that he is flying over fields of golden wheat on a sunny day. Then, in a voice of wonderment, he asks if he is still alive or if he has died. His physician replies that he is still alive. Caleb dies later that day.

Patients who experience altered states at the end of life need supportive treatment. Once this stage has been reached, decisions about artificial hydration and feeding ideally should have already been made and formalized through advance directives. If they have not (as is frequently the case) the designated health care agent or the family, taking into consideration the patient's condition and prognosis, must make a substituted judgment as to what the patient would want. If this cannot be determined, the physician's decision should be based on a consensus among family and providers about what is in the best interest of the patient.

Providing nutrition and hydration through feeding tubes and intravenous lines when the dying patient can no longer eat or drink may appear compassionate, but such practices may inadvertently prolong dying and aggravate suffering. When a person with a terminal illness is actively dying, our acceptance of this fact should guide all treatments in the direction of decreasing the suffering, enhancing the quality of life left, and respecting the patient's dignity.

The Wish to Die

Sometimes, even with the best methods of palliative care, suffering cannot be alleviated to the patient's satisfaction.

If this occurs, the patient may feel that dying is the only way out. The patient may no longer be able to tolerate the pain, humiliation, loss of control, increased dependency, or burden the illness places on the family. Such patients often actively begin to contemplate ending their life.

CASE ILLUSTRATION 7

Marvin is 63 years old; he has amyotrophic lateral sclerosis and has been on a respirator at home for a year. He has lost the ability to use his arms and legs and requires total care. He increasingly resents his life on the respirator and finally requests that it be removed and he be permitted to die. He makes this request repeatedly over the course of a month. His primary care physician sees him several times on home visits and discusses the request with Marvin's family. They agree that the respirator should be stopped. A psychiatrist visits the patient and indicates that he finds Marvin competent, not depressed; he concurs with the patient, family, and primary care physician on removing the respirator. An attempt to remove the respirator without the

sedative effects of morphine leads to air hunger and feelings of suffocation. A morphine drip is instituted and the respirator is turned off. The patient dies comfortably several minutes later, attended by his family and physician.

The ***double effect*** of providing medications intended to relieve suffering and yet could inadvertently shorten the patient's life is an accepted part of medical practice and palliative care, provided the patient's suffering is proportionately severe. Withdrawing life-sustaining but burdensome treatments, even though the withdrawal leads to death, is also an accepted part of practice based on the patient's right to bodily integrity. These practices have widespread legal, ethical, and medical acceptance and should not be confused with the controversy surrounding assisted suicide and voluntary euthanasia. In this case, the patient's wish to die can be acceded to, as a treatment that is life-sustaining but very burdensome could be removed in conjunction with the provision of a high-dose narcotic that is intended to lessen panic and suffering (Table 37-2).

Table 37-2. Euthanasia and assisted death: definitions.

Term	Definition	Legal Status in the United States
Double effect	Administering drugs that are intended to relieve suffering but may unintentionally shorten life. The risk of shortening life must be proportionate to the degree of suffering.	Legal
Withholding or withdrawing life-sustaining treatment	Withholding or withdrawing life-sustaining care that results in the patient's death with the consent of the patient or surrogate. Justification based on the right to bodily integrity.	Legal with the proper consent
Palliative sedation (also called terminal sedation)	With consent from the patient or surrogate, the patient is sedated to unconsciousness to relieve otherwise intractable suffering, and then food and fluids are withdrawn. Generally viewed as a combination of double effect and withdrawal of treatment, but not without moral controversy if viewed in aggregate.	Legal with the proper consent
Physician aid-in-dying (also called physician-assisted suicide)	Physician provides, at the patient's request, the means for the patient to end his or her own life. The patient then takes or does not take the overdose at a future time.	Illegal in most states except for Oregon, but difficult to prosecute
Active euthanasia	Physician administers an intentional lethal overdose of medication with the competent patient's informed consent. The physician is the direct agent causing death at the patient's request.	Illegal, and likely to be successfully prosecuted if discovered

Patients, however, may ask the clinician, sometimes in an off-hand way, as if testing the water, about help in dying (either assisted suicide or euthanasia). This subject has both ethical and legal repercussions, and patients are often as reluctant as their physicians to discuss it.

If the patient has terrible suffering but does not have a life-sustaining treatment that can be withdrawn (e.g., respirator, dialysis, feeding tube) or the kind of pain that can justify high doses of narcotics, the request for help in dying would put the clinician in a more difficult position legally and ethically. Voluntary active euthanasia is the act of intentionally intervening to cause the patient's death, at the explicit request of, and with the full informed consent of, the competent patient. The physician administers a lethal agent, with the intent of both alleviating suffering and causing death. Voluntary active euthanasia is illegal everywhere in the United States and would lead to prosecution if discovered. In assisted suicide, the physician provides the means (such as a prescription for barbiturates) at the request of the patient, but the patient must eventually take (or not take) the potentially lethal medication by his or her own hand. Assisted suicide is illegal in most states, but the underground practice is not actively prosecuted provided it is conducted in secret. A referendum legalizing assisted suicide at the request of a terminally ill patient was passed in Oregon in 1997, and has now withstood several legal challenges. There are now several years of data about the legalized practice in Oregon which can allow for comparison of utilization patterns of assisted dying and other palliative care practices in comparison to other states.

CASE ILLUSTRATION 8

Sara, a bedridden 84-year-old woman with end-stage congestive heart failure, is seen on rounds. She is on multiple medications, including morphine, to relieve her dyspnea and pulmonary edema. Despite intensive treatment, even eating causes her to be dyspneic. She looks up from her bed and asks to be given a lethal dose of medicine so that she can die. When asked why she wants to die now, Sara replies that she has lived long enough—through the deaths of her husband, two of her children, three of her brothers, and both her sisters. Her one remaining son is dying of leukemia and has only weeks to live. She wants to die before him so she won't have to grieve his death. Her request for lethal medication is not granted. Sara leaves the hospital with public health nurses and family to look after her. Her physician agrees to make home visits as Sara is too weak to travel to the office. A few days later, Sara is found dead in bed by the visiting nurse. The physician, called to the house to pronounce
the patient dead, notices several empty pill bottles, including those from the morphine, at the bedside. The physician thinks that this may have been a suicide, but decides not to pursue it and simply completes the death certificate as for a natural death.

A patient's request to hasten death should be explored in detail. At first, it should be considered a cry for help. It may represent the wish to escape from depression, anxiety, uncontrolled physical pain, shame of dependency, and other psychosocial issues. Once the underlying reasons for the request are fully understood, the problem(s) can usually be ameliorated through appropriate techniques of palliative care, and the request is frequently withdrawn. If the request is ignored, minimized, or belittled, the patient is left to deal with these feelings alone, and may (as in this case) take an overdose because of suffering that might have been dealt with by other means.

There are times, however, as in our example, when protracted pain and other debilitating symptoms might make choosing death a plausible alternative to continued suffering. The relationship between the physician, patient, and family as well as the physician's own values determine the response to such requests. Clinicians who refuse to participate in assisted suicide, because of their own moral positions, should make this clear to the patient. In this event, they have an obligation to seek common ground with the patient and to continue to search for other avenues to relieve suffering. Usually such intractable suffering can be addressed with symptom management, withdrawal of all potentially life-sustaining therapies, and terminal sedation if all else fails. In this particular case, if the patient's request was found to be rational and all reasonable alternatives had been explored, the patient could have stopped all of her heart failure medicines except for her morphine, which could have been titrated upward to control emerging shortness of breath. Those clinicians who are considering any last-resort options (whether legally permitted, but especially if legally prohibited) should fully explore the potential personal, professional, and legal consequences and get second opinions from experienced clinicians. Guidelines for assisted suicide have been published, and clinicians confronted with a reasonable request to end life should refer to these, as well as to colleagues experienced in palliative care, for help. In almost all cases, legally permissible and clinically preferable alternatives can be found.

ACCEPTANCE

Some patients are not afraid of dying and come to accept death as a natural step in completing the life cycle. Many such persons are able to die with grace and ease, demonstrating that death does not always have to be feared or denied. Furthermore, some patients experience profound personal growth in the process of dying. For some highly independent persons, this becomes a time to be more accepting and appreciative of the love and care of others.

CASE ILLUSTRATION 9

A 64-year-old veterinarian, Richard, develops headaches so severe that he can no longer carry on his surgical practice. Within 3 months, he is diagnosed with an inoperable brain tumor. Over the ensuing 6 months, he loses the ability to walk and swallow. Because of recurrent aspiration, he is placed on a home ventilator and fed through a gastrostomy tube. In the face of his overwhelming losses, he decides he wants to tape a description of his life and journey to the point at which he is now. Relatives, friends, colleagues, and members of his church come to his home, and joint recollections and reflections are taped. When this process is complete Richard says good-bye to his wife and family and requests that the respirator and fluids be withdrawn. With his physician's consent and instructions to family members, he is given regular doses of morphine and the respirator is turned off. He dies with his loved ones in attendance. His life and death leave a legacy of courage and an acquiescence to fate that touches the hearts of those he knew.

The search for love, a connection to others, and a sense of meaning are essential in helping patients through the dying process. The ability to experience love and meaning can ameliorate considerable suffering. If love and purpose can be found, then fears usually lessen, and dying may be accepted as an adventure and entry into the next phase of existence.

CARE OF THE FAMILY

Terminal illness can help resolve or intensify family conflict. Issues of power, money, allegiances, previous losses, and grief may surface along with unforeseen courage and the noblest sacrifices that family members may ever have made on behalf of one another. Paradoxical feelings of anger and love, fear and bravery, anxiety and compassion, depression and transcendence never seem to be far removed from dying patients and their caregivers.

The physician can be a healing presence in this volatile mix by including the patient's family and other caregivers as part of the treatment team. Such collaboration broadens the patient's network of support, enlisting new allies and more widely distributing the burden of care.

The clinician needs to communicate clearly with family members regarding plans for care, prognosis, complications, and who will make decisions if the patient cannot. Establishing advance directives with the patient and the proxy is essential when it is likely the patient will lose capacity during the illness. The selection of a proxy forces the patient to choose among family members and may trigger old family wounds over who was favored and who has more power. The patient's wishes and choices should take precedence over what family members may want, although in actual practice this is sometimes difficult to achieve. When the patient loses mental capacity, the family becomes the focus of decision making, and processes are brought into play that may create conflict. Family pressures may even influence the decisions of a competent patient. The clinician may need to remind family members that whether the patient is competent or not, the patient's values, beliefs, and preferences need to be honored.

When a family has many members, the clinician may want to meet regularly with a small group and at special times with more members. The family can be asked to designate representatives who can stay in close touch with the physician. If patients have lost the capacity to express their wishes and family members are in conflict about a certain plan, it is best to focus on what the patient would have wanted, applying the ethical principle of substituted judgment. If the patient's wishes are unknown, what is in the patient's best interest must be discussed. Views on what is truly in the patient's best interest may vary widely between family members and clinicians (see Chapter 8).

Unexpected Death

An unexpected death puts a particular strain on the family and the clinician. Sudden or traumatic death sends a shock through the family and, when it occurs in a medical facility, may elicit strong doubt about competence in clinicians. Meeting with the family, expressing sympathy, and answering questions in as straightforward a way as possible may be helpful. Family members should be allowed to view and stay with the deceased; when possible, the eyes and mouth should be closed and the limbs arranged peacefully. Strong emotional reactions should be anticipated and the tears of grief welcomed.

The clinician should recognize each family member present and solicit each person's reaction. Cultural norms may vary widely in the emotional behaviors displayed. The normal reactions to grief in some cultures (screaming, yelling, falling to the ground) may seem inappropriate or embarrassing to a clinician from another, less demonstrative background (see Chapter 12).

Only through experience with various manifestations of grief can the clinician judge what "normal" grief should look like. Physicians and nurses may want to call in clergy and social workers; each may have something to offer a family that is trying to integrate the shock and loss.

When an unexpected death occurs in the context of ongoing medical care, the practitioner should critically examine what, if anything, could have been done to prevent its occurrence. Self-recrimination and blame may initially be part of this process for the clinician, especially if a medical misjudgment was involved. Learning from the experience, discussing it with trusted colleagues, and, if necessary, disclosing it to the family are often appropriate. It is important that clinicians not bear the burdens of these experiences alone (see Chapter 34).

Unresolved Grief

Of all the causes of unremitting grief, one of the most overwhelmingly difficult for families and practitioners is the death of a child, especially when the death is unexpected. The parents' grief must be followed closely for signs of becoming pathologic. The physician should not try to ameliorate the pain of the loss prematurely. Supportive listening, acknowledging and legitimizing the suffering, and expressing empathy may be the best initial approach. Follow-up visits to elicit stories and memories give the parents a chance to talk about the deceased if they choose. Discussing and expressing anger, guilt, and sadness can help the bereavement process. In many other cases, survivors are unable to deal with the loss of a parent, a sibling, a spouse or partner, or a long-time friend. Grief that is unresolved may lead to clinical depression, social isolation, and emotional numbing as well as multiple physical symptoms. Social problems such as drug abuse, marital and work conflicts, and feelings of hopelessness and abandonment may also appear. If the clinician cannot help the family resolve the grief, referral should be made to an appropriate support group or a therapist for counseling.

SELF-CARE

How health care workers take care of themselves when involved in work related to death and dying has not received a great deal of attention. Burnout is common among physicians and nurses who work with patients who are suffering a terminal illness. Having responsibility for dying patients' care and management in a society that denies death exacerbates the problem. From the initial delivery of bad news about a new potentially fatal diagnosis, to discussions about disease recurrence, to the transition to hospice, to decisions about whether to attend the funeral, clinicians are confronted with thoughts and feelings that enmesh them with the

patient and the family. How closely the patient's family resembles their own family dynamics or illness experience may determine how emotionally involved they become. The grief that follows the death of a close patient may be quite profound and requires time and reflection to heal. Unfortunately, most institutions do not have an organized way for caregivers to get and give support during these times. The feelings of loss need to be recognized and discussed. Support or bereavement groups may help in this process. Hospital morbidity and mortality committees review the decedent's medical care, but they rarely reflect on how caregivers felt about the death, or what effect it has on the staff. Setting aside time to review the death from this perspective is likely to be helpful for staff morale, cohesiveness, and healing (see Chapter 6).

Taking care of the dying patient enables clinicians to view death at very close range. Feelings of compassion and love as well as loneliness and vulnerability are frequently stirred up in providers. Healing responses may include turning to music, art, religion, literature, nature, humor, or psychotherapy for solace and understanding. Spiritual questions of purpose and meaning in life become more immediate in the face of impending death. Not only do workers in the realm of death and dying midwife patients through the dying process, but also the dying patient midwifes us into a fuller experience of life.

SUGGESTED READINGS

American Medical Association: Good care of the dying patient. *JAMA* 1996;275:474–478.

Back AL, Arnold RM, Quill TE. Hope for the best, and prepare for the worst. *Ann Intern Med* 2003;138(5):439–443.

Clinical Practice Guideline: Management of Cancer Pain. Agency for Health Care Policy and Research. Publication No. 94-0592. Available through the National Cancer Institute.

Ferris FD, von Gunten CF, Emanuel LL. Competency in end-of-life care: last hours of life. *J Palliat Med* 2003;6(4):605–613.

Hickman SE, Hammes BJ, Moss AH, et al. Hope for the future: achieving the original intent of advance directives. *Hastings Cent Rep* 2005;35:S26–S30.

Meier DE, Back AL, Morrison RS. The inner life of physicians and the care of the seriously ill. *JAMA* 2001;286:3007–3014.

Morrison RS, Meier DE. Clinical practice: palliative care. *N Engl J Med* 2004; 351:1148–1149.

Quill TE, Holloway R, Shah MS, et al. *Palliative Care Primer*, 4th ed. American Academy of Hospice and Palliative Medicine, 2007.

Quill TE. *Caring for Patients at the End of Life: Facing an Uncertain Future Together.* New York, NY: Oxford University Press, 2001.

Rabow MD, Hauser JM, Adams J. Supporting family caregivers at the end of life: *"They don't know what they don't know."* *JAMA* 2004;291:483–491.

Snyder L, Quill TE, eds. *Physician Guide to End-of-Life Care.* Philadelphia, PA: ACP-ASIM Publishing, 2001.

Sulmasy DP. Spiritual issues in the care of dying patients " . . . *It's okay between me and God." JAMA* 2006;296:1385–1392.

Von Gunten CF. Discussing hospice care. *J Clin Oncol* 2002;20: 1419–1424.

WEB SITES

American Academy of Hospice and Palliative Medicine Web site. www.aahpm.org. Accessed October, 2007.

Center to Advance Palliative Care Web site. www.capc.org. Accessed October, 2007.

Compassion and Choices Web site. www.compassionandchoices.org. Accessed October, 2007.

Death with Dignity National Center Web site. www.deathwithdignity.org. Accessed October, 2007.

Education in Palliative and End-of-Life Care Web site. www.epec.net. Accessed October, 2007.

End of Life/Palliative Education Resource Center Web site. www.eperc.mcw.edu. Accessed October, 2007.

National Hospice and Palliative Care Organization Web site. www.nhpco.org. Accessed October, 2007.

National Palliative Care Research Center Web site. www.npcrc.org. Accessed October, 2007.

Palliative Care Policy Center Web site. www.medicaring.org. Accessed October, 2007.

Physician Orders for Life-Sustaining Treatment (POLST) Web site. www.polst.org. Accessed October, 2007.

SECTION VI
Teaching Behavioral Medicine in Medical Settings

Education for Competencies in the Social & Behavioral Sciences

Debra K. Litzelman, MA, MD, Eric S. Holmboe, MD, & Thomas S. Inui, ScM, MD

After each surgery, the surgeon I worked with fully takes off his mask and hair bonnet prior to speaking with the patient's family. Although it only takes seconds to do this, I believe it helps the family feel more at ease and allows them to see the surgeon as a true human not hiding behind anything. Third-year medical student, IUSM 2006

Our team and the ICU team were rounding and we all entered a patient's room. There were at least 15 of us in the room. Our teams spoke about the patient, examined him, adjusted the ventilator setting, and then left—all oblivious to the family member who was in the room the entire time. After we had all left, I noticed that the intern—who had just started the service that morning—kneeled down beside the patient's wife and began explaining what the team had just done. No one else noticed what she had done, but I was very impressed by her behavior. Third-year medical student, IUSM 2006

INTRODUCTION

Across the country, medical training institutions are enhancing traditional formal curricula to develop and assess trainees' competency in a wide range of abilities, including competencies in the social and behavior sciences such as communication, self-awareness, professionalism, and moral reasoning. "Competency" is a complex notion that refers to the capacity, in varying circumstances, to use knowledge, skills, and values in actions that serve a purpose (e.g., promoting or regaining health or various intermediate outcomes on the way to health). The lowest-order competency is the ability to take certain actions successfully without much self-awareness, capacity to reflect, or adaptability. The highest-order competency is to interact with others with mindfulness, awareness, and adaptability, that is, to be what Donald Schön has called a "reflective practitioner." The acquisition of competencies in the social and behavioral sciences (SBS) in undergraduate medical education, indeed throughout the long career in medicine, is a staged process that combines learning of several different types (cognitive, behavioral, and social). Throughout their professional life cycle, physicians learn from formal and informal sources that are both didactic and experiential. The most powerful learning aligns both formal and informal sources while providing opportunities for reflection and feedback.

A useful framework for integrating trainees' formal and informal experiences in the SBS is to focus on their competency. Educators must attend both to the formal curriculum, as well as trainees' learning environment, which comprises the institution's informal or "hidden" curriculum. Using current theories of learning, this chapter illustrates innovative educational methods that integrate formal and informal curricula in teaching and assessing competency in the SBS.

BACKGROUND

The 2004 Institute of Medicine (IOM) report, *Improving Medical Education: Enhancing the Behavioral and Social Science Content of Medical School Curricula*, identifies 26 topics in six SBS domains that are important to the education of future physicians (see Table 38-1). The need for such training in the behavioral and social sciences has been well documented. Nevertheless, several decades of efforts to teach this content have resulted in only mixed success. While many courses have successfully achieved their objectives, many others have been subject to student and faculty criticism, frequent course revision, discontinuation, and faculty turnover. With some exceptions, the same limitations and critiques directed toward undergraduate medical education hold true for graduate medical education as well.

In seeking to understand the difficulties involved in integrating SBS content, researchers have focused almost exclusively on the formal curriculum. Expressions of the formal curriculum include course and clerkship content and format, time blocks, and evaluation and assessment methods. The medical education literature, however, clearly identifies several barriers specific to the teaching of SBS in the formal curriculum, including the marginalization of SBS content and faculty, a multiplicity of learning objectives, timing of teaching the SBS content, mismatch between teaching methods and context of use, and failure of social scientists and clinicians to work together to create effective learning experiences. It is not difficult to find examples of these barriers. SBS content can be marginalized in many ways. Trainees may lack exposure to qualified faculty or may only have exposure to "visiting" faculty who are seen as add-ons to basic science courses. Medical training programs may lack support and incentives for faculty to include SBS content, and career development programs in SBS are frequently absent. Because there is a limited amount of time available to teach a wide range of SBS topics, their inclusion may be superficial or based on the availability of teachers rather than importance. The timing of SBS teaching is often developmentally and methodologically inappropriate. Topics such as death and dying are often covered in small group discussions in the first or second year and not revisited in any formal way in the clerkship years, yet research on knowledge use and acquisition concludes that there is little immediate transfer of learning from one context of use to another. For example, students who discuss death and dying in a classroom (academic context) will be challenged to exhibit professional and humanistic behavior in the presence of real patients (practice context) without formal training in the clinical context. Finally, emphasis on discipline-based knowledge creates another barrier to integration of SBS content. True integration of SBS content requires various

disciplines to work closely together to establish joint responsibility for knowledge creation, development, and dissemination.

Formal Competency Curriculum Initiatives

CASE ILLUSTRATION 1: UNDERGRADUATE MEDICAL EDUCATION: BROWN UNIVERSITY COMPETENCY-BASED CURRICULUM

While many institutions struggle to incorporate social and behavioral content in a comprehensive and integrated way, in 1993 Brown University undertook a significant reform of their formal curriculum explicitly to include the wide range of knowledge and abilities critical to excellent patient care. Brown University's competency-based curriculum focuses on curricular outcomes and criteria for assessing students in many areas identified as underrepresented in our nation's current curricula. The groundbreaking work accomplished by Brown University, as documented in An Educational Blueprint for the Brown University School of Medicine, has proven to be a model for other medical training institutions. The Brown University competencies include: (1) Effective Communication; (2) Basic Clinical Skills; (3) Using Basic Science to Guide Therapy; (4) Diagnosis, Management, and Prevention; (5) Lifelong Learning; (6) Self-awareness, Self-care, and Personal Growth; (7) Social and Community Contexts of Health Care; (8) Moral Reasoning and Ethical Judgment; and (9) Problem Solving. The curriculum is available electronically at: http://biomed. brown.edu/Medicine_Programs/MD2000/Blueprint_ for_the_Web_04.pdf.

CASE ILLUSTRATION 2: GRADUATE MEDICAL EDUCATION: AMERICAN COUNCIL ON GRADUATE MEDICAL EDUCATION OUTCOME

In 2001, the American Council on Graduate Medical Education (ACGME) recognized the need to broaden the curricular focus for residency training and began a stepwise phase-in of competencies deemed essential for residency training into programs around the

Table 38-1. SBS domains with priority topics and learning objectives.[*]

Domain: Mind-Body Interactions in Health & Disease

Biological Mediators Between Psychological and Social Factors and Health

Describe how behavioral and social factors and stress alter physiology to make disease more likely and the interconnectivity of homeostatic systems.
Explain the relationship between chronic stress, affective illness, social support, and health.

Psychological, Social, and Behavioral Factors in Chronic Illness

Understand the interrelationship between psychological, social, behavioral, and lifestyle factors and particular chronic medical conditions (e.g., diabetes, coronary artery disease [CAD], arthritis, cancer).
Understand and predict on-going risky health behaviors.
Describe how to recognize stress in chronically ill patients.

Psychological and Social Aspects of Human Development That Influence Disease and Illness

Recognize the various life-cycle theories (Freud, Piaget, Erikson, Bowlby) in normal development and the Epigenetic Principle of Life Cycle Theory.
Understand the interplay between stages of human development and disease states.

Psychological Aspects of Pain

Understand the wide range of psychosocial and cultural factors that influence the perception and expression of pain.
Be familiar with the classic gate-control and contemporary theories of pain.
Perform a functional analysis of patients with chronic pain.
Describe the multimodal treatments for pain control.
Recognize the physician biases that influence the treatment of pain.

Psychological, Biological, and Management Issues in Somatization

Understand the definition, prevalence, common symptoms, and underlying affective illnesses associated with somatization.
List the diagnostic criteria for somatoform disorders.
Reflect on personal reactions to patients presenting with possible somatoform disorders.

Interactions Among Illness, Family Dynamics, and Culture

Understanding family and cultural influences on patient's interpretation of illness and treatment decisions and the importance of eliciting such information.

Domain: Patient Behavior

Health Risk Behaviors

Understand the psychological factors associated with the development and maintenance of behaviors associated with major causes of morbidity and mortality.
Demonstrate the ability to assess patients for health risk behaviors.
Understand key strategies for prevention and cessation of these behaviors.
Reflect on the role of health care providers in instigating and maintaining changes in these behaviors.
Apply principles of motivational interviewing and counseling for behavioral change to the patient care situations.

Principles of Behavior Change

Demonstrate the ability to apply the various models (classical conditioning, cognitive social learning theory, health belief model, theory of reasoned action, stage-of-change model) available for guiding behavior change.
Understand how behaviors are acquired, maintained, and eliminated in the context of health risk.
Understand patient, family, and sociocultural variables that impact motivation to change behavior.

Impact of Psychosocial Stressors and Psychiatric Disorders on Manifestations of Other Illness on Health Behavior

Recognize the association between and co-occurrence of chronic medical illness and mental disorders.
Know and be able to discuss with patients the range of treatment options when medical and mental illness coexist.
Know the role of a primary care physician and specialist in the treatment when medical and mental illness coexist.
Demonstrate the ability to screen patients for depression.
Understand the pathogenetic relationships between depression and comorbid conditions.

(Continued)

Table 38-1. SBS domains with priority topics and learning objectives.*(Continued)*

Domain: Physician Role and Behavior

Ethical Guidelines for Professional Behavior

Analyze ethical and professional dilemmas faced by health care professionals.
Identify and apply guidelines of ethical decision making.

Personal Values, Attitudes, and Biases as They Influence Patient Care

Describe how the effect of family of origin, cultural background, gender, life experiences, and other personal factors may influence your attitudes toward emotional reactions to patients.
Identify methods for processing the highly emotional encounters that regularly occur in medical care.

Physician Well-being

Recognize risk factors and warning signs for mental health issues in yourself.
Develop personal wellness strategies.

Social Accountability and Responsibility

Engage in activities that foster the development of socially responsible leadership skills.
Recognize the ever-changing health care needs of the community, region, and/or nation you serve.

Work in Health Care Teams and Organizations

Recognize the contribution that each member of the health care team has to offer.
Identify ways to work effectively as a part of the team.

Use of and Linkage With Community Resources to Enhance Patient Care

Identify available community resources in the patient's community.
Demonstrate a working knowledge of the types of interventions offered.

Domain: Physician-Patient Interactions

Basic Communication Skills

Demonstrate basic communication skills including, establishing rapport and building trust, eliciting adequate information to permit a robust differential diagnosis, understanding, and addressing patient.
Understand how to engender (and potential barriers to development of) a therapeutic relationship.
Demonstrate ability to express empathy, actively listen, elicit information about patients' lives and reasons for medical visit.
Demonstrate motivational interviewing techniques and the 5 A's counseling skills.

Complex Communication Skills

Demonstrate ability to communicate effectively in contextual (cultural, translator, family) and developmental (pediatric, adolescent, geriatric) interview situations.
Demonstrate ability to communicate effectively in assessment and counseling situations.
Practice basic skills in communicating effectively in challenging situations using principles of patient-centered interviewing.
Practice basic skills in communicating effectively with colleagues using principles of relationship-centered communication.

Context of a Patient's Social and Economic Situation, Capacity for Self-care, and Ability to Participate in Shared Decision Making

Demonstrate an awareness of the patient's ability to participate in decision making.
Identify necessary resources available to ensure access to care.

Management of Difficult or Problematic Physician-Patient Interactions

Describe approaches to working with patients in difficult situations.
Identify taxonomy of difficult interviews (including personal or sexual history taking; abusive relationships; patients with HIV; breaking bad news).
Identify key characteristics of difficult patient encounters, including personality types and stressful situations.
Identify and use basic skills of patient-centered interviewing to ask sensitive questions and listen respectfully and nonjudgmentally.

Table 38-1. SBS domains with priority topics and learning objectives.*(*Continued*)

Domain: Social & Cultural Issues in Health Care

Impact of Social Inequalities in Health Care and the Social Factors that are Determinants of Health Outcomes

Analyze the intricate relationship that social factors (race, ethnicity, education, income, and occupation) have with patients' health. Reflect on the impact your (students'/physicians') own social views can have on the delivery of effective health care.

Cultural Competency

Describe the impact the cultural context of illness can have on a successful patient-physician relationship.
Recognize ways that cultural competency encompasses language, customs, values, belief systems, and rituals.

Role of Complementary and Alternative Medicine

Describe complementary and alternative medicine treatments available in the local community and within local ethnic/cultural groups.
Recognize and apply required skills for eliciting information from patients seeking or using alternative treatment methods.
Describe to patients the efficacy and safety of alternative methods of treatment.

Domain: Health Policy & Economics

Overview of the U.S. Health Care System

Appreciate the magnitude of the investment in health care services made by individuals and organizations in the United States, the impact of these expenditures on individuals and on organizations, and the limited "return on investment."
Explain why competition and other "market forces" may not work in health care.
Use state-of-the-art utilization controls within the TBL scenario in an attempt to allocate financial resources to critical sectors of care.

Economic Incentives Affecting Patients' Health-related Behaviors

Appreciate how patients' values and life circumstances may affect their motivations for health-supporting behaviors, health care utilization, and preference for outcomes of health care.
Use this understanding to predict a patient's response to a complex and costly plan of care for several concomitant, chronic conditions, including the need to choose among therapeutic alternatives, adherence challenges, and patient-based assessments of risk.
Outline potential physician actions in this situation that might preserve the essential ingredients of effective care.

Costs, Cost-effectiveness, and Physician Responses to Financial Incentives

Appreciate how "delivery system" income is allocated to sectors of cost, using a microsystem model as an exemplar.
Apply this understanding, together with a statement of practice objectives, to develop the key elements of the practice in a financial context—staffing, services provided, in-office equipment, patients accepted, relationship to payers.

Variations in Care

Appreciate how large the variations in practice are, even in the presence of generally accepted evidence-based guidelines for care, and what some of the determinants of those variations might be.
Apply this knowledge to a specific case example, decide what "unwanted" variation means in this situation, and design a plan of action to eliminate this variation.

---

*Social and Behavioral Science Domains with Priority Topics are from a report issued by the Institute of Medicine (2004). Learning Objectives are used with permission from the Office of Medical Education and Curricular Affairs, Indiana University School of Medicine, Indianapolis, Indiana.

nation. The ACGME competencies include: (1) Patient Care; (2) Medical Knowledge; (3) Practice-based Learning and Improvement; (4) Interpersonal and Communication Skills; (5) Professionalism; and (6) Systems-based Practice. See ACGME web site <<http://www.acgme.org/outcome>> for more details.

The behavioral objectives for each of the six domains of behavioral and social science identified by the recent IOM report can be mapped to the existing Brown University and ACGME competencies. As other medical schools across the country develop similar competency curricula and residency training programs respond to the ACGME competency requirements, models are emerging of how behavioral and social science content can be infused, evaluated, and tracked in a competency curriculum structure.

Informal Curriculum

Attention to the formal curriculum, while important, has overshadowed attention to another critical influence on trainees' appreciation of the behavioral and social sciences, experiential learning in the informal curriculum. Research indicates that it is the social environment of the medical training programs, the "informal" curriculum, which guides almost all aspects of a future physician's behavior. It is this powerful role-modeling, where students see what physicians actually do, beyond what they say, that powerfully influences the beliefs, values, and role expectations of physicians-in-training. Despite diligent efforts by many dedicated faculty over the last several decades to revise the formal curriculum in critical areas, many of the attributes we purport to value continue to be lacking in our trainees. Attributes such as social-mindedness and interest in the psychosocial issues embedded in all illness have been found to decline during both undergraduate and graduate medical education, while self-centeredness and cynicism increase. This quandary, and the power of the hidden curriculum, is the focus of much of the seminal AAMC (Association of American Medical Colleges) report, *A Flag in the Wind: Educating for Professionalism in Medicine.* The report illuminates the many ways in which classroom teaching is undermined when trainees observe how faculty actually behaves. For example, talk of cultural competency is quickly undone by comments ridiculing the "peculiar" ideas of a particular patient's culture or religion. The report recommends an action agenda for addressing the incongruence between expressed values and actual behavior: (1) proposed actions should acknowledge **relationships**, (2) emphasis should be placed on individual and organizational **behavior**, (3) medical schools and residency training programs should invest in the processes of personal and professional **formation**, and (4) members of the educational community should engage in open, ongoing **discussion** of individual and organizational values, challenges, and choices.

Integrated Formal & Informal Curricula Initiative

CASE ILLUSTRATION 3: INDIANA UNIVERSITY SCHOOL OF MEDICINE'S RELATIONSHIP-CENTERED CARE INITIATIVE

Indiana University School of Medicine (IUSM) began a process of self-study and organizational development in January 2003 known as the Relationship-Centered Care Initiative (RCCI). The goal of the RCCI is to explore the culture of the faculty, student, staff, and patient community of IUSM and to initiate

small transformative changes into this environment to foster relationship—attentiveness to human interactions—in all aspects of medical school and practice. The desired outcome is a social environment that consistently reflects and reinforces the moral, ethical, professional, and humane values expressed in the school's formal curriculum. The activities of the RCCI have instigated the formation of novel faculty workgroups for innovation, broader engagement of faculty with students, attention to the values of the academic medical center community, and activities formally organized as reflective learning from the "hidden curriculum."

Central to this initiative has been the collection and sharing of stories from students, faculty, and staff that detail their range of experiences of the informal curriculum. Many of these stories describe events that would be effectively illuminated by behavioral and social science perspectives. Key stories from the informal curriculum, mapped to identify behavioral and social science learning objectives, are being used as core content in the formal curriculum, including problem-based as well as team-based learning (TBL) and standardized patient experiences. A curriculum team is intentionally developing teaching and assessment activities for all six SBS domains identified by the IOM report, using student, faculty, and staff narratives as the foundation. These personal stories from IUSM's own community are intended to capture students' attention, integrate the power of the informal curriculum into the formal curriculum in the professional development of a medical student, and deeply engage students in the desire to know and understand the science behind the SBS competencies.

It is anticipated that explicit reflection on SBS issues in the school's own informal curriculum will not only improve student and faculty knowledge and competency in SBS, but will heighten their self-awareness, mindfulness, and attention to role models around them. Ultimately, this should improve their ability to participate in the life of the academic medical center in ways that reflect the highest standards of professionalism and competency in the SBS (see Figure 38-1).

INTEGRATING THE FORMAL & INFORMAL CURRICULA TO TEACH SOCIAL & BEHAVIORAL SCIENCE

Educational Learning Theories Foundational to Creating Social & Behavioral Science Curriculum

As medical training programs seek to integrate their formal and informal curricula to improve SBS education,

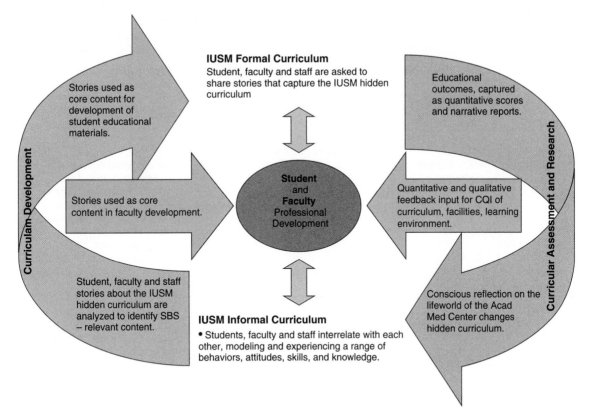

Figure 38-1. Uniting the formal and informal curricula to improve education in the SBS.

current learning theories provide a useful underlying framework. Understanding of the various theoretical orientations will allow educators to address concerns raised in the IOM report about incorporating the most appropriate teaching and assessment methodologies when teaching SBS. The five learning theories described in the adult learning literature include behaviorist, humanist, social learning, cognitivist, and constructivist orientations. An overview of these orientations, associated educational methods, and theoretical principles are briefly summarized in Table 38-2.

Teaching & Evaluation Methods Foundational to Learning Social & Behavioral Sciences

The following is a framework for applying the five theoretical orientations of adult learning theory to methods of teaching and evaluation. We describe each of the suggested methods under each orientation. We have included case illustrations applying the suggested methods in teaching and assessing SBS competencies. In some cases, the examples provided could be categorized under more than one orientation. However, the main

purpose of the illustrations is to provide a wide sampling of educational vignettes that integrate the formal and informal curricula for varying levels of medical trainees.

BEHAVIORIST ORIENTATION

The behaviorist orientation is very useful for teaching and assessing technical, clinical, and psychomotor skills as well as other observable behaviors. Direct observation of trainees with real or standardized patients (SPs), particularly when trained observers utilize well-designed checklists and/or rating forms, provides valuable information about trainees' social and behavioral science competence.

Direct observation: Direct observation of trainees is an important way to assess their basic clinical and communication skills, as well as interpersonal and professional behavior, yet it is infrequently done. Here patient care competency, in the context of everyday interactions within the informal curriculum or institutional culture, is brought into the formal curriculum for purposes of assessment and formative feedback.

Direct observation is itself a skill that requires faculty training and practice. Research has documented the lack

Table 38-2. Learning theories and orientations foundational to teaching and evaluating SBS.

Orientation	Educational Methods/Tools	Useful for Assessing	Theoretical Principles
Behaviorist	Direct observation SPs Checklists Rating forms	Clinical and psychomotor skills Other observable behaviors	Learning results from environmental factors and positive and negative reinforcement that shapes behavior
Humanist	PBL Self-assessment	Self-awareness Autonomy Self-directedness	Learning results from learners' desire to achieve their full potential
Social learning	Role modeling Mentoring Collaborative/cooperative learning (e.g., TBL)	Social adaptability Teamwork	Learning results from learners' interaction with and observation of others in a social context in which creative retrievable cognitive representations are used by learners when they are motivated to act
Cognitivist	Cognitive maps Reflective exercises	Insight Information processing	Learning results from relating new knowledge/experiences to existing knowledge/experiences
Constructivist	Reflective journaling CtC statements Building portfolios	Ability to broaden one's perspective Critical reflection Ability to create meaning from experiences	Learning results from learners' construction of meaning from experiences through critical reflection on their existing assumptions

of faculty observational accuracy in the absence of training. Faculty training should focus on standardizing and accurately identifying trainee behaviors. This is especially important for high inference behaviors, such as those provided below (see "Case Illustration 4," below). For example, in the behaviorist approach, what does nonjudgmental communication about a sexually transmitted disease actually look like? Faculty should spend some time discussing these issues as part of the standardization and calibration process. These discussions help to ensure fairness in the assessment of students, regardless of the faculty member performing the observation.

The American Board of Internal Medicine has emphasized the need for direct observation of residents' clinical skills. The Clinical Evaluation Exercise (CEX) and more recently the mini-CEX (a shortened version of the CEX) are used by a majority of internal medicine residency training programs. Four mini-CEXs possess sufficient reliability for "pass-fail" decisions, but it is important to note that multiple evaluations (as many as 12-14) are needed for high stakes reliability. A larger number of observations are also necessary for improved validity and sampling across multiple types of patient encounters.

Standardized patients: In an effort to standardize training of doctor-patient communication, physical examination skills, and other competency areas, medical schools, residency training programs, and the National Board of Medical Examiners (NBME) have progressively moved toward using SPs, Objective Structure Clinical Exams (OSCE), and the NBME Clinical Skills Exam for training and assessment in curricular units. Unannounced SPs can be inserted into selected clinical care venues as a way of measuring trainees' application of the SBS competencies. Using standardized checklists, SPs rate trainee performance on a variety of behaviors. Studies have shown that trainees cannot reliably distinguish unannounced SPs from actual patients. Videotaped encounters with SPs—whether in OSCEs or other selected experiences—can be used by trainees for self or group reflection, or by trained reviewers for assessment purposes. SPs provide an excellent method to assess the *capability* of a student; assessment of *performance* requires direct observation in the context of actual clinical care.

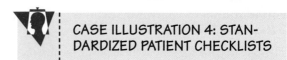

CASE ILLUSTRATION 4: STANDARDIZED PATIENT CHECKLISTS

Depicted here are sample items from IUSM SP checklists mapped to SBS domains (see Table 38-1):
- *Student gave you adequate time to voice your concerns without interrupting. (Physician-Patient Interactions)*

- Student spoke to me in a nonjudgmental way about my sexually transmitted disease. (Health Risk Behaviors)
- Student gave me the name and contact for a clinic for follow-up care for my child. (Use of and Linkage With Community Resources to Enhance Patient Care)
- Student was sensitive to worries about money/ insurance. (Economic Incentives Affecting Patients' Health-related Behaviors)

HUMANIST ORIENTATION

The humanist orientation promotes learners' autonomous, self-directed activities to achieve their full potential. Problem-based learning (PBL) and exercises that promote self-assessment are primary in this model.

Problem-based learning: PBL is a learner-centered method in which cases based on actual patient care vignettes are discussed in small groups. The case discussions generally evolve over several days or weeks with information disclosed to the students upon request or at critical times. Students identify their own learning needs and the resources required to meet those needs. A facilitator guides the process of the small group sessions but does not provide the content. This method promotes autonomous, self-directed, lifelong learning skills. It also prompts learners to reflect on the cultural assumptions or observations that shape their list of learning issues and resources, providing an opportunity for integrating the informal with the formal curriculum.

CASE ILLUSTRATION 5

As part of the first-year medical students' Concepts of Health and Disease PBL course, SBS objectives of addressing principles of behavioral change have been woven into a case covering medical and genetic risk factors for cardiovascular disease (CVD). Students meet Monday, Wednesday, and Friday during 1 week to cover serial aspects of the case of "Robert Richardson's Achilles Tendon."

Sample excerpts from case:

Day 1: Mr. Robert Richardson, a 44-year-old white male, visits his family physician, Dr. Roberts, for a follow-up of his myocardial infarct suffered several weeks ago. Mr. Richardson has been feeling well and continues his prescribed walking program. He is trying to follow his suggested diet and has begun a smoking cessation program. Mr. Richardson tells Dr. Roberts that he has been experiencing pain in his left Achilles tendon for the past several days. Mr. Richardson says that the pain had appeared several times during the past year. The pain usually resolved itself within several days without treatment.

Student instructions: During the week the case is being presented, please make a commitment to change (CtC) the following:

- Engage in some form of aerobic exercise every day for at least 10 minutes.
- Take the provided pill twice a day (each student is given a packet of inert pills).
- Diet—give up one thing that contributes to heart disease that you eat regularly.

Suggestions: salt, red meat, butter, cheese, milk, eggs, fried foods.

At the end of each day write a paragraph or two about the experience of complying with these activities. Did it all go as planned? Rate the amount of effort necessary to do these things (1 being the easiest and 10 being the hardest). What happened if things did not always go as planned? What did you struggle with? What were your successes?

Facilitator notes: The facilitator might also consider doing these things to be able to aid in the discussion.

Guided self-assessment: Self-assessment exercises can be built into a variety of educational activities stimulated by questions posed by medical educators. Creating a safe forum for students to discuss their personal reflections on journal entries can promote self-awareness, personal growth, and professional development. Students are asked in the formal curriculum to reflect on and assess their abilities and performance in both the formal and informal curricula.

To be effective, self-assessment is not performed by the student in isolation. The impact of self-assessment is most valuable when performed with *guidance*, which we define as either externally provided data (e.g., peer observations) or in dialogue with an advisor or mentor.

CASE ILLUSTRATION (CONTD.): "ROBERT RICHARDSON'S ACHILLES TENDON" (PBL)

Sample excerpts from case:

Day 2: Dr. Roberts reports that Mr. Richardson's lipid and enzyme values are improved, that he should continue to follow the prescribed treatment, and that his prognosis will remain improved as long as he follows the diet, exercise, and medication program. He should have semiannual checkups to follow his cholesterol and liver enzyme levels.

Facilitator notes: On the second and last day of the session, ask the following questions of the group.

Guided discussion of journals with prompting questions:

- *What was hardest?*
- *What was easiest?*
- *Any association with your lapses?*
- *How did you feel after you lapsed?*
- *How well did you comply with your journal writing?*

Thinking about Mr. Richardson and what you learned with your own exercise, how could you help Mr. Richardson and his children to comply with these lifelong issues?

A sample of one student's self-assessment logged in her personal dietary/exercise/medicine adherence journal as part of the PBL exercise above.

Overall, this exercise has shown me that it is all too easy for a physician to become annoyed and frustrated with noncompliant patients, and write them off as not caring about their own well-being or progress. Adherence with diet, exercise, and medication is not as simple as it seems. I hope to remember those lessons in the coming years as I struggle with explaining to patients why it is so important, so they don't feel they are just doing something "because the doctor said to." *First-year medical student, IUSM 2010*

SOCIAL LEARNING ORIENTATION

According to the social learning orientation, learners assimilate new information and assume new roles through role modeling, behavioral rehearsal, and attending to observed behaviors. This orientation is central to the importance of the informal curriculum in shaping the professional development of medical trainees. Identifying ways to make stories about role models within a training community more tangible and visible will inevitably lead to a heightened mindfulness about the importance of role modeling. Educational methods that promote collaborative, cooperative approaches such as TBL also highlight the complexities and value of collective problem solving and resourcefulness.

Role modeling: Role modeling shapes the professional culture or informal curriculum of an organization and substantially impacts the professional identity of trainees. The window into the impact of medical educators' role modeling can be seen in the trainees' stories about their learning environment. How the faculty conduct themselves and live their values through their actions can be influenced by looping trainees' stories into the "formal" content of faculty development programs (see Figure 38-1).

CASE ILLUSTRATION 6

Story of a negative role model from a student's professionalism journal maintained during her ambulatory block rotation.

What I observed during my clerkship struck me and made me think about what type of doctor I'm going to be when it comes to drug reps. I do think that they are of benefit. You and your office are provided with new info on drug research, clinical trials, etc. I also think they are of benefit for the pts who cannot afford medications or would just like to sample these drugs before filling the prescription. I do think there comes a time when too many drug reps can be a hindrance to pt care. At the office I was at for each pt there seemed to be a drug rep. It may sound unbelievable but there's a 1 to 1 ratio of patient to rep. It cuts down on the time he has for his pts b/c these reps are standing there also needing to get his signature. But it's just not the signature and off they go it's more like a social scene. This dr. seems to be buddy-buddy with every single drug rep. It also gets in the way of teaching. The time I'm supposed to be staffing with my physician barely exists because the drug rep is staffing with the physician. So there is very little time for teaching. It's unfortunate because at the end of the day the whole office is running behind and the time the patients have with the doctor is cut in half because of the socializing. I think there's a workable medium in there and that's for each one of us to find. *Third-year medical student, IUSM 2005*

CASE ILLUSTRATION 7

Story of positive role modeling from a student's professional journal maintained during his surgery rotation: observations are made on the operating room culture and learning environment.

The operating room (OR) is a strange place. It can be exciting, boring, loud, quiet, tense, laid back and many more opposite things. When a patient comes back, there is a pause, a hush, and everyone turns and follows the patient in with their eyes. Some say hi, some just smile. It's almost a kind of reverence, especially when compared to the easy humorous atmosphere that preceded the patient's entrance. I think it's appropriate. Not the reverence, but the change of focus from whatever task is being done, to the patient. Everyone centers on the patient, and I sense that recentering attention like that sets a tone of patient centered decision-making that should describe the OR. Setting the tone is very important it seems,

because it's easy to forget the patient is a walking, talking person who is scared and alone back in the OR, under anesthesia, under the drapes, with only a small part of him open and worth our attention. The other behavior I find helpful is the description of the history that staff will often provide in the OR about the patient. They'll talk about how he presented, what he thought about surgery, how his family is involved, etc. It's great for learning, but it's also important for the OR nurses and anesthesia to hear about the patient, who is usually unknown and quickly in and out of their scope of attention.
Third-year medical student, IUSM 2006

Team-based learning: TBL promotes active learning and effective team skills without requiring intensive faculty resources for tutoring sessions. TBL develops small groups of students into effective learning teams who not only learn course content but also high-level content application, problem solving, and effective team interaction.

The three-part team-learning instructional strategy puts these principles into action: Part I is the initial exposure to the concepts of an instructional unit through a Readiness Assurance Process. The Readiness Assurance Process begins with individual preclass work (through assigned readings, work on computer modules, and other modalities). It includes students completing an Individual Readiness Assurance Test (IRAT) during the first few minutes of class that covers the preassigned material. Immediately following the IRAT, the teams take the same test (a Group Readiness Assurance Test, or GRAT), which allows for peer discussion of important course content. The IRAT/GRAT tests are reviewed in class to ensure all students have thorough knowledge of foundational content. The instructor provides focused feedback and instruction on areas demonstrated to need additional clarification. Teams have the opportunity to appeal and defend any answers marked incorrect. This allows teams an opportunity to further review and discuss difficult concepts.

Upon completion of the Readiness Assurance Process, teams are ready to begin work on Part II, which involves team application assignments. Team assignments allow students to increase their understanding of the main unit concepts by using them to solve a problem. Assignments generally ask team members to reach a decision on the problem solution (rather than write a report) and thus stimulate a high level of team interaction. At a given point, all teams simultaneously reveal their decisions and begin cross-team feedback and discussion. Team assignments for a given instructional unit usually progress from the simple to the more complex. Individual team members prepare for team assignments outside of class, then work together with their team members in class to reach a consensus conclusion. After sufficient team application practice, the instructor reviews the major course content and application learning points.

In Part III of the TBL process, students are individually assessed on their ability to solve a final application problem.

These team-learning experiences provide a perfect opportunity for learners to move from "stage-to-stage" as part of the process of professional development and role recognition. The experience of being a member of a TBL group will also directly address key SBS learning objectives, including "*identify ways to work effectively as a part of a team*" and "*engage in activities that foster the development of socially responsible leadership skills*" (see Table 38-1 under the Physician Role and Behavior Domain). TBL also formally includes peer assessment in the sessions and can incorporate self-assessment as well.

Student narratives describing their experiences in the informal curriculum can provide opportunities for TBL groups to integrate multiple SBS competencies/domains into a discussion addressing key learning objectives and exploration of the science supporting these objectives. Used in this way, narrative has the potential to utilize personal experiences of the informal curriculum to enhance the relevance and enrich the content related to formal curricular objectives (see Figure 38-1).

CASE ILLUSTRATION 8

See "Multisource Methods and Evaluation" for a case illustration of TBL below.

COGNITIVIST ORIENTATION

The cognitivist orientation suggests that learners use cognitive tools such as insight, information processing, perceptions, and memory to facilitate learning by assigning meaning to events. Use of cognitive maps and reflection exercises are educational methods for promoting the cognitivist orientation.

Concept mapping: Concept mapping exercises provide trainees with a tool to graphically depict their understanding of complex problems or systems. Concept mapping offers a way for learners to incorporate new information into existing knowledge frameworks by associating relationships. As an assessment tool, concept mapping can be used longitudinally to visually represent the progressively more complex neural connections in the developing mind. One can readily see the increasing complexity, hierarchical layers, and growing complexity of cross-linking between the pre- and postfigures when learners' cognitive development is tracked across time.

Analysis and reporting of developmental changes in concept mapping within individuals across time and between groups can be performed. Qualitative analysis of phrases and terms entered onto maps can be performed using software packages (e.g., NVivo) along with some quantitative or semiquantitative measures based on scoring schemes reported elsewhere.

CASE ILLUSTRATION 9

Concept maps: understanding factors influencing CVD risk (Figure 38-2).

CASE ILLUSTRATION (CONTD.)

Concept maps: understanding factors influencing CVD risk (Figure 38-3).

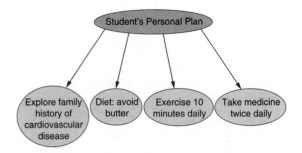

Figure 38-2. Concept maps: prebehavioral and social science curriculum.

Reflective exercise: Medical training programs around the country are increasing the use of 360° (multisource) evaluations for trainees. When accompanied by facilitated one-on-one reviews with mentors

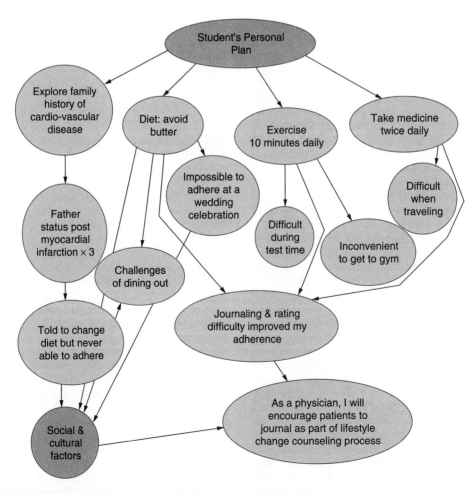

Figure 38-3. Concept maps: postbehavioral and social science curriculum.

and advisors, these sessions offer the opportunity for learners to use a breadth of cognitive tools in an effort to assign meaning to these highly complex and personal data.

CASE ILLUSTRATION 10

A sample of one student's personal reflection stimulated by reviewing his self- and peer-assessment data during his annual meeting with his self-selected self- and peer-assessment advisor.
" . . . the ideal professional physician must be respectful, tolerant, patient, and a good listener. From my peer assessment, I realize I don't need to be the first to speak when I think an underdog is being exploited . . . it is better to first listen to understand before making assumptions about whether a colleague is demonstrating tolerance . . . this will help me be a better doctor." *Second-year medical student, IUSM 2008*

CONSTRUCTIVIST ORIENTATION

The constructivist orientation supports the theory that knowledge is formed within the learner by integrating learning activities and experiences into knowledge and beliefs. The creation of meaning from these experiences emerges through critical reflection on existing beliefs and assumptions. Reflective journaling and active creation of learning or competency portfolios are examples of educational methods used by educators to tap into constructivist learning styles.

Reflective journaling: Medical training institutions around the country are including reflective journaling in their curricula. Journaling exercises can range from brief informal invitations to write one's thoughts about a personal experience from the informal curriculum, to writing annual letters to oneself that are personally reviewed, to more extensive narrative writing exercises that are formally analyzed by faculty with expertise in "Narrative Medicine." Reflective journaling can be solely for personal use and review, for one-on-one review with learner-selected and trusted mentors, for anonymous self-disclosure within small group seminars, or for required carefully evaluated narrative writing courses.

When used for evaluative purposes, reflective journal entries can be analyzed to assess changes in the experiences of trainees from year-to-year and to identify improved understanding of key SBS concepts. A goal can be to make more seamless the experience of the medical

trainees regarding biomedical principles and social/behavioral principles in the context of patient care. Trainees' narratives can provide clear evidence of their ability to integrate these different dimensions of health and disease, in a different and more holistic manner than the knowledge measures or other quantitative measures of student performance. With permission from trainees, their personal reflections (stories) can be used to generate new curricular materials linking informal and formal aspects of their training.

Commitment to change statements: Another approach to help learners integrate knowledge and experience is CtC statements (see student journaling exercise on lifestyle change commitments above under the PBL case illustration). Research has shown the CtC method does enhance the probability of an individual making a change. At the end of an educational experience, the student is simply asked to write down a limited number of things they wish to change or accomplish as a result of the educational experience. In addition to writing what they would like to do differently, they can provide a rating on how motivated they are to make the change and how difficult they believe it will be to make the change. At a predetermined follow-up time, the student's CtC statements can be returned to them for reflection—whether they were successful in making the change and why. If they were not successful, they can also reflect on the barriers to making the change and what the lessons learned from the experience.

CASE ILLUSTRATION 11

Students select anonymous journal entries made by their cohort to discuss in small group facilitated professionalism seminars during the medicine clerkship. In discussing their own narratives in a small group, the students are being professional as they talk and learn about professionalism. Reflection is stimulated by questions posed by the seminar facilitator such as: "What was it about this setting or these individuals that makes this possible?" *As the students examine their experiences together, they are bringing their lived encounters, the informal curriculum, into the explicit, formal curriculum. Students report that the experience of being present to others' stories of professionalism helps them feel less isolated and alone in their own experiences and also helps them name professional issues that might otherwise go unacknowledged and unaddressed.*

A sample from one student's professionalism journal entry made while on her third-year medicine rotation:
During my first week of my first medicine rotation I was lucky enough to have an intern that taught me some valuable lessons about medicine

as well as integrity and accountability. Drug/Pharmaceutical representative lunches are carried out every Wednesday and during the week the representatives show up almost daily with all types of free stuff—from sodas and snacks to promises of dinners at St. Elmo's. These guys and gals spare no expense to gain even a lowly third year's attention and favor. In an unbiased, way my intern challenged me to think about my stance on these representatives, their reason for being in our hospital and what ethical questions were raised by these practices by drug companies. In retrospect he gave me a choice to make my own conscious decision on an ethically-charged issue. It was a great lesson and I'll appreciate it for the rest of my career. I'm sorry his month with our team ended because we enjoyed boycotting the free food last Wednesday after we realized that as young physicians in training we couldn't passively participate in what these unethical solicitations represent. *Third-year medical student, IUSM 2005*

Portfolios: Together trainees and programs can aggregate specially selected as well as predetermined learning products into a portfolio for review by course and residency program directors, for personal review, and/or for evaluation purposes. Medical training programs espousing competency-based curricula have found portfolios to be of high utility in documenting evidence of performance in "less traditional" competency areas such as self-awareness, professionalism, and ethical judgment and moral reasoning. Trainees can populate portfolios with documented experiences or activities from the formal or informal curricula. Given the sensitive nature of some materials entered into trainees' portfolios, several institutions have created ways to allow learners to self-populate both "personal" and "academic" versions of their portfolios. Mentors and advisors can assist trainees in their decisions about artifacts most appropriate for their academic portfolios that might be used for final performance measures and release to residency and fellowship training sites or to future employers. For ease of handling data, electronic portfolio tracking systems are increasingly available.

CASE ILLUSTRATION 12

As part of an electronic portfolio pilot program, 16 first-year medical students from IUSM's Terre Haute campus were asked to self-populate fields to document students' performance in each of the core competency areas. Four students chose to populate their academic portfolios with their reflective narratives written following their observations of an autopsy. One student mapped his narrative into the "Using

Science to Guide Diagnosis, Management, Therapeutics, and Prevention" competency, explaining that the experience helped him better understand the anatomy important for performing future procedures. One student added her story to the "Self-awareness, Self-care, and Personal Growth" competency stating that, although she would never want to be a coroner, she now has a new appreciation for the important role these health care providers play as members of the larger health care team. Two students logged their entries into the "Moral Reasoning and Ethical Judgment" competency. One student reflected on the inappropriate behavior of the health care providers in handling human body remains of a deceased patient for whom some family members were likely still grieving. The second ethics entry included the student's reflection about how providers choose to deal with medical errors that resulted in a child's death. This demonstrates how a single curricular exercise can provide highly varied educational experiences for trainees uncovered through self-categorization based on the personal meaning these experiences had for the individual student. Portfolios can help document broad curricular exposure to all core competency areas as perceived by trainees.

MULTISOURCE METHODS & EVALUATION

Although curricular teaching and assessment methods for each of the theoretical orientations have been described above, in practice it is appropriate and often desirable to combine a variety of orientations within teaching exercises for a more comprehensive view of a trainee's competence in several areas.

CASE ILLUSTRATION 13: ANNOTATED WITH THE THEORETICAL ORIENTATIONS EMPLOYED AND THE SBS LEARNING OBJECTIVE ADDRESSED

The following is an example of how narrative and TBL methodology can address SBS-specific learning objectives for the "Psychological Aspects of Pain" priority topic as part of the Mind-Body Interactions Domain (see Table 38-1).

IUSM student narratives provide opportunities for TBL groups to integrate multiple competencies/domains of the SBS into a discussion addressing key learning objectives and exploration of the science supporting these objectives. Used in this way, narrative has the potential to utilize personal experiences of the informal curriculum to enhance the relevance and enrich the content related to the SBS formal curricular objectives.

A sample set of TBL materials, based on a story from a third-year IUSM medical student's current professionalism journal, illustrates how these naturalistic "critical incident events" with high heuristic value will be used to create SBS education modules.

• Constructivist (looping informal and formal curriculum):

One of my patients complained of severe chronic leg pain that resembled sciatica but the pain was not reproducible. She was writhing in pain and crying. However, when the physician couldn't reproduce the pain, he decided she was making it up. The patient had some discrepancies in her story and she wasn't well known to the physician. She didn't have anything in her chart to suggest that she was drug seeking. However, the physician didn't think her pain was real so he did not work it up. Third-year medical student, IUSM 2006.

• Traditional knowledge content:

TBL Preparation Phase
Objective: "Be familiar with the classic gate-control and contemporary theories of pain."
Objective: "Describe the multimodal treatments for pain control."

Prestudy materials: Review web module and take imbedded prepost test on classical gate-control and contemporary theories of pain and the multimodal etiologies and treatments (traditional and alternative) for pain control.

• Social learning (team work):

Readiness Assurance Test (RAT—individual and group): Complete a multiple-choice exam covering content from prestudy materials; grade immediately; discuss result with team members; retake the test as a group.

• Behavioral (SP)/Social (team work):

TBL Application
Objective: "Understand the wide range of psychosocial and cultural factors that influence the perception and expression of pain."
Objective: "Perform a functional analysis of patients with chronic pain."

Application exercise: Employing a trained SP to simulate the above case, students will take turns interviewing and examining the patient in the simulated patient care area of the TBL classroom. They will be expected to elicit the psychosocial and cultural factors that influence the perception and expression of pain and perform a functional analysis of this patient with chronic pain. Students will observe, discuss, and debrief with one another as each student takes a turn with the SP.

• Humanist (SA):

TBL Self- and Peer Assessment
Objective: "Identify ways to work effectively as a part of a team."
Objective: "Engage in activities that foster the development of socially responsible leadership skills."

Self- and peer assessment: Student will complete self- and peer assessment on surveys programmed into IUSM's competency database. Figure 38-4 shows sample questionnaire items.

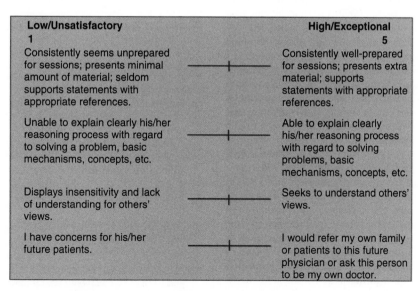

Low/Unsatisfactory 1		High/Exceptional 5
Consistently seems unprepared for sessions; presents minimal amount of material; seldom supports statements with appropriate references.	———┼———	Consistently well-prepared for sessions; presents extra material; supports statements with appropriate references.
Unable to explain clearly his/her reasoning process with regard to solving a problem, basic mechanisms, concepts, etc.	———┼———	Able to explain clearly his/her reasoning process with regard to solving problems, basic mechanisms, concepts, etc.
Displays insensitivity and lack of understanding for others' views.	———┼———	Seeks to understand others' views.
I have concerns for his/her future patients.	———┼———	I would refer my own family or patients to this future physician or ask this person to be my own doctor.

Figure 38-4. Sample questionnaire items from the University of Rochester School of Medicine and Dentistry's Peer Assessment Intstrument. Modified with permission from Blackwell Publishing with reference to: Danneter EF, Henson LC, Bierrer SB, et al. Peer assessment of professionalism competence.

• *Cognitivist (concept map):*

Conceptual mapping exercise: Students will be asked to draw a picture (web) of all the possible contributing factors to this patient's pain and possible therapeutic options.

• *Constructivist (reflective journaling):*

TBL Assessment
Objective: "Recognize the physician biases that influence the treatment of pain."

Reflective exercise: Before leaving the session, the students will be asked to reflect on physician biases that influence the treatment of pain and write a paragraph or two in their electronic competency portfolio tracker as part of the "Self-awareness, Self-care, and Personal Growth" competency for review by the competency director. Alternatively, students can write a story about a personal experience they have had with a patient with chronic pain and what new understanding they have based on the TBL experience.

SUMMARY

Medical training programs have employed a variety of organizational and theoretical frameworks as vehicles for expanding education in the SBS. Case illustrations demonstrate how some schools, as well as the ACGME, have implemented competency-based frameworks that identify and make explicit important abilities of physicians, such as communication, self-awareness, or professionalism, that in the past were not formally represented in the curriculum. These efforts, while important, are an incomplete solution. Attention to trainees' learning environment, and their experiential learning in the informal curriculum, is also critical. The authors suggest that educators consider learning experiences and assessments that draw upon and integrate both formal and informal curricular content and experiences. They provide examples of educational activities within a range of theoretical orientations that accomplish this integration. Examples illustrate how narratives, generated by trainees and other members of the academic community about personal experiences and perceptions of the organizations' professional culture, can be creatively integrated into the formal curriculum in a variety of contexts. This strategy promotes personal and organizational reflection and mindfulness and reinforces the importance of lessons learned in the informal curriculum. This cyclical process promotes awareness of the individual community members' roles in the creation of a culture conducive to learning and caring for patients.

SUGGESTED READINGS

Benbassat J, Bauman R, Borkan JM, et al. Overcoming barriers to teaching the behavioral and social sciences to medical students. *Acad Med* 2003;78:372–380.

Branch WT, Kern D, Haidet P, et al. Teaching the human dimensions of care in clinical settings. *JAMA* 2001;286:1067–1074.

Charon R. *Narrative Medicine: Honoring the Stories of Illness.* New York, NY: Oxford University Press, 2006.

Committee on Quality of Care in America, IOM. *Crossing the Quality Chasm: A New Health System of the 21st Century.* Washington, DC: National Academy Press, 2001.

Cuff PA, Vanselow NA, eds. *Improving Medical Education: Enhancing the Behavioral and Social Science Content of Medical School Curricula.* Institute of Medicine of the National Academies. Washington, DC: National Academy Press, 2004.

Hafferty FW. Beyond curriculum reform: confronting medicine's hidden curriculum. *Acad Med* 1998;73:403–407.

Hilton SR, Slotnick HB. Proto-professionalism: how professionalism occurs across the continuum of medical education. *Med Educ* 2005;39:58–65.

Holmboe ES, Hawkins RE. Effects of training in direct observation of medical residents' clinical competence: a randomized trial. *Ann Intern Med* 2004;140:874–881.

Holmboe ES, Hawkins RE. Methods for evaluating the clinical competence of residents in internal medicine: a review. *Ann Intern Med* 1998;129:42–48.

Hsu LL. Developing concept maps from problem-based learning scenario discussions. *J Adv Nurs* 2004;48(5):510–518.

Inui TS. A Flag in the Wind: Education for Professionalism in Medicine. Washington, DC: Association of American Medical Colleges, 2003. Available at: https://services.aamc.org/Publications/.

Kern DE, Branch WT, Jackson JK, et al. Teaching the psychosocial aspects of care in the clinical setting: practical recommendations. *Acad Med* 2005;80:8–20.

Litzelman DK, Cottingham A. The new formal and informal curricula at Indiana University: overview and five year analysis. *Acad Med* 2006, in press.

Schön D. *The Reflective Practitioner: How Professionals Think in Action.* Aldershot, England: Ashgate Publishing Limited, 1995.

Suchman A, Williamson P, Litzelman D, et al. Toward an informal curriculum that teaches professionalism: transforming the social environment of a medical school. *J Gen Intern Med* 2004; 19:501–504.

Torre DM, Daley BJ, Sebastion JL, et al. Overview of current learning theories for medical educators. *Am J Med* 2006;119:903–907.

West DC, Gerstenberger EA, Park JK, et al. Critical thinking in graduate medical education: a role for concept mapping assessment? *JAMA* 2000;284:1105–1110.

WEB SITES

ACGME Outcomes Project Web site. http://www.acgme.org/outcome. Accessed October, 2007.

Brown University School of Medicine Competency-based Curriculum Blueprint Web site. http://biomed.brown.edu/Medicine_Programs/MD2000/Blueprint_for_the_Web_04.pdf. Accessed October, 2007.

Improving Medical Education: Enhancing the Behavioral and Social Science Content of Medical School Curricula, 2004.

Institute of Medicine Web site. http://www.iom.edu/CMS/3775/3891/19413.aspx. Accessed October, 2007.

Team-based Learning Users Web site. http://aspen21.webcrossing.com. Accessed October, 2007.

The Indiana Initiative: Physicians for the 21st Century: IUSM's Competency-based Curriculum Web site. http://meded.iusm.iu.edu/programs/comptmanual.pdf. Accessed October, 2007.

Professionalism

39

Richard M. Frankel, PhD

INTRODUCTION

PROFESSION:
The place where
your deep gladness meets the
world's deep needs

Frederick Buechner

CASE ILLUSTRATION 1

A basic science course director is concerned that a second-year medical student is "heading for trouble" because he has made verbal statements in class such as, "I hate this course" and "The course instructor is really stupid."

CASE ILLUSTRATION 2

Several male residents are overheard by a female medical student talking at the nurse's station about sexually explicit matters, most of which are unrelated to medicine. A group of male medical students on service join in the conversation.

CASE ILLUSTRATION 3

A surgical resident who has been asked to begin a procedure refuses because the attending surgeon is not present and he has never done the procedure before. When the attending arrives (30 minutes late) he proceeds to scream and publicly humiliate the resident for not having followed his orders.

What do these three cases have in common? They are all about professionalism. Case 1 involves a student who expresses emotion inappropriately. Case 2 involves male residents who are unable to recognize appropriate boundaries for when and where to talk about patients and private matters. Case 3 involves a question of hierarchy and power. The cases also involve different levels of training and responsibility (medical student, resident, attending physician). Finally, all three cases involve the so-called "hidden" or informal curriculum of medical education (see Chapter 38).

Our goals in this chapter are to: (1) provide a broad overview of the current state of professionalism in medical education; (2) describe the competency curriculum in professionalism at one institution using the cases above; and (3) suggest some unifying themes and activities to teach professionalism in undergraduate, graduate, and continuing medical education.

Background

Codes of ethical and professional conduct for physicians have been in existence for millennia. Hippocrates, for example, counseled physicians to, "first, do no [biological] harm." Some 2500 years later, the first code of medical ethics published by the American Medical Association in 1847 recognized that harm could stem from communication as well as physical acts and opined that, "The life of a sick person can be shortened not only by the acts, but also by the words or the manner of a physician. It is, therefore, a sacred duty to guard himself carefully in this respect, and to avoid all things which have a tendency to discourage the patient and to depress his spirits." One hundred and sixty years later, in 2007, the idea that physicians should hide the truth, assuming that it will invariably depress the patient's spirits and shorten life, has largely been replaced by the principle of patient autonomy and the duty of physicians to tell the truth and support patients as they deal with its implications. In sum, definitions of professionalism and ethical conduct change over time, reflecting the fact that "*Professionalism is the basis of medicine's contract with society,*" and as such reflects society's norms and values.

In his seminal essay, "A Flag in the Wind: Educating for Professionalism in Medicine," Inui suggests that the current interest in medical professionalism is multifactorial and has its basis in economic, social, and technological developments over the past half century. He goes on to assert that there is widespread agreement among accrediting agencies, professional societies, educators, and policy makers about the qualities and characteristics that make up professional behavior. Although there are variations in emphasis and content, it is generally agreed that the competent professional must be knowledgeable, skillful, altruistic, and dutiful.

While there is common agreement on the qualities, characteristics, and expectations of the *ideal* professional physician, there is much less emphasis on the lived experience of becoming or being a physician and the very real dilemmas and constraints trainees and practitioners feel in the moment—the so-called informal or hidden curriculum of medicine. Inui's paper is one of the few that systematically moves back and forth between the author's narratives of his personal experience and the ideals he had committed to uphold.

In addition to focusing on professionalism as an ideal type, the literature tends to focus on particular phases of training or practice. Undergraduate, graduate, and continuing medical education are viewed as separate containers or silos with separate competencies and modes of evaluation. As a result, there is little guidance about how to approach and integrate professionalism education across the spectrum of experience that makes up a physician's professional life cycle.

One might reasonably ask if there is any evidence that connects professionalism issues within and between stages of training. In other words, is there any greater likelihood that a first-year student who castigates his instructor publicly is more likely to wind up in trouble as a practicing physician? The answer is "yes," and its implications for professionalism education are significant. Writing in the December 22, 2005, issue of the *New England Journal of Medicine*, Papadakis and colleagues described a study of 235 graduates of 3 medical schools who had been disciplined between 1990 and 2003 by a state board of medicine for unprofessional behavior. Using data from these individuals' medical schools and a matched set of controls, the investigators sought to understand whether such predictors as the presence or absence of narratives describing unprofessional behavior, grades, standardized test scores, and demographic characteristics were associated with having been disciplined in later career. The investigators found that disciplinary action by a medical board was strongly associated with prior unprofessional behavior in medical school.

In sum, the rationale for developing an overarching approach to medical professionalism is that the same behaviors which are problematic at the undergraduate level have salience and relevance at each stage of professional development. Identifying and dealing with professional development issues early may be the best deterrent currently available for avoiding later sanction. Current approaches to develop professionalism education at the undergraduate, graduate, and continuing education levels are still largely uncoordinated.

The Professionalism Competency at Indiana University School of Medicine

In February of 1999, the Accreditation Council for Graduate Medical Education (ACGME) took the bold step of recommending that all residency programs adopt a competency-based approach to residency education. This is now a requirement for all programs. In March of 1999, the curriculum council of Indiana University School of Medicine (IUSM) adopted one of the first competency-based undergraduate curricula in the United States. The curriculum, modeled on the ACGME competencies, was designed to educate and assess students in 9 areas: (1) effective communication; (2) basic clinical skills; (3) using science to guide decisions; (4) lifelong learning; (5) self-awareness, self-care, and personal growth; (6) the social and community contexts of health care; (7) moral reasoning and ethical judgment; (8) problem solving; and (9) professionalism and role recognition (see Chapter 38).

The professionalism competency, in particular, focuses on the development of professional *character*, exemplified by the qualities of **excellence** in medical knowledge and patient care; high standards of **accountability**, including accepting responsibility for one's own behavior as well as the behavior of peers, colleagues, and other health care professionals; **humanism** in all dealings with patients, colleagues, learners, and others; and **altruism**—putting the interests of the patient before self-interest.

In terms of logistics, each competency in the curriculum has a statewide competency director (CD) who is responsible for overseeing the activities of their competency in the curriculum. The nine CDs also work together as a learning community, sharing information and teaching strategies with one another on a regular basis. Each CD is appointed by the dean and is supported for 20% of their salary.

Evaluation

In addition to an academic transcript, each student at IUSM carries a competency transcript. Failure to satisfactorily pass the competency curriculum means that a student is not qualified to graduate from the medical school.

Students are evaluated at three different levels of competency. At **Level 1**, students are, in principle, able to:

1. Describe to others the core behavioral abilities of the IUSM competency in professionalism—excellence, humanism, accountability, and altruism.

2. Understand the acquisition of professional abilities as *phronesis* (practical wisdom).

3. Identify professional behaviors ranging from exemplary, to expected, to unprofessional in the IUSM formal and informal curriculum.

4. Demonstrate the core skills of professionalism as specified for Level 1 in all IUSM-related interactions with fellow learners, faculty, staff, administrators, patients, the health care team, and others.

By the time of graduation students will have achieved **Level 2** and have:

5. Mastered skills of professionalism in teams.

6. Engaged in at least three formal dialogues (Intersessions, STEP, and Surgery) and discussion sessions about professionalism and professional challenges and be able to articulate the elements of professional behavior in difficult or challenging circumstances.

7. Demonstrate the core abilities of professionalism in all IUSM-related interactions with colleagues, faculty, staff, administrators, patients, the health care team, and others.

To achieve **Level 3** in Professionalism, students select a topic that will affect their learning in future stages of their career, for example, residency or practice. Working together with a faculty mentor, students seeking Level 3 credit do library research or observe the faculty in one or more actual settings, keeping a log of what they encounter. The log is then used as data for analyzing formal and informal elements of professionalism in the chosen setting(s).

Remediation

There are two primary routes for dealing with students who exhibit unprofessional behavior. The first is a "competency concern" which is designed as an informal method for a course or clerkship director to bring a question or concern about a student's performance to the attention of the CD. As an informal method of communication, any actions taken do not appear on a student's transcript. Case 1 above is an example of a "competency concern."

An "isolated deficiency" is issued when there is evidence that a student has acted in an unprofessional manner and needs to either "show cause" before the Student Promotions Committee as to why he or she should be permitted to continue in medical school, and/or remediate the deficiency in an agreed upon program devised in concert with the CD.

The goal of the competency curriculum is to catch students as early in their medical school training as possible and provide them with opportunities to correct their behavior in a positive constructive way. The idea is not to punish students into compliance but rather to allow them to discover the threads that connect professional behavior early and later in training.

Case 1 above is based on a competency concern I received from a basic science course director. A narrative account of what happened when the student in question and I met follows:

CASE ILLUSTRATION 1 (CONTD.)

Todd Welsh (a pseudonym) came into my office full of bravado and bluster explaining that his conflict with the course director was just the way he was, plain and simple. Born in Israel and raised on the East coast, he asserted that he really didn't care much about what others thought of him as long as he got his work done and didn't fail any courses.

I listened carefully to the student, trying to figure out what might have an effect on his view of himself and his worldview. Rather than give him a lecture on professionalism which I thought would be unlikely to have any effect, I suggested that he read Maxine Papadakis' recent paper in the New England Journal on the link between physicians who come before state medical boards for unprofessional behavior and performance in medical school, and that we talk again in the next 2–3 weeks.

I didn't have long to wait, as it turned out. Less than 24 hours later I got an e-mail from Todd wondering if we could meet "soon." Todd came into my office a different person. He said that he had read the Papadakis article the night before and had been "shocked" to discover that the article described him to a tee, which really scared him. What could he do, he wondered out loud, to keep his dream of becoming a physician and serving society alive in the face of his self-defeating behavior?

We talked about various options that might be available, including psychological counseling. Todd was eager to pursue this course of action and confessed that he had thought of this a year earlier but rejected the idea as "weak minded." After some discussion, we settled on a cognitive-behavioral therapist who works extensively with medical professionals. This is still a story in evolution. Todd may or may not succeed in bringing his impulses under control and adopting a professional persona. Whatever happens, he has reached an important crossroads early in his professional development, a challenge that he now understands from the inside out.

Professionalism Teaching at IUSM

In addition to working with individual learners, the professionalism curriculum at IUSM attempts to raise questions of professionalism in small group and community settings across the 4 years of medical school (see Tables 39-1 through 39-4). Our methods of teaching about professionalism rely heavily on storytelling and attempts to locate professionalism as embodied action. Thus, in addition to teaching professionalism as a content area with theories and facts to learn, we operate on the assumption that students often bring with them into

Table 39-1. IUSM Indianapolis, year 1.

| Course | 2006/2007 | | Projected 2007/2008 | |
	Activity	Assessment	Activity	Assessment
MS 1, week 1	First-year students review, third-year student descriptions of professionalism experiences and reflect on their own positive traits of character.	S/N* based on participation		
Introduction to Clinical Medicine	Students are evaluated by preceptors & small group facilitators using checklists of professional behavior.	S/N based on facilitator checklist evaluation		
Session 12	Students review key articles on professionalism and, with this background, write a paper that reflects their vision of themselves as a "good doctor."	S/N based on quality of paper		
Concept of Health & Disease	Students are evaluated by preceptors & small group facilitators using checklists of professional behavior. Students explore issues of professional self-regulation in one problem-based learning (PBL) experience.	S/N based on facilitator checklist evaluation		
Biochemistry Cell and molecular biology Physiology Myers-Briggs Type Indicator (MBTI) Gross anatomy Immunology Microbiology Evidence-based medicine Histology				

*S/N refers to satisfactory or nonsatisfactory.

medical school the core values we hope to see them exercise in medicine. They lack, however, experience in being mindful of these values while pursuing the work of medicine. They do not yet know how to sort out confusing situations, make decisions, and take actions derived from these values in the situations they will face during their careers. Learning about professionalism through storytelling allows students to develop a vocabulary for describing their joyful and challenging professional experiences "in community." It also takes positive advantage of the informal curriculum and underscores its importance in professional development.

Funded by an initial STEP (Strategic Teaching and Evaluation of Professionalism) grant from the American Medical Association (AMA), we have developed a series of storytelling activities that occur in medicine, surgery, OB/GYN, and during 3 intersession days between the third and fourth year. During these rotations, students keep a running electronic narrative journal of their professionalism experiences (both positive and negative). In the third-year medicine clerkship, the stories are used as a point of departure for a small group conversation about professionalism. All of the student stories from each month's rotation are de-identified, copied, and given to the students to read during a small group session. Students are encouraged to choose a story (typically not their own) that speaks to them in one way or another, read it to the group, and have a facilitated small group discussion based on 1 or 2 of the stories.

Table 39-2. IUSM Indianapolis, year 2.

| Course | 2006/2007 | | Projected 2007/2008 | |
	Activity	Assessment	Activity	Assessment
Pathology	Students are evaluated using a Likert scale to rate behaviors listed in the competency description.	S/N based on evaluation		
Introduction to Clinical Medicine (ICM) 2				
Medical Genetics				
ICM-Radiology				
Neuroscience/ Neurology				
Pharmacology			Small group session on conflicts of interest pertaining to dealing with pharmaceutical representatives	

Table 39-3. IUSM Indianapolis, year 3.

| Course | 2006/2007 | | Projected 2007/2008 | |
	Activity	Assessment	Activity	Assessment
Intersession 1	Students write professionalism narrative.	S/N based on participation		
Intersession 2	Students reflect on professionalism narrative.	S/N based on participation		
Intersession 3	Students reflect again on professionalism narrative.	S/N based on participation		
Jr. Objective Structured Clinical Exam (OSCE)	OSCE cases include professionalism abilities.	S/N based on evaluation		
Medicine Clerkship	Students keep electronic diary of experiences (minimum of 1/month) with elements of professionalism observed. Discussed in small groups.	S/N based on participation; Medicine also evaluates professionalism with its clinical evaluation form.		
Neurology Clerkship				
Psychiatry Clerkship				
Family Medicine	Evaluate using a checklist of behaviors.	None now		
Pediatric Clerkship	Evaluated using list of behaviors & parent comments.	None now		
Surgery Clerkship	Three didactic sessions on professionalism & electronic journal.	None now		
Anesthesia OB/GYN Clerkship				

Table 39-4. IUSM Indianapolis, year 4.

		2006/2007		Projected 2007/2008	
Course	**Activity**	**Assessment**		**Activity**	**Assessment**
Emergency Medicine Subinternship	Level 3 is optional.	Professionalism evaluated with clinical performance evaluation form.			
Radiology					
Electives	17 electives offer professionalism level 3 attainment.	S/N based on course director and/or compentency director evaluation of project.			

CASE ILLUSTRATION 2 (CONTD.)

Case 2 is based on a story contributed by one of the students. Her journal entry follows:

"This incident happened on a ward floor at [hospital name] in the area where all the computers are—I was working on one of the computers and a Neurology resident and his students were sitting across from me. It was a real good ol' boys club. The resident was talking about sexually explicit matters (not at all medically related) and just didn't seem to want to stop. All the students joined in as well and were having a great time. I know that guys talk about this stuff but I completely lost respect for everyone sitting across from me—there is a time to leave it in a locker-room or bar and not in a professional setting with colleagues and nurses all around. Or maybe a time to just grow up."

In the small group discussion that followed, the students discussed boundaries and where it is and is not appropriate to talk about intimate or private matters. Both male and female students used the story as a point of departure for talking about their own experiences of being harassed by peers or superiors. There was also a discussion of appropriate ways of dealing with stress and boredom short of turning to "locker room" tactics. Finally, the students brainstormed methods they could have used in this or similar situations to express their attitudes and values without causing an escalation of the unprofessional behavior. At the conclusion of the session the students acknowledged that they were grateful for the opportunity to talk about a "difficult" subject in a nonjudgmental way and to discover that there was general agreement across genders that the behavior described by the student was unprofessional.

Mindfulness in Medicine

Many of the professionalism experiences reported by undergraduate medical students involve residents and attending physicians. While it is useful to discuss cases of positive or negative professional behavior in small groups of students it leaves the larger community out of the picture and unaffected by the students' experiences. To address this gap, IUSM instituted an occasional column in SCOPE, the weekly newsletter of the medical school that goes out to the entire faculty, students, and staff.

Mindfulness in Medicine is an attempt to bring forward issues of professionalism that affect the entire community. Stories are solicited from a variety of sources: faculty, students, and staff. An editorial board reviews submissions and makes decisions on which ones to put forward for publication. The stories are generally short and focus on a topic of general concern to the community. In addition to the story, a commentary is often included. The commentaries are generally from senior faculty, but medical students and residents have also contributed commentaries as well.

Case 3 is a story that was submitted by a medical student who was present when the surgical resident first refused to begin a procedure and then was yelled at by the attending surgeon. The twist in his story was that after several minutes spent berating the surgical resident, the attending surgeon stopped and apologized to the resident, stating that it was his anxiety and his issue around the operating schedule that had prompted his outburst. The fact that an attending surgeon apologized to a trainee impressed the student so much that he was moved to first share it in a mentoring group meeting and then submit it to SCOPE.

The story, as it appeared in SCOPE is reproduced below along with a commentary by the new Chairman of Surgery.

M&M: Mindfulness in Medicine

CASE ILLUSTRATION 3 (CONTD.)

A Surgery Story

The following story was shared at a meeting of one of IUSM's vertical mentoring groups. The response was written by Keith Lillemoe, chairman of the IUSM Department of Surgery.

A student reports: A surgery resident was to begin a surgical procedure and have the patient ready for the attending to take over when he arrived. When he didn't arrive on time, the resident told those assembled that he would wait since he had never done this procedure before and was uncomfortable starting it without supervision. Although this decision created discomfort for some, the resident held firm. When the attending arrived, he publicly "bawled out" the resident. After he had calmed down and reflected for a bit, he said that the resident had, in fact, made the right decision and apologized for making a scene. He admitted that his strong reactions were due to his own discomfort and embarrassment at being late. The attending's admission of responsibility left a positive impression on the student and everyone involved agreed that the attending's admission of responsibility was a model of "conducting oneself professionally."

Response: Unfortunately, the event described here happens far too commonly on the surgical service and most frequently in the operating room. Contributing factors include the stress associated with the life and death nature of some surgeries, the technical and cognitive complexity of the environment, and the surgeon feeling that he or she is the "captain of the ship." Being late to the operating room would obviously create a domino effect for the rest of the surgeon's day, a stressful situation for anyone. Upon discovering that the resident had not made progress to help him "catch up," his frustration led to a public display of displeasure directed toward the resident. Regrettably, many surgeons have learned such behavior having seen it modeled by their own teachers.

Regardless of the causes, a lot went wrong in the case described above, but the outcome ended up right. A surgical resident, regardless of his or her level of experience, is still a trainee. While there are certainly aspects of an operation that a resident can proceed with safely and confidently, at no time should a resident be asked to proceed without supervision in a setting in which he or she feels uncomfortable. The decision of the resident in this case was clearly the correct one. Having been there myself on a number of occasions, I am sure that the attending realized within minutes that the resident had done the right thing and that it was the attending's reaction that was inappropriate. Rather than try to save face and continue to show "command" of the situation, he made the effort to publicly apologize for his error and affirm that the resident had made the right decision.

It is important for surgeons to remember that there is no one–resident, scrub nurse, anesthesia team member, or other–who is not trying to do his or her best. Even when a strong response seems justified at the time, recognizing and acknowledging difficult interpersonal dynamics can go a long way to soothing any hard feelings, and the day may still be salvaged with a brief apology and a thank you to everyone involved. This incident shows that we surgeons are learning to better deal with frustrating situations. It is my hope that my surgical colleagues will continue to maintain this progress in the future.

CONCLUSION

If profession is indeed the place where your deep gladness meets the world's great needs, then being a professional is about the joy of doctoring and being called to work in a demanding yet rewarding field. Some might say that the recent focus on medical professionalism is a sign that medicine has lost its way and its moral compass. Others might say that in a field with newly emerging technological, social, and economic horizons, medicine needs to adjust its boundaries and refocus its priorities. Whatever the case may be, renewed interest and emphasis on medical professionalism creates the conditions for physicians in training and physicians in practice to recall and renew their commitments to professionalism with patients, colleagues, and themselves. Such an opportunity ought not to be squandered, but viewed as a gift. The call of medicine is a call to personal awareness, deeply held values, and a lifetime's commitment that will be played out on a moment-by-moment basis. By recognizing how much professionalism is embedded in the narratives of lived experience, and how liberating the telling of those narratives can be, we can approach the ideals of the profession in a much more realistic and humane way.

ACKNOWLEDGMENTS

The author wishes to acknowledge Ann Cottingham from the Dean's Office for Medical Education and Curriculum and Assessment and the Statewide Professionalism Team for their efforts to build a strong professionalism competency at Indiana University School of Medicine.

SUGGESTED READINGS

American Medical Association. *Code of Medical Ethics of the American Medical Association.* Chicago, IL: American Medical Association,1847.

Buechner F. *Now and Then.* New York, NY: Harper and Row, 1983.

Education ACGME. *Toolbox for the Evaluation of Competence*, 2002.

Hafferty FW, Franks R. The hidden curriculum, ethics teaching, and the structure of medical education. *Acad Med* 1994;69:861–871.

Haidet P, Stein H. The role of the student-teacher relationship in the formation of physicians: the hidden curriculum as process *J Gen Intern Med* 2006;21:S16–S20.

Hundert EM, Hafferty F, Christakis D. Characteristics of the informal curriculum and trainees' ethical choices. *Acad Med* 1996; 71:624–642.

Husser WC. Medical professionalism in the new millennium: a physician charter. *J Am Coll Surg* 2003;196:115–118.

Inui TS. *A Flag in the Wind: Educating for Professionalism in Medicine.* Washington, DC: Association of American Medical Colleges, 2003. Available at: http://www.aamc.org/members/facultyaffairs/publications/start.htm. Accessed October, 2007.

Papadakis MA, Teherani A, Banach MA, et al. Disciplinary action by medical boards and prior behavior in medical school. *N Engl J Med* 2005;353:2673–2682.

Stern DT. *Measuring Medical Professionalism.* New York, NY: Oxford University Press, 2006.

Connections & Boundaries in Clinical Practice

Sarah Williams, MD & Richard M. Frankel, PhD

Imagine two neighbors, leaning over a backyard fence chatting. The scene looks comfortable, perhaps somewhat intimate if they have known each other a long time. Possibly, they are discussing their latest difficulties with their respective teenage children, or their feelings about the upcoming local elections. Now consider the fence that separates them—what purposes does it serve? Most obviously, it provides something to lean on, however, it also defines a geographic boundary that marks a recognizable "territory," for example, house, yard, driveway for each.

There are also less obvious "boundaries" operating in this exchange that delineate each person's rights, duties, and obligations. These are neighbors, perhaps close friends; perhaps not. They are not lovers, doctor, and patient, relatives, or teacher and student. They could become these things, but if they did, the boundaries defining their relationship would change. In addition, there are boundaries around the kind of information and emotions they will share, based, in part, on their past history, who they are as people, and what feels comfortable and appropriate to each given the nature of their relationship.

Boundaries are the lines we draw between and around things. They can be physical, defining where one country begins and another one ends; biological, differentiating cells, organs, and organisms from one another; or social; delineating norms or rules for what is appropriate or relevant in a particular relationship, conversational exchange, or individual behavior.

Boundaries are necessary, but must be flexible enough to adapt to different situations, different cultures, and other factors. For example, there is a general social convention that limits or prohibits physical contact between strangers. The rule or norm applies in some but not all situations. In a crowded elevator or subway car at rush hour physical contact is the norm, and strangers must manage social relations while in bodily contact (e.g., by pulling in personal boundaries

and avoiding eye contact). Boundaries allow for relationships to form, but if too rigid, can be inhibiting. Likewise, where boundaries are too porous and unclear, they can make relationships unsafe and conflicted. Confusion arises when boundaries are unclear, participants disagree on what they should be, multiple relationships with the same person (e.g., physician and friend) exist simultaneously and require different boundaries, or when one or both participants do not feel entitled to, or do not know how to create and maintain healthy boundaries.

As in the crowded subway, providers and patients must be able to adapt and manage boundaries to maintain optimal relationships. For example, providers are permitted to ask intimate questions of relative strangers, and to touch and manipulate parts of the body that are generally thought to be "private" during the physical examination (especially genital and rectal examinations). Such acts would be serious boundary violations in other settings. To protect the patient (and ourselves) from boundary confusion it is important to be more careful about the other boundaries that allow for safety and comfort in the provider-patient relationship. Finally, boundaries are generally enacted tacitly, one doesn't become aware of them until there is some confusion, crossing, or violation. This means that boundaries are often left open to interpretation on both sides of the stethoscope.

Learning to create and maintain appropriate boundaries, while developing meaningful and caring doctor-patient relationships is a significant challenge for many health care trainees. The medical student or intern who becomes over involved with his or her suffering, needy (and sometimes manipulative) patient, and becomes overwhelmed, is an archetypal story in medicine. So too are stories about physicians who cope by erecting rigid walls between themselves and their patients. These physicians find themselves cut off from some of the major rewards of doctoring. They often feel a lack of work satisfaction and are vulnerable to early burnout. In addition, they may find themselves dealing with unco-operative, dissatisfied, and possibly litigious patients.

While the challenges of dealing with boundary diffi-culties may feel most acute during training and the early years of practice, these challenges are ongoing, and the habits and patterns developed during training may remain in place for a professional lifetime. Minor boundary challenges are ubiquitous in the day-to-day work of doctoring. Most providers have met a patient in the supermarket, or at a school board meeting or other nonmedical setting. Many have wondered whether it would be ok to ask one's financially savvy stockbroker/patient for a few tips, or one's car mechanic/patient for some free advice about the strange noise the transmission has been making lately. And who hasn't been asked by a friend or relative to write a pre-scription refill for a skin cream they've been "using for ages" to save a trip to the doctor? Are these actions truly "boundary violations?" Why not just relax and say a warm hello or give a hug to your patient when you meet him or her in the checkout line? Why not get your free financial or mechanical advice, and make your patient feel useful? Why not just write that prescription for aunt Bessie, and save her a day off from work and the expense of a doctor's visit?

In this chapter, we focus on some of the more chal-lenging boundary issues in medical practice: "The limits of caring," "Sexuality in the provider-patient relation-ship," and "Medical advice for family members." Each section is built around a case example or provider narra-tive, followed by a discussion of the issues it raises. We then offer guidelines for the reader/practitioner to understand, assess, and manage challenging boundary dynamics.[1]

CASE EXAMPLES & DISCUSSION

Boundary Challenges 1: The Limits of Caring

 CASE ILLUSTRATION 1

Dr. M was a young, smart, and extremely dedicated and caring intern midway though her first year of training. One night on call, she admitted a young diabetic woman, Ms. R, (just a few years younger

than herself) who was in severe ketoacidosis from not taking her insulin for the past several days. Dr. M stayed up with Ms. R throughout the night, mon-itoring her fluids and electrolytes, and carefully calibrating her insulin dose. When she entered the room early the next morning after checking on some lab results, she was greeted by a breakfast tray thrown at her by Ms. R, who was unhappy with her restricted calorie meal!

Over the next few days Ms. R's diabetes proved difficult to control, and it became clear that she was a very brittle diabetic. What probably should also have become clear, but did not, was that she was also suffering from a severe borderline person-ality disorder. In fact, a number of her diabetic crises had been precipitated by self-destructive behavior, such as stopping insulin abruptly, eating high sugar foods, or overdosing on insulin. Ms. R seemed to have an uncanny knack for knowing just how far she could go with these dangerous maneu-vers before actually putting her life at risk.

As the team worked to get her glucose under control, Dr. M struggled to build a relationship with Ms. R despite her assaultive behavior on the first morning. As her trust grew, Ms. R shared with her young doctor the story of her difficult life, which was marked by neglect and abuse in childhood, and ongoing struggles with depression, loneliness, and a feeling that people she depended on always disappointed or betrayed her. Dr. M felt her heart go out to Ms. R, and vowed that she would not be another in the long line of disappointing caretakers.

When Ms. R finally stabilized, she was discharged to be followed up in Dr. M's clinic. Things went pretty well for a short while, but trouble soon began to creep in. Dr. M began receiving phone calls, infrequently at first, but then steadily increas-ing in number. At first Ms. R would call the clinic and pester the clerks, particularly after missing a scheduled appointment, which she began doing more frequently. She then discovered the page operator, and began paging Dr. M at all times of the day and night. Dr. M was annoyed, but felt help-less to stop the phone calls without hurting the patient; she understood Ms. R's emotional distress and her aloneness, and wanted to be able to be there for her. One day, in a moment of weakness, Dr. M gave the patient her cell phone number, ask-ing her to only use it in serious emergencies. Unfor-tunately, Ms. R was unable to limit her calls and continued to call Dr. M for both medical and emo-tional problems.

One night, when she called Dr. M at 1 A.M. to tell her she had just broken up with her boyfriend and was desperate, Dr. M exploded. She berated Ms. R for call-ing her at that hour (and all the other inappropriate times), told her in no uncertain terms that this was

---

[1]Examples and case studies in the "Caring" and Prescriptions" sec-tions are derived from the personal experiences of the authors and their colleagues, friends, and students. Narratives and quotes for the "Sexuality" section come from workshops conducted by the authors. All are used with permission.

not an emergency and to please stop calling and leave her alone. She turned off her phone and went back to bed, tossing and turning for the rest of the night. The next day she turned on her phone (with much trepidation) to find a message from Ms. R telling Dr. M that she did not need to worry about her anymore, she would never see her or hear from her again, now that she had disappointed her like all the others. She would try to manage her diabetes on her own, and if that didn't work—"don't worry, I won't come to the hospital and bother you— I thought you were different, but you're the same as all the others!" Dr. M was mortified and guilt stricken; she tried numerous times to call Ms. R to apologize and ask her to come back in for care, but to no avail. The patient never answered her phone, or the letter Dr. M sent to her home.

CASE DISCUSSION

While the case of a borderline patient may illustrate an exaggerated spectrum of behavior, it provides an excellent opportunity for thinking about the boundaries of caring behavior (see Chapter 26). At first glance, what went wrong seems to be that Dr. M allowed herself to care too much for a difficult patient. We suggest that the problem was *not* due to the amount of caring, but rather to the lack of appropriate boundaries or limits set by Dr. M in her relationship with Ms. R. Thinking back to the concept of boundaries as demarcating a set of behaviors appropriate to a given relationship, we can see that both the doctor and her patient acted in ways that exceeded the bounds of what was safe, comfortable, and appropriate for even the most caring doctor-patient relationship.

An important function of boundaries in the physician-patient relationship is to create a sense of "safe space" (partly physical and partly felt or conceptual), within which each person feels protected, autonomous, and comfortable. When this space is mutually understood and respected, it is possible for interaction to be trusting and reciprocal. When relationship boundaries are violated, most people go into defensive mode, putting their efforts toward strengthening and protecting their own personal boundaries rather than connecting with others. Dr. M let Ms. R's incessant and inappropriate demands continue to escalate over time without bringing them to light as a problem, or setting limits. In the end it caused her to "explode," destabilizing the relationship and making it unsafe for herself and her patient. As this case also illustrates, changes in patient behavior (e.g., increasing numbers of calls, no-shows, demands for care, asking personal questions, or being sexually provocative) often indicate a shift or confusion in boundaries

Fortunately, Dr. M got another chance and this time was prepared. . .

CASE ILLUSTRATION 1 (CONTD.)

About a year after having been "fired" by Ms R, Dr. M, who was by then a seasoned second-year resident, walked into her clinic and was very surprised to find Ms. R listed as the first patient of the day. After getting her feelings under control, she called the patient into the examining room where they both took the opportunity to apologize and express regret over the previous year's debacle. Ms. R stated that while she had initially been deeply hurt and angry, she also realized how hard she had pushed Dr. M, who was the only doctor who really had cared for her. Now, she wondered whether Dr. M would take her back.

Dr. M was deeply touched and said so. She replied that she would be happy to resume caring for Ms. R, but that this time there would need to be "rules" for the relationship, particularly regarding the frequency and nature of their communication, and the delineation of responsibilities for Ms. R's health. They created a written contract outlining these rules and responsibilities in a way that was comfortable for both.

While the subsequent doctor-patient relationship was not without its stormy moments, it was maintained. Ms. R's diabetes came under increasingly good control, and Dr. M eventually came to feel that this was one of her most meaningful and rewarding patients.

Finally, this case poignantly illustrates the dynamic nature of boundary confusion and difficulties. Fortunately, there is (almost) always potential for repair even in the most difficult circumstances.

BOUNDARY CHALLENGES 2: SEXUALITY & PROFESSIONALISM

Sexuality and sexual feelings are a normal part of being human. Sexual feelings between a doctor and patient are not abnormal, but they can sometimes be confusing and troublesome. When acted upon, they can be dangerous to the relationship and potentially exploitative. In previous research based on the narratives of students, residents, and practicing physicians, we found that the majority of situations in which providers' sexual feelings came into play involved boundary confusion on the physician's part. These situations typically involved their recognition of a sexual attraction or the potential for becoming aroused during the medical visit. Very infrequently, the feelings led to a boundary crossing where physician and patient mutually disclosed their feelings of attraction to one another. Much more frequently, the physician took steps to avoid the feelings by fleeing the encounter or skipping portions of the physical examination. Both male and female physicians described failing to do rectal, genitourinary (GU), and breast examinations in order to avoid boundary confusion. The following narrative from a third-year resident in internal medicine graphically illustrates the effect sexual feelings and assumptions about others' behavior can have on the medical encounter.

> I was sitting in the conference room when the assistant came in and said, 'You have a patient in the exam room who is going to make your day.' I walked in and this woman is dressed in like a wet tee shirt, no bra, very good looking and very shapely. I started talking to her and she was giggling at every other word and acting more inappropriately than I'm used to ... And it was very uncomfortable because I was sitting in that room looking at her and I couldn't divert my attention from looking at her breasts. I tried to spend a lot of time looking down at her chart, but every time I looked up my eyes zoomed in on her breasts. She was controlling my eyes ... jiggling those things around so that her already prominent breasts were more prominent ... She was just too flirtatious for me. I was really uncomfortable.

It is clear from this narrative that the patient's appearance and manner of interacting (inappropriately described by the assistant as "a patient who's going to make your day") led the resident to "sexualize" the situation and make some assumptions about the patient, her behavior, and her intentions. He then became caught and confused between the nature and boundaries of the doctor-patient interaction, and those of an encounter between himself as a sexually interested man, and an attractive woman. It is interesting to note that the resident did not recognize his own role in nonverbally encouraging the very behavior that made him so uncomfortable. He reported that each time he looked up his eyes zoomed in on her breasts, the result of which he felt was to make her display them even more prominently. The resident was clearly stuck, attracted to his patient and at the same time struggling to distance himself sufficiently to maintain an appropriate professional boundary. He knew something was wrong, but wasn't sure what it was, or what to do about it. This sense of helplessness and lack of clarity is typical of confusing boundary situations.

As it happens, our resident is not alone in feeling a confusing attraction to his patient. Research conducted with Psychiatry residents found that most men and about half of the women reported sexual attraction to one or more patients, and 1% acknowledged sexual contact with patients. Another study found that 57% of medical students had sexual feelings about patients, and that males had them more frequently than female

students. Twenty-one percent of the students surveyed thought it was okay to have sex with patients. The same study reported that there was no teaching in the undergraduate curriculum about sexual boundaries in medical care (see "Suggested Readings," below).

TIPS FOR DEALING WITH BOUNDARY THREATS

- Take a breather: excuse yourself, get out of the room, and take a few minutes to clear your head and think about what's happening.
- Get immediate advice: find a nurse, or a colleague or supervisor you trust, tell them what's happening and get another, hopefully clearer, perspective.
- Bring a third person (supervisor, nurse, patient family member) into the room to diffuse the situation (the resident in our story brought in a nurse, which was very helpful).
- Consider changing your physical position in relation to the patient (e.g., put more distance between you or put a barrier like a desk between you). For example, the resident in our example might have stood up, so that when he raised his eyes from the chart they would be level with the patient's face, rather than her chest.
- Try to disentangle your own assumptions and feelings (sexual or otherwise) from what you actually observe in a patient. Was the patient in the story actually being sexually provocative, or was our resident just interpreting her behavior this way?
- Finally, re-establishing (in one's own mind and perhaps with an appropriate question or statement) the interaction as a doctor-patient encounter may help. Similarly, try reminding yourself that the patient to whom you are attracted (or toward whom you have other confused feelings) is actually a person in need who has sought your professional help.

BOUNDARY CHALLENGES 3: MEDICAL ADVICE FOR FAMILY MEMBERS

Dr. B is a family doctor who lives and practices in the small town where she grew up and where most of her extended family still lives. Seeing her patients at many local events, Dr. B has become pretty good at separating her work from her social relationships, but recently she experienced a difficult boundary challenge when a family member asked for her medical opinion.

Dr. B had taken a rare afternoon off to watch her daughter's soccer game when she ran into her cousin whose daughter played on the same team. As they sat watching and chatting, her cousin suddenly asked: "Do you mind if I ask you a doctor question?" Without waiting for an answer, she pushed up her pant leg and proceeded to report that her leg, somewhere around the calf, had been hurting for the past day or so. She thought it was probably a pulled muscle, but had put ice on it and it hadn't gotten better . . . her doctor was away for the week, so in order to get it looked at, she'd have to go to the emergency room, which would mean missing work, and "you know I can't afford to do that, what with Jimmy (her husband) out of work and all."

Dr. B peered at the leg that was thrust in front of her, but couldn't see much in the dim light of a fall afternoon. She squeezed the calf gently, eliciting only minor tenderness. Mentally, she ran down the list of risk factors for a deep vein thrombosis (DVT) (smoking, recent travel, pregnancy . . .), and asked her cousin all of them, getting a negative response to each. When she got to the last item on the list, she hesitated: she knew that birth control pills were probably the most common risk factor for a DVT in a woman of her cousin's age. She also knew that her cousin and her family were very devout and belonged to a religion that did not accept artificial birth control. Dr. B was afraid to offend her cousin by asking, especially as her worried husband was attending carefully to the conversation.

Dr. B felt the familiar sense of being pulled in different directions: should she be a careful, compulsive doctor and insist that her cousin go to the emergency room (ER) and miss a day of work she could ill afford? Or, was she going overboard—maybe it was just a pulled muscle, and how would she feel putting her cousin through all that for nothing? After all, she didn't have any risk factors . . . or did she?

In the end, being a good family member won out; she told her cousin to go home, put her leg up, put more ice on it, and see the doctor if it didn't get better. Dr. B slept uneasily that night and wasn't surprised when the phone rang at 5 o'clock the next morning. It was her cousin's husband, calling from the ER; the leg pain had gotten steadily worse, so they had gone to the hospital. Dr. B's cousin had just been diagnosed with a large DVT, apparently caused by the birth control pills she had been taking without her husband's, or anyone but her doctor's, knowledge.

This case illustrates several important themes:

1. Boundary confusion often results when two different relationships exist simultaneously. In this case, Dr. B was torn between her familial relationship to her cousin and her professional role, so she was unable to be either the family member and refuse to "treat" her cousin, or to be the physician, whatever uncomfortable questions and recommendations this might have involved.

2. Often when boundaries become unclear, there is a temptation to go against one's better judgment and ignore that little voice that whispers "maybe that's not such a good idea. . . . " Somehow it's easier to justify questionable beliefs and actions to oneself than to risk offending or making the other person

uncomfortable. In the case above, Dr. B's desire to save her cousin a trip to the ER and the potential embarrassment of discussing oral contraception with her husband in earshot led her to minimize the risks of the situation; a faulty judgment which could have had fatal consequences.

Similar situations in which boundaries become unclear and judgment becomes clouded include prescribing antibiotics, or refilling pain medicine or benzodiazepines without insisting that the patient come in for re-evaluation. Even if the odds of an untoward outcome are small, there's always the chance that doing the patient "a favor," that is, stretching a professional boundary, will put them, or ourselves, at risk. It is always a good idea to stop and ask yourself: what are the potential risks and benefits of stretching (or not stretching), the boundaries in this situation? (See "Guidelines," below.)

GUIDELINES FOR PRACTITIONERS

There is no set formula for setting and working with boundary issues. Different practitioners find different boundaries issues difficult based on past history, personality, and so on. Similarly, different types of patient and physician personalities create different physician-patient relationships. However, here we present some guidelines to help physicians develop an individualized approach to dealing with boundaries in practice:

1. Learn to recognize the warning signs of boundary confusion, including:
   - Difficulty thinking as clearly as usual, judgment feels clouded.
   - A request or demand by the patient that doesn't feel quite right.
   - Changes in patient behavior, such as increasing numbers of calls, no-shows, demands for care, asking personal questions, or being sexually provocative which may indicate a shift or confusion in boundaries.
   - A change in the practitioners' usual behavior may also indicate impending Boundary confusion.
   - Fear of hurting or angering the patient, or not wanting to be "the bad guy."

2. Be aware of your own feelings and needs, and take care of them as much as possible; remembering that:
   - Creating safe and healthy boundaries is your right as well as your responsibility to yourself and your patient.
   - Provider feelings and needs which are unmet, or unrecognized, are much more likely to spill over into the doctor-patient encounter and cause boundary confusion. For example, a physician who is single and perhaps feeling lonely may be more likely to develop sexual or romantic feelings toward a patient.

- Honesty with oneself and others (where appropriate) helps ensure healthy boundaries.

3. Get together with colleagues and/or teachers to share concerns in a safe, supportive, nonjudgmental atmosphere. Balint[2] or personal awareness groups are ideal for this activity.

4. Practice the skills involved; setting clear and appropriate boundaries requires practice. Workshops and courses devoted to boundary setting can be found on the American Academy for Communication in Healthcare (AACH) web site; cases for discussion can be found on the American Board of Internal Medicine (ABIM), Association of American Medical Colleges (AAMC), and American Medical Association (AMA) web sites.

5. Consider professional counseling. Brief counseling or psychotherapy may be a useful tool for defining personal boundaries in particularly challenging situation.

GUIDELINES FOR TEACHERS

Faculty development and modeling:

- There is currently little in the medical literature on teaching about appropriate boundaries for medical students and residents. Regarding sexual boundaries, a study by Gartrell in 1998 found that 3.9% of males and 6.3% of females acknowledged sexual contact with their educators, clinical supervisors, course instructors, advisors, and administrators. The fact that a small number of trainees have sexual contact with their instructors, and the parallel finding that a small number of physicians in practice have sexual contact with their patients suggests the need for faculty development in the area of setting appropriate boundaries with learners and patients.

- Begin early in training. As trainees learn the expectations of their professional role it is useful to engage them in discussions about boundaries, both preclinical and clinical.

- Use literature and the arts as a way in. Films like "Lovesick," "The Prince of Tides," and "The Doctor" serve as powerful stimuli for discussion of boundary confusion, crossing, and violation.

CONCLUSION

Boundary confusion is common and challenging, whether it arises from the patient, the provider, or both. Until recently, the development of healthy boundaries was considered to be part of the "informal" or "hidden" curriculum of medical school and residency training. Rather than engage in specific learning tasks around boundary and relationship formation it was assumed that trainees would learn these skills by seeing, doing, and teaching. However, much of what trainees learned through the informal curriculum about healthy boundaries and relationships was often highly variable and idiosyncratic. Over the past three decades, clinical and educational research evidence has confirmed the need for training in this area, the earlier in training the better.

We invite those reading this chapter to take the time to learn more and practice the skills outlined in this chapter. In much the same way that fences make physical reality obvious "at a glance," healthy boundaries between patients and physicians lead to relationships that engender comfort, trust, satisfaction, and clarity. Some aspects of doctoring are just too important to be left to happenstance; teaching and learning about healthy boundaries is one that should be on every health care professional's list.

EPILOGUE

We close with an experience of one of us (SW) in which stretching traditional boundaries led to a meaningful, shared experience for the doctor and her patient and his family:

"As a junior medicine attending, I cared for a young man with AIDS who was declining and clearly going to die soon (this was before the development of effective treatments for HIV). In the course of caring for him, I became close to the patient and to his devoted mother, both lovely, interesting people.

At the end he had a rapid downhill course and died while I was on vacation. I made the decision to be in touch with the patient and his mother by phone during this process. Upon my return, I attended my patient's funeral, at his mother's invitation. It was a new and deeply meaningful experience for me to meet my patient's family and friends, and see how much he was loved and admired.

Later, his mother sent me a very touching thank you note along with the gift of a necklace. Although this happened close to 20 years ago, I still treasure this necklace, and never wear it without thinking of my patient and his mother and the powerful experience we shared."

SUGGESTED READINGS

Frankel RM, Williams S, Edwardsen E. Sexual issues and professional development: a challenge for medical education. In: Feldman MD, Christensen JF, eds. *Behavioral Medicine in Primary Care*, 2nd ed. New York, NY: Appleton and Lange, 2003.

---

[2] Note: Balint groups are case-based discussion groups focusing on the personal and interpersonal aspects of difficult doctor patient situations and interactions.

Gartrell N, Herman J, Olarte S, et al. Psychiatric residents' sexual contact with educators and patients: results of a national survey. *Am J Psychiatry* 1988;145(6):690–694.

Hafferty FW, Franks R. The hidden curriculum, ethics teaching, and the structure of medical education. *Acad Med* 1994;69: 861–871.

La Puma J, Stocking CB, La Voie D, et al. When physicians treat members of their own families. Practices in a community hospital. *N Engl J Med* 1991;325(18):1290–1294.

Levinson W. Mining for gold. *J Gen Intern Med* 1993(8):172–173.

Peterson MR. *At Peronal Risk: Boundary Violations in Professional-Client Relationships.* New York, NY: W.W. Norton, 1992.

Pfifferling JH, Gilley K. Overcoming compassion fatigue. *Fam Pract Manag* 2000;7(4):39–44.

Smith RC, Zimny GH. Physician's emotional reaction to patients. *Psychosomatics* 1988;29:392–397.

White GE. Medical students' learning needs about setting and maintaining social and sexual boundaries: a report. *Med Educ* 2003;37(11):1017–1019.

Training of International Medical Graduates

41

H. Russell Searight, PhD, MPH, Jennifer Gafford, PhD, & Vishnu Mohan, MD

INTRODUCTION

This chapter will review issues involved in the training and education of international medical graduates (IMGs), including differing views of psychiatric conditions and treatment; differences in educational experiences; clinical issues involving interactions with patients and nonphysician staff; technology and documentation; psychosocial issues; and medical ethics. General suggestions are offered regarding possible modifications to residency education to address the special needs of these trainees. As in any discussion of cross-cultural differences, the tremendous variability in the backgrounds of IMGs must be acknowledged. Generalizations will always be qualified and may not reflect the experience of all IMGs.

CASE ILLUSTRATION 1

The primarily U.S.-trained family medicine residency faculty meets one last time to review candidates before submitting their final rank order list to the National Resident Matching Program (NRMP). With few exceptions, the rank order begins with the U.S. medical graduates (USMGs) and ends with IMGs, who comprise two-thirds of the total list. Visa issues further complicate the selection process. "She is a strong applicant, but her visa status is likely to cause some administrative difficulties." Thoughtful, sensitive discussions sort out which applicants, particularly among the IMGs, appear genuinely interested in family medicine; which applicants are more familiar with the U.S. medical system; which applicants might effectively relate to and communicate with this residency's low-income, urban population; and which applicants might appreciate and attend to psychosocial issues in patient care.

One faculty member comments, "The ranking process was more straightforward when we considered only USMGs." Another adds, "So was residency education!" A third retorts, "Don't forget, some of our strongest residents have been IMGs!"

GROWING NUMBER OF IMGS IN U.S. RESIDENCY PROGRAMS

International medical graduates are filling an increasing proportion of the U.S. family medicine residency positions. The results of the 2005 NRMP indicate that 24.3% of all matched positions in family medicine were filled by the non-U.S. citizens educated internationally, marking the seventh consecutive year when more positions in family medicine were filled with non-U.S. citizen IMGs than the previous year. These changes in family medicine residencies parallel those in medicine in general. Twenty-five percent of all pediatrics and 35% of internal medicine residency positions were filled with IMGs in 2005, with the majority of these IMGs being non-U.S. citizens (69.8% and 78.6%, respectively). The top 10 countries for medical school training include: India, the Philippines, Mexico, Pakistan, Dominican Republic, Russia and other former eastern block countries, Grenada, Egypt, Italy, and South Korea. One in four physicians in the United States is an IMG; that is, 185,234 physicians coming from 127 different countries. IMGs are well represented in primary care professions (family medicine, internal medicine, pediatrics), and they provide a disproportionate share of health care in medically underserved areas.

With the anticipated physician shortage and distribution of the U.S. physician workforce away from primary care, the increase in IMGs entering primary care specialties is likely to continue. Previous assumptions about the prior training of first-year residents no longer apply to a large percentage of incoming residents, requiring changes in how faculty evaluate and train residents.

PRIOR TRAINING IN THE BIOPSYCYHOSOCIAL MODEL

In the United States, the biopsychosocial model is at the foundation of primary care and community medicine. While the diverse backgrounds of IMGs are valuable in caring for a multiethnic and increasingly diverse U.S. population, the extent to which IMGs have been trained in the biopsychosocial model differs tremendously depending on the country in which the resident was trained. For instance, with a few exceptions, such as Canada, England, Australia, South Africa, and the Netherlands, applied behavioral science and psychology is much better developed in the United States than elsewhere in the world. One recent study examined whether differences in medical training affected IMGs' recognition of late-life depression in standardized vignettes of older patients. Among 178 primary care physicians and 321 psychiatrists, IMGs were significantly less likely than USMGs to make the correct diagnosis of depression or recommend treatment with a first-line antidepressant. These findings remained significant even after controlling for factors such as specialty, board certification, other physician characteristics, and patient race and gender. The authors proposed that the decreased diagnosis and treatment of late-life depression by IMGs may be attributable to decreased familiarity with depressive symptoms due to different training or cultural paradigms of depression.

Our experiences in family medicine residency training and semistructured interviews with IMGs support this hypothesis. As our programs matched greater numbers of IMGs, physician faculty increasingly commented that many of these residents did not appear to appreciate the psychological and social components of family medicine's biopsychosocial foundation. For example, without prompting and perhaps even with direct modeling, an IMG resident might interview a 17-year-old pregnant patient without inquiring about the patient's feelings about the pregnancy; the father of the child; parental/family support; whether and how she plans to continue her education; and the availability of other social supports. Moreover, comments by the IMGs with whom we worked suggested that many of the common mental health conditions seen in the United States were not commonly diagnosed or treated in their home countries. Many described little exposure to behavioral science in their preresidency education. Attention deficit hyperactivity disorder (ADHD), for example, was perceived as misbehavior rather than a medical condition requiring medication. These differences in practice appeared to

stem both from differences in previous training (i.e., limited education in behavioral medicine) as well as acculturation factors (i.e., the way mental health was conceptualized in the resident's home country).

DIFFERENCES IN EDUCATIONAL EXPERIENCES PRIOR TO U.S. RESIDENCY TRAINING

While medical schools vary widely internationally, residents from non-Western countries describe differing educational experiences than the typical U.S. graduate. First, in many Asian countries, entrance into medical school occurs directly after completion of high school. While there are some 6-year medical school programs in the United States that take students at a similar point in their educational career, most U.S. students earn a bachelor's degree before applying to medical school. Of note, the undergraduate major may not be directly related to medicine. While meeting medical school requirements in the sciences, many U.S. medical school applicants major in fields such as English literature, history, psychology, foreign language, or even art history. In contrast, in those countries in which students enter medical school at age 17, a direct career trajectory heavily loaded with education in the biological sciences precludes broadening the student's scope of knowledge and intellectual exploration in the humanities.

Approaches to teaching and evaluation of students' knowledge also frequently differ by country. In many international schools, rote memorization of information from textbooks and lectures is the principal learning style. In the United States, there is more emphasis on the application of medical knowledge and on small group learning experiences such as "problem-based learning" (PBL), rather than pure memorization of information. The current U.S. medical school emphasis on evidence-based medicine (EBM), combined with PBL, encourages critical analysis of knowledge and its applicability to a given context rather than retention of facts. Ironically, however, the United States relies heavily on multiple-choice exams to evaluate medical students, residents (in training exams), and practicing physicians (board exams)—thereby reinforcing the memorization of facts. Because of the demands for mass assessment, a multiple choice examination format has become the norm, making it difficult to assess critical thinking. Outside of the United States, essay and oral exams are more commonly used to assess medical students' knowledge.

IMGs often come from societies in which there is a rigid boundary between student and teacher. International graduates often demonstrate much greater deference toward faculty than their U.S.-trained counterparts. In many countries, social encounters between residents and faculty are rare. In these countries, two-way exchanges of ideas are also very rare—the learner would not consider being impolite by openly questioning a faculty member. In the United States, faculty may view themselves as educators, but also as mentors and sometimes as friends of their residents and students. These differences are particularly evident when learners are asked to evaluate their teachers. The U.S.-trained residents and students have considerable experience evaluating faculty; student evaluations are commonly used for promotion and tenure decisions in undergraduate colleges and universities. IMGs often indicate that they are very uncomfortable evaluating their U.S. faculty and consider it inappropriate. This reticence to speak up in the presence of authority often extends to rounds and precepting interactions, frequently leading the U.S.-trained faculty member to conclude erroneously that the IMG has a deficient knowledge base.

CLINICAL ISSUES

Patient Care & Physician–Patient Interaction

Many IMGs come from third world countries and have a wealth of experience with diseases that their U.S. counterparts rarely see. For example, early childhood death due to diarrhea and parasitic diseases are relatively uncommon in the United States compared with the developing world. The physician–patient relationship also differs across cultures. Many IMGs come from countries in which patients simply do what their physician tells them and neither seek nor expect an explanation of their medical condition. Medicine in the United States has moved away from a paternalistic physician-centered model to more of an egalitarian relationship. Under the basic tenets of informed consent, patients have a right to know what is wrong with them, what treatments are being recommended, the risks and benefits of the treatment(s), and alternatives—including no treatment. The ultimate decision maker is the patient with the physician acting more as an expert facilitator. This model is in stark contrast to the approach in India described by a family medicine resident from that country:

In India, the doctor is God-like. "The doctor cured me, saved my life, my God." Whatever the doctor says, that's enough.... Patients don't ask questions, they don't doubt. That wouldn't be taken very nicely. "I am the physician. If you are coming to me, my rule goes."

IMGs from this background are likely to be disoriented and perhaps offended by American patients coming to them requesting specific tests or medications that they have seen on television and the Internet, or that have been recommended by friends. Because much of primary care in the United States emphasizes chronic disease management rather than treatment of acute illness, patient adherence has become a particularly challenging issue. Some IMGs were brought up in systems that have little respect for patients who do not take their antihypertensive medications or follow their diabetic regimen. The idea of a difficult patient, requiring specialized interpersonal management skills, may not have been viewed as part of the physician's responsibility. Health behavior change requires active listening, negotiation, setting initially small goals, and providing social support for the patient. These skills are unlikely to be taught outside the United States, nor are health behavior models that provide a conceptual framework for counseling these patients. IMGs may have a particularly frustrating time as they learn that instruction from an authority is often not enough to generate adherence.

Even if the IMG begins practice with an appreciation of the American patient as a consumer, there are still concrete challenges, such as language barriers. Often IMGs who have spoken English much of their lives still find conversations with U.S. patients challenging:

"My first day in clinic in the U.S., I couldn't understand most of my patients. My entire education has been in English but these patients could have been from Mars."

Particularly those IMGs who have learned English as a second language find it confusing that their patients don't speak "proper" English. American English is strongly impacted by regional and ethnic factors influencing word choice, idioms, intonation, and emphasis. Similarly, U.S. patients may be unfamiliar with the accent and terminology (some of which includes British words) of IMGs who acquired much of their English outside the United States.

Interactions with Nonphysician Staff

U.S. medical care is multidisciplinary. IMGs need to learn to work with and respect social workers, pharmacists, nurses, care managers, nurse practitioners, physicians' assistants, physical therapists, and other professions who are all involved in the care of patients. Physicians frequently manage patients as a member of a complex team, and though in many cases they coordinate care, in other instances (e.g., hospice care), nonphysician providers take the lead in many aspects of patient care. As one IMG said: "I can't believe the number of people who tell me how to do things their way—and I'm the one who went to medical school."

In many countries, the interdisciplinary nature of health care is not as well developed, if recognized at all. Physicians are the lead decision makers, and their orders are obeyed unquestioningly. Additionally, in countries with social and economic distinctions, ancillary workers are typically from different social strata than physicians. In U.S. outpatient settings, the easy familiarity existing between staff, including calling physicians by their first names, is often seen as uncomfortably disrespectful and overly familiar by those trained in a more formal, hierarchical system.

Medical Ethics

Many IMGs come from societies where physician paternalism is still the rule. This power differential between doctor and patient may lead to significantly different views of ethical principles, such as informed consent. Ethical dilemmas can be evaluated from the perspective of four principles: autonomy, benevolence, nonmaleficence (do no harm), and justice. Over the past 50 years, U.S. health care has de-emphasized beneficence and increasingly valued autonomy as a pre-eminent principle. Changes in disclosing a cancer diagnosis to patients clearly illustrate this historical shift. In 1961, 90% of American oncologists indicated that they would not disclose a cancer diagnosis to a patient. Twenty years later, this pattern had been reversed, in that oncologists routinely informed patients of their condition. The U.S. emphasis on autonomy, which takes the form of giving patients choices about how to treat their condition (e.g., "You could take any of these three medicines; which one would you like to try?") is likely to be disorienting to IMGs from countries where the physician remains an unchallenged authority.

Every year the first author routinely polls groups of internal medicine residents (comprised of approximately 75% IMGs) about whether physicians in their home countries routinely disclose serious or terminal conditions to patients. Many, if not most, residents from India, Pakistan, and Eastern Europe respond "no." Cross-cultural research suggests that beneficence typically guides nondisclosure. In these societies, it is seen as cruel to inflict emotional distress on an already ill person through such a disclosure. To paraphrase an Eastern European physician: "It's cruel to take away the patient's hope."

In societies in which patients are kept from knowing their diagnosis, the locus of decision making is likely to differ from the U.S. norm. Family members, often within a network that includes the physician, make medical decisions for the patient. For example, among ethnic groups within the United States, Korean Americans and Mexican Americans were more likely than African Americans and European Americans to see the family as the appropriate health care decision maker. In Pakistan, where family decision making is common, the physician may become adopted into the family and addressed as "parent," "aunt," "uncle," or "sibling."

This collectivist value may conflict with U.S. laws and ethics that emphasize individual autonomy. IMGs from traditional cultures, particularly when treating a patient in the United States from their own background, may feel caught between the legal requirements for disclosure and their own societal ethics about proper physician conduct.

Technology

Many IMGs are from countries with far less access to sophisticated laboratory and radiologic testing. As a result, they often have particularly well-developed skills in obtaining maximum information from the history and physical examination, since other data sources are limited. The educational system in many international medical schools rewards acumen in physical exam skills, which is heavily emphasized in evaluating the competence of medical students and residents. The routine of ordering multiple tests is initially surprising to many IMGs: "When I first started my training in the U.S., I was stunned by the number of tests that we ordered. I wish I had the luxury of ordering an echocardiogram for every heart murmur or a CT scan for every head injury back home!"

Recently, the influence of technology has spread to the medical record, commonly used pharmaceutical reference sources, and treatment guidelines—all of which are increasingly digitized in the United States. Personal digital assistants (PDAs) and electronic medical records further challenge physicians trained in systems with significantly less technology.

Documentation & Litigation

Depending on their training, IMGs have varying degrees of exposure to medical documentation formats common in the United States. While some are aware of the SOAP (Subjective, Objective, Assessment, and Plan) format, others, once exposed to this approach, cannot understand its significance. The vast majority indicate that the amount of detail required in patient notes far exceeds customary practice in their home countries. Additionally, the presence of third parties "looking over the physician's shoulder" through the chart notes creates some anxiety. One IMG resident observed: "Documentation is a huge issue here. Not just documenting in a professional way, but in a legal way. Every word is important."

Malpractice litigation is a relatively new concept in many developing countries. Concerns such as patient abandonment, negligence, and the dictum "if it isn't written in the chart, it didn't happen," are new to many IMGs. Some report frequently being worried that they have "missed something" in a patient's care that could lead to a lawsuit.

PSYCHOSOCIAL & MENTAL HEALTH ISSUES

IMGs Views of Psychiatric Conditions

IMGs often have different views of psychiatric conditions compared to the U.S.-trained residents and faculty. In a qualitative study investigating the behavioral science training of IMG residents prior to coming to the United States, the majority of respondents commented that rates of mental disorders appeared to be higher in the United States than in their home countries. IMG residents will sometimes attribute these higher rates to differences in the U.S. social structure—such as the widespread use of nursing homes, elders without visitors in the hospital, and mothers raising several children alone—as the primary reasons there is more depression in the United States. These residents perceive family support to be stronger in their home countries, buffering against mental illness.

IMGs also tend to perceive strong religious faith to be a resource in coping with difficult life events. These residents suggest that Americans often become "depressed" in response to chronic or daily struggles, in contrast with their international counterparts who may be more likely to accept their fate:

> "It is a religious society (India), so if there is a difficult life event, people accept it and move on... The strong belief in God means that if something bad happens, that's because of God."

Other cultures share with the United States the belief that psychiatric mental disorders are a form of illness, but the perceived causes of mental illness may differ. For example, in Karachi, Pakistan, 30% of primary care patients believed that psychiatric illness was caused by supernatural powers and spirits. These patients commonly sought treatment from a Hakim (12%), spiritual healer (12%), and family support (2.5%).

The stigma of mental illness also affects how these issues are addressed by IMG residents in primary care. In many cultures, mental health issues are viewed as shameful and taboo: "You practically never do this... [in my country]...psychiatry is for the mad man." Due to their own culturally based misgivings about mental health issues, many residents fear they will offend patients and therefore avoid such questioning.

Views of Mental Health Treatment

Not surprisingly, many IMGs report minimal exposure to behavioral medicine prior to residency education in the United States. Many medical schools throughout the world do not provide sufficient training in the management of common mental disorders, preferring to emphasize schizophrenia and other severe mental disorders. Clinical training often involves observerships or walking rounds in institutions for patients with severe mental illness. One resident from India reported:

> I had minimal training or no training in anxiety and depression. I was in a mental hospital and I had one month. It was in my fourth year. We had lectures for two weeks and two weeks in an institution. We looked at locked-up people all the time. We did not interview patients; we just walked through. It was like looking at specimens.

Even in countries in which primary care physicians inquire about and treat psychiatric symptoms, there may be little diagnostic specificity. For example, one IMG from Bosnia stated:

> Mental health does not look the same there as it does here. In my country, our people are simply "nervous." All psychiatric problems, depression, posttraumatic stress disorder, everything, it is just "nervous."...People in my country, they come to the office and say they are nervous, so we just give them some benzodiazepines.

The sociopolitical history in the IMGs home country may influence how they approach mental disorders. One study explored the perceptions and experiences of 10 Russian family physicians regarding the practice of behavioral medicine. Through a series of semistructured interviews, these physicians revealed a reluctance to refer for mental health care, in part due to recent history in which psychology and psychiatry was used by the State to control political dissidents rather than for treatment. In the Stalinist era it was said, "No person, no problem." Diagnoses such as schizophrenia meant that there was "no person," and the "patient" could be locked up indefinitely in a mental hospital, which was little different than a prison. People became afraid of psychiatrists. As one of the interviewees said, "The fear of that kind of specialist is probably somewhere in the genetic code."

Family Life

International medical graduates, particularly from East Asian countries and the Philippines, are startled by many aspects of U.S. family life, including single parent families, cohabiting relationships, and serial monogamy. Before beginning residency, IMGs obtain their knowledge about U.S families from several sources, including TV "talk" shows as well as from listening to the discussions of the personal lives of office staff in settings where they were completing observerships.

Usually, IMGs are stunned by the permissive parenting practices in the United States and the childhood behavior problems that they believe result from this approach. Many find it odd that conditions like childhood ADHD, not commonly diagnosed in their home countries, are so common in the United States. As one resident from Eastern Europe said:

> Parents in this country, they let the kids do whatever they want ...ADHD is not diagnosed in my country— it's simply a matter of discipline. Here it seems to

calm down parents and teachers when you give the kids medicine.

IMGs tend to view parental discipline, even when physically harsh, as important for preventing oppositional and disrespectful behavior among children. The notion of child physical abuse is new to many IMGs. They are surprised that the state becomes involved when parents physically discipline their children. Child protective services' power to remove children from their parents' custody is very troubling to many of these residents. What is considered abusive in the United States may be seen as responsible parenting that builds character in their home countries. A resident from India noted that the children of strict parents do very well in school and college.

Sexual Behavior

Early sexual experiences are particularly troubling to those raised in traditional societies. They often react in one of two ways. One approach is to avoid discussing sexuality with adolescents seen in the office. Preceptors often need to remind residents repeatedly to raise these issues. Even then, residents often appear uncomfortable with the topic—speaking awkwardly while looking at the floor rather than the patient. The other approach is to accept that the West is a sexually permissive society. The resident may address sexuality in a matter-of-fact, almost business-like manner. For example, an IMG seeing a 12-year-old girl who recently had her first sexual intercourse approached the patient in much the same way as an adult. A PAP and pelvic examination were conducted, and customary guidance about pregnancy, contraception, and safe sex provided. There was no discussion about the circumstances under which the girl had intercourse (e.g., was it coerced?), the age of the partner, or the patient's perspective on the experience. Despite research evidence that early sexual activity is associated with sexual abuse history, smoking cigarettes, and using marijuana, the resident raised none of these issues until some of them were suggested by the behavioral scientist observing the encounter.

Nonmarital cohabitation is also a unique experience for many IMGs. In one instance, a resident from the Asian-Pacific region was seeing a hospitalized patient with injuries reportedly sustained through an assault by her boyfriend. The supervising physician had urged the resident to address the issue with the patient and provide her with resources for victims of domestic violence. The IMG was confused and didn't follow through at first. When asked about her reluctance, she responded: "It's not domestic violence. They are just boyfriend and girlfriend; they're dating. Each of them has their own house." The resident was surprised to learn that adult "boyfriends" and "girlfriends" often live together, and domestic violence can indeed occur in these situations.

The increased nuclearization and isolation of generations among U.S. kinship networks is troubling for IMGs from non-Western cultures, where extended families are common. Many types of individual and interpersonal distress are seen as arising from the absence of a multigenerational kinship network. To those from East Asia, for example, domestic violence in their home country was not a dyadic event with a perpetrator and a victim, but a situation in which the wife's family members would rightfully intrude into the marriage to protect her. The family should handle this problem rather than the medical–legal system:

> *Back home, if I hit my wife, they would not take that to the doctor. There is family support. Women are abused here, and they often do not want to do anything about it. Back home, women are hit and their dad says: "Come home." Here, women get put out on the street.*

Caring for geriatric patients in institutional settings contributes to a view of American families as isolated and cut-off from their extended kinship network. Residents from societies that care for aging family members at home have difficulty comprehending the practice of placing senior family members in impersonal nursing homes: "Nursing homes do not exist in India—because no son or daughter would ever lose the honor of caring for his or her elders, especially a parent." Similarly, hospitalized patients receiving no visitors—even when family members live nearby—are troubling to IMGs. One resident commented that he could now understand why he saw so many depressed patients here in the United States compared with his home country: "Back home families are crucial. Here, people are left alone. You have a chance to get depressed much more here."

Challenges in Learning Behavioral Science

At the most fundamental level, many IMGs are challenged by the inclusion of psychiatry and psychosocial aspects of the patient's life as a significant component of primary care. Coming from societies where diagnosis of mental health problems was often less common and those syndromes that were diagnosed were typically severe, many resident IMGs initially feel inadequate to diagnose and treat these conditions. Early in residency some IMGs respond by referring nearly all depressed and anxious patients to psychiatrists. It is important that preceptors establish early in training that diagnosis and treatment of common mood and anxiety disorders, dementias, childhood behavior and adjustment problems, as well as sexual dysfunction, are expected competencies. Unless the case is complicated and beyond the scope of a non-specialist (e.g., schizophrenia), the resident should learn to manage the patient.

Diagnostic interviewing for mental health conditions is particularly challenging for IMGs. After taking the United States Medical Licensing Exam (USMLE), most IMGs are familiar with the DSM-IV (Diagnostic and

Statistical Manual of Mental Disorders, Fourth Edition) system and the use of explicit criteria for diagnosis. It was very difficult for them, however, to convert these dimensions to conversational questions. Often the questions tend to be verbatim recitations of the DSM-IV criteria and have a stilted quality that is confusing to the patient (e.g., "Are you having feelings of worthlessness or inappropriate guilt?" Or "Do you have chronic feelings of emptiness?"). IMGs often recognize that they do not know how to ask about these types of symptoms and consequently omit them. This reluctance may be particularly pronounced for questions about self-harm, suicide, abuse, and illegal acts. One IMG resident describes his experience of learning how to ask sensitive questions:

> *First, you are very uncomfortable, then you feel better and better ... how to ask questions, how to ask about suicide. For me, that was very embarrassing. I was surprised people responded normally to these questions. "How will this influence her relationship with me?"*

Another IMG said:

> *"In my country, if I asked a woman with a child if she was married, she'd get mad at me."*

In our residency training program during the supervised month in behavioral science and mental health, we have noticed unspoken discomfort when IMG residents are asked to interview, for example, a 14-year-old unwed mother, an openly lesbian couple, or divorced parents—each with their new spouse. The resident who has done quite well interviewing other patients often seems at a loss about how to proceed with these family configurations. After sensing that they are uncomfortable asking the patient(s) further questions, the behavioral science faculty member will take over the interview for awhile. Later in the interview, we typically try to turn it back over to the resident who often at this point appears less confused and can follow the faculty member's lead. After the encounter, when asked about their reaction and reason for not continuing the interview, a common response is something like:

> *"I know these relationships exist in America, but I have never seen them face-to-face. I don't know what to say to these people."*

RECOMMENDATIONS FOR IMPROVING THE EDUCATION & TRAINING OF INTERNATIONAL MEDICAL GRADUATES

General Suggestions

International medical graduates would benefit from early acclimatization. Instead of the typical July 1 start date, it would be helpful if some preparatory experiences could begin at least 8–12 weeks before the formal residency year begins. English immersion experiences would be helpful for IMGs with uneven abilities in written and/or spoken English. For those residents who learned English late in life and whose accent is a barrier to understanding, there are specialists in accent reduction who can be quite helpful.

In particular, it is helpful for the instructor to include local idioms. There are CD-ROMs and other resources for learning specialized medical terminology.

Other areas that could become part of a preresidency curriculum include medical documentation, the mechanics of ordering lab work and radiographic studies, writing prescriptions, and how to use a PDA. An overview of the U.S. health care system including legal, ethical, and insurance issues would also be valuable. Basic medical interviewing skills can be taught through use of videotapes, simulated patients and role-plays. One resource that may be helpful is the *Doc.com* interactive web-based curriculum on clinician–patient communication, produced by the American Academy on Communication in Healthcare (see "Other Resources," at the end of chapter). The general "style" that a primary care physician uses when relating to patients, however, is difficult to reduce to a set of skills. IMGs might benefit from shadowing faculty or seasoned primary care physicians as they see patients.

The individualist-collectivist distinction that plays a significant role in ethics and determining moral responsibilities should be discussed explicitly in the context of ethical decision making, end-of-life care, and other relevant areas in medicine. For both U.S.-trained physicians as well as IMGs, an open exploration of these issues, including their cultural and religious background, would allow all physicians to be more sensitive with a broader cultural array of patients.

When IMG residents are having apparent difficulty meeting performance criteria, faculty should consider both cultural and language issues. As anyone who has learned a second language knows, people can appear to understand even if they are only picking up bits and pieces of what is being said. The deference that IMGs show towards faculty may be misinterpreted as a lack of assertiveness, an absence of independent thinking, inadequate knowledge base, or poor motivation. Before drawing conclusions, it would be helpful to have several supportive, noncritical conversations with these residents to better understand their background. During observation of clinical interactions with patients, we noted that an IMG from Pakistan never sat down during any of four to five encounters. In our discussion afterward, the resident indicated that she knew that sitting was the correct thing to do in terms of carrying out an effective interview, but thought it would be disrespectful to sit while the supervisor was present. If we had not clarified this point, we would have "graded" her interview skills as much less than optimal.

Suggestions for Teaching Psychiatry & Psychosocial Medicine

Psychosocial content should be introduced early in the first year of residency. To address educational and training needs in behavioral science, a formal block rotation can be scheduled during the resident's first year. At our program, we added a first-year rotation in addition to the second-year rotation that had been in place for many years. The first-year behavioral science rotation focuses more on effective interview skills and several common psychiatric conditions, while the second-year block focuses exclusively on diagnosing and treating mental disorders.

To help residents with wording questions about psychiatric symptoms, we heeded their advice and developed a series of "cheat sheets." Specifically, we made up a series of laminated cards (they easily fit into a lab coat) with helpful questions to elicit symptoms for many common psychiatric disorders. These became very popular among residents.

Faculty should be aware that patients with diverse backgrounds, customs, and family configurations are likely to be somewhat disconcerting to the IMG resident. In an individual discussion with a resident, the faculty member may want to begin by asking: "How often have you had the experience of ... interviewing an openly gay male, a teenager being raised by foster parents, or a patient who requests a specific test that you don't think is indicated? Would physicians see patients or situations like these in your home country? Why do you think it's different here?" The faculty member should demonstrate genuine interest in the resident's experiences, respect, and intellectual curiosity during this exchange. These conversations can be useful learning experiences for both parties. Next, the clinical instructor should provide some focused information on the topic (e.g., "In the inner city, up to 50% of children are being raised by grandparents. Research shows that raising grandchildren has a negative effect on the grandparents' health compared to grandparents not raising grandchildren.")

We typically do joint patient interviews with residents as part of their behavioral science training. This allows observational learning of the faculty's unspoken acceptance of patients and a way of responding to them "like anyone else." In discussing these issues with IMGs, faculty should appreciate the extent to which patterns of family organization, views of the physician role, and so forth, are culturally relative. For example, many Westerners who automatically accept the norm of "companionate marriage"—a product of an extended friendship, dating relationship, and often a period of cohabitation—may be disturbed by the East Asian custom of arranged marriage. However, the teacher's genuine, noncritical interest in the background of arranged marriages often creates a climate in which the IMG is receptive to learning about the U.S. relationship variations.

As many seasoned clinical faculty know, patients can be great teachers. IMGs who have been successful in understanding U.S. patients in a cultural context, approach them with respect, intellectual curiosity, concern, and a genuine desire to learn. While obtaining pertinent historical and symptomatic information, these physicians can also encourage patients to "tell their story," and in so doing provide meaning and satisfaction for both doctor and patient.

SUGGESTED READINGS

Buyck D, Floyd M, Tudiver F, et al. Behavioral medicine in Russian family medicine. *Patient Educ Couns* 2005;59(2):205–211.

Goldberg D. Psychiatry and primary care. *World Psychiatry* 2003; 2(3):153–157.

Kales HC, DiNardo AR, Blow FC, et al. International medical graduates and the diagnosis and treatment of late-life depression. *Acad Med* 2006;81:171–175.

Novack DH, Plumer R, Smith RL, et al. Changes in physicians' attitudes towards telling the cancer patient. *JAMA* 1979;241: 897–900.

Pugno PA, Schmittling GT, Fetter GT, et al. Results of the 2005 National Resident Matching Program: family medicine. *Fam Med* 2005;37:555–564.

Qidwai W, Azam SI. Psychiatric morbidity and perceptions on psychiatric illness among patients presenting to family physicians, in April 2001 at a teaching hospital in Karachi, Pakistan. *Asia Pac Fam Med* 2002;1:79–82.

Searight HR, Gafford J. Cultural diversity at the end of life: issues and guidelines for family physicians. *Am Fam Physician* 2005; 71:515–22.

Searight HR, Gafford J. Behavioral science education and the international medical graduate. *Acad Med* 2006;81:164–170.

Shah RG. In: Pories S, Jain SH, Harper G, eds. *The Soul of a Doctor: Harvard Medical Students Face Life and Death*. New York, NY: Algonquin Books, 2006.

Singhal K, Ramakrishnan K. Training needs of international medical graduates seeking residency training: evaluation of medical training in India and the United States. *The Internet Journal of Family Practice* 2004;3(1).

Sobel RK. MSL-Medicine as a second language. *N Engl J Med* 2005;352(19):1045–1046.

Whelan GP. Commentary: coming to America: the integration of international medical graduates into the American medical culture. *Acad Med* 2006;81(2):176–178.

World Health Organization World Mental Health Survey Initiative. Prevalence, severity, and unmet need for treatment of mental disorders in the World Health Organization World Mental Health Surveys. *JAMA* 2004;291:258–259.

OTHER RESOURCES

Novack DH, Clark W, Saizow R, et al., eds. *Doc.com: An Interactive Learning Resource for Healthcare Communication*. American Academy on Communication in Healthcare Web site. http://aachonline.org. Accessed September, 2007.

WEB SITES

Data tables from National Resident Matching Program—2005 Match. American Academy of Pediatrics Web site. http://www.aap.org/gme. Accessed September, 2007.

International medical graduates in the U.S. workforce: a discussion paper. American Medical Association Internal Medical Graduate Governing Council Web site. http://www.ama-assn.org/amal/pub/upload/mm/18/workforce2006.pdf. Accessed September, 2007.

International medical graduates in the U.S. workforce: a discussion paper. American Medical Association International Medical Graduate Governing Council Web site. http://www.ama-assn.org/amal/pub/upload/mm/18/workforce2006.pdf. Accessed September, 2007.

International medical graduates by country: The top 20 countries where IMGs received medical training. American Medical Association International Medical Graduate Governing Council Web site. http://www.ama-assn.org/ama/pub/category/1550.html. Accessed September 10, 2006. Accessed September, 2007.

Trainee Well-being

John F. Christensen, PhD & Mitchell D. Feldman, MD, MPhil

Behavioral medicine education for health professionals entails paying close attention to the well-being of trainees. The demands of professional training are enormous, and trainees often neglect their own physical, emotional, relational, and spiritual health. A central component of professionalism, however, is awareness of one's own limits, and mindfulness about the wise allocation of one's energy in providing quality patient care (see Chapters 6 & 7). Neglect of this awareness may sow the seeds of burnout and lead to poor quality care and medical error (see Chapter 34). Close attention to maintaining well-being, however, can enhance satisfaction with medicine as a career and optimize the clinician-patient relationship. Given that trainees are vulnerable to pressures to postpone their own well-being until training is completed, it is paramount to include promotion of self-care in the formation of health professionals.

CASE ILLUSTRATION 1

Jill Rayburn hadn't slept in 30 hours. She had been studying for her pathophysiology exam for a week, and still she felt ill prepared. As a second-year medical student she was beginning to wonder whether she was cut out for medicine, in spite of the fact that she was in the upper 20% of her class. Many of her classmates seemed to be on top of the material and to be unthreatened by the huge domain of the material to be mastered for this exam. Some of them had even gone for a hike yesterday afternoon. Last night she declined an invitation to play indoor soccer. It was mid-January and cold outside, and she was tired of being stuck in the library. She was beginning to resent the professor who invited her to coauthor a paper, even though at the time she felt flattered that he had singled her out for this honor. Now she didn't feel up to the task, and she wished she had started preparing for this exam earlier

rather than working on the paper. She looked back to her days of high school and college, when she was consistently at the top of her class, and remembered many carefree days. She wondered what had happened to that teenager with the sense of humor and the time to hang out with friends. Now as she looked ahead to the remainder of the winter, all she saw were more deadlines and isolated days in the library without respite. She wondered if she would ever have fun again.

A common trait of many physicians is compulsivity. Although many attributes of compulsivity—thoroughness, accuracy, second guessing, monitoring changes—are beneficial to patient care and success in medical training, this trait may also erode the personal health, satisfaction, and well-being of the physician. Early in her training, Jill is manifesting many of the associated characteristics of compulsivity that if unchecked by reflection can lead to cynicism and burnout by the time she is a resident. She is beginning to question her competence, in spite of the fact that she is in the top fifth of her class. Ultimately, she is at risk of developing what has been labeled the "imposter syndrome," in which the individual feels that she has fooled others into thinking she is competent, but the threat of being unmasked lurks at every turn. Jill is also feeling guilt about not having been wiser in her allocation of time. No matter how hard she has worked, it does not seem to be enough. In addition to self-doubt and guilt, Jill is also carrying a burden of responsibility for meeting all her obligations, and she feels alone with that burden. She thinks about her peers enjoying an outing together and envisions continued isolation for herself in the library. This triad of doubt, guilt, and an exaggerated sense of responsibility has been described by Gabbard as constituents of the compulsivity that is a "normal" trait in most physicians.

Jill's discontent has its roots in the early conditioning of many bright young people in American society that implies that our value or worth as persons is linked to academic success or outward performance. Most of us have an inherent need for love and acceptance, and when children are repeatedly told that they are special and valued only when they are "exceptional," that is, at the top of their class in grades and stars in various performance endeavors, they begin to link their personal worth to meeting these standards of excellence. This high need for achievement collides with the reality that many of one's peers in medical school also came from the top of their class and consequently being smart and performing well are not so exceptional. They must work harder to stand out. Being less than outstanding is construed as having failed to meet an essential marker of their worth and value as a person. They are left with the dilemma of backing off from overwork and consequently carrying the self-stigma of being "second best," "ordinary," "mediocre," and unconsciously feeling less lovable; or of working harder to stand out. Paradoxically, these efforts to excel and "stand out" can lead to the very isolation and loneliness from which they are trying to escape.

Some trainees may have the nagging thought that overwork is not good for them, that taking care of themselves by getting enough sleep, exercise, eating well, having fun, and spending time with friends are all important; but in the "psychology of postponement" they think, "As soon as this exam is over, then I can unwind." In addition, their elevated expectation of themselves multiplies this self-bargaining: "As soon as I get into the residency I want, then I can relax;" "as soon as I get accepted for a fellowship, then I can start working out;" "as soon as I start my first real job, then I can have a life." Thus, early in professional training a habit of postponement can develop that if unchecked can lead to neglecting many of one's most valued relationships and activities throughout one's career. Sir William Osler in a commencement address to graduating medical students in 1889 had these words to say about postponement:

> Engrossed late and soon in professional cares ... you may so lay waste that you may find, too late, with hearts given way, that there is no place in your habit-stricken souls for those gentler influences which make life worth living.

Jill's story also illustrates the insidious manner in which the system of medical education with its overt and covert rewards and punishments can reinforce the student's inherent compulsivity. Her exceptional performance has been noticed by one of her professors, who asks her to work with him as coauthor on a paper for publication. It is natural for teachers to ask top performers to do more, yet neither the teacher nor the student pauses to reflect on the potential toxicity of rewarding overwork. Medical school traditionally is better at channeling students into ever refined strata of academic and professional success then at mentoring them into building a career in which

their professional endeavors unfold within a context of a healthy life well lived. Unless Jill were to encounter a mentor that has this broader grasp of personal and professional well-being, her role models and professors will continue unwittingly to provide a "hidden curriculum," in which being a successful physician entails putting one's own life on hold.

 CASE ILLUSTRATION 1 (CONTD.)

Jill was walking across the quadrangle after her pathophysiology exam and failed to notice Dr. Ann Bennington, her teacher from the previous term in a class on the medical interview. Dr. Bennington noticed Jill's hunched over posture and drawn facial expression. "Jill, you look like you have the weight of the world on your shoulders and haven't slept in days. How are you doing?" Jill managed a smile and protested, "I'm fine. I just finished the pathophys exam." Ann confronted her mildly, "Well you look exhausted. When's the last time you had an evening off?"

When she noticed a tear forming in Jill's eyes, Ann replied, "Jill, I suspect you're carrying more of a burden than you let on to others. I'd really like to talk with you more about this." She then suggested they meet later that afternoon in her office. At the meeting later in Dr. Bennington's office, after some initial hesitation Jill opened up with the self-doubt, emptiness, fatigue, and isolation she had been feeling the last few weeks. After a pause, Ann replied, "You know, Jill, you remind me of myself when I was a medical student." Noticing Jill's tears, she continued, "The fact that you are one of the brightest people in your class doesn't seem to matter to you now, and I think I know why. Like me you are perfectionist, and there are reasons too numerous for us to go into now why we are that way. But one of the effects of that perfectionism is that we never feel we can get enough praise or external validation for our worth. That's because we weren't taught to value ourselves from within, that we are lovable and have immense worth before we ever set out to do great things." She paused to observe Jill's response. Since she was breathing more freely and seemed curious, Ann continued: "There's nothing wrong in striving for excellence. In fact that's desirable. But what we mean by 'excellence' needs to be challenged. Your work as a physician, like your work as a student, will always occur within a real world context of the various values you hold and commitments you have made, as well as the limitations of time, personal energy, and competing tasks. Bumping up against these limits can be humbling, but ultimately accepting those limits and allowing your excellence to be contextualized into your life will give you wisdom. Your body, mind, and spirit are giving you feedback that you ignore only at your peril. Rather than anesthetizing yourself to this pain, let it teach you more about yourself and the full context of joy of which you are capable. To the extent you can let your awareness of the origin of this pain lead you to greater self-acceptance, you will be an excellent physician and a healing presence for others."

Jill's chance encounter with Dr. Bennington, along with Ann's willingness to mentor Jill about the importance of honoring life values in becoming a doctor, shows the powerful influence of senior physicians who have struggled themselves to attain life wisdom in revising the "hidden curriculum" of medical training. In choosing mentors, students would do well to seek out physicians who tolerate the tension of keeping their personal and professional lives in balance and who explicitly honor a variety of values beyond their professional lives, including family relationships, friendships, recreational pursuits, hobbies, and personal self-care. Having a mentor is a critical component of career satisfaction and success in medicine. The mentoring relationship has been described as one of the most complex and developmentally important in a person's life. Mentors act as teachers, exemplars, and guides for their mentees, and most importantly, according to Levinson in his book on mentoring, can help facilitate the realization of the mentee's dream. On a practical level, medical students and residents who have a mentor report better career preparation than do those without a mentor. Ideally, the mentoring relationship provides some benefits to both mentor and mentee, such as opportunities for collaboration, mutual teaching and learning, and the promotion of self-reflection as illustrated by the above vignette.

Among the perspectives worth cultivating is the awareness that becoming a health professional is a process that occurs over several years and that self-perceived imperfection is an inherent part of that process. It is helpful to think of ourselves as "becoming" rather than insisting on holding an image of what we have not yet become, then unfavorably comparing ourselves to that image. Given the continual pressures inherent in medical training to evaluate one's performance and judge one's own competence, it is important to cultivate the equally important capacity for "appreciation." When we respond to a sunset, to the first flower blooming in the garden in spring, or to the final movement of Beethoven's *9th Symphony*, this is typically not an act of judgment, but one of appreciation. It is impossible to engage the "judgment" and "appreciation" centers of our minds at the same time.

The exaggerated sense of personal responsibility that is part of the compulsive triad is often reinforced by the competitive climate of getting into medical school and advancing through training. This attitude is frequently carried into residency training and subsequent practice, in which the illusion is maintained that one is a self-sufficient professional, that asking for help is a sign of weakness, and that competency is distinguished by the ability to "go it alone." Nothing could be further from the way health care is actually delivered, in which systematic attempts to improve quality and reduce error now demand that teams of professionals from various disciplines work cooperatively to provide patient care and promote the health of the community. The best medical schools are beginning to train for this, and the Accreditation Council of Graduate Medical Education (ACGME) states that "systems-based practice," which largely involves working as part of a team, is one of the core competencies to be mastered during residency (see Chapter 38). Whether or not teamwork is reinforced by one's medical school or residency, cultivating the practice of working cooperatively with others and committing oneself to helping colleagues succeed can contribute enormously to one's personal and professional satisfaction.

CASE ILLUSTRATION 1 (CONTD.)

In April of her fourth year of medical school, Jill dropped by Dr. Bennington's office to let her know she would be going to a family medicine residency in the South. "How are you feeling about the match?" Ann asked. "Well, to tell you the truth," Jill replied, "my first choice was another program where I could have pursued some work in epidemiology based on that paper I coauthored a couple of years ago. Since the match, however, I've thought more about the program I'm going to, and especially about one physician on the faculty there who interviewed me. I was struck by the pictures he had on his wall of his wife and children, his children's poems and drawings, and what he shared with me about how much their training program valued both professionalism and the personal growth and life satisfaction of their residents." Ann smiled and nodded. Jill went on, "I have you to thank for reaching out to me at a critical moment a couple of years ago and helping me realize there was more to me than trying to be a star. You helped me realize the value of humility, which includes appreciation of my gifts as well as acceptance of my limitations. You also gave me the greatest gift, which was affirming my own capacity for appreciating my life and for letting that be the ground from which to appreciate others." In June, after her white coat ceremony Jill opened a card from Dr. Bennington, which contained this poem by Derek Walcott:

Love After Love
The time will come
when, with elation
you will greet yourself arriving
at your own door, in your own mirror,
and each will smile at the other's welcome,
and say, sit here. Eat.
You will love again
the stranger who was yourself.

Give wine. Give bread. Give back your heart
to itself, to the stranger who has loved you
all your life, whom you ignored
for another, who knows you by heart.
Take down the love letters from the bookshelf,
the photographs, the desperate notes,
peel your own image from the mirror.
Sit. Feast on your life.

CASE ILLUSTRATION 2

Bill Trimmell was shaking as he sat in the resident's room wondering why he had yelled at the patient he had just admitted to the hospital, scolding her about not doing enough to monitor her blood sugars and therefore contributing to her hyperglycemia and subsequent infection. As he reflected on the unpleasant conversation with her, he suddenly asked himself, "What am I doing?" This was only the second admission of the day, and already he couldn't wait to go home. He had had a busy morning caring for a patient he had admitted to the Intensive Care Unit, leaving him only 10 minutes over the noon hour to eat a stale bagel left over from the morning conference. Bill was only a third of the way through his second year of internal medicine residency, and he found himself more often than not resenting many of his patients and wondering what had happened to the altruistic dream of helping people that had led him into medical school. Why did he feel like he no longer cared?

Bill is showing the classic signs and symptoms of *burnout*, which consists of emotional exhaustion (including compassion fatigue and dissociation from feelings in general), depersonalization in relationships (treating oneself, patients, coworkers, and family members as objects),

and a perceived clinical ineffectiveness. Burnout has been described as "an erosion of the soul," and it spreads gradually and continually over time, sending people into a downward spiral in which it is difficult to recover if one remains in the circumstances that generated it. Burnout has been associated with impaired job performance and poor health, including headaches, sleep disturbance, irritability, relationship difficulties, fatigue, hypertension, anxiety, depression, myocardial infarction, and chemical dependency. For physicians, the seeds of burnout may be sown in medical school and residency training, where fatigue and emotional exhaustion are often the norm. By midcareer, the momentum of this condition is maintained by the subtle reinforcements in the work setting for being a hard worker and placing service to others before self-care.

All too often residents are confronted with the reality of patients who for one reason or another are nonadherent to medical regimens, or who have chronic health problems that are refractory to interventions (see Chapter 4). Unremitting exposure to cases in which one's own efforts appear futile can engender frustration and cynicism. Without the opportunity to discuss these common experiences with their peers and faculty, trainees may begin to experience the early symptoms of burnout.

Ward residents like Bill may begin to view their work in terms of the tasks involved in admitting and discharging patients, rather than in terms of the patient's experience of illness. Terry Mizrahi, a medical anthropologist, spent several months observing teams of ward residents in one training hospital, and through observation of what they did and what they communicated among themselves, she concluded that the job of the ward resident is "getting rid of patients."

Frequently, underlying this detached attitude is "compassion fatigue," in which an overload of suffering threatens to run our emotional tank dry and lead to *dissociation*, characterized by a withdrawal of attention from emotions and somatic sensations as we focus cognitively and visually on complex patient care problems or get absorbed in our "to do" list. We become anesthetized to feelings and cannot relate to family and friends once we leave work. The cognitive correlate of dissociation is *decontextualization*. This involves a habit of thinking of others (and even ourselves) in a utilitarian way that abstracts and constructs persons into categories that have usefulness for our jobs and getting our tasks done in a timely way. This habit of thinking ignores the full life context in which others (and we ourselves) are embedded. Thus, we relate to patients as diagnoses or appointments on the schedule, to coworkers as facilitating or impeding our work, to family and friends as intruding or placing unrealistic demands on our time, and to ourselves as task-processing machines.

Bill understandably feels a disconnect between the sense of vocation he once felt about medicine and the sense of futility about how he spends his working hours. In the absence of time to reflect on what is happening or discuss it with others, he finds himself slipping into disillusionment and cynicism. His job as a resident has begun to feel meaningless.

CASE ILLUSTRATION 2 (CONTD.)

In January of his second year, Bill attended a resident well-being retreat offered three times a year to all residents in his program. This particular retreat was focused on finding personal renewal in the work of caring for patients. During a small group discussion, one of the senior residents shared that she had felt burned out and uncaring by the middle of her second year. This led to a discussion about burnout and the vulnerability most residents have to this phenomenon. Another resident stated that what had helped him was observing an attending at the bedside of a dying patient showing considerable patience and compassion and asking him how he did that. This attending had replied that he kept a journal of memorable events from the day that gave him an opportunity for reflection. As the group talked, it became clear to Bill that he was not alone with this erosion of meaning and that there were personal and group strategies for renewing his enthusiasm for medicine.

Carl Rogers once said that "what is most personal is most universal." Nothing can be so personally isolating as the perception that one has lost one's way professionally. It is reminiscent of the poignant lament of Dante at the opening of the *Divina Comedia*:

In the middle of the road of my life I awoke in a dark wood where the true way was wholly lost.

Nothing can be so healing and reassuring as to know that others have traveled the same road and have emerged as colleagues to admire and emulate. The value of retreats, support groups, or even impromptu discussions during lulls in the pace of work to share common experiences and struggles is to remind trainees that they are part of the human community and that they have the capacity for renewal and change.

Emotional Intelligence

Among the strategies that trainees can use for restoring a capacity for compassion and enjoyment of work is the cultivation of "emotional intelligence." Developing self-awareness is essential to emotional intelligence. This is a challenge for clinicians who have been trained to dissociate from their feelings as a way of being "objective" in their professional role with patients. Since the quality of clinicians' relationships with their patients is a major component of the therapeutic process as well as a major contributor to their own well-being, developing self-awareness to maximize this process is essential (see Chapter 7). Emotional intelligence includes developing a language for one's emotions and a capacity of self-disclosure to others. The mirror of this process of self-awareness and self-expression is the capacity to recognize emotions in others. We can use our own emotions to develop hypotheses about what the other is feeling. We can learn to check out feelings with others, reflect feelings, comment on what we are observing, and receive the emotional disclosure of others without judgment. It can be helpful to regard emotions as value-neutral information that is passing through our awareness like weather systems, which in themselves are neither right nor wrong. Thus, we can think of attending to the patient's feelings as getting a "weather report" and awareness of our own feelings as "checking the weather." Accepting our own emotions and those of others can be liberating and allow us to be fully present to others and ourselves (see Chapter 2).

Other components of emotional intelligence include controlling impulses, especially by delaying our response in conflict situations, delaying gratification for the sake of achieving goals, and using cognitive reframing and self-instructional statements to regulate our moods. We can enhance our emotional intelligence by naming internally what we're feeling at the moment, keeping a journal that captures the predominant feelings we have experienced on a given day, practicing using emotional words with friends and intimate partners, reflecting the feelings that others disclose to us, and in some cases by engaging in psychotherapy to enhance our emotional literacy.

Bill's feeling of futility in caring for patients who did not get better in spite of his best efforts emanated from his own beliefs and expectations about control. Gaining clarity about the extent to which control is possible in the events of our lives, and in the profession of medicine in particular, is essential to satisfaction with the work of being a doctor. Although people tend to be more satisfied when they perceive a greater control over the events that impact them, most of the outcomes of patient care are multidetermined and to a large extent dependent on many forces beyond the physician's control, including patient choices as well as genetic and environmental variables. Thinking in terms of "influence" rather than "control" may be more realistic. Within the large array of factors that contribute to illness and health, physicians can have enormous influence, but medical care is only one of several events that contribute to the eventual outcome. Assuming a Zen approach of focusing on "right action" in the moment—whether it is the exercise of empathy, conducting a careful physical examination, engaging clinical reasoning, or performing a procedure—and releasing the need to have the outcome be a marker of one's competence, can provide a helpful cognitive framework for self-assessment. Other strategies for inoculating ourselves against futility may include finding meaning in small victories, such as preventing a hospitalization for a patient with chronic emphysema; using a recurrent worsening of a condition, such as a patient repeatedly admitted for diabetic ketoacidosis, as an opportunity to learn more about clinical medicine; regarding "difficult patients" as visiting professors because of the learning they can provide about how to manage such patients; focusing on the quality of the relationship with the patient whose condition is worsening; and spending some reflective time recalling the positive connections with patients who appreciate the work we do.

Common to several of the unhealthy habits described above (compulsiveness, the psychology of postponement, dissociation from feelings, and tolerating conditions of burnout) is the notion of work as *energy depletion*. Hence, many physicians, nurses, administrators, and others view weekends, vacations, and time with family as the opportunity to recharge and recapture a more expansive awareness. Some seek to expand the time available for recharging by working part-time. The converse of protected "personal time" is the intense compression of "work time" and the density of tasks to be processed in a given day. During this surreal pursuit of the processing of tasks in which "productivity" is equated with "being good," an altered state of consciousness emerges (see Chapter 5). This is a trance that one enters in the presence of certain ritualistic cues (the door to the office, turning on the computer, checking the schedule, retrieving voice mails) and may include running an incessant "to do" list, looking for brief tasks to process in an illusory pursuit of "closure," a shortened attention span, irritability in the presence of lengthy or labored conversations, a habit of checking and rechecking one's work, stewing about difficult interactions in the past, and worrying about future events.

Renewal, Reflection, & Mindfulness

Steve McPhee, a professor of medicine at University of California, San Francisco (UCSF), has used the metaphor of solar-powered versus gasoline-powered automobiles to contrast different approaches to human energy in our daily lives. The notion of work as a locus of energy depletion (requiring a leaving of work to find energy renewal) is similar to the nonrenewable dependence of industrial societies on fossil fuels. In the long run such a view of one's own energy is unsustainable. An alternative perspective is that *energy renewal* is continually available as one moves through the day, whether at work or away from work. This is analogous to the solar-powered car, which requires the opening of panels to draw on the renewable energy from the sun. Such a fundamental shift in our thinking about energy may entail re-evaluating our notion of who we are. The fossil fuel model represents a view of oneself as an individual source of productivity and accomplishment, acting with agency upon the material world and upon people's lives to achieve outcomes. The solar panel model suggests a view of oneself as a medium of energy exchange, a self-organizing system much like a candle flame that gives off light in the process of continuous transformation, a system that is embedded within, and a part of, larger self-organizing systems such as a doctor-patient relationship, a health care system, a society, the earth itself.

Trainees should ask themselves: how can we open ourselves to renewal as we move through our days, both at work and at home? What is the psychological equivalent of "opening our solar panels?" One approach is the cultivation of *mindfulness*, which is the practice of being present to where we are and what we're doing. It is the discipline of living an intentional, conscious life (see Chapter 7). Our stream of consciousness often includes thoughts about the past, sometimes accompanied by regret or resentment, and thoughts and images of the future, sometimes threatening, sometimes escapist. Mindfulness is a counterweight to this enchantment with the "there and then" by increasing our skill at being present in the "here and now." Mindfulness involves nonjudgmental attention to our emotional and mental states as they pass through awareness. We learn to see ourselves as vessels through which the various feelings of joy, sorrow, anger, affection, peace, and agitation flow without defining who we are in any moment of intensity. Twenty minutes a day practicing mindfulness meditation can enhance our capacity for mindful attention. This practice can help physicians be present to patients without interference from what happens before or after that encounter. Mindfulness is also the gateway to accessing opportunities for personal renewal in the midst of work, where in addition to expending energy, we are also receiving energy from personal interactions or the satisfaction of work well done.

The process of approaching each day with mindfulness and openness to the uncertainty of who will walk in the door next, and nonjudgmental attention to the "weather" of our own emotions and those of others, is captured in this poem by Rumi, the thirteenth century Sufi mystic whose verses reach across the centuries and cultures to speak to our own experience:

The Guest House

This being human is a guest house.
Every morning a new arrival.

A joy, a depression, a meannness,
some momentary awareness comes
as an unexpected visitor.

Welcome and entertain them all!
Even if they're a crowd of sorrows,
who violently sweep your house
empty of its furniture,
still, treat each guest honorably.
He may be clearing you out
for some new delight.

The dark thought, the shame, the malice,
meet them at the door laughing,
and invite them in.

Be grateful for whoever comes,
because each has been sent
as a guide from beyond.

Incorporating a brief period of reflection at the end of each day is one way of conditioning ourselves to perceive the opportunities for personal renewal and meaning contained in various encounters of the day. Using a journal or simply reflecting back for a few minutes on the events of the day can offer a transitional time to let go of the day and absorb the gifts that came our way. Angeles Arrien suggests that we ask ourselves three simple questions: "What surprised me today? What moved me today? What inspired me today?" Sometimes we may find that there has been great meaning in our encounters with the full panoply of human experience, including suffering. A related practice is that of keeping a "gratitude journal," which can be done at the end of the week. This involves writing down a few things from the week for which one is thankful, from simple events like watching a particularly beautiful sunrise to more profound ones like a satisfying encounter with a patient with whom one had a previous troubling relationship.

 CASE ILLUSTRATION 2 (CONTD.)

In the weeks following the resident retreat, Bill experimented with keeping a journal. Gradually, he found himself noticing sources of energy boost during his day—a joke shared with the nursing staff, the satisfaction of having been present to a patient's distress with compassion, learning a new way of working up patients for certain illnesses, being able to guide an intern in managing a difficult admission, observing a faculty preceptor facilitate a difficult family meeting about end-of-life

care. He read a little each day in an introductory book on mindfulness meditation and on some days was able to take 5 minutes to practice meditation before his day began. Some days were incredibly busy, and he was still confronted with uncertain medical dilemmas and difficult patients, but he seemed to take it more in stride. He found himself more frequently centering himself before walking into the next patient's room by taking a couple of breaths and letting go of what went before, while embracing the unknown of the encounter awaiting him. Most helpful to him were some discussions with fellow residents in which he found himself more willing to share the stresses and uncertainties of his work and to enjoy the comradeship of knowing he was not alone.

Intimacy & Value Clarification

The "psychology of postponement" mentioned above finds a poignant expression in this poem by Rabindranath Tagore:

For the Goddess of Love

There is a ruined temple near here. . . . No one sings now for the Holy One who was once praised there. The air is motionless and heavy above the altar.

The odor of flowers no long pulled for you floats in through the door.

One of your old worshippers goes out every day into the cities, hoping to receive the good things that he used to ask for from you. And every day at dusk he returns five thousand miles to his temple, his shoelaces untied, his face tired.

How many good days go by! How many nights useful for worship go by, and not one candle is lit or one poem sung!

How many sculptors work the whole day with large shoulders and hair whitened with stone dust making a statue of you, and then as dusk comes carry it to the river and throw it in.

She is still in the temple, but no one gives Her food or takes food from Her, in this ignorance that never ends.

If our relationship commitments are consistently subordinated to work demands, a review and clarification of our values is in order. Although humbling, we can get a glimpse into our value hierarchy by examining how we actually spend our time and energy in any given week. We may find that what our practice reveals is at variance with what we tell ourselves and others about our deepest values. We also may find that much of the way we spend our time is in response to urgent demands that are not that important in the long run.

In addition to the challenge of nurturing our relationships with family and friends when constrained by professional demands, another barrier is posed by a fear of intimacy or the lack of skill in sharing our inner selves with others. Since clinicians spend much of their time on the receiving end of other's confidences and disclosures, they may have less practice in self-disclosure. It is in relationship with others, however, that we deepen our identity and sense of who we are as persons. This requires not only the presence of close relationships, in and out of medicine, but also time spent with them and the capacity for self-disclosure and intimacy.

- *Friends.* Given the general erosion of community in American life, we must actively seek connections with others. Sometimes opportunities for forming friendships will arise in the work setting, and there it depends on our willingness to take the initiative. We also can develop hobbies and interests outside of medicine that form natural settings for people with similar interests coming together, whether it is through the arts, volunteer work, political action, a faith community, sports, or engaging in outdoor activities. It is not sufficient to have a network of friends without developing our capacity for self-disclosure. Learning to confide in trusted friends is an essential counterbalance to long hours of receiving the confidences of patients in our professional roles.

- *Intimate partners.* A love relationship sustained over time can be one of the great spiritual paths to our growth and development as persons. A long-term and even lifelong journey with an intimate partner is a cauldron which both tests our identity and expands our capacity to embrace life and endure its stresses and challenges. It is in such a relationship that we can learn acceptance of ourselves with all our flaws and virtues. We also can learn the art of compassion through nurturing our beloved and seeking their well-being. Building and maintaining a successful partnership requires scheduled time. Enhancing our interpersonal communication skills—especially the art of active listening, disclosure of feelings, and negotiating respectfully when there are differences and conflict—is central to an enduring relationship. Other key ingredients include awareness of our family of origin influences on couple communication and expectations; learning to tolerate differences in tastes and preferences; clarifying mutual values as a couple; and negotiating time, sex, money, space, division of labor, and whether and how to raise children. Romance and sex may occur spontaneously in the early stages of a relationship, but over time require our intentional planning to create the time and conditions for this vital component of a relationship to be a lasting source of mutual renewal. Sometimes couples get stuck in stagnating patterns or impasses in their communication, and at such times couple counseling can be a valuable resource.

Another barrier to giving ourselves the needed time to honor personal values and relationships is our concern about money. Many physicians at the beginning of their career are understandably concerned with paying off medical school debt. This may lead to working longer hours in the earlier years, or even moonlighting, which diminishes time and energy for family, friends, and hobbies. Sometimes material aspirations and the consumer mentality of our culture lead us to encumber more debt than is necessary, and we end up trading valuable time for more money to service those debts. The way money flows through our lives and whether it is a burden or a useful tool will depend on our core philosophy about wealth. Engaging in a process of clarifying our life values and financial goals, either through consultation with a financial planner or through some of the self-help literature in this area can provide a framework for making wise decisions about what we need to sustain our lives and how much time and energy we will expend in generating an income to support those needs. One physician couple reported a process of reflection they used when they realized they were "sacrificing precious time and earning money to support a lifestyle not worth living." They engaged in a process of value clarification and financial assessment that eventually led to downsizing their material possessions, eliminating debt, and embracing a path of "voluntary simplicity." They traded financial wealth for the time to travel, spend more time with their families, and pursue other interests.

Organizations & Trainee Well-being

Although it is vital that we engage in self-reflection, value clarification, and behavior change to move our own lives toward renewal and sustainability, viewing this solely as a personal project will not be sufficient to make meaningful changes. Well-being is not only an individual process, but a political process as well. With the best of intentions we may begin a practice of mindfulness, enhancement of our intimate relationships, and caring for ourselves physically—only to have those intentions evaporate at the next attending rounds or faculty meeting where overwork is reinforced and rewarded with admiration, the esteem of colleagues, and the imperatives of meeting productivity expectations. For the well-being of trainees to thrive, the organizations in which they are trained and work (hospital systems, group practices, academic medical centers, and government institutions) must be sustainable enterprises that value the health and well-being of all their workers. Each of us has a responsibility not only to ourselves but to our colleagues and the sustainability of our profession to engage in the difficult work of changing our organizations—medical schools, residencies, health care systems, and practice settings—so that they allow time and energy for "those gentler influences which make life worth living."

We can learn from models of excellence where health care organizations have developed work environments and policies that honor the values of their clinicians. Making these changes is a collective enterprise, and we will create healthy work environments only to the extent that we can work collaboratively with others and where necessary exert political pressure through group efforts.

CONCLUSION

Training health professionals in this complex, information-rich and choice-rich era of human society requires new skills that were not required of previous generations. At the same time, doing so in a way that sustains both educators and trainees as persons requires drawing upon the "practical wisdom" of previous generations. This practical wisdom, what Aristotle called *phronesis*, incorporates the cognitive, emotional, behavioral, and interpersonal skills to expand our capacity as persons and reduce or eliminate the nonimportant and unnecessary loads that erode our spirits. We also need to develop a practical wisdom of working within health care systems that is mindful of the factors that promote sustainability, such as expanding our capacity for service through teamwork, clarifying the organization's values, and establishing structures and processes that promote the well-being of health care workers. This perspective is the responsibility of trainees and faculty alike. Developing the practical wisdom to engage in this work in a sustainable way is our personal and collective challenge.

SUGGESTED READINGS

Barks C. *The Essential Rumi, Trans.* Edison, NJ: Castle Books, 1997.

Chodron P. *When Things Fall Apart.* Boston, MA: Shambhala, 1997.

Christensen JF, Feldman MD, eds. *Recapturing the Spirit of Medicine.* Special issue on physician well-being. *Western J Med* 2001; 174:1–80. Available at: http://www.pubmedcentral.nih.gov/tocrender.fcgi?iid=116276/.

Dunn PM, Rosson CL. Medicine and money: how much is enough? *Western J Med* 2001;174:10–11.

Elgin D. *Voluntary Simplicity: Toward a Way of Life That is Outwardly Simple, Inwardly Rich.* New York, NY: William Morrow, 1993.

Gabbard GO, Menninger RW. The psychology of postponement in the medical marriage. *JAMA* 1989;261:2378–2381.

Gabbard GO. The role of compulsiveness in the normal physician. *JAMA* 1985;254:2926–2929.

Hanh TN. *The Miracle of Mindfulness: A Manual on Meditation.* Boston, MA: Beacon Press, 1987.

Kabat-Zinn J. *Wherever You Go There You Are: Mindfulness Meditation in Everyday Life.* New York, NY: Hyperion, 1994.

Kinder G. *Seven Stages of Money Maturity.* New York, NY: Dell, 1999.

Levinson DJ, Darrow CN, Klein EB, et al. *The Seasons of a Man's Life.* New York, NY: Knopf, 1978.

McPhee SJ. Letter from the abbey. *Western J Med* 2001;174:73–75.

Mizrahi T. *Getting Rid of Patients.* New Brunswick, NJ: Rutgers University Press, 1986.

Osler W. Address to students of the Albany Medical College, February 1, 1899. *Albany Med Ann* 1899;261:307–309.

Ratanawongsa N, Wright SM, Carrese JA. Well-being in residency: a time for temporary imbalance? *Med Educ* 2007;41:237–280.

Spickard A, Gabbe SG, Christensen JF. Mid-career burnout in generalist and specialist physicians. *JAMA* 2002;288:1447–1450.

Walcott D. *Collected Poems 1948–1984.* New York, NY: Farrar, Strauss, and Giroux, 1987.

OTHER RESOURCES

Christensen JF. Balance & Self-Care. Web-based Learning Module in *Doc.com: An Interactive Learning Resource for Healthcare Communication.* American Academy on Communication in Healthcare Web site. http://aachonline.org. Accessed October, 2007.

WEB SITES

New Road Map Foundation Web site (Based on *Your Money or Your Life*). www.newroadmap.org. Accessed October, 2007.

Resident well-being resources. Professional Association of Interns and Residents of Ontario (PAIRO) Web site. http://www.pairo.org/Content/Default.aspx?pg=1009. Accessed October, 2007.

Resources on medical student well-being. American Medical Student Association Web site. http://www.amsa.org/well/. Accessed October, 2007.

Seligman M, Aspinwall L, Fredrickson B, et al. Positive Psychology Annotated Bibliography. University of Pennsylvania: Center for Positive Psychology Web site. http://www.ppc.sas.upenn.edu/ppappend.htm. Accessed October, 2007.

The Foundation for Medical Excellence Web site. www.tfme.org. Accessed October, 2007.

Index